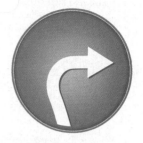

Resident Readiness®
Internal Medicine

Second Edition

Debra L. Klamen, MD, MHPE

Senior Associate Dean for Education and Curriculum
Professor and Chair
Department of Medical Education
Southern Illinois University School of Medicine
Springfield, Illinois

Susan Thompson Hingle, MD

Associate Dean for Human Organization and Potential
Professor and Chair, Department of Medical Humanities
Southern Illinois University School of Medicine
Springfield, Illinois

Mc
Graw
Hill

Resident Readiness®: Internal Medicine, Second Edition

1 2 3 4 5 LBC 28 27 26 25 24

ISBN 978-1-264-86355-6
MHID 1-264-86355-1

This book was set in Minion Pro by Thomson Digital.
The editors were Bob Boehringer and Kim J. Davis.
The production supervisor was Richard Ruzycka.
Project management was provided by Sonali Kumari, Thomson Digital.
The designer was Eve Siegel; the cover designer was W2 Design.

This book is printed on acid-free paper.

Library of Congress Cataloging-in-Publication Data

Names: Klamen, Debra L., editor. | Hingle, Susan Thompson, editor.
Title: Resident readiness. Internal medicine / [edited by] Debra L Klamen,
    Susan Thompson Hingle.
Other titles: Internal medicine
Description: Second edition. | New York : McGraw Hill, [2025] | Includes
    bibliographical references and index.
Identifiers: LCCN 2023049878 (print) | LCCN 2023049879 (ebook) |
    ISBN 9781264863556 (paperback ; alk. paper) | ISBN 9781264865475 (ebook)
Subjects: MESH: Diagnosis | Therapeutics | Internal Medicine--methods |
    Case Reports
Classification: LCC RC71.3 (print) | LCC RC71.3 (ebook) | NLM WB 141 |
    DDC 616.07/5--dc23/eng/20240207
LC record available at https://lccn.loc.gov/2023049878
LC ebook record available at https://lccn.loc.gov/2023049879

McGraw Hill books are available at special quantity discounts to use as premiums and sales promotions, or for use in corporate training programs. To contact a representative, please visit the Contact Us pages at www.mhprofessional.com.

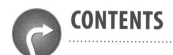

CONTENTS

CONTRIBUTORS

Dorcas Adaramola, MD, MPH
Assistant Professor of Clinical
Psychiatry and Internal
Medicine Chief, Division of
Medicine/Psychiatry
Department of Psychiatry
Southern Illinois University School of
Medicine
Springfield, Illinois
Chapters 5, 10, 35

**Bemi (Oritsegbubemi)
Adekola, MD**
Nephrology and Clinical
Hypertension Assistant Professor of
Internal Medicine Southern Illinois
University School of Medicine
Springfield, Illinois
Chapters 2, 4, 15, 33

Mohammed Al Hosaini, MD
Southern Illinois University School of
Medicine
Springfield, Illinois
Chapter 15

Basma Al-Bast, MD
Southern Illinois University School of
Medicine
Springfield, Illinois
Chapter 6

Mariam Murtaza Ali, MD
Assistant Professor of Medicine
Division of Endocrinology
Southern Illinois University School of
Medicine
Springfield, Illinois
Chapter 49

Yasser Al-Kadra, MD
Southern Illinois University School of
Medicine
Springfield, Illinois
Chapter 3

Zainab Alnafoosi, MD
Assistant Professor of Clinical
Medicine Division of
Infectious Diseases
Southern Illinois University
School of Medicine
Springfield, Illinois
Chapter 14

Satyam Arora, MD
Southern Illinois University School of
Medicine
Springfield, Illinois
Chapter 29

Muhammad Farooq Asghar, MD
Southern Illinois University School of
Medicine
Springfield, Illinois
Chapter 14

M. Haitham Bakir, MD, FCCP, DABSM
Associate Professor, Department
of Internal Medicine Pulmonary
Critical Care and Sleep Medicine
Southern Illinois University School of
Medicine
Springfield, Illinois
Chapter 31

Priyanka Bhandari, MD
Southern Illinois University School of
Medicine
Springfield, Illinois
Chapters 17, 40

Mukul Bhattarai, MD, MPH, FACC
Assistant Professor of Clinical
Medicine, Cardiology Division
Southern Illinois University School of
Medicine
Springfield, Illinois
Chapter 3

Stephanie Bitner, PharmD, CACP
Assistant Professor of Clinical
Internal Medicine
Southern Illinois University School of
Medicine
Springfield, Illinois
Chapter 48

Cheryl Burns, RDN, CDCES
Clinical Dietitian
Division of Endocrinology
Southern Illinois University School of
Medicine
Springfield, Illinois
Chapter 20

Rexanne Lagare Caga-anan, MD, FACP
Associate Professor of
Clinical Medicine
Southern Illinois University School of
Medicine
Springfield, Illinois
Chapters 32, 41

Youssef Chami, MD, FACC, FSCAI
Associate Professor of Medicine
(Retired)
Southern Illinois University School of
Medicine
Springfield, Illinois
Chapters 3, 6, 9

Asad Cheema, MD
Cardiology Fellow
Southern Illinois University School of
Medicine
Springfield, Illinois
Chapters 17, 40

Beaux Cole, PharmD
Director of Pharmacy
Standards and Operations
Office of Correctional Medicine
Southern Illinois University School of
Medicine
Springfield, Illinois
Chapter 47

Edgard Cumpa, MD
Southern Illinois University School of
Medicine
Springfield, Illinois
Chapter 10

Wael Dakkak, MD
Southern Illinois University School of
Medicine
Springfield, Illinois
Chapters 7, 27

Alan J. Deckard, MD
Associate Professor of Clinical
Medicine (Retired)
Southern Illinois University School of
Medicine
Springfield, Illinois
Chapter 21

John M. Flack, MD, MPH
Professor of Medicine
Southern Illinois University School of
Medicine
Springfield, Illinois
Chapters 17, 40

Nathalie Foray, DO, MS
Assistant Professor of Clinical
Medicine
Southern Illinois University School of
Medicine
Springfield, Illinois
Chapter 26

Ruchika Goel, MD, MPH, CABP
Associate Professor of Internal
Medicine and Pediatrics
Associate Vice Chair of Research
Department of Internal Medicine
Division of Hematology/Oncology
Simmons Cancer Institute
Southern Illinois University School of
Medicine
Springfield, Illinois
Adjunct Faculty
Department of Pathology
Division of Transfusion Medicine
Johns Hopkins University School of
Medicine
Baltimore, Maryland
Chapter 29

Zak Gurnsey, MD, SFHM, FACP
Associate Professor of
Clinical Medicine
Southern Illinois University School of
Medicine
Springfield, Illinois
Chapters 16, 18

Se Young Han, MD
Southern Illinois University School of
Medicine
Springfield, Illinois
Chapters 5, 7

Ashley Hill, DNP
Hypertension Specialist
Southern Illinois University School of
Medicine
Springfield, Illinois
Chapters 17, 40

Susan Thompson Hingle, MD
Associate Dean for Human
Organization and Potential
Professor and Chair, Department of
Medical Humanities
Southern Illinois University School of
Medicine
Springfield, Illinois
Chapters 7, 28, 43

Martha L. Hlafka, MD
Associate Professor of
Clinical Medicine
Southern Illinois University School of
Medicine
Springfield, Illinois
Chapters 25, 28

Sonaina Imtiaz, MD
Assistant Professor of Medicine,
Division of Endocrinology,
SIU School of Medicine in
Springfield, Illinois
Chapter 11

Sayeeda Azra Jabeen, MD, FACP
Southern Illinois University School of
Medicine
Springfield, Illinois
Chapters 1, 13

Michael Jakoby, MD, MA
Professor of Medicine Chief
Division of Endocrinology
Vice Chair of Research
Department of
Medicine
Southern Illinois University School of
Medicine
Springfield, Illinois
Chapters 11, 12, 20, 36, 39, 49, 51

Ramprasad Jegadeesan, MD
Assistant Professor of
Clinical Medicine
Department of Gastroenterology and
Hepatology
Southern Illinois University School of
Medicine
Springfield, Illinois
Chapter 13

Ahmed Khan, MD
Southern Illinois University School of
Medicine
Springfield, Illinois
Chapter 42

Akshay Kohli, MD
Southern Illinois University School of
Medicine
Springfield, Illinois
Chapter 8

**Tiffany I. Leung, MD, MPH, FACP,
FAMIA, FEFIM**
Adjunct Associate Professor
Southern Illinois University School of
Medicine
Springfield, Illinois
Chapters 35, 47, 48

Morton Machir, MD
Southern Illinois University School of
Medicine
Springfield, Illinois
Chapter 42

Noupama N. Mirihagalle, MD
Southern Illinois University School of
Medicine
Springfield, Illinois
Chapters 38, 43

Muralidhar Papireddy, MD
Southern Illinois University School of
Medicine
Springfield, Illinois
Chapters 7, 43

Sanober Parveen, MD
Assistant Professor of
Clinical Medicine
Division of Endocrinology
Southern Illinois University School of
Medicine
Springfield, Illinois
Chapter 51

Raj Patel, MD
PGY VI Cardiology Fellow
Division of Cardiology
Department of Internal Medicine
Southern Illinois University School of
Medicine
Springfield, Illinois
Chapter 6

Zafar Quader, MD, FASGE
Associate Professor of Clinical
Internal Medicine
Chief, Division of Gastroenterology
Southern Illinois University School of
Medicine
Springfield, Illinois
Chapter 16

**Harini Rathinamanickam, MD,
FACP**
Transplant Hepatology Fellow
Mayo Clinic
Jacksonville, Florida
Chapters 44, 50

Alyssa Ray
Southern Illinois University School of
Medicine
Springfield, Illinois
Chapter 42

Robert Robinson, MD, MS, FACP
Professor of Clinical
Internal Medicine
Southern Illinois University School of
Medicine
Springfield, Illinois
Chapters 22, 23, 30

Stacy Sattovia, MD, MBA
Professor of Clinical Medicine
Hospitalist Medical Director
Office of Continuing Professional
Development
Co-Director, Professional
Development Pillar, Center for
Human and Organizational
Potential
Director, Culinary Medicine
Southern Illinois University School of
Medicine
Springfield, Illinois
Chapters 34, 50

Keivan Shalileh, MD
Indiana University Health
Lafayette, Indiana
Chapter 24

Mingmar Sherpa, SBB
Chapter 29

Omar Siddiqui, MD
Assistant Professor of
Clinical Medicine
Southern Illinois University School of
Medicine
Springfield, Illinois
Chapter 9

Mingchen Song, MD, PhD
Associate Professor of
Clinical Medicine
Southern Illinois University School of
Medicine
Springfield, Illinois
Chapter 8

Sheryll Mae C. Soriano, MD
Southern Illinois University School of
Medicine
Springfield, Illinois
Chapter 42

Raj Sreedhar, MD
Professor of Medicine
Division of Pulmonology and
Critical Care Medicine
Southern Illinois University School of
Medicine
Springfield, Illinois
Chapter 19

Vidya Sundareshan, MD, MPH
Professor and Chief, Infectious
Diseases Program Director,
Infectious Diseases
Southern Illinois University School of
Medicine
Springfield, Illinois
Chapter 14

**Abdul Monem Swied, MD,
FASGE, MACG**
Associate Professor of Clinical
Medicine-Gastroenterology
Southern Illinois University School of
Medicine
Springfield, Illinois
Chapter 1

Vajeeha Tabassum, MD, FACP
Southern Illinois University School of
Medicine
Springfield, Illinois
Chapter 37

Christine Y. Todd, MD, FACP, FHM
Professor Emeritus of Internal
Medicine
Southern Illinois University School of
Medicine
Springfield, Illinois
Chapters 44, 45, 46

Jacob Varney, MD
Assistant Professor of Clinical
Medicine
Southern Illinois University School of
Medicine
Springfield, Illinois
Chapters 21, 34, 37

Peter White, MD
Professor of Clinical Internal
Medicine
Southern Illinois University School
of Medicine
Springfield, Illinois
Chapter 26

Vanessa Williams, MD
Assistant Professor of Clinical
Medicine
Southern Illinois University School
of Medicine
Springfield, Illinois
Chapters 12, 36

Siegfried W. B. Yu, MD, FACP
Southern Illinois University School of
Medicine
Springfield, Illinois
Chapter 38

ACKNOWLEDGMENTS

The Resident Readiness series evolved from ideas that a talented educator and surgeon, David Rogers, had about preparing senior students interested in going into surgery through a resident readiness course. This course was so successful at Southern Illinois University School of Medicine that it spread to other core clerkships, and resident readiness senior electives now exist throughout them. The idea for this book series was born by watching the success of these courses, and the interest the senior students have in them. It has been a great joy working with Susan Hingle, a singularly devoted physician who retains her humanity for others and passion for education, as well as with the other contributors to this book. We are grateful to the Dean, Dr. Jerry Kruse, whose dedication to education and innovation allowed us to carve out time in our work to be creative. We would like to thank the many contributors to this book, whose commitment to medical education undoubtedly led to long nights writing and editing in its service. Lastly, we appreciate our husbands' forbearance for the hours we spent in front of the computer at home; their patience and understanding are unparalleled.

Debra L. Klamen
Susan Thompson Hingle

INTRODUCTION

Facing the prospect of an internship is an exciting, and undoubtedly anxiety-provoking, prospect. Four years of medical school culminate in, after graduation, a rapid transition to someone calling you "Doctor" and asking you to give orders and perform procedures without, in many cases, a supervisor standing directly over your shoulder.

This book is organized to help senior medical students dip their toes safely in the water of responsibility and action from the safety of reading cases, without real patients, nurses, families, and supervisors expecting decisive action. The chapters are short, easy to read, and "to the point." Short vignettes pose an organizing context to valuable issues vital to the function of the new intern. Emphasis on the discussion of these cases is not on extensive basic science background or a review of the literature; it is on practical knowledge that the intern will need to function well in the hospital and "hit the ground running." Many of the cases include questions at the end of them to stimulate further thinking and clinical reasoning in the topic area discussed. References at the end of the cases are resources for further reading as desired.

HOW TO GET THE MOST OUT OF THIS BOOK

Each case is designed to simulate a patient encounter (or nurse request for a patient encounter in some instances) and is followed by a set of open-ended questions. Open-ended questions follow and are used purposefully, since the cued nature of multiple-choice questions will certainly not be available in a clinical setting with real patient involvement. Each case is divided into four parts.

Part 1

1. **Answers** to the questions posed. The student should try to answer the questions after the case vignette before going on to read the case review or

other answers, in order to improve his or her clinical acumen, which, after all, is what resident readiness is all about.

2. A **Case Review:** A brief discussion of the case presented in the vignette will be presented, helping the student understand how an expert would think about, and handle, the specific issues at hand with the particular patient presented.

Part 2

Topic Title followed by **Diagnosis** and **Treatment** discussions: In this section, a more generalized, though still focused and brief, discussion of the general issues brought forward in the case presented will be given. For example, in the case of a patient presenting with coma and a significantly elevated glucose, the case review might discuss the exact treatment of the patient presented, while this part of the book will discuss, in general, the diagnosis and treatment of DKA. Of note, not all of the cases in the book will fit entirely into this model, so variations do occur as necessary. (For example, in the case of a patient in need of palliative care.)

Part 3

Tips to Remember: These are brief, bullet pointed notes that are reiterated as a summary of the text, allowing for easy and rapid review, such as when preparing a case presentation to the faculty in morning rounds.

Part 4

Comprehension Questions: Most cases have several multiple-choice questions that follow at the very end. These serve to reinforce the material presented, and provide a self-assessment mechanism for the student.

Section I.
Inpatient Medicine

Patients With Abdominal Pain

Abdul Monem Swied, MD, FASGE, MACG
and Sayeeda Azra Jabeen, MD, FACP

A 75-year-old Woman with Epigastric and Periumbilical Pain

Ms. Jones is a 75-year-old woman with medical history of type 2 DM, HTN, and CAD admitted with a 2-day complaint of fever, cough, and shortness of breath. She was diagnosed with community-acquired pneumonia and started on levofloxacin. On admission her vitals were stable. The on-call intern received a call at 2:00 AM from the hospital ward nurse, stating that Ms. Jones has been complaining of excruciating constant abdominal pain (epigastric and periumbilical pain) radiating to the flank for the past 15 to 20 minutes. Her pain is associated with nausea and vomiting but no fever or chills, hematuria, dysuria, or chest pain. She had a normal bowel movement earlier today. Medical history includes no h/o renal or gallstones. Social history is significant for smoking, but no alcohol use. Medications include levofloxacin, hydrochlorothiazide, aspirin, metoprolol, and lovastatin; no NSAID use is noted. On physical examination, she looks to be in moderate distress. Blood pressure lying down is 120/60, heart rate is 100, and the patient is afebrile. Heart and lung examinations are unremarkable. Abdominal examination reveals obese abdomen with moderate, diffuse tenderness without guarding or rigidity; bowel sounds are present but hypoactive. Pulses are diminished in the lower extremities. Rectal examination reveals normal with no blood.

1. What should be included in your differential diagnosis (DDx)?

Answer

1. Acute pancreatitis
2. Acute diverticulitis (although pain would be expected more in the left lower quadrant [LLQ])
3. Peptic ulcer disease unless associated with perforation with signs of peritonitis (rebound tenderness and rigidity)

4. Abdominal aortic aneurysm (AAA) dissection or rupture

5. Urinary tract infection (UTI)

6. Ovarian torsion

CASE REVIEW: ABDOMINAL AORTIC ANEURYSM

The classic presentation of AAA complication is a woman with a history of HTN who has the triad of severe abdominal pain, a pulsatile abdominal mass, and hypotension. Physical examination is not sufficiently sensitive to rule out AAA. Although atherosclerosis is the most common cause for AAA, there are a number of nonatherosclerotic causes, which include cystic medial necrosis, and infections such as syphilis and *Salmonella*. Aneurysms also occur with diseases such as Marfan syndrome or Ehlers-Danlos syndrome. Risk factors include smoking, male sex, family history, advanced age, and uncontrolled hypertension. Complications include aortic aneurysm rupture. Rates of rupture rise as the aneurysm increases in diameter size. Mortality with rupture is 70% to 90%. Bedside emergent ultrasound has been demonstrated to be highly accurate with a sensitivity of 96% to 100% and a specificity of 98% to 100%. For screening, ultrasound is preferred. Treatment may be surgical or medical. Urgent surgical management is used when the AAA has ruptured. For an asymptomatic AAA, repair is recommended when an aneurysm is greater than or equal to 5.5 cm, is tender, or has increased in size by more than 1 cm in 1 year. For smaller aneurysms that have not ruptured, medical management with smoking cessation, statin therapy, and optimal blood pressure control is initiated.

Alternative diagnoses to consider include nephrolithiasis, diverticulitis, ovarian torsion, and UTI.

Nephrolithiasis

The classic presentation is acute onset of severe back and flank pain that may radiate to the abdomen or groin. Pain may be associated with nausea, vomiting, or dysuria. Abdominal tenderness is unusual and, if present, should raise the possibility of other diagnoses.

Diverticulitis

A diverticulum is a sac-like protrusion of the colonic wall. A low-fiber diet and constipation are believed to cause diverticula to form by decreasing stool bulk and increasing intraluminal pressure. Diverticulitis develops secondary to microscopic or open perforation of the diverticula. Some 85% to 90% of acute diverticulitis develops in the sigmoid or descending colon. The classic presentation is gradually increasing LLQ pain. Fever is often present. Patients may present with diarrhea and/or constipation. Guarding and rigidity may be seen. Diverticulitis can be complicated with abscess formation, peritonitis, colonic obstruction, fistula formation, and sepsis. Computed tomographic (CT) scanning of the abdomen with IV and oral contrast is the diagnostic test of choice. If the patient has no fever or elevated white blood cell count and is able to tolerate oral antibiotics, then start ciprofloxacin and metronidazole for 7 to 10 days. Encourage oral liquid intake. For moderate to severe attacks, broad-spectrum IV antibiotics should be started. Keep the patient NPO (nothing by mouth) and start IV fluids. If there is an abscess (5 cm or larger), obtain CT-guided drainage. Emergent surgery is indicated only in cases of frank peritonitis, uncontrolled sepsis, clinical deterioration, obstruction, or large abscesses.

ABDOMINAL PAIN

Abdominal pain is one of the most common causes for hospital admission in the United States. It is caused by conditions that range from trivial to life-threatening.

An uncommon but serious condition called ovarian torsion occurs in women when the ovary and/or the fallopian tube twist around the tissues that support them. When this happens, the blood supply to the ovary is cut off; if not treated promptly, this can cause tissue in the organ to become ischemic and potentially infarct.

Diagnosis

The first pivotal step in diagnosing abdominal pain is to identify the location of the pain. The DDx can then be narrowed to a subset of conditions that cause pain in that particular quadrant of the abdomen (see Figure 1-1).

There is an overlap among the differential diagnoses in the various quadrants, and there are some different concerns based on age and sex.

History

The character and acuity of the pain are pivotal features that help prioritize the DDx. Other important historic points include factors that make the pain better or worse (eg, eating), radiation of the pain, duration of the pain, and associated symptoms (nausea, vomiting, poor appetite, inability to pass stool and gas, melena, hematochezia, fever, chills, weight loss, altered bowel habits, orthostatic symptoms, or urinary symptoms). Pulmonary symptoms or a cardiac history can be clues to pneumonia or myocardial infarction (MI) presenting as abdominal pain. In women, sexual and menstrual histories are very important. The patient should be asked about alcohol consumption as well.

Physical Examination

A few points about the physical examination are worth emphasizing. Vital signs such as hypotension, fever, tachypnea, and tachycardia are pivotal clinical clues

Right upper quadrant

Appendicitis (retrocecal)
Biliary colic
Cholangitis
Cholecystitis
Hepatitis
Hepatic abscess
Perforated duodenal ulcer
Pneumonia (right lower lobe)
Pulmonary embolism

Left upper quadrant

Gastric ulcer
Gastritis
Myocardial ischemia
Pancreatitis
Pneumonia (left lower lobe)
Pulmonary embolism
Splenic congestion or rupture

Right lower quadrant

Aortic aneurysm
Appendicitis
Crohn disease
Diverticulitis (cecal)
Ectopic pregnancy
Endometriosis
Incarcerated inguinal hernia
Ischemic colitis
Ovarian cyst
Ovarian torsion
Pelvic inflammatory disease
Psoas abscess
Testicular torsion
Ureteral calculi

Left lower quadrant

Aortic aneurysm
Diverticulitis (sigmoid)
Ectopic pregnancy
Endometriosis
Incarcerated inguinal hernia
Ischemic colitis
Ovarian cyst
Ovarian torsion
Pelvic inflammatory disease
Psoas abscess
Testicular torsion
Ureteral calculi

Diffuse pain

Aortic aneurysm
Aortic dissection
Appendicitis (early)
Bowel obstruction
Gastroenteritis
Mesenteric ischemia
Metabolic disorders (diabetic ketoacidosis, uremia)
Narcotic withdrawal
Pancreatitis
Perforated bowel
Peritonitis
Sickle cell crisis
Volvulus

Figure 1-1. DDx of abdominal pain.

that must not be overlooked. The HEENT examination should look for pallor or icterus. Careful heart and lung examinations can suggest pneumonia or other extra-abdominal causes of abdominal pain.

Treatment

Acute abdominal pain frequently requires urgent investigation and management. Some patients require assessment of their airways, breathing, and circulation, followed by appropriate resuscitation. Many patients will require analgesics, which can be administered judiciously without compromising the physical assessment of peritoneal signs.

Patients with a suspected surgical abdomen must be transferred to an acute care facility where surgical consultation and management are available.

Acute versus chronic pain: while an arbitrary interval, such as 12 weeks, can be used to separate acute from chronic abdominal pain, there is no strict time period. Pain in a sick or unstable patient should generally be managed as acute pain.

A 26-year-old Man With Diffuse Abdominal Pain for the Past 12 Hours

Mr. Smith is a 26-year-old man with no significant past medical history who presents with diffuse abdominal pain that began 12 hours ago and is described as a pressure sensation, most intensely in the mid-abdomen. He has a decreased appetite but no nausea or vomiting. His last bowel movement was 2 days ago. He denies fevers and chills, hematuria, dysuria, or chest pain. The patient has no known history of gallstones, kidney stones, or abdominal surgeries. He takes no medications (no aspirin or NSAIDs) and reports occasional use of alcohol. Vitals are stable. Patient is afebrile. Cardiac and lung examinations are normal. Abdominal examination reveals a flat abdomen with hypoactive bowel sounds. There is mild, diffuse tenderness present. No guarding or rigidity is present. Rectal examination is normal with normal stool color.

1. What should be included in your DDx?

Answer

1. Appendicitis (always to be considered in young adults)
   Peptic ulcer disease
   Acute pancreatitis (may present with epigastric or mid-abdominal pain)
   Early bowel obstruction

CASE REVIEW: ACUTE APPENDICITIS

The classic presentation is diffuse abdominal pain that migrates to the right lower quadrant (RLQ) to McBurney point (1.5–2 in from the anterior superior iliac crest toward the umbilicus). The pain is associated with nausea, vomiting, fever, and anorexia. Appendicitis develops due to obstruction of the appendiceal orifice with secondary mucous accumulation, swelling, ischemia, necrosis, and perforation. Complications include perforation and abscess formation. The risk of perforation increases steadily with increasing age (50% in patients >75 years old). Fever, tenderness, guarding, and rebound may be absent in patients with appendicitis. Nonetheless, when present, they increase the likelihood of appendicitis. Some 80% of patients with appendicitis have a WBC >10,000 with a left shift. Urinalysis may reveal pyuria and hematuria due to reactive bladder inflammation from adjacent appendicitis. CT of abdomen and pelvis with IV and oral/rectal contrast is the test of choice. Although ultrasound is inferior to CT scan, it is the test of choice in pregnant patients. Frequent clinical observation is critical in patients with an unclear diagnosis. One should start IV fluids and broad-spectrum antibiotics and obtain a surgical consult without delay, as urgent appendectomy is the treatment of choice.

Other diagnoses to consider in patients with RLQ pain include cecal diverticulitis, Meckel diverticulitis, acute ileitis, Crohn disease, and gynecologic conditions.

Cecal Diverticulitis

Cecal diverticulitis usually occurs in young adults and presents with signs and symptoms that are virtually identical to those of appendicitis.

Meckel Diverticulitis

A Meckel diverticulum is a congenital remnant of the omphalomesenteric duct. It contains all layers of the intestine and may have ectopic tissue present from either the pancreas or stomach. It is located on the small intestine 2 ft from the ileocecal valve and is about 4 to 5 cm length. The small bowel may migrate into the RLQ and mimic the symptoms of appendicitis.

Acute Ileitis

Acute ileitis is due most commonly to an acute self-limited bacterial infection (*Yersinia, Campylobacter, Salmonella,* and others) and should be considered when diarrhea is a prominent symptom.

Crohn Disease

Crohn disease can present with symptoms similar to appendicitis. Fatigue, chronic diarrhea with abdominal pain, weight loss, and fever, with or without gross bleeding, are the hallmarks of Crohn disease. Crohn disease should be suspected in patients who have persistent pain after surgery, especially if the appendix is histologically normal.

Gynecologic Conditions

A number of gynecologic conditions, most notably ectopic pregnancy and pelvic inflammatory disease (acute salpingitis), should be considered in the DDx. Always rule out pregnancy in women of childbearing age who complain of abdominal pain.

A 55-year-old Woman with Crampy Epigastric Pain

Mrs. Hampton is a 55-year-old female who presents to the emergency department with crampy epigastric pain that woke her up in the middle of the night. She has had similar attacks over the past several months that generally last for 3 to 4 hours. Heavy meals worsen the pain. She denies nausea and vomiting, has normal bowel movements, no fever or chills, and no hematuria, dysuria, or chest pain. Patient medical history is remarkable for type 2 DM, HTN, and atrial fibrillation. Medications include metoprolol, insulin, and aspirin; she occasionally takes acetaminophen for knee pain. She reports no alcohol use. On physical examination vitals are normal. The patient is afebrile. Sclera is anicteric. Cardiac and lung examinations are normal except for the presence of an irregularly irregular cardiac rhythm. Abdominal examination shows a slightly obese abdomen. Bowel sounds are present. Abdomen is soft, with mild epigastric tenderness present. No guarding or rigidity is present. Murphy sign is negative. Rectal examination is normal with normal stool color.

1. What should be included in your DDx?

Answer

1. Biliary-type abdominal pain (cholelithiasis)

    Peptic ulcer disease

    Acute pancreatitis

    Irritable bowel syndrome (IBS)

    Mesenteric ischemia

CASE REVIEW: BILIARY-TYPE ABDOMINAL PAIN

The classic presentation of biliary-type abdominal pain is a deep, sharp, severe, gnawing episodic pain that is localized to the right upper quadrant (RUQ) or the epigastrium. It may radiate to the back and can be associated with nausea and vomiting. Patients are pain-free between the episodes. Biliary-type abdominal pain occurs when a gallstone becomes lodged in the cystic duct and the gallbladder contracts against the obstruction, at times in response to a fatty meal. Complications include acute cholecystitis, acute pancreatitis, choledocholithiasis, and ascending cholangitis. A RUQ ultrasound is the diagnostic test of choice due to its high sensitivity and specificity. Cholecystectomy is recommended. Dissolution therapies (e.g., ursodiol) are reserved for nonsurgical candidates.

Alternative possible diagnoses include peptic ulcer disease (PUD), acute pancreatitis, IBS, ischemic bowel, mesenteric ischemia, and ischemic colitis.

Peptic Ulcer Disease

PUD presents with dull or hunger-like pain in the epigastrium that is either exacerbated or improved by food intake. Most ulcers are due to NSAID use, *Helicobacter pylori* infection, or both. The best predictor of PUD is a history of NSAID use and *H. pylori* infection. A significant number of patients with NSAID-induced ulcers do not experience pain. Anemia, GI bleeding, early satiety, or weight loss may be the only symptoms of PUD. Zollinger-Ellison syndrome is a rare cause of PUD. An esophagogastroduodenoscopy (EGD) should be considered with symptoms of significant bleeding, anemia, weight loss, early satiety, dysphagia, recurrent vomiting, or a family history of GI cancer, or in patients who do not respond to initial therapy with proton pump inhibitors (PPIs). Gastric ulcers always warrant biopsy to rule out adenocarcinoma. *H. pylori* testing should be done via the biopsied tissue.

One can also test for *H. pylori* with a urea breath test and *H. pylori* stool antigen in patients not undergoing EGD. A rapid urease test on biopsy and histology are preferred in patients undergoing EGD. Serology does not distinguish active from prior infection (avoid the use of serology on a routine basis). Active bleeding from PUD decreases the sensitivity of a rapid urease test. Patients with bleeding and a negative rapid urease test and negative histology should undergo a urea breath test or *H. Pylori* stool antigen several weeks after completing PPI therapy.

Treatment goals include eradication of *H. pylori*, symptom alleviation, and ulcer healing. The regimen most commonly recommended for first-line treatment of *H. pylori* is triple therapy with a PPI (lansoprazole 30 mg twice daily, omeprazole 20 mg twice daily, pantoprazole 40 mg twice daily, rabeprazole 20 mg twice daily, or esomeprazole 40 mg once daily), amoxicillin (1 g twice daily), and clarithromycin (500 mg twice daily) for 10 to 14 days. Metronidazole (500 mg twice daily) can be substituted for amoxicillin, but only in penicillin-allergic individuals. An increased incidence of *H. pylori* resistance has led to the recommendation of posttreatment testing to confirm eradication. Appropriate testing includes stool antigen or urea breath test 4 to 6 weeks after completion of therapy. Before testing for *H. pylori* and to lower false negative results, PPI should be held for 2 weeks and antibiotics held for 4 weeks. Don't forget to discontinue NSAIDs in these patients.

Acute Pancreatitis

The classic presentation of acute pancreatitis is a constant, boring abdominal pain of moderate to severe intensity in the epigastrium that may radiate to the back. Pain is often associated with nausea, vomiting, low-grade fever, and abdominal distention. Alcohol abuse and choledocholithiasis cause 80% of acute pancreatitis cases. Other causes include idiopathic, post–endoscopic retrograde cholangiopancreatography (ERCP), and medications (hydrochlorothiazide, azathioprine, corticosteroids, sulfonamides, furosemide, etc). Less common causes are trauma, marked hypertriglyceridemia (>1000 mg/dL), hypercalcemia, and pancreatic divisum. Regardless of the inciting cause, trypsinogen is activated to trypsin that activates other pancreatic enzymes resulting in pancreatic autodigestion and inflammation. Patients with pancreatitis may develop pseudocysts, abscesses, or pancreatic necrosis. Systemic complications include hyperglycemia, hypocalcemia, acute respiratory distress syndrome, acute renal failure, and disseminated intravascular coagulation (DIC). Death may occur in patients with infected pancreatic necrosis and multiorgan system failure. Several predictive scores have been developed. These include Ranson criteria, the BISAP score, and the APACHE II score. The American Gastroenterological Association (AGA) recommends the use of the APACHE II system. Hemoconcentration (Hct ≥50%) on admission predicts severe pancreatitis. C-reactive protein >150 mg/dL at 48 hours also can predict severe pancreatitis. Diagnostic testing should include amylase and lipase. Transabdominal ultrasound is ideal to image the gallbladder and biliary tree to look for gallstones. CT scan is the test of choice to look for complications and assess severity.

Treatment is generally supportive care with IV fluids. It is recommended, after initial fluid resuscitation with 20 cm^3/kg IV fluids over 60 to 90 minutes, to give approximately 250 to 300 cm^3/h IV fluids for 48 hours if the patient's cardiac status permits. One should closely monitor vital signs, renal function, hematocrit, and fluid status. Patients are kept NPO, unless they are hungry and can take PO. Prophylactic antibiotics are not routinely indicated and only given if there is strong evidence of infected necrosis (fever, leukocytosis, clinical deterioration, or CT scan findings). Acute necrotizing pancreatitis or fluid collections are not indications for IV antibiotics by themselves. ERCP and sphincterotomy can be therapeutic and only recommended in patients with gallstone pancreatitis with persistent biliary obstruction or cholangitis.

Irritable Bowel Syndrome

IBS is characterized by intermittent chronic abdominal pain accompanied by diarrhea, constipation, or both. The diarrhea is often associated with cramps relieved by defecation and passing flatus. Pain cannot be explained by structural or biochemical abnormalities. Symptoms of IBS are due to a combination of altered motility, visceral hypersensitivity, autonomic function, and psychological factors. Symptoms are often exacerbated by psychological or physical stress.

Diagnosis

The diagnosis is usually made by a combination of (1) fulfilling the Rome criteria, (2) the absence of alarming features, and (3) a limited workup to exclude other diseases.

1. Rome criteria: Recurrent abdominal pain or discomfort (of ≥6 months' duration) at least 3 days per month for the past 3 months, associated with 2 or more of the following:

   A. Improvement with defecation

   B. Onset associated with a change in frequency of stool

   C. Onset associated with a change in form (appearance) of stool

2. Alarm symptoms suggest alternative diagnoses and necessitate evaluation

   A. Positive fecal occult blood test or rectal bleeding

   B. Anemia

   C. Weight loss >10 lb

   D. Fever

   E. Persistent diarrhea causing dehydration

   F. Severe constipation or fecal impaction

   G. Family history of colorectal cancer

   H. Onset of symptoms at age 50 years or older

   I. Major change in symptoms

   J. Nocturnal symptoms

   K. Recent antibiotic use

3. Workup

   A. Common recommendations for patients fulfilling Rome criteria without alarm symptoms include the following:

      - CBC
      - Test stool for occult blood
      - Serologic tests for celiac sprue (eg, IgA tissue transglutaminase or IgA EMA) in patients with diarrhea as the predominant symptom
      - Routine chemistries (recommended by some experts)

   B. Colonoscopy with biopsy (to rule out microscopic colitis) is recommended in patients with chronic diarrhea, alarm symptoms, age ≥50 years, and a marked change in symptoms.

   C. There is no evidence that flexible sigmoidoscopy or colonoscopy is necessary in young patients without alarm symptoms.

D. In addition to the above testing, the following should be evaluated in patients with alarm symptoms:

- Thyroid function levels
- Basic chemistries
- Stool for *Clostridium difficile* toxin and presence of ova and parasites

A variety of serum and fecal markers, including ASCA, p-ANCA, fecal cal-protectin, and fecal lactoferrin, are useful in selected patients(not routinely) and can suggest bowel inflammation or inflammatory bowel disease (IBD).

Treatment

Treatment of IBS includes avoiding certain foods (milk products, caffeine, alcohol, fatty foods, gas-producing vegetables, etc) that may worsen symptoms. Specific therapy is based on predominant symptoms. When abdominal pain is a predominant symptom, medications such as anticholinergics (dicyclomine or hyoscyamine) and/or smooth muscle relaxants may be beneficial. Cognitive behavioral therapy also is useful. When diarrhea is the predominant symptom, medications such as loperamide, diphenoxylate, and cholestyramine may be useful. Alosetron, a 5-HT3 receptor antagonist, is also useful with diarrhea but is generally only prescribed by gastroenterologists, as serious complications such as bowel obstruction and ischemic colitis may occur with its use. When constipation is the predominant symptom, a change to a high-fiber diet and osmotic laxatives such as lactulose and polyethylene glycol are used.

Ischemic Bowel

There are 3 distinct subtypes of ischemic bowel, including chronic mesenteric ischemia (chronic small bowel ischemia), acute mesenteric ischemia (acute ischemia of small bowel), and ischemic colitis (ischemia of the large bowel).

Mesenteric ischemia

This is a life-threatening condition that virtually always presents with the abrupt onset of acute, severe abdominal pain that is typically out of proportion to a relativity benign physical examination. It may be associated with nausea and vomiting. This ischemia usually occurs due to a superior mesenteric artery embolism (50%) that is frequently due to a dislodged thrombosis from the left atrium, left ventricle, or cardiac valves. Mesenteric arterial thrombosis (15%–25%) occurs due to progressive atherosclerotic stenosis of the involved artery. Mesenteric venous thrombosis occurs often due to portal hypertension, hypercoagulable states, and intra-abdominal inflammation. Nonobstructive mesenteric ischemia (NOMI) (20%–30%) often occurs in elderly patients with atherosclerotic disease and superimposed hypotension (MI, heart failure, cardiopulmonary bypass, dialysis, or sepsis). Mortality is high at 30% to 65%. Complications include bowel infarction and peritonitis. Lactic acid level is typically elevated. Although CT angiography and magnetic resonance angiography have been used, direct mesenteric angiography is the gold standard diagnostic test.

Treatment consists of emergent revascularization via thromboembolectomy, thrombolysis, vascular bypass or angioplasty, and surgical resection of necrotic bowel. Broad-spectrum IV antibiotics, volume resuscitation, and preoperative and postoperative anticoagulation to prevent thrombosis propagation also are essential. Intra-arterial papaverine has been used to block reactive mesenteric arteriolar vasoconstriction and improve blood flow.

Ischemic colitis

Ischemic colitis presents with left-sided abdominal pain that is frequently associated with bloody or maroon-colored stools and/or diarrhea. It occurs due to a nonocclusive decrease in colonic perfusion (hypotension, MI, sepsis, CHF, etc). It typically involves the watershed area of the colon, most commonly the splenic flexure, descending colon, and rectosigmoid junction. Lactic acid level is elevated. Colonoscopy and biopsy are the preferred diagnostic test. CT scan may demonstrate segmental circumferential wall thickening (nonspecific) or appear normal. Treatment is generally supportive with bed rest, IV fluids, and broad-spectrum antibiotics. Colonic infarction occurs in a small percentage of patients and requires surgical intervention.

A 55-year-old Woman With a Diagnosis of Biliary-type Pain, Now Presenting With Constant RUQ Pain, Fever, and Chills

Mrs. Hampton's history suggests biliary-type pain. A RUQ ultrasound reveals multiple small gallstones with no acute cholecystitis and normal bile ducts. CBC and liver profile are normal. Serum lipase and liver enzymes were normal. Urea breath test for *H. pylori* was negative. After surgical consultation, elective cholecystectomy was planned 2 weeks later. Unfortunately, Mrs. Hampton returned to the emergency department prior to her scheduled surgery with constant pain in her RUQ associated with fever and chills. She appeared in acute distress. She reports dark urine. Vitals are stable except for the presence of fever at 38.3°C. Sclera were icteric. Abdominal examination reveals RUQ tenderness with a positive Murphy sign.

1. What should be included in your DDx?

Answer

1. Common bile duct (CBD) obstruction (also known as choledocholithiasis)
   Ascending cholangitis
   Acute cholecystitis
   Acute hepatitis

CASE REVIEW: CHOLEDOCHOLITHIASIS AND ACUTE ASCENDING CHOLANGITIS

The classic presentation is RUQ pain, fever, and jaundice, also known as Charcot triad. This occurs due to CBD obstruction, most commonly from a slipped gallstone. Complications include obstruction, jaundice, fever, leukocytosis, sepsis, and acute pancreatitis. ERCP is both diagnostic and therapeutic. It is the preferred test of choice in patients with a high pretest probability of CBD stone with obstruction. It allows direct cannulation of CBD and relieves obstruction via simultaneous sphincterotomy and stone extraction. In patients who are less likely to have a CBD stone, a less invasive test such as magnetic resonance cholangiopancreatography (MRCP) or endoscopic ultrasound (EUS) would be appropriate as an initial study to examine the CBD. Treatment includes IV hydration, IV broad-spectrum antibiotics, and decompression of the biliary system (via ERCP in patients with persistent pain, hypotension, altered mental status, persistent high fever, WBC ≥20,000, and bilirubin >10 mg/dL and electively in more stable patients), followed by cholecystectomy.

Alternative diagnoses to consider include acute cholecystitis and acute hepatitis.

Acute Cholecystitis

Acute cholecystitis presents as persistent dull RUQ or epigastric pain associated with fever, nausea, and vomiting. Murphy sign may be present (sensitivity 65% and specificity 87%). Acute cholecystitis is caused by persistent obstruction of the cystic duct with stones resulting in gallbladder inflammation and pain. It may be complicated with necrosis, infection, and gangrene. The test of choice is a RUQ ultrasound. Cholescintigraphy (HIDA scan) is useful when the pretest probability is high and ultrasound is nondiagnostic. Nonvisualization of the gallbladder suggests cystic duct obstruction and is highly specific for acute cholecystitis. Treatment includes IV hydration, IV antibiotics, and cholecystectomy.

Acute Hepatitis

Viral or alcoholic hepatitis should be considered in a patient presenting with abdominal pain, jaundice, anorexia, nausea, malaise, hepatomegaly, or hepatic tenderness. Liver enzymes are very high in acute hepatitis. If suspected, appropriate serologies should be ordered.

A 70-year-old Man With Crampy Mid-abdominal Pain

Mr. Lantern is a 70-year-old man with a history of hypertension, type 2 DM, and coronary artery disease who presents with intermittent, crampy, mid-abdominal pain that started 2 days ago and is associated with nausea, vomiting, constipation, and an unintentional weight loss of 10 lb over the past 2 months. The patient denies fever or chills, hematuria, dysuria, or chest pain. There is no history of gallstones, kidney stones, or abdominal surgeries. Current medications are lisinopril, aspirin, metoprolol, simvastatin, and insulin. He reports no alcohol use. On physical examination the patient looks moderately distressed. Vitals are significant for orthostasis with the heart rate increasing by 20 beats/min and blood pressure dropping by 20 mm Hg when the patient sits up. The patient is afebrile. Sclerae are anicteric. Cardiac and lung examinations are normal except for an irregularly irregular rhythm. Abdominal examination reveals a distended abdomen with hyperactive bowel sounds. Rectal examination is normal.

1. What should be included in your DDx?

Answer

1. Large bowel obstruction (LBO)
    Small bowel obstruction (SBO)

CASE REVIEW

Large Bowel Obstruction

LBO typically presents with severe, diffuse, crampy abdominal pain that appears in waves associated with vomiting. Abdominal pain and the absence of bowel movements or flatus suggest bowel obstruction. Initially, patients may have several bowel movements as the bowel distal to the obstruction is emptied. Obstruction can be due to cancer, volvulus, diverticular disease, or external compression from metastatic cancer, etc. LBO may be complicated by bowel infarction, perforation, peritonitis, and sepsis. Plain x-rays of the abdomen may show air-fluid levels and distension of large bowel (>6 cm) and also free air under the diaphragm in the case of perforation. CT scan of the abdomen and pelvis is also accurate in the diagnosis of LBO (91% sensitive and 91% specific). Hypaque enema (water-soluble enema) is 96% sensitive and 98% specific and is highly accurate for larger bowel obstruction. It can be both diagnostic and therapeutic. It can also exclude acute colonic pseudo-obstruction (Ogilvie syndrome, distension of the cecum and colon without mechanical obstruction). Colonoscopy can decompress pseudo-obstruction and prevent cecal perforation. Treatment of LBO includes aggressive hydration, broad-spectrum antibiotics, and a surgical consultation. Emergent surgical indications include perforation or ischemia. Nonemergent indications include increasing abdominal distension and failure to resolve with conservative management.

Small Bowel Obstruction

SBO presents similarly to LBO, except that the patient typically has a history of prior abdominal surgeries. It is usually caused by adhesions, malignant obstruction, hernias, IBD strictures, or radiation-induced strictures. SBO complications include bowel infarction, perforation, peritonitis, and sepsis. Plain x-rays of the abdomen may show 2 or more air-fluid levels or dilated loops of bowel proximal to the obstruction (>2.5 cm diameter of small bowel). Complete obstruction is unlikely if air is seen in the rectum or in the colon. CT scan of the abdomen is the diagnostic test of choice. It may delineate the etiology of the obstruction as well. Obstruction is suggested by a transition point between bowel proximal to the obstruction, which is dilated, and bowel distal to the obstruction, which is collapsed. A small bowel series may be useful when CT is nondiagnostic. SBO treatment includes aggressive IV hydration, keeping the patient NPO with a nasogastric tube to suction, careful frequent observation, repeated physical examinations over the first 12 to 24 hours, and frequent plain radiographs. Broad-spectrum IV antibiotics are typically initiated. Surgical indications include signs of ischemia, infarction on CT scan, and obstruction due to hernia.

TIPS TO REMEMBER

- DDx of abdominal pain may be very expansive.
- History and physical examination are the most important elements in developing and refining your list of diagnostic possibilities.
- Localizing the pain to a quadrant helps to refine and narrow your DDx.
- Not all abdominal pain is of gastrointestinal origin.
- Workup should be targeted based on the history and physical examination.

SUGGESTED READINGS

Chung J. *Natural history abdominal aortic aneurysm*. In: Eidt J, Mills J, Creager M, eds. *UpToDate*. 2022.

Jim J. *Management of abdominal aortic aneurysm*. In: Mills J, Eidt J, eds. *UpToDate*. 2022.

Kamboj A, Oxentenko A, Wang T, et al. *Approach to the patient with abdominal pain, gas and bloating*. In: Wang TC, Camilleri M, Lebwohl B, et al, eds. *Yamada's Text Book of Gastroenterology*. 7th ed. Hoboken: Wiley-Blackwell; 2022.

Penner R, Fishman M. *Differential diagnosis of abdominal pain in adults*. In: Auerbach A, Aronson M, eds. *UpToDate*. 2022.

A Review of Acid-base Disorders

Bemi (Oritsegbubemi) Adekola, MD

CASE 1

A medical consult was called for persistent elevated bicarbonate and hypokalemia in a 63-year-old male. The patient underwent emergent partial gastrectomy 4 days ago for a perforated gastric ulcer. His hospital course was complicated by early wound infection and ileus. For the last 3 days the patient has received IV potassium supplements and lactated Ringer's solution at 50 cc/h. Continuous gastric suctioning via nasogastric (NG) tube is in place. His vital signs are as follows: BP 105/60 mm Hg, HR 90 bpm, RR 10.

> Laboratory findings:
> ABG: pH 7.47, Po_2 85, Pco_2 48
> Sodium 138 mEq/L, potassium 2.8 mEq/L, chloride 88 mEq/L, bicarbonate 40 mEq/L
> BUN 15 mg/dL, creatinine 0.8 mg/dL, glucose 120 mg/dL, calcium 8.5 mg/dL, albumin 3.0 g/dL

Which of the following is the best next step in addition to potassium repletion?
   A. Acetazolamide
   B. Potassium citrate
   C. Potassium chloride
   D. Start IV saline infusion and proton pump inhibitor (PPI)

Discussion

The patient has hypokalemia and chloride-sensitive metabolic alkalosis. This scenario of persistent loss of gastric fluid—which can be up to 1–2 L per day containing sodium and chloride losses (up to 400 mEq/d), potassium (minimal <15 mmol/L), and water and hydrogen ions (H^+) (200 mmol/mEq in 1 day)—results in volume depletion, hypokalemia, and increasing metabolic alkalosis. A similar case would be seen in a patient with persistent vomiting.

The initiation phase of metabolic alkalosis is as follows:

1. Loss of sodium, water, and chloride from gastric fluid from NG suctioning or vomiting results in decreased extracellular volume. This triggers the renin-angiotensin-aldosterone system, which first causes sodium and water reabsorption.

2. The gastric parietal cells secrete H^+ at the luminal H^+ ATPase, leaving $HCO3^-$ to be reclaimed at the basolateral membrane and resulting in increased plasma pH.

3. The presence of alkalosis causes shifts of potassium into the cells, resulting in hypokalemia.

4. The normal buffering that occurs by the respiratory system is hypoventilation causing retention of CO_2 (hypercapnia). This is why the P_{CO_2} noted in the ABG is >40.

Maintenance Phase of Metabolic Alkalosis
If corrective measures are not put in place, the metabolic alkalosis is perpetuated by increased renal bicarbonate reabsorption and synthesis (primarily in the proximal tubule) brought about by the above-mentioned triggers—namely, hypercapnia, hypokalemia, and the renin-angiotensin-aldosterone system. They cause an increase in tubular bicarbonate reabsorption (T_{max}), further increasing plasma bicarbonate.

Clinical Consequences of Metabolic Alkalosis
Metabolic alkalosis rarely has clinically significant adverse effects. If serum bicarbonate is increased to more than 50 mmol/L, serious complications may occur.

- Seizures and delirium can be caused by alkalosis-induced hypocalcemia.
- Hypoxia may occur secondary to hypoventilation.
- Serious cardiac arrhythmia may occur secondary to hypokalemia.

Treatment

Replacing the chloride with IV normal saline will treat the alkalosis in most patients with vomiting or NG tube suctioning. Rarely, normal saline will not be enough and hydrogen chloride solution is needed.

Holding loop or thiazide diuretics can be enough to treat diuretic-induced metabolic alkalosis (another cause of chloride-sensitive metabolic alkalosis).

Hypokalemia should always be treated aggressively and concurrently with volume repletion with isotonic normal saline, which will turn off the renin-angiotensin system and the upregulated bicarb reabsorption threshold, and the serum bicarbonate gradually will start to decrease to normal levels. Additionally, a PPI (if able to administer) will decrease the production of chloride and mitigate the initiation phase of metabolic alkalosis.

Lastly, in these cases of chloride-sensitive metabolic alkalosis, the urine sodium is usually less than 10 mol/L.

The answer is D.

Another type of metabolic alkalosis is chloride-resistant metabolic alkalosis. Consider a patient with uncontrolled hypertension (170/100 mm Hg) on losartan

100 mg daily, amlodipine 10 mg daily, metoprolol 100 mg twice daily, and hydralazine 50 mg twice daily. Blood chemistry is as follows: sodium 138 mEq, potassium 3.4 mEq, bicarbonate 29 mEq/L, and urine chloride 25 mmol/L.

Given the uncontrolled stage II hypertension, workup for resistant hypertension is ordered and reveals an elevated aldosterone–renin ratio suggesting primary hyperaldosteronism as the cause of metabolic alkalosis and resistant hypertension. In this case the metabolic alkalosis is chloride-resistant, and urine chloride is >20 mmol/L. Other causes of chloride-resistant metabolic alkalosis are Cushing syndrome, licorice ingestion, and Bartter and Liddle syndromes. Lastly, there is an important etiology of metabolic alkalosis that occurs mainly in ICU patients with severe respiratory acidosis, as in the case of severe COPD exacerbation or ARDS. There is observed renal compensation with metabolic alkalosis. When the respiratory acidosis resolves. The metabolic alkalosis with elevated bicarbonate may persist for a few days. If symptomatic, acetazolamide may be administered.

CASE 2

A 50-year-old female patient with a history of immunodeficiency syndrome requiring intravenous immunoglobulin (IVIG) infusions and type 1 diabetes mellitus (DM) presents to the ED with nausea, epigastric discomfort, and generalized weakness of 2 days' duration. The patient reports respiratory tract infection for the last 4 weeks, which she noted to be getting worse.

Laboratory findings:
Sodium: 136
Potassium: 5.4
Chloride: 109
Bicarbonate: 15
BUN: 25
Creatinine: 0.9
Glucose: 300
Calcium: 7.3
Albumin: 2.0
ABG: pH 7.25, Po_2 95, and Pco_2 31. CXR shows a right lower-lobe infiltrate.

What is the most likely etiology of this patient's acid-base abnormality?
A. Diarrhea
B. Diabetic ketoacidosis
C. Acute kidney injury
D. Renal tubular acidosis type IV

Discussion and answer to Case 2 follows Case 3.

CASE 3

A 55-year-old man with a history of multiple myeloma recently started chemo-therapy. He presented to his oncologist for follow-up and complains of diarrhea and lethargy. Routine labs reveal the following:

Sodium: 140
Potassium: 3.3
Chloride: 110
Bicarbonate: 13
BUN: 25
Creatinine: 1.2
Glucose: 100
Calcium: 10.1
Albumin: 3.3
ABG: pH 7.28, Po_2 95, and Pco_2 29.

What other labs would you send to help make the diagnosis? What is the diagnosis based on the above lab work, and what is the underlying etiology? Reviewing the renal pathophysiology of this condition, what is the treatment?

A. Diarrhea
B. Diabetic ketoacidosis
C. Acute kidney injury
D. Renal tubular acidosis type II

Discussion for Case 2

The answer is **B**. The patient's anion gap is 12 mEq/L. Because her albumin is only 2.0, her expected normal anion gap should be lowered by 5 mEq/L more than the usual normal range (usual normal anion gap is 10–12 mEq/L; this patient's expected normal anion gap is around 5–7 mEq/L). After correcting the anion gap, it is clear that this patient has high anion gap metabolic acidosis (HAGMA). The only listed etiology that can cause HAGMA is diabetic ketoacidosis. Acute kidney injury (AKI) will cause normal anion gap metabolic acidosis (NAGMA) most of the time. Severe AKI may cause HAGMA, but there is no evidence that this patient has severe AKI.

Discussion for Case 3

The answer is **A**: type 2 renal tubular acidosis causing a non anion gap metabolic acidosis.

Non Anion Gap Metabolic Acidosis

Remember this mnemonic: HARDUP

H: Hyperalimentation (e.g., starting TPN) or dilutional acidosis following saline infusion

A: Acetazolamide use

R: Renal tubular acidosis (type I = distal; type II = proximal; type IV = hyporeninemic hypoaldosteronism)

D: Diarrhea

U: Ureterosigmoid fistula (because the colon will waste bicarbonate)

P: Pancreatic fistula (because of alkali loss—the pancreas secretes a bicarbonate-rich fluid)

NAGMA is caused either by bicarbonate loss (diarrhea, renal tubular acidosis [RTA] type II) or by inability of the kidney to excrete hydrogen (RTA type I, RTA type IV, and mild to moderate renal failure).

Diagnosis

Most of the time, a history and simple workup will be sufficient to determine the etiology (Table 2-1). If you are still not sure of the etiology, urine anion gap (UAG) will help narrow the differential diagnosis. UAG is calculated by the following formula: UAG = urine [Na] = urine [K] – urine [Cl]. Normal urine anion gap is 0 to <10 mmol/L.

Treatment of Normal Anion Gap Metabolic Acidosis

1. Acidosis secondary to diarrhea is corrected by treating the diarrhea. If that is not possible or the acidosis is severe, alkali may be used. Potassium should always be replaced, as alkali treatment will worsen hypokalemia.

2. Renal failure–related acidosis should be treated with oral bicarbonate (see above).

3. RTA type II (proximal RTA) may be treated with a thiazide diuretic. The volume contraction induced by thiazide will decrease the bicarbonate losses.

4. RTA type I is treated by alkali administration. Potassium citrate is preferred because of the associated hypokalemia in RTA type I. Additionally, the underlying etiologies of the RTA (as noted in Table 2-1) should be treated.

5. RTA type IV treatment is directed mainly toward hyperkalemia. Achieving normal potassium levels will help in controlling the acidosis. Low-potassium diet and loop diuretics are usually tried first. If there is no response, fludrocortisone can be tried to induce urinary potassium secretion.

Table 2-1. Renal Tubular Acidosis

	Defect	Urine Chemistry Finding	Electrolyte Abnormality	Etiology
Distal RTA (type 1 RTA)	Defective secretion of hydrogen ions in distal tubule	Urine pH usually >5.5	Hypokalemia	• Collagen vascular diseases like Sjögren syndrome • Nephrocalcinosis • Lithium • Multiple myeloma
Proximal RTA (type 2 RTA)	Decreased bicarbonate reabsorption in proximal tubule	Urine pH usually <5.5	Hypokalemia	• Drugs: sulfonamide, topiramate • Heavy metals • Amyloidosis • Multiple myeloma • Hereditary • Fanconi syndrome
Type 4 RTA	Decreased aldosterone, from decreased renin, impairs distal potassium secretion	Urine pH usually <5.5	Hyperkalemia	• Reduced aldosterone production (hyporeninemic hypoaldosteronism) as seen in DM, NSAIDs, calcineurin inhibitors Aldosterone resistance as seen with potassium-sparing diuretics

Overview of Metabolic Acidosis

How to approach a patient with low serum bicarbonate

Along with a thorough history, the first step in the evaluation includes an arterial *blood gas analysis* to assess for respiratory compensation. Winter's formula can help calculate the degree of respiratory compensation expected for metabolic acidosis: $Pco_2 = 1.5 \times Hco_3 + 8 \pm 2$ mm Hg.

1. If measured Pco_2 = calculated Pco_2, the respiratory compensation is appropriate.
2. A measured Pco_2 < calculated Pco_2 suggests associated respiratory alkalosis.
3. If measured Pco_2 > calculated P_{CO2}, there is likely an underlying, coexisting respiratory acidosis with poor compensation.
4. The next step is calculating the *serum anion gap (AG)* [serum sodium – (serum chloride + serum bicarbonate)] and correcting the AG for serum albumin. (Uncorrected AG increases by 2.5 mmol/L for every 10-g/L decrease in serum albumin from a normal value of 40 g/L.) This helps in differentiating the two important categories of metabolic acidosis: normal anion gap (4–12 mmol/L) and anion gap metabolic acidosis (>12 mmol/L)

Once the anion gap is noted, the delta gap should be calculated. This is the ratio of delta AG to delta bicarbonate and helps in determining coexisting NAGMA or the presence of metabolic alkalosis.

- Ratio = 1 is due to uncomplicated HAGMA.
- Ratio <1 is seen in combined NAGMA and HAGMA
- Ratio >1 is due to coexisting metabolic alkalosis in addition to metabolic acidosis

For example, this patient's AG is 18 mEq/L and bicarbonate is 14 mEq/L (with 12 mEq/L being the normal AG and 24 mEq/L being the normal bicarbonate level). The delta AG is 18 – 12 = 6 mEq/L, and delta bicarbonate is 24 – 4 = 10 mEq/L. The delta gap/ratio in this case is 6/10 = 0.6 (<1 and thus concurrent NAGMA and AGMA).

Lastly, always calculate the *serum osmolar gap* (measured serum osmolality – calculated serum osmolality). It is important to diagnose toxic alcohol ingestion. Calculated osmolality is the sum of serum sodium, serum glucose, and serum urea (all in mmol/L) as follows:

Serum sodium (mEq/L) + serum glucose (mg/dL)/18 + blood urea (mg/dL)/2.8

Elevated osmolal gap (>10 mOsm/L) suggests the presence of other substances and is associated with ethylene glycol, methanol, or propylene glycol toxicity.

Anion Gap Metabolic Acidosis

High anion gap metabolic acidosis (HAGMA/AGMA) is caused simply by adding exogenous acid to the serum. The excessive hydrogen ions will be buffered by bicarbonate, so bicarbonate concentration will decrease. Chloride concentration will stay the same because the negatively charged anion part of the added acid will compensate for the loss of bicarbonate. The low bicarbonate and the normal chloride concentrations will result in a high anion gap.

The most clinically important acids that cause HAGMA and their etiologies are listed in the mnemonic GOLDMARK, replacing the old mnemonic MUDPILES.

G: Glycols (propylene glycol and ethylene glycol)

O: 5-oxoproline (associated with acetaminophen use)

L: L-lactate

D: D-lactate (short bowel syndrome)

M: Methanol

A: Aspirin

R: Renal failure

K: Ketoacidosis (diabetic/alcohol/starvation)

Rationale for New Mnemonic

- Metabolic acidosis due to excessive paraldehyde or phenformin use has become very rare.
- Iron and isoniazid are just two of many drugs and toxins that can cause hypotension and lactic acidosis. Isoniazid can also generate a component of ketoacidosis.
- Three new organic acids and acid precursors have been recognized as causes of HAGMA: D-lactate, 5-oxoproline, and propylene glycol.

Different Causes of Anion Gap Metabolic Acidosis

Advanced Renal Failure
Advanced chronic kidney disease (CKD) is commonly associated with AGMA when the estimated glomerular filtration rate decreases to <20 mL/min. Metabolic acidosis promotes protein catabolism and worsens bone disease in this group. Patients not on hemodialysis may need sodium bicarbonate to keep serum bicarbonate above 22 mEq/L. The starting dose is usually 650 mg three times a day. Loop diuretics are frequently added to avoid volume overload.

L-Lactic Acidosis
Lactic acidosis treatment should be directed at the underlying cause. Type A lactic acidosis occurs when lactic acid is overproduced in ischemic tissues as a byproduct of anaerobic generation of ATP during oxygen deficit. Overproduction usually occurs during global tissue hypoperfusion in hypovolemic, cardiogenic,

or septic shock and is worsened by decreased lactate metabolism in the poorly perfused liver. It may also occur in primary hypoxia due to lung disease and various hemoglobinopathies. Type B lactic acid is less ominous and occurs in states of local tissue hypoxia—eg, vigorous muscle use during exertion, seizures, hypothermic shivering, certain cancers, toxic ingestion of certain drugs like metformin. In these cases, metabolism may be decreased due to hepatic insufficiency. Bicarbonate should be avoided because it may have an adverse effect on cardiac function and may even worsen the acidosis (how?). When the pH is less than 7.1, bicarbonate may be used. The goal is to get the pH above 7.1 and not to the normal range.

Ketoacidosis
Ketoacidosis is caused by diabetes, starvation, or ethanol. Diabetic ketoacidosis is treated with fluids and insulin. Starvation and alcohol ketoacidosis should be treated with glucose administration. (Inducing insulin release will decrease lipolysis in adipose tissue as well as keto acid production from the liver.) Again, bicarbonate should be used only if the pH is less than 7.1.

The test to send is serum beta-hydroxybutyric acid—this is positive in alcoholic ketoacidosis and diabetic ketoacidosis and less pronounced in starvation ketoacidosis.

Toxic Alcohol Ingestion
Ethanol dehydrogenase is responsible for producing formic, oxalic, and formic acids from ethylene glycol and methanol. Inhibition of ethanol dehydrogenase by IV fomepizole or IV ethanol is an essential part of treatment. In contrast to lactic acidosis and ketoacidosis, IV bicarbonate should be used in HAGMA secondary to ethylene glycol or methanol intoxication (as a higher pH makes these toxins water soluble and unable to cross the blood–brain barrier). Emergent hemodialysis should be done if the ethylene glycol or methanol intoxication is confirmed and the patient has AKI, metabolic acidosis, or very high serum toxin levels (>50 mg/dL of methanol or >8.1 mmol/L of ethylene glycol).

Lastly, isopropyl alcohol (rubbing alcohol) ingestion causes confusion and slurred speech. Toluene causes headache, dizziness, and drowsiness. Both do not cause elevated anion gap acidosis for up to 6 h after ingestion. The key to diagnosis is the elevated osmolar gap.

Salicylate Poisoning
Salicylate poisoning should be treated by increasing blood and brain pH. It is usually associated with mixed acid-base disorder—namely, HAGMA and respiratory alkalosis. IV bicarbonate will increase the negatively charged fraction of salicylic acid. This ionized fraction will have less ability to cross the blood–brain barrier and higher solubility in urine. The end result will be less CNS toxicity and higher urinary excretion. When the serum concentration is above 80 mg/dL, hemodialysis is an option.

D-Lactic Acidosis

D-Lactic acidosis is a rare cause of metabolic acidosis. It is seen in patients who have a history of small intestine resection. If such a patient ate a high-carbohydrate meal, more carbohydrate will reach the colon. In the colon, bacteria will produce D-lactic acid from carbohydrate metabolism. The typical presentation is confusion, ataxia, and acidosis after a meal rich in carbohydrate. The symptoms and the acidosis improve after discontinuation of the meal. The serum lactic acid test is normal in this condition because the test detects only the more common L-lactic acid. If you have a suspicion of D-lactic acidosis, ask the lab to check it specifically. Low-carbohydrate meals and antibiotic use to decrease bacterial overgrowth in the colon are the main measures used to prevent the acidosis episodes.

A second uncommon cause of HAGMA is pyroglutamic acidosis (also known as 5 oxoproline). This is usually seen in critically ill patients who have been ill for a long period of time and who are on acetaminophen. Both chronic critical illness and acetaminophen (even at therapeutic levels) decrease glutathione. The low glutathione in turn will cause the accumulation of pyroglutamic acid. Diagnosis is confirmed by checking urine pyroglutamic acid levels. Acetaminophen should be stopped in these patients. N-Acetylcysteine may be used to increase glutathione production.

The final uncommon cause of AGMA to note is propylene glycol accumulation, which for example can be seen in prolonged use of IV lorazepam for sedation mostly in ICU patients. Propylene glycol is the carrier fluid for lorazepam.

Positive UAG is found in renal etiologies (AKI, RTA), and negative UAG is found in extrarenal etiologies (such as diarrhea). The UAG will be positive if the urine [Cl] is low and will be negative if the urine [Cl] is high. Lower urine [Cl] is associated with lower urine ammonium [NH_4]. Urine ammonium reflects the kidney's ability to acidify the urine, so low urine ammonium in the setting of acidosis indicates an inappropriate response of the kidney to the acidosis (so the kidney is the cause of the acidosis). Higher urine [Cl] is associated with higher urine ammonium and indicates appropriate response of the kidney to the acidosis (so the kidney is not the etiology of the acidosis). The major characteristics of the different RTA types are summarized below.

Intravenous Bicarbonate Replacement in Metabolic Acidosis

Isotonic bicarbonate solution can be made by adding 3 ampules of sodium bicarbonate (50 mEq each) to 1 L of D5W.

A bicarbonate deficit can be calculated by the following formula:

$$\text{Deficit } HCO_3 = (0.5 \times \text{lean body weight [kg]}) \times (24 - \text{current } HCO_3 \text{ levels})$$

Keep in mind that the above formula underestimates the deficit if there is edema or if the HCO_3 level is <5 mmol/L. The first part in parentheses on the right-hand side of the formula may need to be increased in situations like this.

Only half of the bicarbonate deficit should be corrected over the first 24 h. After 24 h, bicarbonate level and the patient's condition should be evaluated again before any further bicarbonate treatment.

CASE 4

A 60-year-old man presented to the ED complaining of shortness of breath that began that morning. He has a history of hypertension, COPD, and colon cancer for which he had received chemotherapy and was in remission. He had returned from a 5-h road trip the day before. On examination, his BP is 140/80 mm Hg. His oxygen saturation is 85% and respiratory rate is 25. His CXR shows hyperinflation. Lab work is as follows: sodium 140 mEq/L, potassium 4 mEq/L, bicarbonate 20 mEq/L, chloride 114 mEq/L, calcium 9 mg/dL, and creatinine 1.5 mg/dL. ABG: pH 7.46, Pco_2 30 mm Hg, Po_2 80 mm Hg, HCO_3 20 mEq/L.

What is the acid-base disorder? Is the compensation appropriate?

A. Compensation is appropriate with rise in bicarbonate. The patient has chronic respiratory acidosis.

B. Compensation is appropriate with fall in bicarbonate. The patient has metabolic acidosis.

C. Compensation is appropriate with fall in bicarbonate. The patient has acute respiratory alkalosis.

D. Compensation is inappropriate with degree of fall in bicarbonate. The patient has respiratory alkalosis.

Answer to Case 4: C

DISCUSSION: RESPIRATORY ALKALOSIS

Respiratory alkalosis results from hypocapnia. Hyperventilation is the underlying mechanism of hypocapnia. It is induced by signals from the lungs, the peripheral ventilation chemoreceptors (peripheral stimulation), or the central ventilation chemoreceptors (central stimulation). Maladjusted mechanical ventilation is another common cause of respiratory alkalosis. See Table 2-2 for etiologies of respiratory alkalosis.

The clinical manifestations of respiratory alkalosis usually start when the Pco_2 drops to less than half the normal range. Usual symptoms include lightheadedness, circumoral numbness, chest discomfort, and paresthesia of the extremities. Hypocapnia causes cerebral vasoconstriction that can have serious neurologic complications in patients with a history of traumatic brain injury or acute stroke. Respiratory alkalosis can cause cardiac arrhythmia as well.

Table 2-2. Causes of Respiratory Alkalosis

Central Stimulation	Peripheral Stimulation
Fever from infection or inflammation causing tachypnea	High altitude
Anxiety	Severe anemia
Cerebrovascular accident (ischemic or hemorrhagic stroke)	Pulmonary diseases like pulmonary embolism, pulmonary edema, asthma
Pain	Hypoxemia
Drug induced (eg, salicylates)	Congestive heart failure
Pregnancy (progesterone)	

Metabolic encephalopathies also stimulate respiratory alkalosis by unknown mechanisms.

Treatment

Hypocapnia is not a benign finding and can cause long-term brain injury. Therefore, respiratory alkalosis should always be taken seriously and treated. Treatment should be directed toward the underlying etiology.

CASE 5

A 45-year-old man presents to the ED, brought in by friends who found him unresponsive. There is no known medical history. On examination, he is obese (BMI 50). His BP is 120/80 mm Hg, oxygen saturation is 84%, and respiratory rate is 10. His pupils were normally reactive. He was unresponsive to verbal or tactile stimulation. His head CT was negative for an intracranial process. Lab work is as follows: sodium 138 mEq/L, potassium 3.5 mEq/L, bicarbonate >40 mEq/L, chloride 108 mEq/L, calcium 10.1 mg/dL, and creatinine 1.8 mg/dL. ABG: pH 7.31, Pco_2 90 mm Hg, Po_2 80 mm Hg, Hco_3 44 mEq/L.

What is the acid-base disorder? Is the compensation appropriate?

   A. Compensation is appropriate with rise in bicarbonate. The patient has acute respiratory acidosis.

   B. Compensation is inappropriate with degree of rise in bicarbonate. The patient has chronic respiratory acidosis.

   C. Compensation is appropriate with degree of rise in bicarbonate. The patient has chronic respiratory acidosis.

D. Compensation is appropriate with rise in bicarbonate. The patient has respiratory alkalosis.

ANSWER to case 5: C

DISCUSSION: RESPIRATORY ACIDOSIS

The lungs are responsible for keeping Pco_2 within the normal range by exhaling co_2. The exhalation process increases or decreases depending on the production of co_2 by the body. Alveolar hypoventilation occurs when the lung fails to exhale the normal production of co_2 or fails to increase this process in response to higher co_2 generation. Alveolar hypoventilation will cause an increase in the Pco_2, and respiratory acidosis may develop. Causes of this failure may be divided into central nervous system–related etiologies, neuromuscular etiologies, and lung etiologies (Table 2-3).

Most hypercapnic symptoms are related to the CNS. Confusion is common, and coma may occur in untreated cases. Tremor, myoclonic jerks, or seizures may occur.

The hypercapnia-induced CNS vasodilation can be severe and can cause increased intracranial pressure. Less commonly, the cardiovascular system can be affected with arrhythmia, decreased cardiac output, and labile blood pressure.

Treatment

Inappropriate use of O_2 is common and is an easily preventable precipitator of respiratory acidosis. In patients with chronic CO_2 retention status, correcting

Table 2-3. Causes of Respiratory Acidosis

CNS Etiology	Neuromuscular Disorders	Chest Wall Abnormalities	Pleural Abnormalities	Airway Obstruction	Parenchymal Lung Disease
Medications/ drugs like opioid analgesics	Neuropathy	Kyphoscoliosis	Pneumothorax	Foreign body	Pulmonary edema
Cerebral ischemia/ trauma	Myopathy		Pleural effusion	Tumor	Pulmonary embolism
Sleep disorders				Severe asthma	Interstitial lung disease
Pickwickian syndrome				COPD	

hypoxia to a normal range will further increase the Pco_2 by three mechanisms. First, O_2 will reverse the hypoxia-induced pulmonary vasoconstriction, which in turn will increase the perfusion to the lung areas that have minimum ventilation—and thus the dead space ventilation will increase. Second, O_2 will increase CO_2 release from red blood cells by decreasing hemoglobin's affinity for CO_2. Third, respiratory drive in chronic CO_2 retainers depends on hypoxia, and O_2 administration will suppress this drive.

Another preventable cause of respiratory acidosis in hospitals is discontinuing the use of CPAP or BiPAP machines. Very often, patients with sleep apnea do not tolerate the hospital machines and prefer to use their home machines. Patients should always be encouraged to bring their home machines to the hospital as soon as possible. If that is not possible, try machines with lower pressure, autotitrated pressure, or a nasal-only mask. This may make it easier for patients to use the hospital machine.

If respiratory acidosis develops, management depends largely on the Po_2 level and the patient's mental status. If Po_2 is >60 mm Hg and the patient is alert, careful observation is recommended. If Po_2 is <55 mm Hg and the patient is alert, you may try a small dose of O_2 until you get the Po_2 to >60 mm Hg (do not try to get saturation greater than 90%–92%). If the patient respiratory status does not improve, noninvasive positive-pressure ventilation may be tried. Arterial blood gases should be drawn 2 h after starting noninvasive ventilation. If there is no improvement in the Pco_2 level, intubation should not be delayed. Any time a patient starts to become confused, intubation should be considered. Noninvasive ventilation in confused patients is a relative contraindication because of the higher risk for aspiration.

Table 2-4. System for Acid-base Compensation

Acid-base Disorder	Expected Compensation
Metabolic acidosis	Winter's formula $Pco_2 = (1.5 \times HCO_3) + 8 \pm 2$ *Compensation takes 2–24 h.*
Metabolic alkalosis	$Pco_2 = HCO_3 + 15$ or $\Delta HCO_3 \uparrow 1 \rightarrow$ expect $\Delta Pco_2 \uparrow 0.7$ *Starts in 30 min and completes in 24 h.*
Acute respiratory acidosis	$\Delta Pco_2 \uparrow 10 \rightarrow \Delta HCO_3 \uparrow 1$ or $\downarrow$ pH 0.08
Chronic respiratory acidosis	$\Delta Pco_2 \uparrow 10 \rightarrow \Delta HCO_3 \uparrow 4$ or $\downarrow$ pH 0.03
Acute respiratory alkalosis	$\Delta Pco_2 \downarrow 10 \rightarrow \Delta HCO_3 \downarrow 2$ or $\uparrow$ pH 0.08
Chronic respiratory alkalosis	$\Delta Pco_2 \downarrow 10 \rightarrow \Delta HCO_3 \downarrow 4$ or $\uparrow$ pH 0.03

SUGGESTED READINGS

Adrogué HJ, Madias NE. Secondary responses to altered acid-base status: the rules of engagement. *J Am Soc Nephrol*. 2010;21(6):920–923.

Cervantes CE, Menez S, Monroy Trujillo JM, Hanouneh M. Clinical approach to a patient with an acid-base disturbance. *Am J Kidney Dis*. 2021;77(2):A9–A11

Floege J, Johnson RJ, Feehally J. *Comprehensive Clinical Nephrology*. 4th ed. Philadelphia: Mosby; 2007.

Mehta AN, Emmett JB, Emmett M. GOLD MARK: an anion gap mnemonic for the 21st century. *Lancet*. 2008;372(9642):892.

Renal Fellow Network. www.renalfellow.org.

A 72-year-old Man With Altered Mental Status

Yasser Al-Kadra, MD, Mukul Bhattarai, MD and Yousef Chami, MD

A 72-year-old man presented to the emergency department with altered mental status. The patient resides in a skilled nursing facility where he was noted to have a temperature of 102.1°F with increased urination frequency for the past 4 days. The patient was diagnosed with a urinary tract infection and was admitted for administration of IV antibiotics. During his second day of hospitalization, the patient complained of substernal chest pain radiating to his left arm. The patient had associated shortness of breath as well as diaphoresis. Blood pressure was 132/76, heart rate 106 bpm, temperature 101.1°F, respiratory rate 22/min, and oxygen saturation 92%.

The patient's past medical history included hypertension, hypercholesterolemia, type 2 diabetes on insulin therapy, and stage IIIa chronic kidney disease. The patient has no history of tobacco abuse. Physical examination shows the patient to be alert and in moderate distress. An ECG was ordered immediately. See Figure 3-1.

1. What is your differential diagnosis?

2. What should you do next?

3. What is your final diagnosis?

Answers

1. Differential diagnosis for a hospitalized patient with acute onset of chest pain includes acute coronary syndrome, pulmonary embolism, and anxiety attack.

2. Check an ECG and cardiac enzymes.

3. This is a 72-year-old patient with classic symptoms of and risk factors for coronary artery disease. The ECG is consistent with an inferior acute coronary syndrome.

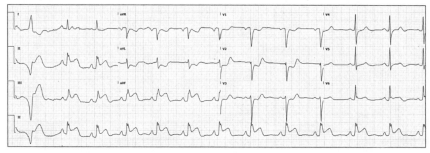

Figure 3-1. Patient's ECG at the time of presentation.

ACUTE CORONARY SYNDROME

Diagnosis

Chest pain is a common complaint for patients in the United States, accounting for 7.6 million annual visits to the emergency room. About 10% to 20% of these chest pain visits are attributed to acute coronary syndrome (ACS), which usually results from acute disruption of an atherosclerotic plaque due to rupture or erosion of the thin fibrous cap. Myocardial injury in the absence of plaque rupture is known as type 2 myocardial infarction (MI) or demand-related MI. Accurately identifying this high-risk population and steering the management in the right direction is critical for improving outcomes.

ACS can be divided into two major subcategories: ST-elevation myocardial infarction (STEMI) and non-ST-elevation acute coronary syndrome (NSTE-ACS). ST elevation can be defined as ≥2-mm elevation of the ST segment of 2 contiguous leads in the precordial leads and ≥1 mm in all other leads. If no overt ST segment elevation is identified, the diagnosis of NSTE-ACS is considered. NSTE-ACS can

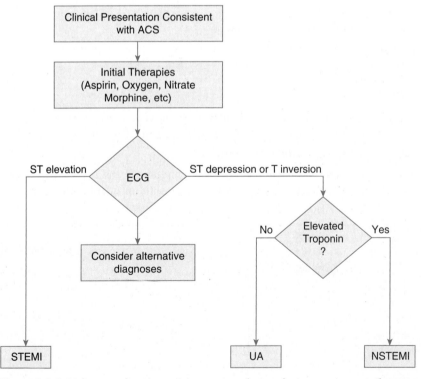

Figure 3-2. Initial approach to managing a suspected case of acute coronary syndrome.

be further stratified into two categories: non-ST-elevation myocardial infarction (NSTEMI) and unstable angina (UA).

The 2021 American College of Cardiology/American Heart Association (ACC/AHA) guidelines advised avoiding the use of the term *atypical chest pain*, as it was thought to imply noncardiac pain etiologies. The term that is proposed now is *possible cardiac* chest pain. The guidelines also list descriptions of chest pain, which in their presence increase the likelihood of ischemia: central, pressure, squeezing, gripping, heaviness, tightness, exertional/stress-related, and retrosternal. Obtaining a detailed history is key for identifying the cause of the chest pain and is considered an important initial step in the risk stratification process for these patients.

Physical examination is usually normal, although there is a need to carefully examine for chest wall tenderness, positional changes of pain, and peripheral pulses (unequal pulses or bruits, aortic dissection). Also assess for the hemodynamic consequences from ischemia, such as an S3 gallop, jugular vein distention, right heart failure signs, and murmurs, perhaps secondary to ventricular septal defect/papillary muscle ruptures.

ECG is the second pillar in the assessment of ACS. Detecting the presence of ST elevation will steer management in a drastically different manner compared with absence of ST elevation or an equivalent of ST elevation. ST segment deviations or T wave inversions are important, as dynamic ECG changes indicate a change in the clinical scenario, indicating progression of the coronary lesion and dictating a different course of action.

The third tool to be used when myocardial ischemia is suspected is cardiac biomarkers including troponin I and high-sensitivity troponin. Troponin is an amino acid that is found only in cardiac tissue, making it highly specific for detecting myocardial injury. The latest ACC/AHA guidelines suggest repeating troponin I between 3 and 6 hours and high-sensitivity troponin between 1 and 3 hours for optimal sensitivity. Elevated troponin should be analyzed in a clinical context. For example, modest elevation of troponin may occur in the setting of underlying sepsis, anemia, kidney injury, arrythmia, stress cardiomyopathy, etc, and not necessarily due to acute coronary syndrome. This is referred to as type 2 MI, as mentioned above (Table 3-1). Cardiac biomarkers are very useful for diagnosis and help in guiding therapeutic interventions.

Many scored tools have been devised to aid in risk stratification and clinical decision-making for patients presenting with chest pain. The first is the HEART score (Table 3-2). The HEART score has been validated by multiple studies. The score consists of aspects of clinical presentations, ECG changes, age, risk factors, and troponin levels. A score of 0 to 3 has a 1.6% chance of cardiac events, 4 to 6 has a 13% chance, and ≥7 has a 50% chance of major cardiac events within 6 weeks of follow-up.

The Thrombolysis in Myocardial Infarction (TIMI) score is a widely validated score for use in unstable angina and non-ST-elevation myocardial infarction

Table 3-1. Causes of Type 2 Myocardial Infarction

Secondary to ischemia due to increased oxygen demands or decreased oxygen supply

Causes

Cardiac	Non-cardiac
Arrythmias	Hypotension
Coronary vasospasm	Hypertension
Coronary thromboembolism	Anemia
Coronary artery dissection	Hypovolemia
Aortic dissection	Hypoxia
Sever aortic valve disease	Pulmonary embolism
Heart failure	

Reproduced with permission from Thygesen K, Alpert JS, Jaffe AS, et al. Third universal definition of myocardial infarction. *Circulation*. 2012;126:2020–2035, Table 1.

(Table 3-3). It has been used to identify the need for early intervention in patients with high risk. A score of 0 to 1 indicates a low risk of cardiac events. The score has similar elements to the HEART score, with the addition of the use of aspirin within the 7 days prior to hospitalization.

The third score is the Global Registry of Acute Coronary Events (GRACE) score. The score has been devised to predict the all-cause mortality risk within 6 months after discharge from an ACS admission. Nevertheless, the score has been utilized to predict both in-hospital and postdischarge mortality and myocardial infarction. The score consists of age, heart rate, systolic blood pressure, creatinine, cardiac arrest on admission, ST deviation on ECG, elevated cardiac enzymes, and Killip class. The European Society of Cardiology (ESC) has specified a GRACE score of less than 140 to indicate low risk for mortality.

Once the clinical picture is more refined, a diagnosis of ACS can be made. Furthermore, utilizing one of the validated scoring systems, risk stratification can be used, based on the clinical picture and the risk derived from the selected model. From there, a management plan is initiated.

Management

Any possible ACS needs prompt evaluation and treatment, which is primarily driven by clinical presentation, ECG changes, cardiac biomarkers, and the history

Table 3-2. Heart Score for Chest Pain Patients

History (anamnesis)	Highly suspicious	2
	Moderately suspicious	1
	Slightly suspicious	0
ECG	Significant ST deviation	2
	Nonspecific repolarization disturbances/LBBB/PM	1
	Normal	0
Age	≥65 Years	2
	45–65 Years	1
	≤45 Years	0
Risk factors	≥3 Risk factors or history of atherosclerotic disease	2
	1–2 Risk factors	1
	No risk factors	0
Troponin	≥3 × Normal limit	2
	1–3 × Normal limit	1
	≤ Normal limit	0
Total		

Risk factors:

Hypercholesterolemia	Cigarette smoking
Hypertension	Positive family history
Diabetes mellitus	Obesity (BMI >30)

Table 3-3. The TIMI Risk Score for Unstable Angina/NSTEMI

Age ≥65 years?	Yes: +1
≥3 Risk factors for CAD?	Yes: +1
Known coronary artery disease?	Yes: +1
ASA use in past 7 days?	Yes: +1
Severe angina (≥2 episodes within 24 h)?	Yes: +1
ST changes ≥0.5 mm?	Yes: +1
Positive cardiac marker?	Yes: +1

of risk factors of developing coronary artery disease such as diabetes, tobacco use, hypertension, prior history of CAD, etc.

ECG is the first test that needs to be performed within 10 minutes of first medical contact in any individual suspected for ACS. Patients with ST elevation, presumed new LBBB, or posterior STEMI should be considered for immediate heart catheterization. In suspected cases of posterior MI, an ECG with posterior leads V7–V9 should be obtained. In patients with inferior STEMI, it is recommended to obtain an ECG with right-sided leads (V3R and V4R) to evaluate right ventricular involvement. Medications at this stage can include aspirin, dual antiplatelet therapy, or nitroglycerine.

Early risk stratification needs to be conducted in all patients with NSTE-ACS, assessing them clinically, and analyzing ECG findings and cardiac biomarkers. High-risk features including ongoing ischemia refractory to medical therapy, high-risk features in the ECG or telemetry monitoring, and hemodynamic instability; these all warrant early coronary angiogram and critical care unit admission. TIMI risk score and GRACE risk score are clinically validated algorithms that may help guide clinical decision-making, including decisions regarding coronary angiography. In the absence of high-risk features, patients with NSTE-ACS are generally admitted to the telemetry floor with continuous ECG monitoring and bed rest for 24 hours.

Treatments for Use in Patients With ACS

Oxygen therapy
Only hypoxic patients (O_2 saturation <90%) or those in respiratory distress need supplemental oxygen.

Antiplatelet therapy
Aspirin has an antithrombotic property due to irreversible acetylation of the platelet COX-1 enzyme. Non-enteric-coated, chewable aspirin is recommended in all cases of suspected ACS without contraindications as soon as ACS is suspected. A P2Y12 inhibitor is given with aspirin as dual antiplatelet therapy (DAPT), but the timing of administration of a P2Y12 inhibitor is variable, depending on clinical circumstances such as prior and during PCI, or in a post-fibrinolytic state. Usually, DAPT is continued for up to 12 months in all patients with ACS. Prasugrel is not recommended in patients with a history of stroke or transient ischemic attack, or in patients of 75 years or older.

Dosing
Aspirin: non-enteric-coated, 300–325 mg followed by 81 mg daily P2Y12 inhibitors:

> Clopidogrel: 600 mg load, 75 mg daily
> Prasugrel: 60 mg load, 10 mg daily
> Ticagrelor: 80 mg daily loading, 90 mg BID
> Cangrelor: 30 µg/kg × body weight (kg)/200 µg/mL

Glycoprotein IIB/IIIA receptor inhibitors
GP IIb/IIIa inhibitors such as abciximab, eptifibatide, and tirofiban are reserved for high-risk patients in whom coronary angiogram is delayed, and they are usually started during intervention when a large thrombus burden is present. The decision to start this class of medication should be discussed with a cardiologist before administration.

Anticoagulant therapy
Unfractionated heparin (UFH), low-molecular-weight heparin (LMWH), bivalirudin, and factor Xa inhibitors constitute anticoagulant therapy. UFH is monitored by aPTT or ACT and is not renally cleared. LMWH is to be avoided in patients with kidney injury, with a creatinine clearance cutoff of <30.

Dosing
UFH: 60 IU/kg, infusion 12 IU/kg/h
LMWH: 1 mg/kg SC BID
Bivalirudin: 0.75 mg/kg, infusion 1.75 mg/kg/h

Nitrates
Nitrates dilate the coronary vascular beds and act as an effective anti-ischemic treatment in ACS. They also reduce cardiac preload. They should be avoided in hypotension and in recent use of phosphodiesterase inhibitors, and they must be avoided in patients with RV infarction and severe aortic stenosis. They are usually recommended in ongoing chest pain, hypertension, and heart failure. Tolerance is common after 24 hours of use.

Beta blockers
By inhibiting the beta-1 adrenergic receptors in the heart, these medications reduce cardiac work and myocardial oxygen demand. The early start of oral beta blockers within 24 hours is recommended (if not contraindicated) because it has been shown to reduce ischemia or reinfarction and improves overall long-term survival. Avoid its use in acute heart failure, in hypotension, in second- and third-degree heart block without a pacemaker, and in the presence of signs of cardiogenic shock. Metoprolol, carvedilol, and bisoprolol are preferred beta blockers.

Calcium channel blockers (CCBs)
CCBs in NSTE-ACS are used as second-line therapy, mainly limited to symptom control. They cause coronary and peripheral vasodilation leading to antihypertensive and antianginal effects. Diltiazem and verapamil, which are nondihydropyridines, are recommended in ACS because of their negative inotropic and chronotropic effects. They should not be used in patients with significant heart failure with reduced ejection fraction (HFrEF) (LVEF ≤35%), as they increase risk of cardiogenic shock. These medications also need to be avoided in patients with high-grade conduction disease without a pacemaker present. CCBs are the first line treatment in Prinzmetal angina, which is characterized by transient epicardial coronary vasospasm and ST-segment elevation.

Analgesic agents

Morphine is a potent analgesic. It may mask ongoing myocardial ischemia, potentially delaying a coronary reperfusion procedure. It is usually considered only in patients with ongoing ischemic symptoms despite maximally tolerated anti-ischemic therapy with beta blockers and nitrates.

Avoid nonsteroidal anti-inflammatory agents that potentially block endothelial prostacyclin production, resulting in platelet aggregation, and mediate adverse remodeling.

Cholesterol management

High-potency statin use (atorvastatin, rosuvastatin) with an early initiation is recommended after ACS. These HMG-CoA reductase inhibitors reduce LDL-cholesterol production from the liver, resulting in reduction of recurrent MI, coronary death, coronary revascularization, and stroke in patients with ACS.

Dosing

Rosuvastatin: 20–40 mg daily
Atorvastatin: 40–80 mg daily

Renin-angiotensin-aldosterone system (RAAS) inhibitors

This class of medications is particularly useful in a select group of patients, particularly those with LV dysfunction. It is recommended that ACE inhibitors or ARBs be started and/or continued in patients with ACS and LV dysfunction and/or those with hypertension, diabetes mellitus, or stable chronic kidney disease (class I). Aldosterone antagonists are recommended for ACS patients without contraindication in the setting of adequate ACE inhibition and beta blockade who have LV dysfunction, diabetes mellitus, or heart failure (class I). A RAAS inhibitor is usually considered only after the first 24 hours of presentation, and they need to be avoided in significant hypotension or shock. Aldosterone antagonists should be avoided in renal impairment (creatinine >2.5 mg/dL in men and >2.0 mg/dL in women) or hyperkalemia (>5.0 mEq/L).

Optimal medical management and heart catheterization

Any patient with ACS needs to be started on appropriate medical therapy, including antiplatelet and anticoagulant therapy, anti-ischemic therapy, cholesterol management, and RAAS antagonism. The determination of the appropriateness and timing of coronary angiography in NSTE-ACS is critical. Immediate invasive strategy (within <2 h) is recommended for the following:

1. Persistent or recurrent angina despite optimal medical treatment

2. Hemodynamic instability, acute heart failure, cardiogenic shock

3. Arrhythmia (sustained VT, V fib)

Early invasive therapy (within 24 h) is usually recommended for GRACE score >140, temporal changes in cardiac biomarkers, TIMI score ≥2, or new ECG changes such as ST-segment depression.

Delayed invasive strategy (within 25–72 h) is considered in the absence of the above features in the setting of LV dysfunction (EF <40%), prior PCI within 6 months, history of CABG, or GRACE score of 109 to 140.

Low-risk patients with TIMI score 0 or 1, or GRACE <109, may not need invasive testing. Noninvasive testing prior to discharge, such as echocardiography and a stress test, is usually recommended, guiding further management.

TIPS TO REMEMBER

- For any hospitalized patient with acute onset of chest pain, consider ACS as differential diagnosis.

- Management is driven primarily by clinical presentation, ECG changes, cardiac biomarkers, and the presence of risk factors of atherosclerosis.

- Medical therapy includes antiplatelet and anticoagulant therapy and anti-ischemic therapy. The determination of coronary angiography in ACS is critical in high-risk patients.

SUGGESTED READINGS

Braun M, Kassop D. Acute coronary syndrome: management. *FP Essent.* 2020;490:20–28.

Gulati M, Levy PD, Mukherjee D, et al. 2021 AHA/ACC/ASE/CHEST/SAEM/SCCT/SCMR Guideline for the Evaluation and Diagnosis of Chest Pain: A Report of the American College of Cardiology/ American Heart Association Joint Committee on Clinical Practice Guidelines. *Circulation.* 2021;144(22):e368–e454. Erratum in: *Circulation.* 2021;144(22):e455.

Smith JN, Negrelli JM, Manek MB, et al. Diagnosis and management of acute coronary syndrome: an evidence-based update. *J Am Board Fam Med.* 2015;28(2):283–293.

Switaj TL, Christensen SR, Brewer DM. Acute coronary syndrome: current treatment. *Am Fam Physician.* 2017;95(4):232–240.

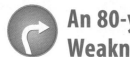

An 80-year-old Man With Generalized Weakness

Bemi (Oritsegbubemi) Adekola, MD

An 80-year-old male was transferred from his nursing home to the emergency room for generalized weakness of 3 days' duration. His weakness got worse to the extent that he found it difficult to go to the bathroom unassisted. He also mentioned worsening dysuria and difficulty passing urine for the last week. There was no chest pain, fever, cough, abdominal pain, back pain, hematuria, diarrhea, melena, or rash. The patient has a history of dementia, benign prostatic hypertrophy (BPH), congestive heart failure (CHF) with an ejection fraction of 40% via transthoracic echocardiogram measured 6 months ago, chronic kidney disease (CKD) stage III, diabetes mellitus type 2, and hypertension.

His medications include donepezil, memantine, tamsulosin, finasteride, lisinopril, metoprolol, amlodipine, torsemide, and metformin. The patient is a widower who has lived at the nursing home for the last 4 years. He has never smoked or drunk alcohol.

On presentation to the ED, his vital signs were as follows: blood pressure 100/60, heart rate 100, and respiratory rate 20. He had a normal temperature and oxygen saturation on room air.

On physical examination, the patient's mucosa looked dry. Neck, heart, and lung examinations were unremarkable. There was mild abdominal tenderness in the hypogastric area with dullness to percussion. He had a 1+ bilateral pitting edema. Neurologic examination was within normal limits. Void collector on the bedside contained 30 cm³ of dark yellow urine.

Initial workup:

WBC: 9000 with normal differential

Hemoglobin: 10 g/dL

Platelet count: 200,000

Sodium: 130

Potassium: 5.1

Chloride: 103

Bicarbonate: 16

Blood urea nitrogen: 95

Creatinine: 8.5 (patient's baseline is 1.8; last check was 1 month ago)

Glucose: 220 mg/dL

CXR: mild bilateral interstitial infiltrates and cardiomegaly

ECG showed sinus tachycardia with peaked T waves in the anterior leads

1. What is the most important next step?
2. How would you work up the patient's acute kidney injury (AKI)?

Answers

1. The physical examination reveals a patient who has volume depletion as well as urinary retention elicited from percussion dullness in hypogastric region. This is likely from prostate enlargement in this elderly man. A urinary catheter should be inserted immediately to relieve the obstruction. If any resistance to placing the catheter is encountered, urology should be consulted for catheter placement—this is both therapeutic and diagnostic.

2. The lab work is consistent with severe AKI and metabolic acidosis. Due to the history of decreased oral intake, tachycardia, and mild hypotension, intravenous normal saline should be started. Continuous oximeter and serial lung examinations are important in such patients with low ejection fraction. Once the urinary obstruction is relieved, the patient's urine output is expected to improve in 1 to 2 days.

   On initial medication reconciliation, do not forget to hold medications like antihypertensives, RAAS blockers, metformin, and other oral hypoglycemic agents. Insulin is the hypoglycemic agent of choice in this case.

PATHOPHYSIOLOGY OF OBSTRUCTIVE UROPATHY

By 24 to 48 hours after obstruction sets in, renal plasma flow decreases by up to 60%.

Increased intratubular pressure results in increased pressure in Bowman's capsule and decreased filtration pressure causing decreased intraglomerular blood flow. This in turn leads to an increase in vasoconstrictor activity, namely thromboxane A2 and angiotensin II.

Thromboxane A2 and angiotensin II cause vasoconstriction of afferent and efferent arterioles, respectively, and a decrease in GFR.

Eventually renal blood flow decreases by up to 60% to 70%, and this is associated with extensive tubular and interstitial damage. Animal studies with dissection at ~8 weeks show extensive vascular damage that is thought to precede the tubular and interstitial injury. Extensive tubular brush epithelial loss also has been described. This explains the nonrecovery of renal function after patients' have had prolonged urinary obstruction.

A renal tubular acidification defect explains the presence of metabolic acidosis and hyperkalemia in patients with obstructive uropathy.

An arterial blood gas measurement will help confirm the presence of metabolic acidosis.

Discussion

AKI is very common in the inpatient setting (0.5%–13%). The wide incidence range can be explained by the different definitions of AKI among different authors and physicians. Because of its reversibility in the early stages and its impact on morbidity and mortality, we suggest having a low threshold to diagnose AKI. An increase in serum creatinine of 0.3 mg/dL or by 1.5 times the baseline should raise your suspicion of AKI. A more important, but not widely used, criterion is the decrease in urine output (UOP) to less than 0.5 mL/kg/h for at least a 6-hour duration. The decrease in UOP actually precedes the decrease in glomerular filtration rate (GFR) and the increases in serum creatinine. UOP criteria are more practical in the intensive care unit, where more accurate UOP measurement is conducted.

There is ongoing research to evaluate urinary biomarkers that can detect AKI at much earlier stages. None of these biomarkers is used in practice yet. Commonly, baseline creatinine will not be available for comparison. In situations like this, it becomes hard to differentiate between CKD and AKI when faced with elevated creatinine.

Anemia, hypocalcemia, and hyperphosphatemia are abnormalities seen in CKD, and their presence makes CKD more likely than AKI. Small kidney size and thinning of the cortex on renal ultrasound are the most accurate markers that can differentiate CKD from AKI. Keep in mind that the kidney size is normal in diabetic nephropathy, amyloidosis, and polycystic kidney disease. The easiest way to approach AKI is by dividing the etiologies into 3 categories: prerenal, renal, and postrenal (Table 4-1).

It is important to remember that overlap among different etiologies is a common scenario.

Detailed history and a careful physical examination are an essential part of the diagnostic process.

Mild to moderate AKI secondary to volume depletion, or secondary to decreased intravascular effective circulation, is a very common scenario in the inpatient setting. In situations like this, volume status assessment is crucial.

There is commonly failure in accurately assessing the volume status because of the ongoing loss of physical examination skills and the limited predictive values of these signs.

Simple urine tests and renal imaging will often identify the etiology of the AKI. In the majority of cases, they are the only needed workup.

Urine tests

Urinalysis is an inexpensive and valuable test that can help narrow the differential diagnosis of AKI. Urine tests should include the following: dipstick test, microscopic and sediment evaluations, osmolality, fractional excretion of sodium (FeNa) (or urea), and ratio of urine creatinine to serum creatinine. Dipstick and microscopic tests should be reviewed carefully. In acute tubular necrosis (ATN),

Table 4-1. Acute Kidney Injury Etiologies

Prerenal (hypoperfusion of the kidney)	Renal (tubular or glomerular injury)	Postrenal (obstruction of the urinary tract)
1. Volume depletion (diarrhea, vomiting, bleeding, burns, pancreatitis, hyperglycemia, excessive diuresis, sepsis)	1. Acute tubular necrosis	1. Urinary retention
	2. Vascular causes: various vasculitis—polyarteritis nodosa, ANCA vasculitis, hemolytic uremic syndrome, TTP, cholesterol emboli	2. Urologic malignancies
		3. Pelvic masses
		4. Obstructing nephrolithiasis
2. Decreased intravascular effective circulation (CHF, cirrhosis)	3. Glomerulonephritis	
	4. Acute interstitial nephritis	
3. Renal artery thrombosis	5. Cast nephropathy	
	6. Contrast nephropathy	
4. Renal artery dissection	7. Myoglobin nephropathy	
	8. Tumor lysis syndrome	

the kidneys' acidification function can be impaired, and urine pH of more than 6.5 is seen sometimes in these patients. Hematuria is seen in obstructive AKI—like prostate pathology, nephrolithiasis, or urologic malignancy. A positive blood dipstick with only a few red blood cells should raise the suspicion of myoglobinuria.

Proteinuria
This is common in AKI. The ratio of protein to creatinine in a random urine spot is a quick and easy test that can give you an idea about the 24-hour protein urine. Trace to mild proteinuria is seen in prerenal etiologies. Moderate proteinuria (<1 g in 24 h) is seen with ATN.

Proteinuria that is more than 1 g in 24 hours should make one think of a nephritic syndrome or cast nephropathy, and it is more helpful in narrowing the differential diagnosis than just mild to moderate proteinuria.

Identification of casts
Hyaline casts can be seen in normal persons, so their presence or absence is of little value. Muddy brown casts and cellular debris are seen in ATN; however, their absence doesn't rule it out. Red blood cell casts are pathognomonic for glomerulonephritis (GN). White blood cell casts are seen with acute interstitial nephritis (AIN). Again, the absence of red blood cell casts or white blood cell casts

Table 4-2. Volume Status Signs

Heart rate and blood pressure	Tachycardia is more sensitive for hypovolemic states than for hypotension, but both are sometimes absent in hypovolemic patients
	Patients on beta blockers may not have reflex tachycardia when they are hypovolemic
	Tachycardia is not specific for hypovolemia (it can be seen in euvolemic and hypervolemic states)
Orthostatic hypotension	Good specificity for hypovolemia (>90%) but low sensitivity (22%)
	Common mistakes when checking for orthostatic hypotension: not having the patient stand up long enough (at least 2 min) and not counting the heart rate
Dry mucosa and diminished skin turgor	Both of these signs do not necessarily mean hypovolemia in the elderly; mouth breathing, a common problem in the elderly, can cause dry mouth regardless of the volume status; skin turgor diminishes in the elderly
CVP	Low CVP has a modest positive predictive value (47%) in detecting volume-responsive patients
Jugular venous distention (JVD)	Good specificity for hypervolemia but low sensitivity
	JVD in pure right heart failure can be seen even if the patient is hypovolemic
	Carotid pulsation should not be mistaken for JVD; carotid pulsation is faster and brisker than JVD; it has only 1 phase, while JVD has multiple phases; carotid pulsation is synchronized with the radial pulsation
Third heart sound	Good specificity for hypervolemic state (80%–90%) but low sensitivity (30%–40%)
Bilateral pitting edema	Peripheral edema is seen in hypervolemic states, but it is also seen in low albumin states and venous stasis states regardless of volume status
Rales	Elderly can have fine crackles in the lower parts of the lung fields regardless of volume status (age-related crackles)

does not rule out GN or AIN, respectively. Cast identification needs good skills and practice. Experienced nephrologists examine the urine themselves looking for casts. We encourage residents to learn this important skill during their nephrology elective.

Urine osmolality

Urine osmolality can help differentiate between prerenal AKI and ATN. Osmolality of more than 500 mOsm/kg is more consistent with prerenal etiologies. Urine osmolality of less than 400 mOsm/kg is seen with ATN. Keep in mind that elderly patients, CKD patients, and patients on diuretics have impaired water reabsorption, so they have low urine osmolality even when they are volume depleted. Having high osmolality in these groups indicates a severe volume contraction state.

Urinary electrolyte excretion

FeNa is a useful test that helps differentiate prerenal from renal AKI. In volume depletion states, the FeNa will be less than 1% due to excessive sodium reabsorption. FeNa of more than 2% is consistent with intrarenal injury. However, a number of intrarenal AKI etiologies are associated with FeNa of less than 1% (contrast nephropathy, myoglobin nephropathy, GN, and early stages of ATN1). On the other hand, high FeNa is seen in prerenal AKI secondary to excessive vomiting. This is because the consequent bicarbonaturia is associated with excessive urinary sodium loss. The high urine sodium seen in patients taking diuretics makes FeNa less helpful. In this situation, the fractional excretion of urea (FeUrea) is the best alternative. FeUrea of less than 35% is suggestive of prerenal etiologies, while values more than 50% suggest ATN.

During early nonoliguric ATN, the intact tubules will face large loads of water and sodium and they will try to preserve the body's sodium by excessive reabsorption. In this situation the overall result will be a low FeNa.

In oliguric ATN, the intact tubules will face small loads of water and sodium. To avoid significant sodium retention, the intact tubules will reabsorb less sodium and the FeNa will be high.

The take-home message is that FeNa is most likely to be useful in oliguric AKI.

Imaging

Renal ultrasound is a helpful tool when you suspect obstructive AKI or when you are not sure of the diagnosis. Pelvicalyceal dilation is a very sensitive sign for obstruction.

In obstruction, dilation may not appear. Also, in some malignancies, there will be ureteral encasement and retroperitoneal fibrosis, and dilation will not appear. Because of that, in cases of high suspicion for obstruction with negative ultrasound or CT scan, retrograde or anterograde pyelography is recommended due to its improved accuracy.

Renal biopsy

Biopsy is rarely needed for diagnosis. Think about getting a biopsy when you suspect GN, vasculitis, or AIN. It can also be done in cases of persistent elevated creatinine when prerenal and postrenal etiologies have been ruled out and the etiology of the intrinsic AKI is still unclear.

General management

After an AKI diagnosis, avoidance of further injury is a main goal for all patients. Contrast materials, kidney-insulting medications, and hypotension should be avoided as much as possible. Most patients with volume depletion–induced AKI improve with hydration or/and blood transfusion if it is caught early. If there is no improvement after fluid administration, reevaluate the patient for ATN or other diagnoses.

In CHF patients, the differentiation between AKI caused by acute exacerbation of CHF and AKI caused by excessive diuresis is sometimes tough. The best strategy is a diuretic trial. Diuretics will improve the renal function if the injury is caused by a CHF exacerbation, and they will make it worse if excessive diuresis is the cause. This should be apparent in the first 24 hours after adequate diuretic dose. In the latter case, diuretics should be stopped and a small fluid challenge should be tried. Remember to look at the patient as a whole; the decision of holding diuretics and giving fluid to improve the renal function should be weighed against worsening of the cardiac condition. Thorough discussion with the cardiology service is important in such cases.

The balance between fluid administration and diuresis is more complicated in ICU patients. As mentioned earlier, volume status assessment is a challenging task especially in the ICU. Echocardiogram is probably the most accurate tool available now to help in making the decision to give or restrict fluids. If the cardiac output of a patient is expected to increase with fluids, the patient is called volume responsive (organ perfusion will increase by fluids). If the cardiac output of a patient is expected to be the same after fluid administration, the patient is called volume nonresponsive (organ perfusion will not increase by fluids), and fluid restriction or diuretics will be beneficial if the patient has poor cardiac function. Echocardiogram helps estimate the cardiac output by measuring the stroke volume. In patients who are not on a ventilator, the change in stroke volume is measured when the patient is flat and after the patient raises the legs 45°. Raising the legs will increase the venous return and the preload to the heart, an effect that is similar to fluid bolus. If the cardiac input variation is more than 15% with this maneuver, the patient is considered volume responsive.

Echocardiogram is also useful in ventilated patients. During mechanical ventilation, the positive pressure with inspiration will increase the pressure in the chest. This will decrease the venous return to the right ventricle. The venous return will increase during expiration. This variation of the venous return will cause variation of the stroke volume, and hence the cardiac input. Respiratory variation of more than 20% in the stroke volume predicts positive response to fluid expansion.

Management of hepatorenal syndrome, GN, AIN, and cast nephropathy is beyond the internist level, and a nephrology consult is recommended when you suspect these diagnoses.

Benign prostate hypertrophy–induced urinary retention and AKI is a common scenario. This is discussed in an earlier clinical scenario.

Other AKI management considerations

Dietary modification should always be considered in AKI patients. In oliguric AKI, water and sodium excretion is limited and restriction of both is important to prevent any pulmonary edema. Potassium and phosphorus dietary restriction is also recommended because of impaired excretion in AKI. The potassium level should always be observed to prevent any cardiac complications from hyperkalemia.

In the polyuric phase of AKI, potassium and phosphorus depletion may occur. Close monitoring and replacement are required. Patients with AKI are at risk for protein-energy malnutrition and should be on at least 1.5 g/kg of protein daily. Renal recovery after AKI usually takes place during the first 2 weeks after diagnosis. Renal recovery after ATN and in CKD patients is a long and incomplete process. Even after creatinine normalization, it is better to avoid any nephrotoxic medication whenever this is possible. If there is no improvement after 8 weeks of onset, end-stage renal disease becomes very likely.

Management of complications

AKI complications are life threatening and need quick intervention. A nephrology consult is a must anytime you suspect the patient needs dialysis or specialist management.

Fluid overload patients with oliguric AKI are at high risk for pulmonary edema. Mild to moderate pulmonary edema can be treated with loop diuretics. Oxygen, morphine, and nitroglycerine can be helpful too. Patients with severe pulmonary edema or those who don't respond to diuretics may need to have emergent hemodialysis.

Remember the ABC rule in resuscitation, and consider intubation before diuresis or hemodialysis when indicated.

Hyperkalemia

This has a major effect on the cardiac conduction system and includes bradycardia and asystole. Once hyperkalemia is discovered, immediate medical treatment should be started. Unresponsive and persistent hyperkalemia should be treated with hemodialysis.

Acid-base abnormalities

Metabolic acidosis is the most common acid-base complication of AKI. Contributing factors include decreased bicarbonate regeneration, decreased ammonium excretion, and accumulation of other unmeasured anions. Anion gap stays normal in 50% of acidosis cases. Bicarbonate may be replaced when it is lower than 15 mmol/L or the pH is less than 7.20 (see Chapter 2 to learn bicarbonate replacement principles). Keep in mind that sodium bicarbonate administration can induce volume overload. Refractory acidosis should be treated with hemodialysis.

TIPS TO REMEMBER

- AKI has significant morbidity and mortality in patients.
- Urinalysis, urine osmolality, random protein to creatinine ratio, FeNa, and renal ultrasound are enough to diagnose the etiology of the AKI in most cases.
- Volume depletion–induced AKI is easily reversed with volume resuscitation.
- AKI secondary to acute CHF improves with diuresis.
- Obstructive AKI warrants a urology consult.
- Pulmonary edema resistant to diuretics, refractory hyperkalemia or metabolic acidosis, and symptomatic uremia are indications for hemodialysis in AKI.

COMPREHENSION QUESTIONS

1. A 75-year-old female presents to the emergency department with vomiting, high-grade fever, and left flank pain of 2 days' duration. Prior to that, the patient started having dysuria a week ago and her primary care doctor started her on ciprofloxacin. The dysuria did not improve. The patient has a history of CHF with an ejection fraction of 35% (measured 1 month ago), and coronary artery disease status post–coronary bypass surgery 5 years ago. Home medications include aspirin, carvedilol, lisinopril, ciprofloxacin, furosemide, and spironolactone. The patient mentioned that a CT of the chest was done 10 days prior to this presentation for follow-up of a pulmonary nodule found incidentally on CXR 6 months ago. On examination, the patient is lying in bed and sweating. Vital signs are as follows: temperature 39°C, blood pressure 100/60, heart rate 110 bpm, respiratory rate 22/min, and oxygen saturation 97% on room air. Positive findings on clinical examination include bilateral fine crackles in both lung bases, a systolic ejection murmur at the heart base rated 3/6 with radiation to the carotids, and left costophrenic tenderness. CXR showed an enlarged cardiac silhouette and a 3-cm nodule in the right middle lobe. Initial labs are as follows: WBC 18,000 with 15% bands, Hg 12, HCT 36, platelets 250,000, Na 131, K 3.7, Cl 99, HCO_3 28, BUN 80, Cr 2.8 (last Cr was 0.7 ten days ago), glucose 95, Ca 8.0, BNP 300, and lactic acid 3.0 (normal is up to 2.0). Urinalysis showed elevated white blood cells, trace protein and blood, bacteriuria, and many hyaline casts. Urine sodium was 8 mmol/L. FeNa was <1%.

What is the most likely cause of the patient's AKI?
- A. Contrast nephropathy
- B. Acute interstitial nephritis
- C. AKI secondary to volume depletion
- D. AKI secondary to CHF
- E. Acute tubular necrosis

2. An 80-year-old female with a history of advanced CHF is admitted to the hospital with acute on chronic systolic heart failure. The patient was started on a high dose of IV furosemide twice a day. The next day, she made a good amount of urine and her shortness of breath improved slightly. Her creatinine increased to 2.1 (baseline is 1.5). On hospital day 3, the patient's creatinine increased to 2.4. Her respiratory rate is 24/min and her saturation is 92% on 6 L by nasal cannula. On examination, her estimated jugular venous pressure is 15 and she has bilateral fine crackles heard diffusely in both lung fields. Her input in the last 24 hours was 1500 cm^3, and her UOP was 2700 cm^3.

What would you do next?

A. Hold furosemide and repeat BMP the next day

B. Continue IV furosemide

C. Switch to oral furosemide

D. Hold furosemide, give 250 cm^3 of normal saline, and repeat BMP

E. Call nephrology for hemodialysis

Answers

1. C. The patient's presentation is consistent with severe sepsis and pyelonephritis. She was vomiting for 2 days. She is tachycardic and sweating. Her lactic acid is elevated. These are likely from sepsis and volume depletion. Urine sodium concentration is low even though the patient is on furosemide and spironolactone, which means the kidney is reabsorbing a higher fraction of urine sodium because of the severe prerenal state. Patients with AKI secondary to CHF are usually in clear fluid overload state—not so here. It is not uncommon to see mild edema in the lower extremities and fine crackles on pulmonary examination of elderly patients with stable CHF (New York Heart Association Functional Class I).

BNP should be interpreted very carefully in low GFR states (serum BNP level will be high with poor kidney function). The CXR did not show any pulmonary edema. After contrast administration, the vast majority of contrast nephropathy patients will have an elevated creatinine within the first 72 hours, and it usually comes back to normal in 5 to 7 days. This patient had contrast given 10 days ago, which makes contrast nephropathy a very unlikely cause of her AKI.

The patient was started on ciprofloxacin a few days ago, and this put her at risk for AIN. Some 50% to 60% of AIN patients have proteinuria (<1 g in 24 h urine), pyuria, and hematuria. Leukocyte casts are also seen with AIN. However, because it is a much less common etiology of AKI than prerenal causes, AIN is usually a diagnosis of exclusion. This patient has only trace proteinuria and hematuria. More importantly, the patient's presentation and initial workup is very consistent with prerenal AKI.

If the renal function doesn't improve after fluid resuscitation, the patient should be evaluated for other etiologies including AIN. ATN is an important differential diagnosis in this case. Prolonged dehydration and sepsis are risk factors for ischemia and subsequent ATN. The low FeNa in this case does not rule out ATN. That is because FeNa is less than 1% during the early stages of nonoliguric ATN. The only way to differentiate between the two conditions is by fluid challenge. If there is no improvement, ATN becomes more likely.

2. **B.** The patient's kidney function got worse with an IV diuretic. However, she is still in acute heart failure (saturation is 92% on 6 L of oxygen, high JVP, diffuse crackles on chest auscultation). An IV diuretic—in this case, furosemide—should be continued at this point in order to improve cardiac function. Pay close attention to urine output, daily weight, and daily serum creatinine trend as well as attention to onset of other conditions that can complicate recovery from AKI. Recall that when patients are hospitalized, several conditions can be occurring at the same time.

Holding the furosemide with or without fluid bolus, at the stage when the serum creatinine appears to have trended up, may appear to be in the interest of the kidney function—but this is bad for the heart as the patient is still in fluid overload state, increasing risk for acute respiratory failure that has a higher mortality than mild to moderate AKI. Before switching from IV to oral diuretics, patients should be back to their baseline volume status with minimal or no symptoms of heart failure. Some CHF patients will be resistant to diuretics. In situations like this, increasing the dose of the loop diuretic or adding a thiazide diuretic should be tried. If this doesn't work and the kidney function worsens with low UOP, hemodialysis should be considered.

In the above clinical vignette, IV furosemide improved her symptoms slightly and she is still making a good amount of urine. Continuing the IV furosemide will most likely improve her volume status.

SUGGESTED READINGS

McPhee S, Papadakis M. *Current Medical Diagnosis & Treatment*. New York: McGraw-Hill Companies; 2011:869–878.
Szerlip H. Acute kidney injury. In: *Internal Medicine Essentials for Students*. Philadelphia: American College of Physicians and RR Donnelly Publishing; 2011:231–235.

A 48-year-old Man With Restlessness, Tremulousness, and Hypertension

Dorcas Adaramola, MD, MPH and Se Young Han, MD

A 48-year-old man is admitted to the hospital because of pneumonia. On the second day of his hospitalization, the patient becomes agitated and restless. Heart rate is 115/min and BP is 155/102. RR is 24/min. There is a mild fever of 100.4°F. On physical examination, the patient is noted to be alert but anxious, tremulous, and disoriented to place and time, and these findings are new compared with those on examination at admission. His alcohol history is significant as he reports drinking a fifth of vodka daily for several years. His most recent alcohol intake occurred the day before coming to the hospital. There is no known history of alcoholic liver disease. On physical examination, there are no changes from admission except those noted above. He does not appear to be in worsening respiratory distress, and repeated CXR is unchanged from admission. Lab investigations including CBC show mild anemia with Hb 12.4, and CMP showed moderate hyperglycemia. ECG shows sinus tachycardia.

1. **What is the next step to determine the treatment? Once you start medications, how do you adjust their dose? And before deciding how to give them, what should you consider first?**

Answer

Patients with a history of alcohol use may develop autonomic instability as signs of withdrawal within 48 hours of their last drink of alcohol. It is important to anticipate this and order the Clinical Institute Withdrawal Assessment (CIWA) protocol to be utilized for benzodiazepine-managed alcohol withdrawal. Familiarity with the scoring of the CIWA scale is valuable. The initiation of benzodiazepine use for withdrawal symptoms is indicated when a score is 8 or above on the CIWA protocol. (Since the use of the protocol relies on the ability of patients to communicate their symptoms, it is appropriate only in patients who are conscious and able to communicate verbally.)

CASE REVIEW

Given his history of alcohol use disorder and symptoms, the patient is likely demonstrating signs of alcohol withdrawal and delirium tremens (DTs).

APPROACH TO ALCOHOL WITHDRAWAL PROBLEMS

Screening

The Prediction of Alcohol Withdrawal Severity Scale (PAWSS) is a key tool for determining a patient's likelihood to experience clinically significant alcohol withdrawal. A score of 4 or higher indicates a patient at risk for withdrawal and should trigger the anticipatory ordering of the CIWA protocol.

Alcohol-related problems are estimated in up to 20% of patients in community teaching hospitals. Internal medicine is frequently asked to manage these problems in a patient who has been admitted to the hospital for other medical or surgical illnesses. Although DTs have a mortality rate as high as 20% in the untreated, early recognition of a patient at risk and initiation of appropriate treatment can lower the mortality significantly.

Diagnosis

Currently, CIWA-Ar (a shortened, improved version of CIWA) is recommended for guiding benzodiazepine dosing and administration in patients with clinically significant alcohol withdrawal. In general, a score of 8 or more indicates the need for benzodiazepine-managed withdrawal from alcohol.

CLINICAL INSTITUTE WITHDRAWAL ASSESSMENT FOR ALCOHOL SCALE

Scoring

The cumulative score provides the basis for treatment of patients undergoing alcohol withdrawal (Table 5-1).

Assessment Tool

Nausea and vomiting
Ask: "Do you feel sick to your stomach? Have you vomited?" (See Table 5-2.)

Table 5-1. CIWA Scoring Interpretation

Cumulative Score	
0–7	No medication is necessary
8–14	Medication is optional for patients with a score of 8–14
15–20	A score of ≥15 requires treatment with medication
>20	A score of >20 poses a strong risk of delirium tremens
67	Maximum possible cumulative score

Table 5-2. Nausea Scoring

Score	
0	No nausea and no vomiting
1	Mild nausea with no vomiting
2	
3	
4	Intermittent nausea with dry heaves
5	
6	
7	Constant nausea, frequent dry heaves, and vomiting

Tremor
Arms extended and fingers spread apart (Table 5-3).

Paroxysmal sweats
See Table 5-4.

Anxiety
Ask: "Do you feel nervous?" (See Table 5-5.)

Agitation
See Table 5-6.

Tactile disturbances
Ask: "Have you any itching, pins-and-needles sensations, burning sensations, or numbness, or do you feel bugs crawling on or under your skin?" (See Table 5-7.)

Table 5-3. Tremor Scoring

Score	
0	No tremor
1	Not visible, but can be felt fingertip to fingertip
2	
3	
4	Moderate, with patient's arms extended
5	
6	
7	Severe, even with arms not extended

Table 5-4. Sweating Scoring

Score	
0	No sweat visible
1	Barely perceptible sweating, palms moist
2	
3	
4	Beads of sweat obvious on forehead
5	
6	
7	Drenching sweats

Table 5-5. Anxiety Scoring

Score	
0	No anxiety, at ease
1	Mildly anxious
2	
3	
4	Moderately anxious, or guarded, so anxiety is inferred
5	
6	
7	Equivalent to acute panic states as seen in severe delirium or acute schizophrenic reactions

Table 5-6. Activity Scoring

Score	
0	Normal activity
1	Somewhat more than normal activity
2	
3	
4	Moderately fidgety and restless
5	
6	
7	Paces back and forth during most of the interview, or constantly thrashes about

Table 5-7. Neurologic Scoring

Score	
0	None
1	Very mild itching, pins and needles, burning, or numbness
2	Mild itching, pins and needles, burning, or numbness
3	Moderate itching, pins and needles, burning, or numbness
4	Moderately severe hallucinations
5	Severe hallucinations
6	Extremely severe hallucinations
7	Continuous hallucinations

Auditory disturbances
Ask: "Are you more aware of sounds around you? Are they harsh? Do they frighten you? Are you hearing anything that is disturbing to you? Are you hearing things you know are not there?" (See Table 5-8.)

Visual disturbances
Ask: "Does the light appear to be too bright? Is its color different? Does it hurt your eyes? Are you seeing anything that is disturbing to you? Are you seeing things you know are not there?" (See Table 5-9.)

Headache, fullness in head
Ask: "Does your head feel different? Does it feel as if there is a band around your head?" Do not rate for dizziness or light-headedness. Otherwise, rate severity (Table 5-10).

Table 5-8. Auditory Disturbance Scoring

Score	
0	Not present
1	Very mild harshness or ability to frighten
2	Mild harshness or ability to frighten
3	Moderate harshness or ability to frighten
4	Moderately severe hallucinations
5	Severe hallucinations
6	Extremely severe hallucinations
7	Continuous hallucinations

Table 5-9. Visual Disturbance Scoring

Score	
0	Not present
1	Very mild sensitivity
2	Mild sensitivity
3	Moderate sensitivity
4	Moderately severe hallucinations
5	Severe hallucinations
6	Extremely severe hallucinations
7	Continuous hallucinations

Orientation and clouding of sensorium

Ask: "What day is this? Where are you? Who am I?" (See Table 5-11.)

Besides patient's history on alcohol, what clues may alert us to the patient's alcohol use and risk of developing withdrawal symptoms?

Physical examination findings that may provide clues to the presence of an alcohol disorder include mild elevations of blood pressure, history of repeated infections such as pneumonia (particularly aspiration pneumonia), and unexplained cardiac arrhythmias such as atrial fibrillation (so-called "holiday heart syndrome").

When present, abnormalities of liver function tests such as an AST:ALT ratio >2:1 are helpful clues. Among other laboratory tests, elevated carbohydrate-free transferrin (>20 U/L) and gamma-GT (>35 U) are the most sensitive and specific (>70%) to make a diagnosis of alcohol use disorder; the combination of the 2 is likely to be more accurate than either alone. These tests are also useful in monitoring

Table 5-10. Headache Scoring

Score	
0	Not present
1	Very mild
2	Mild
3	Moderate
4	Moderately severe
5	Severe
6	Very severe
7	Extremely severe

Table 5-11. Orientation Scoring

Score	
0	Oriented and can do serial additions
1	Cannot do serial additions or is uncertain about date
2	Disoriented for date by no more than 2 calendar days
3	Disoriented for date by more than 2 calendar days
4	Disoriented for place and/or person

abstinence as well. Other than the aforementioned tests, a high MCV (>91 μm^3) and serum uric acid (>7 mg/dL) can be useful in identifying heavy users of alcohol.

Once a patient is determined to be at risk for clinically significant alcohol withdrawal, interventions may be initiated to prevent alcohol withdrawal syndromes.

The primary effect of alcohol on the CNS is depression of excitability and conduction, so patients with alcoholism seem to have compensated for the depressant effect because the brain has been exposed repeatedly to high doses of alcohol. When alcohol intake is terminated or the alcohol level in the CNS decreases, withdrawal symptoms occur. Since withdrawal is a form of rebound overactivations from the suppression, many of these withdrawal symptoms are the opposite of those produced by intoxication. That is, symptoms of increased CNS activity, particularly agitation, and autonomic hyperactivity such as an increase in heart rate, respiratory rate, and temperature are seen. Patients may develop various withdrawal signs and symptoms depending on the time from the last alcohol use.

Alcoholic hallucinosis develops 12 to 48 hours after discontinuing alcohol use. Patients typically have distinctive visual, auditory, and/or tactile hallucinations without autonomic instability. This is in contrast to the autonomic instability in DTs, which may or may not be accompanied by symptoms of hallucinosis.

Alcohol withdrawal seizures (often a single generalized tonic-clonic seizure) may occur within 48 hours after last use of alcohol and usually do not require prophylactic antiseizure medications.

DTs refers to delirium associated with a tremor and autonomic hyperactivity and generally occur 2 to 4 days after last alcohol use. This is seen in approximately 5% of alcohol-dependent individuals. The chance of DTs during any single withdrawal is <1%. DTs are more likely to develop in patients with concomitant severe medical disorders, history of sustained drinking, previous history of DTs or alcohol withdrawal seizures, withdrawal symptoms with positive BAL, and age over 30.

Treatment

The goals of treatment are amelioration of symptoms and prevention of complications.

Mild symptoms can be managed supportively (ie, CIWA protocol score <8). If a patient progresses symptomatically despite supportive measures, pharmacologic treatment should be instituted. Most withdrawal symptoms are caused by the rapid removal of a CNS depressant (in this case, alcohol). The symptoms can be controlled by administering any CNS depressant in doses that decrease agitation, and gradually tapering the dose over 3 to 5 days.

Among CNS depressants, benzodiazepines have the highest margin of safety and lowest cost and are, therefore, the preferred class of drugs. All benzodiazepines are effective in the treatment of alcohol withdrawal symptoms. Benzodiazepines with a short half-life are especially useful for patients with serious liver impairment or preexisting encephalopathy. However, short-acting benzodiazepines such as lorazepam can produce rapidly changing drug blood levels and must be given every 4 hours to avoid abrupt fluctuations that may increase the risk of seizures. Therefore, most clinicians use drugs with longer half-lives, such as diazepam or chlordiazepoxide.

A key point in treating alcohol withdrawal is to begin with a larger dose of benzodiazepines than that typically prescribed for anxiety. The patient's response should be observed, and the dosage needs to be adjusted accordingly. Previously, fixed-dose schedules were used, but multiple studies have shown that a symptom-triggered approach may be as efficacious as the fixed one and result in less drug use.

Prerequisite to start CIWA-Ar protocol

Before implementing a symptom-triggered protocol, two factors should be considered: first, is the patient at risk of developing alcohol withdrawal syndrome? (A remote history of alcoholism does not increase the risk of symptom development and therefore doesn't need a treatment protocol.) Second, does the patient have intact verbal communication? Since this protocol is a symptom-triggered treatment, it is ineffective if the patient is not able to communicate.

In addition to alcohol withdrawal syndrome, there are other medical problems complicating the treatment of patients with alcohol withdrawal, especially nutritional deficiencies:

1. Thiamine deficiency:

   A. Wet beriberi (aka beriberi syndrome) is characterized by high-output heart failure (alcoholism is one of the reversible causes of dilated cardiomyopathy).

   B. Dry beriberi (either Wernicke syndrome or Korsakoff psychosis).

      In Wernicke syndrome, patients typically manifest ataxia, ophthalmoplegia (diplopia with nystagmus due to lateral gaze palsy, often affecting the sixth cranial nerve, the abducens nerve), and confusion.

      In Korsakoff psychosis, patients may develop a combination of anterograde and retrograde amnesia, confabulation, or the presence of spur cells on peripheral blood smear. It is associated with a poor prognosis.

Management: give thiamine first before replacing glucose in patients with alcoholism. Thiamine is a vital cofactor for glucose metabolism; therefore, giving glucose prior to thiamine would worsen the status of the patient.

2. Refeeding syndrome (phosphate deficiency): Patients who chronically use alcohol are phosphate-depleted as well. If they are fed a high-carbohydrate diet without correcting hypophosphatemia, it will lead to the depletion of more phosphate because the body's phosphate will be used to make ATP and phosphate-bound glucose in the liver and muscles. Consequently, patients may develop hemolysis, muscle breakdown, and respiratory distress.

3. Vitamin B_{12} and folate deficiency: Clinically, vitamin B_{12} results in both hematologic and neurologic sequelae while folate deficiency causes only hematologic problems.

Biochemically, the level of vitamin B_{12} and folate can be measured directly. However, the folate level can be affected by a recently consumed folate-rich diet, making it appear normal. Moreover, vitamin B_{12} levels are often borderline low (250–500 pg/mL). If these levels are normal but clinical suspicion is high, measure the indirect metabolites of vitamin B_{12} and folate: MMA and homocysteine. If both are elevated, there is a vitamin B_{12} deficiency, and if only homocysteine is high, a folate deficiency is likely present.

In vitamin B_{12} deficiency, neurologic complications come first before hematologic manifestations such as megaloblastic anemia (MCV often higher than 110). Therefore, even without hematologic findings, dementia or an abnormal gait such as a "high stepping gait," in a clinical context, may be indicative of a vitamin B_{12} deficiency.

4. Miscellaneous: hyponatremia (beer potomania), magnesium deficiency, and calcium deficiency.

TIPS TO REMEMBER

- Alcohol-related problems are common in the hospital. Early recognition of a patient at risk and initiation of appropriate treatment can lower mortality significantly.

- PAWSS is recommended for determining the risk of alcohol withdrawal, while benzodiazepine-assisted management of clinical withdrawal should be guided by a validated tool such as the CIWA-Ar protocol.

- Many alcohol withdrawal symptoms observed are due to increased CNS activity, particularly agitation and autonomic hyperactivity such as an increase in heart rate, respiratory rate, and temperature.

- DTs refers to delirium associated with a tremor and autonomic hyperactivity and generally occur 2 to 7 days after stopping the use of alcohol.
- Benzodiazepines are the preferred class of drugs to treat moderate clinically significant alcohol withdrawal syndromes in the hospital.

COMPREHENSION QUESTION

1. A 42-year-old man was admitted for hematemesis. On admission, his examinations including vital signs were unremarkable. Initial laboratory tests showed mild macrocytic anemia on CBC, normal LFT, and a negative alcohol level. The next day, he started to see "spiders hanging from the ceiling." Examination revealed temperature 97.8°F, heart rate 74/min, respiratory rate 12/min, and blood pressure 130/80 mm Hg. There was mild tremulousness. His past medical history was significant for alcohol abuse. CIWA-Ar protocol was started.
   What is the most likely diagnosis?
   A. DTs
   B. Minor withdrawal symptoms
   C. Acute withdrawal seizure
   D. Alcoholic hallucinosis
   E. Korsakoff psychosis

Answer

1. **D.** Lack of autonomic hyperactivity in addition to an atypical time course (onset <48 hours from last drinking) makes DTs highly unlikely. Patients with DTs typically show disorientation, and their hallucinations are tactile rather than visual. Patients may develop minor withdrawal symptoms such as tremulousness, mild anxiety, and nausea usually within 6 hours of cessation of drinking. Alcohol withdrawal seizures, often a single generalized seizure, may occur within 48 hours after stopping alcohol. Based on the development of distinctive visual hallucination without autonomic instability, the patient with withdrawal symptoms is diagnosed with alcoholic hallucination, which happens in 12 to 24 hours after discontinuing alcohol. This patient does not have features of Korsakoff psychosis.

SUGGESTED READINGS

Fauci AS, Braunwald E, Kasper DL, et al. Alcohol and alcoholism. In: *Harrison's Principles of Internal Medicine*. 17th ed. New York: McGraw-Hill Professional; 2008:2725–2728.

Hecksel KA, Bostwick JM, Jaeger TM, Cha SS. Inappropriate use of symptom-triggered therapy for alcohol withdrawal in the general hospital. *Mayo Clin Proc.* 2008;83(3):274–279.

Lohr R. Treatment of alcohol withdrawal in hospitalized patients. *Mayo Clin Proc.* 1995;70(8):777–782.

Maldonado JR, Sher Y, Das S, et al. Prospective validation study of the Prediction of Alcohol Withdrawal Severity Scale (PAWSS) in medically ill inpatients: a new scale for the prediction of complicated alcohol withdrawal syndrome. *Alcohol Alcohol.* 2015;50(5):509–518.

Saitz M, Mayo-Smith MF, Redmond HA, et al. *Individualized treatment for alcohol withdrawal. A randomized double-blind controlled trial. JAMA* 1994;272:519–523.

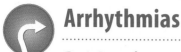

Arrhythmias

Raj Patel, MD, Basma Al-Bast, MD and
Youssef Chami, MD

Introduction

Arrythmias can be organized into the following categories: supraventricular tachyarrhythmias, ventricular tachyarrhythmias, bradyarrhythmia, and conduction blocks (Figure 6-1).

A thorough clinical history and physical examination, as in any other case, are particularly important. Clinically significant arrhythmias may produce symptoms of palpitations, lightheadedness, syncope, or dyspnea. Look for any triggering factors such as infection, pulmonary embolism, pericarditis, myocardial ischemia, surgery, drug toxicity, excess use of caffeine, excessive alcohol intake, thyroid abnormalities, or electrolyte imbalances as potential causes.

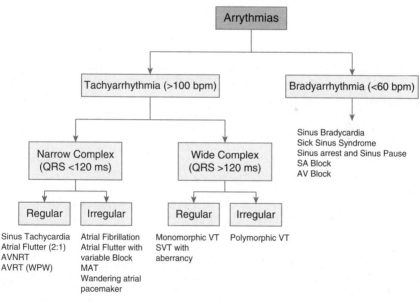

Figure 6-1. Classification of arrythmia.

Supraventricular tachyarrhythmias

A 50-year-old Man With Palpitations and lightheadedness

A 50-year-old male presents for evaluation of palpitation and lightheadednes. He has been having similar episodes for 2 years. These episodes occur irregularly, several times every week, lasting for 1 to 15 minutes. The nurse reports the patient's BP is 130/70 with a heart rate of 150 bpm. The ECG is shown in Figure 6-2.

1. What is the most likely diagnosis and treatment for thispatient.

Answer

1. The ECG reveals SVT with HR of 150 bpm. The best step to perform next is carotid sinus massage. If there is no response, try IV adenosine.

Paroxysmal Supraventricular Tachycardia

Paroxysmal supraventricular tachycardia (PSVT) is a subset of SVT evidenced by intermittent episodes of narrow complex tachycardia with sudden onset and termination. Most SVTs have a narrow QRS complex on ECG, but SVT with aberrant conduction can produce a wide complex tachycardia that may mimic ventricular tachycardia (VT). These tachycardias commonly occur as a result of a precipitating illness or drug interaction.

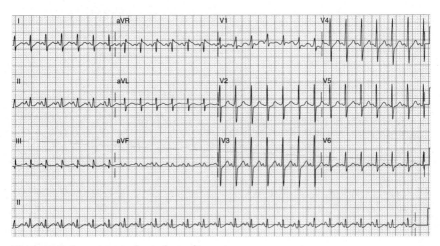

Figure 6-2. Supraventricular tachycardia.

If the patient is hemodynamically stable, vagal maneuvers including carotid massage and Valsalva can be performed. It is important to remember that carotid sinus massage should be avoided in patients with increased risk of carotid artery disease and stroke. Pharmacologic therapy includes adenosine, beta blockers, and/or calcium channel blockers. Adenosine is given via peripheral IV access as a 6-mg dose followed by 20-mL saline flush. Additional 12-mg doses can be given if not effective within 1 to 2 minutes. If the patient is hemodynamically unstable, proceed to synchronized cardioversion.

A 69-year-old Man With Tachycardia and Wheezing

A 69-year-old man is admitted with pneumonia and COPD exacerbation. The nurse calls you saying the patient has developed tachycardia and active wheezing, and his rhythm is irregular. She is worried and wants you to look at the ECG (Figure 6-3). The nurse shows you the following 12-lead ECG from the patient:

1. What is the most likely diagnosis and treatment for this patient.

Answer

The ECG shows multifocal atrial tachycardia (MAT). The patient's underlying lung disease must have precipitated MAT. Treating the COPD exacerbation with beta-2 adrenergic agonist inhalation is the therapy of choice. Make sure to correct hypomagnesemia or hypokalemia if present.

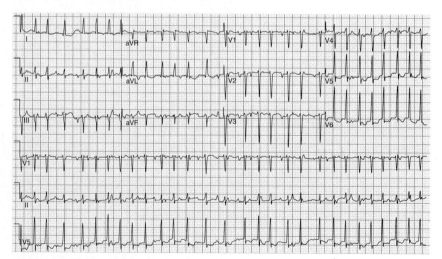

Figure 6-3. MAT with an irregular rhythm and with at least 3 different morphologic P waves and tachycardia.

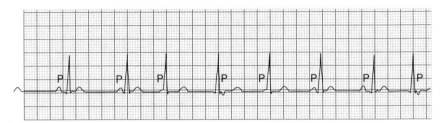

Figure 6-4. Irregular rhythm with 3 morphologically distinct P waves with a heart rate of less than 100 bpm.

Multifocal Atrial Tachycardia

MAT is an irregular SVT with a heart rate of >100 bpm distinguished by at least 3 P-wave morphologies (Figure 6-4). It arises from multiple atrial foci and is often associated with COPD, heart failure, and electrolyte abnormalities (hypokalemia, hypomagnesemia).

Therapy in patients with MAT should be aimed at treating the underlying disease. Medical therapy is reserved for symptomatic MAT requiring ventricular rate control; a nondihydropyridine calcium channel blocker (verapamil, diltiazem) or beta blocker can be used. Beta blockers are preferred in the absence of heart failure exacerbation or bronchospasm.

Wandering Atrial Pacemaker (Multifocal Atrial Rhythm)

This disorder is similar to MAT in that there are 3 morphologically distinct P waves but the heart rate is less than 100 bpm (Figure 6-4). This rhythm is irregularly irregular and can be confused with atrial fibrillation. This is a benign condition, and there is no need for treatment.

A 55-year-old Man With Fatigue and Decreased Exercise Tolerance

A 55-year-old male with a past medical history of hypertension, hyperlipidemia, and obesity presents to the outpatient internal medicine clinic with a 3-day history of fatigue and decreased exercise tolerance. He used to be able to walk 2 blocks without shortness of breath, but now he gets winded even walking in from the parking garage. He feels as though his heart is beating fast but denies palpitations. He has no chest pain, dizziness, visual changes, edema, or orthopnea. His medications include chlorthalidone, lovastatin, and aspirin.

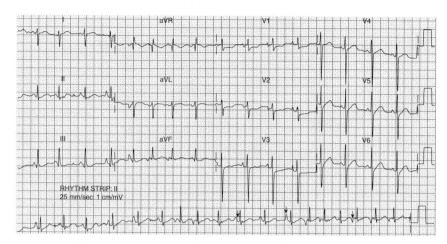

Figure 6-5. Wandering atrial pacemaker.

On physical examination, his blood pressure is 120/60 mm Hg, pulse is 100 bpm, respiratory rate is 16/min, and pulse oximetry is 96% on room air. He is alert and answers questions appropriately. His lungs are clear to auscultation. His cardiac examination reveals an irregularly irregular rhythm that is tachycardic. Extremities reveal no edema. ECG is shown in Figure 6-6.

1. What is the diagnosis?

Answer

1. Atrial fibrillation, a form of supraventricular tachycardia (SVT).

Atrial Fibrillation

Atrial fibrillation is diagnosed with irregularly irregular rhythm on ECG with absence of discrete P waves. It is the most diagnosed arrythmia.

Initial therapy for atrial fibrillation is almost always directed at rate control with a goal of less than 110 bpm. Rate control is achieved with beta blockers, non-dihydropyridine calcium channel blockers, or digoxin. Calcium channel blockers should be avoided in patients with decreased LV function (ejection fraction <35%) due to their negative inotropic effects. Multiple studies comparing rate control versus rhythm control strategy have shown no difference in short-term outcomes, but recent data suggest catheter ablation of AF might be reasonable in patients with heart failure to reduce mortality and readmission. Anticoagulation is recommended for patients with atrial fibrillation and high risk for stroke as determined by elevated CHA2DS2-VASc score (≥2 in men, ≥3 in women) (Table 6-1). Direct oral anticoagulants are recommended over warfarin (except in

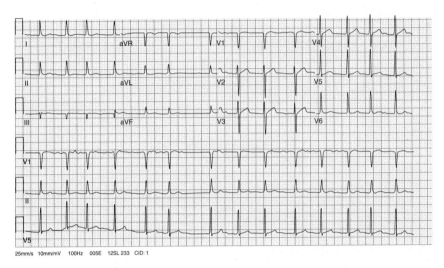

25mm/s 10mm/mV   100Hz   005E   12SL 233   CID: 1

Figure 6-6. Atrial fibrillation with an irregularly irregular rhythm with no P waves. Note the fibrillatory or F waves.

Table 6-1. CHA2DS2-VASc criteria

CHA2DS2-VASc Risk	Score	CHA2DS2-VASc Score	Adjusted Stroke Rate (%/year)
CHF or LVEF <40%	1	1	1.3
Hypertension	1	2	2.2
Age >75	2	3	3.2
Diabetes	1	4	4
Stroke/TIA/ thromboembolism	2	5	6.7
Vascular disease	1	6	9.8
Age 65–74	1	7	9.6
Female	1	8	6.7
		9	15.2

CHF, congestive heart failure; TIA, transient ischemic attack; LVEF, left ventricular ejection fraction.

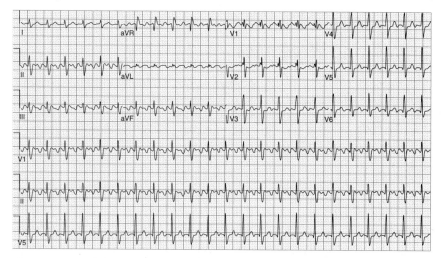

Figure 6-7. Atrial flutter with sawtooth pattern and 2:1 AV conduction.

patients with moderate to severe mitral stenosis or a mechanical heart valve). Synchronized cardioversion is recommended in AF patients with intractable symptoms, hemodynamic instability, or inadequate rate control. For cardioversion, the anterior pad is placed on the right side below the clavicle at the fourth intercostal space lateral to the sternum. The posterior pad is placed on the left side, subscapular and lateral to the spine. Next, administer appropriate sedative medications and secure the airway. Press the "SYNC" button on defibrillator and observe ECG syncing with R wave on the monitor. A starting dose of 100 J of biphasic energy will be successful in the majority of patients; however, if unsuccessful, proceed with 200 J biphasic energy. Antiarrhythmics such as amiodarone also can be used in certain situations.

Atrial Flutter

Atrial flutter results from a single reentrant circuit around a functional or structural barrier to conduction within the atria (Figure 6-6). The 12-lead ECG has a characteristic "sawtooth" pattern with an effective atrial rate of 250 to 350 bpm. There is typically 2:1 (flutter waves:QRS response) conduction across the AV node. As a result, the ventricular rate is usually one-half the flutter rate in the absence of AV node dysfunction.

The clinical presentation and treatment strategies are similar to those of atrial fibrillation, which include rate control and anticoagulation. There is a high rate of success with radiofrequency ablation for typical atrial flutter.

A 75-year-old Man With Sudden Shortness of Breath and Weakness

A 75-year-old male with a medical history significant for hypertension, diabetes, and coronary artery disease presents to the emergency department with a 1-hour history of sudden shortness of breath and generalized weakness.

On examination, he is noted to have a blood pressure of 90/58. He is clammy and diaphoretic. His lungs are clear to auscultation. His heart examination reveals tachycardia.

His ECG is shown in Figure 6-8.

1. What is your diagnosis?

Answer

1. VT.

Ventricular Tachycardia

VT is a wide complex tachycardia (QRS >120 ms) defined as a series of 3 or more ventricular complexes that occur at a rate of >100 bpm and are independent of atrial or AV conduction. It can be difficult to distinguish VT from SVT with aberrancy. Clues to help diagnose VT on ECG include the following: (1) positive or negative concordance of the QRS complexes in the precordial lead; (2) AV dissociation (no relationship between the P wave and QRS complex); (3) presence of capture or fusion beat; and (4) northwest ECG axis (lead 1 and lead aVF both negative). It is important to remember that the majority of wide complex

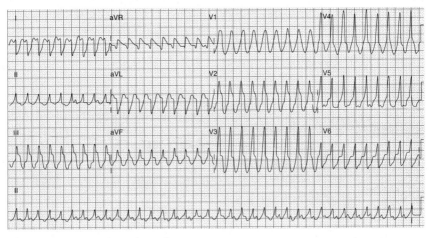

Figure 6-8. Ventricular tachycardia.

tachycardias are VT, so when in doubt treat rhythm as VT. It can be sustained (>30 s) or nonsustained based on duration, or monomorphic or polymorphic based on ECG morphology. Polymorphic VT is characterized by continuously variable QRS complex. Torsade de pointes is a form of polymorphic VT associated with prolonged QT interval. Myocardial ischemia is the most common cause of polymorphic VT with normal baseline QT interval. Other causes of VT include electrolyte abnormalities and congestive heart failure. This is a potentially life-threatening arrhythmia because it may lead to ventricular fibrillation (VF), asystole, and sudden death.

Patients suffering from pulseless VT or unstable VT are hemodynamically compromised and require immediate unsynchronized cardioversion (per ACLS protocol with 200 J). For patients who are hemodynamically stable, antiarrhythmic agents such as amiodarone (150-mg bolus followed by 1-mg/min IV infusion), lidocaine, procainamide, or sotalol should be used.

A 80-year-old Male Presents With Recent Anterior STEMI With Stent Placement

A 80-year-old male with history of hypertension, type 2 diabetes, congestive heart failure, and coronary artery disease was admitted with an acute ST-elevation MI. He underwent successful percutaneous coronary intervention (PCI) of a proximal left anterior descending artery (LAD) stenosis. In recovery, his BP is 110/70, HR is 80 bpm, and ECG is showing the following findings (Figure 6-9).

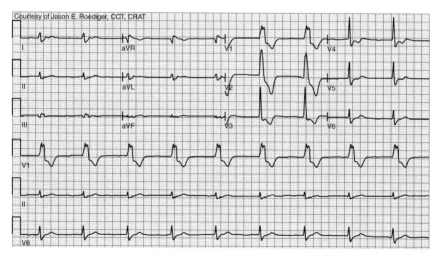

Figure 6-9. Accelerated idioventricular rhythm. (Reproduced with permission from Jason E. Roediger, CCT, CRAT. AIVR from the LV by Jer5150, licensed under CC BY-SA 3.0.)

Diagnosis

Accelerated idioventricular rhythm (AIVR).

Accelerated Idioventricular Rhythm (AIVR)

AIVR is defined as enhanced ectopic ventricular rhythm with at least 3 consecutive ventricular beats with rate between 40 and 100 bpm. It is benign, self-resolving, and rarely symptomatic. It is commonly seen in the reperfusion phase of myocardial infarction, digoxin toxicity, or cardiomyopathy.

AIVR is usually well tolerated and does not require treatment. Patients with AIVR should be treated mainly for its underlying causes. In rare instances, atropine can be used to increase the underlying sinus rate to inhibit the AIVR.

A 75-year-old Man Status Post–Myocardial Infarction With Stent Placement

A 75-year-old male with HTN, type 2 diabetes, ESRD, PVD, and CAD with a CABG in the past is admitted with an acute ST-elevation MI status post–cardiac stent placement. He has a BP of 90/50 and a heart rate of 110 bpm early in the morning. You are at the nurses' station, and the telemetry monitor goes off showing the rhythm in Figure 6-10.

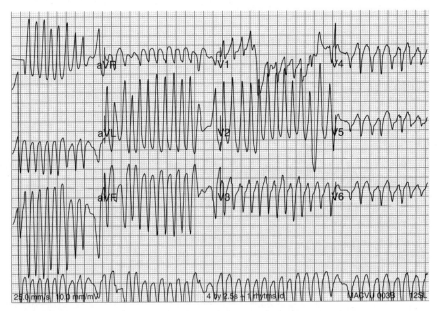

Figure 6-10. Ventricular fibrillation with disorganized rhythm.

1. What is the diagnosis?

Answer

Ventricular fibrillation.

Ventricular Fibrillation

VF is the most frequent mechanism of sudden cardiac death (SCD). It is a rapid, disorganized ventricular arrhythmia resulting in no uniform ventricular contraction, no cardiac output, and no recordable blood pressure. The electrocardiogram in VF shows rapid (300–400 bpm), irregular, shapeless QRS complexes with variable amplitude, morphology, and intervals. Over time, these waveforms decrease in amplitude. Ultimately, asystole occurs.

Immediate unsynchronized cardioversion is the treatment of choice with 120 to 200 Joules for biphasic defibrillation or 360 Joules for monophasic, followed by IV antiarrhythmics such as amiodarone.

HEART BLOCKS

A 65-year-old Woman With Syncopal Episodes

A 65-year-old woman comes in for her Welcome to Medicare examination. She has a history of hypertension and type 2 diabetes. On questioning, she says she has had 2 syncopal episodes in the past week. On physical examination, her blood pressure is 138/78 mm Hg, her pulse is 80 bpm, and her respiratory rate is 14/min. Lungs are clear to auscultation. Cardiovascular examination reveals a regular rate and rhythm with no murmurs, gallops, or rubs. Her extremities have no edema.

Her ECG is shown in Figure 6-11.

1. What is the diagnosis?

Answer

1. Mobitz type II AV block.

First-degree AV Block

First-degree AV block usually results from a conduction delay within the AV node in which the PR interval is lengthened beyond 200 milliseconds. The most common causes include increased vagal tone (athletes), drug effect, electrolyte abnormalities, ischemia, and conduction system disease.

Asymptomatic patients require no therapy. Stop or decrease the dose of AV node–blocking medications such as beta blockers or calcium channel blockers if these are being used (Figure 6-12).

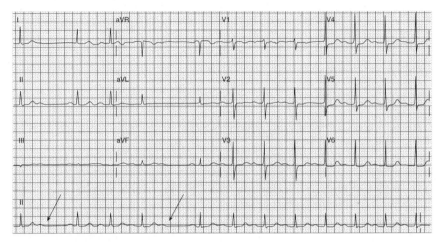

Figure 6-11. Mobitz type II block.

Second-degree AV Block

There are 2 types of second-degree AV blocks. These are recognized based on their pattern of impulse conduction, and the distinction between type I and type II is important, as the 2 types carry different prognostic implications.

Mobitz Type I (Wenckebach) Block

Mobitz type I heart block is characterized by the progressive prolongation of the PR interval on consecutive beats followed by a blocked P wave (Figure 6-13). This is recognized as a dropped QRS complex. After the dropped QRS complex, the PR interval resets and the cycle repeats. The RR interval progressively shortens before a blocked P wave.

Reversible causes of heart block should be first recognized and treated if possible, such as discontinuation of offending medication (beta blocker or calcium channel blocker).

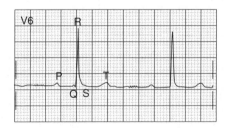

Figure 6-12. First-degree AV block.

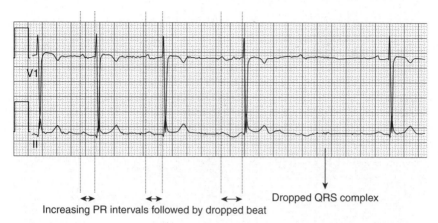

↔ ↔ ←→ Dropped QRS complex
Increasing PR intervals followed by dropped beat

Figure 6-13. Mobitz type I block.

Mobitz type I block is a fairly well-tolerated rhythm and does not require treatment if the patient is asymptomatic. However, if the patient develops symptoms, atropine and transcutaneous pacing should be used—and if symptoms persist, permanent pacemaker is indicated.

Mobitz Type II Block

Mobitz type II block is characterized by an abrupt AV conduction block without evidence of conduction delay in preceding conducted impulses (Figure 6-14). The ECG demonstrates no change in the PR interval preceding conducted impulses. This type of AV block may progress rapidly to complete heart block.

The definitive treatment for this form of AV block is an implantable pacemaker, but transcutaneous pacing can be used to bridge the patient to implantation.

2:1 AV Block

This is a form of second-degree AV block in which every other beat is nonconducted. The ECG will show only 1 PR interval before the blocked beat, and P wave not followed by QRS wave. A 2:1 block cannot be differentiated into Mobitz type I or II. It is associated with higher risk of progressing to complete heart block. Treatment is usually similar to that for Mobitz I block.

Third-degree (Complete) AV Block

Complete heart block occurs when all the atrial impulses fail to conduct to the ventricle and the prevailing ventricular escape rhythm is slower than the atrial rhythm (Figure 6-15). The PR interval will be variable, and the hallmark of complete heart block is no apparent relationship between P waves and QRS complexes.

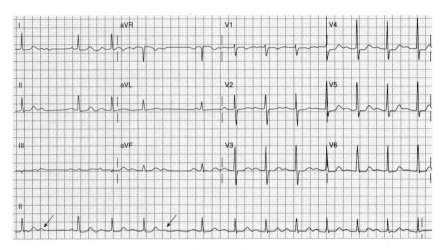

Figure 6-14. Mobitz type II with consistent PR interval and an unpredictable blocked P wave.

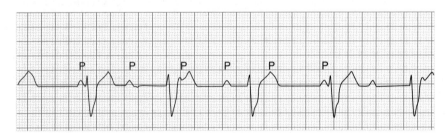

Figure 6-15. Third-degree heart block. Note P waves marching through and QRS complexes without a correlating P wave.

Therapy for complete heart block begins by looking for and correcting reversible causes such as myocardial ischemia, increased vagal tone, and AV-blocking medication. If no reversible causes are present, treatment is a permanent pacemaker for most patients.

SUGGESTED READINGS

Ahya SN, Flood K, Paranjothi S. *Cardiac Arrhythmias. The Washington Manual of Medical Therapeutics.* 30th ed. Philadelphia: Lippincott Williams & Wilkins; 2001:153–167.

A 40-year-old Man With Chest Pain

Wael Dakkak, MD, Muralidhar Papireddy, MD, Se Young Han, MD and Susan Thompson Hingle, MD

A 40-year-old man presented to the emergency department with a 2-day history of chest pain. He also has a 1-week history of sore throat, runny nose, dry cough, and generalized body aches. Yesterday, he woke up with chest pain, which he describes as severe, sharp, substernal chest pain that is aggravated by cough, deep breathing, and lying down. No dyspnea, orthopnea, paroxysmal nocturnal dyspnea, palpitations, or syncope are noted. He is physically active and is training for a 20-mile marathon. He has a history of hypertension, type 2 diabetes, and dyslipidemia. No medication allergies are noted. He drinks 1 glass of red wine on most nights. No history of tobacco or illicit drug use. He is on hydrochlorothiazide, metformin, and lovastatin. On examination, he appears to be in moderate distress from the chest pain. Vitals signs are within normal limits. Cardiac examination shows normal heart sounds with a pericardial rub. The remainder of the physical examination is unremarkable. Complete blood count is normal; basic metabolic profile is within normal range. Cardiac enzymes are normal. Electrocardiogram done in the emergency room shows diffuse ST-segment elevation without reciprocal changes and PR-segment depression in the limb leads. Chest radiograph is within normal limits.

1. What is the diagnosis and treatment of this condition?

Answer

1. Acute pericarditis.

CASE REVIEW

This patient's symptoms and signs are typical for acute pericarditis. The patient had chest pain for 2 days, which is sharp, constant, and worsened by position and deep breathing. Electrocardiogram shows diffuse ST elevation without reciprocal changes, which help to differentiate it from myocardial infarction, where you will find reciprocal ST depression with evolution of Q waves. Normal cardiac enzymes make acute coronary syndrome unlikely. Most cases of pericarditis are idiopathic or viral in etiology. Treatment is to begin nonsteroidal anti-inflammatory medication.

APPROACH TO CHEST PAIN

Chest pain is one of the most common presenting complaints in the emergency department, in clinics, and even in hospital inpatients. Several conditions can present as chest pain, and the challenge is in identifying the life-threatening causes from benign conditions.

In patients with chest pain who are not having a myocardial infarction, 50% to 60% of them have musculoskeletal and gastroesophageal disorders as the etiology of their chest pain. Unknown causes and psychiatric conditions account for another 8% to 35% of the cases. Realizing this, it is also important to recognize that chest pain is a symptom of some life-threatening conditions that require further investigation and management. It is recommended to use the terms *cardiac* and *noncardiac* chest pain rather than typical and atypical. Patients who are discharged with a diagnosis of noncardiac chest pain of unknown origin have survival rates of 94% at 10 years and 88% at 20 years.

A thorough history and physical examination can identify the etiology of the chest pain in most cases. In some cases, though, we may need additional testing to confirm or refute a clinical diagnosis.

History

Characteristics of the pain tell a lot about the underlying process. Every detail may have significance. Classic teaching with the mnemonic OLD-CA^{2}R^{2}T (*o*nset, *lo*cation, *d*uration, *c*haracter, *a*ggravating factors/*a*ssociated symptoms, *r*adiation/*r*elieving factors, *t*iming of the pain) can be applied to help one acquire all critical and specific history.

> Onset: Information on the onset of the pain may provide a great deal of information in the evaluation of patients with chest pain. With aortic dissection, pneumothorax, and pulmonary embolism, the onset of the pain is sudden. Myocardial ischemia is usually gradual in onset.
>
> Location: If a patient points with a finger to the apex or sternal border of the heart, the etiology of the pain is probably musculoskeletal. Describing the pain with a closed fist or palm suggests ischemia.
>
> Duration: If the pain is characterized as constant and lasts weeks, or just a few seconds; the pain is probably not from myocardial ischemia. Stable angina generally lasts 2 to 10 minutes, unstable angina (UA) 10 to 20 minutes, and myocardial infarction >30 minutes.
>
> Character: Pain is described as sharp in pneumothorax, aortic dissection, pleurisy, and pericarditis. Pain in myocardial ischemia is described as discomfort, pressure, tightness, heaviness, or squeezing. Burning pain is most likely from esophageal reflux.

Aggravating factors: Exertion, cold weather, or stress aggravation suggests ischemia. Cough and deep breathing aggravation suggest pleurisy. In esophageal reflux and pericarditis, the pain worsens with lying down. Movement and rotation worsen chest pain in patients with musculoskeletal pain. Swallowing worsens the pain in esophageal disorders, but with postprandial pain, do not forget to think about myocardial ischemia as a possibility.

Associated symptoms: Chest pain with dyspnea suggests pulmonary embolism, pneumonia, myocardial ischemia, pneumothorax, or eroding lung tumors. Nausea, vomiting, and diaphoresis may be associated with myocardial ischemia. Cough may be present with a pulmonary process or GERD. Syncope may occur concomitantly with aortic dissection, massive PE, or critical aortic stenosis.

Radiation: If the chest pain radiates to the neck, jaw, shoulders, back, or arms, this may suggest myocardial ischemia or aortic dissection. In pain that radiates down the neck and then causes chest pain, one should think about cervical radiculopathy. Pericarditis pain radiates to the trapezius area.

Relieving factors: Leaning forwards improves pain in pericarditis. Sitting up improves the pain in esophageal reflux disease. Resting improves chest pain in myocardial ischemia from stable angina. Improvement with antacids and eating suggests gastroesophageal problems. Pain relieved by nitroglycerin does not rule out acute coronary syndrome (ACS).

Timing of the pain: Early morning pain may occur in myocardial ischemia. If chest pain occurs at night while sleeping, think about gastroesophageal reflux or myocardial ischemia. Chest pain that happens after heavy exercise, weight lifting, or moving furniture suggests cardiac ischemia or musculoskeletal sources. Chest pain after recurrent retching or vomiting should make you think about esophageal rupture. If the pain occurs while swallowing, think esophagitis or spasm.

Also important is gathering information on the risk factors for different conditions in consideration of your differential diagnostic hypothesis list. Knowledge of the risk factors may give you pertinent information regarding disease likelihood. It is also important to remember that having no cardiac risk factors in patients presenting with acute chest pain does not rule out ACS.

Physical Examination

Examination should focus on palpation of the upper- and lower-extremity pulses, bilateral upper-extremity blood pressure measurements, a thorough cardiac and respiratory examination, an abdominal examination, and, last but not least, examination of the musculoskeletal system.

Table 7-1. Life-threatening Causes of Chest Pain

Acute coronary syndrome
Pulmonary embolism
Pneumothorax
Aortic dissection
Esophageal rupture

ECG and Chest Radiograph

An ECG should be ordered as a part of an acute evaluation of chest pain. A chest radiograph may help evaluate nonischemic causes of chest pain.

Rapid Evaluation

A rapid evaluation should be carried out on presentation to identify patients who may be having one of the life-threatening conditions (see Table 7-1). These conditions may result in death if ignored. Once we know that the chest pain is not from one of these life-threatening conditions, the next question to ask is the following: does this patient need admission to the hospital for further management or can the patient be managed as an outpatient? The algorithm in Figure 7-1 can help us make decisions regarding further care. We will discuss life-threatening causes of the chest pain and end with a discussion of the common causes of chest pain.

Acute coronary syndrome

Unstable angina (UA), non–ST-elevation myocardial infarction (NSTEMI), and ST-elevation myocardial infarction (STEMI) are all considered to be ACSs. For the convenience of the readers, UA and NSTEMI are discussed together as they are closely related conditions with a similar management strategy.

UA is defined as an ischemic pain occurring at rest that lasts for more than 10 to 20 minutes, new-onset chest pain, or increasing angina that is more frequent, lasts longer, or occurs at a lower threshold, with negative cardiac enzymes and ECG showing ST depression or T-wave inversion. In myocardial infarction pain, the pain lasts longer than 30 minutes and is more intense. It is classified as STEMI or NSTEMI based on the presence or absence of ST segment elevation, respectively.

Symptoms and signs Chest pain is often described as pressure-like pain, chest tightness, squeezing, heaviness, indigestion, or chest discomfort that radiates to the jaw, neck, arms, or shoulder. The classic description of pressure-like chest pain, however, has poor utility in predicting ACS. Pain similar to a previous MI, radiation to one or both shoulders/arms, and exertional pain have better predictability for ACS.

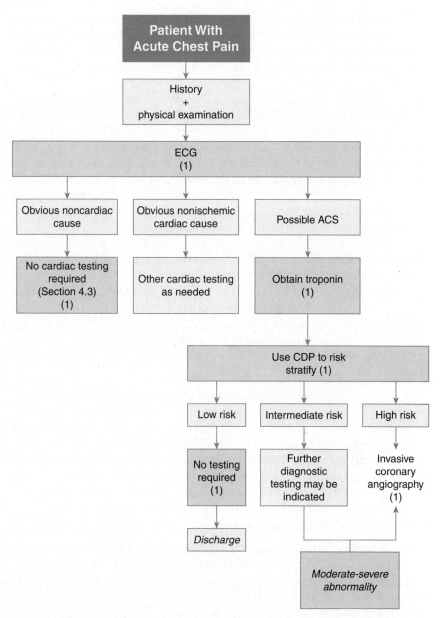

Figure 7-1. Approach to chest pain. (Reproduced with permission from Gulati M, Levy PD, Mukherjee D, et al. 2021 AHA/ACC/ASE/CHEST/SAEM/SCCT/SCMR Guideline for the Evaluation and Diagnosis of Chest Pain: A Report of the American College of Cardiology/American Heart Association Joint Committee on Clinical Practice Guidelines. *Circulation.* 2021;144(22):e368–e454, Figure 8.)

Cardiac ischemia is often associated with dyspnea, diaphoresis, weakness, nausea, or vomiting. Patients often show the painful area by placing a palm or a closed fist over the chest. Obtaining a history of comorbid conditions such as hyperthyroidism, gastrointestinal bleeding, and renal and pulmonary diseases may be important. On physical examination, attention should be paid to general appearance, vitals, pulses, cardiac, lung examination, musculoskeletal examination, signs of heart failure, and fluid overload.

Chest pain that is sharp, pleuritic, positional, lasts only a few seconds, radiates to the lower extremities, and is reproduced with movement or palpation of the chest is less likely to be ischemic. If the pain is constant and lasts for hours, with negative ECG and cardiac enzymes, then the chest pain is probably from some cause other than cardiac ischemia. A word of caution, however: patients with ACS may have sharp/stabbing pain (22%), pleuritic chest (13%), or reproducible chest pain on palpation (7%).

In patients with classic symptoms of ACS, traditional risk factors for CAD are less important than the symptoms, ECG findings, and cardiac enzymes. In other words, risk factors may have no role in diagnosing ACS. Elderly patients, women, and diabetic patients may present with dyspnea alone in ACS. Medication response also has been a poor predictor of cardiac chest pain; nitroglycerin provides relief for cardiac and noncardiac chest pain such as that due to esophageal spasm. Relief of angina with nitroglycerin does not rule out ACS. Also, relief of chest pain with a GI cocktail (mixture of viscous lidocaine, antacids, and an anticholinergic) does not rule out ACS either.

ECG ECG is n important tool to risk stratify patients on presentation. ST elevation seen on an ECG needs emergent cardiology consultation for immediate reperfusion therapy. ST depression of more than 0.5 mm and symmetric T-wave inversions during symptoms suggest ischemia. Patients with ST-segment deviation of less than or equal to 0.5 mm are at increased risk of death and new MI at 1 year compared with isolated T-wave changes or no ECG changes. ECG provides just a single snapshot of a dynamic process; therefore, as many as 53% and 62% of acute MI and UA may have a normal or nondiagnostic ECG on presentation, respectively. Serial ECG monitoring may identify an additional 16% of acute MIs missed in the initial ECG.

Cardiac biomarkers Cardiac troponins should be always a part of the workup for ACS due to their high sensitivity in detecting myocardial injury. If they are negative, serial enzymes should be done for up to 12 hours after the symptom onset. Cardiac troponins are elevated as early as 2 hours and may be delayed for up to 8 to 12 hours. They remain elevated for 5 to 14 days. Troponin levels provide a prognosticator beyond what is known from ECG and predischarge stress tests. There is a quantitative and positive relationship with risk of death. High-sensitivity troponin is now preferred to conventional troponin because of its higher diagnostic accuracy.

CK-MB is not as sensitive or specific for myocardial injury. The levels of CK-MB become elevated at the same time as cardiac troponins but remain elevated for only 1 to 2 days because of a short half-life. They may be elevated with skeletal muscle injury as well. CK-MB may be useful to determine the extension of the infarct or to diagnose a periprocedural MI in the hospital.

Cardiac troponin may be elevated in other conditions too. Therefore, in making the diagnosis of MI, there should be a characteristic rise and fall of cardiac troponin along with an ischemic description of chest pain and/or ECG changes. See Chapter 3 for the new definition of MI.

Brain natriuretic peptide and C-reactive protein have no role in diagnosing ACS but may have prognostic value.

Coronary computed tomography angiography (CCTA) is a noninvasive method to assess the presence of CAD with a high negative predictive value (97% to 100%). Thus, it is recommended for patients who present to the ED with intermediate-risk chest pain—especially those without prior history of CAD.

Initial risk stratification STEMI must be ruled out with ECG, history and, physical exam. If the ECG shows ST elevation, then patients should be treated as STEMI. When STEMI is ruled out, patients with suspected ACS are further classified into high, intermediate, and low risk based on many clinically validated risk stratification pathways such as HEART score, TIMI score, and measurement of cardiac troponins (Table 7-2).

Table 7-2. Unstable Angina/NSTEMI Early Risk Stratification

Extremely high-risk features requiring urgent coronary angiography and revascularization
Ongoing chest pain despite optimal medical management
Hemodynamic instability/shock
Electrical instability (sustained ventricular tachycardia)
Pulmonary edema/new-onset or worsening heart failure/severe ventricular dysfunction
New or worsening mitral regurgitation
TIMI risk score: 7 variables
Age >65
>2 episodes of chest pain in the last 24 h
>3 risk factors (hypertension, diabetes, dyslipidemia, smoker, and significant family history of early MI)
Known coronary artery disease with >50% stenosis
ST-segment deviation on admission ECG
Positive cardiac biomarkers
On ASA for the preceding 7 days

High-risk patients should go for urgent coronary intervention. Low-risk patients (negative cardiac troponins, HEART score ≤3, low TIMI score) have a low 30- day risk for major adverse cardiac events, and no additional cardiac testing is warranted. For those with intermediate risk, additional testing is warranted: exercise ECG, stress echocardiography, stress nuclear testing, or coronary CCTA.

For STEMI, the time from first medical contact to percutaneous coronary intervention (PCI) should be less than 90 minutes (also known as *door to balloon time*). If the patient is transferred from a non-PCI center, the time to PCI should be no more than 120 minutes. If a PCI center is not accessible, then fibrinolytics should be given within 30 minutes of arrival and can be given within 12 hours of symptom onset.

In cases with symptoms suspicious for ACS but not confirmed based on negative initial ECG and cardiac troponin, the patient needs to be admitted to a chest pain unit or a monitored bed to obtain serial ECGs and cardiac enzymes. Remember that cardiac troponin may take up to 8 to 12 hours to rise. Low-risk patients should undergo a stress test within 72 hours.

Detailed management is discussed in Chapter 3.

Pulmonary embolism

The incidence of pulmonary embolism is rising, presumably due to improved quality of imaging and widespread availability of CT scanners. Not all pulmonary embolisms are life-threatening, but proximal ones may pose a significant risk of death and morbidity. PE is responsible for 10% of all in-hospital deaths and more than 200,000 deaths yearly.

Symptoms and signs Pulmonary embolism without infarction may present with dyspnea at rest or exertion. Pleuritic chest pain suggests pulmonary infarction from pulmonary embolism. Patients may complain of cough, wheezing, and calf or thigh pain. Examination may be significant for respiratory distress, sinus tachycardia, and an S3. Massive PE may present with right-sided heart failure, cardiovascular collapse, and fulminant shock.

Diagnosis Before ordering imaging, pretest probability should be assessed to avoid unnecessary investigations and cost burden. The Wells score is a well-validated prediction model. A modified Wells criterion provides a pretest probability for PE. Based on the score, patients are categorized into two groups: PE likely (score >4) or PE unlikely (score ≤4).

For the PE unlikely category, if the D-dimer is negative, PE is essentially ruled out. For the PE likely category and the PE unlikely category with positive D-dimers, CT pulmonary angiogram (CT-PA) should be ordered, unless contraindicated. If CT-PA is negative, it should be followed up with lower-extremity ultrasound to rule out DVT, if there is clinical suspicion.

D-dimer levels increase in pregnancy and cancer, so the marker has limited utility in such populations. Age-adjusted D-dimer (age in years × 10) when using the fibrinogen equivalent units is useful in the elderly population.

If a CT is contraindicated, a V/Q scan should be ordered. The traditional Wells score should be used in conjunction with V/Q scan results to confirm or refute the diagnosis of PE. Normal V/Q scan with any clinical probability rules out PE. With a low clinical probability and low-probability V/Q scan, PE is ruled out. High clinical probability and high-probability V/Q scan confirms PE. Any other combination should be followed up with traditional pulmonary angiogram or serial lower-extremity Doppler to rule out DVT.

ECG most commonly shows sinus tachycardia, nonspecific ST- and T-wave changes, or signs of right heart strain. S1Q3T3 is a rare finding but may signify massive PE. Chest radiograph has limited utility in the diagnosis of PE.

Treatment For hemodynamically stable patients, anticoagulation is the mainstay of treatment. It should be continued at least for 3 to 6 months or indefinitely depending on the risk of recurrence. An IVC filter is placed in patients who have contraindications for anticoagulation.

For hemodynamically unstable patients such as those with massive PE with associated hypotension (SBP <90 mm Hg or a drop in SBP of >40 mm Hg from baseline for >15 minutes), thrombolytic therapy is indicated. Surgical embolectomy and catheter-directed thrombolysis are used in those with contraindication to thrombolysis.

Pulmonary embolism is further discussed in Chapter 29.

Aortic dissection
Aortic dissection is another life-threatening condition that requires prompt diagnosis and urgent intervention. It starts as an intimal tear or as a hematoma within the aortic wall and may extend both proximally and distally. Marfan syndrome, bicuspid aortic valve, coarctation of the aorta, previous cardiac surgery, uncontrolled hypertension, cystic medial degeneration in connective tissue disorders, and pregnancy are some of the etiologies of aortic dissection. Anatomically, aortic dissection is divided into Stanford type A and type B. Type A involves the ascending aorta and type B elsewhere.

Symptoms and signs Aortic dissection presents with sudden, severe, sharp, tearing anterior chest pain (in ascending aortic dissection) and similar posterior chest and back pain (in descending aortic dissection). Thirteen percent of the cases with ascending aortic dissection may have associated syncope. In the International Registry of Acute Aortic Dissection, 73% reported chest pain, and of these, 85% had an abrupt onset and 91% described it as the worst pain ever. Patients present in severe distress with diaphoresis. A pulse deficit and focal neurologic deficits have a good likelihood ratio but poor sensitivity. Aortic insufficiency murmurs may be noted in up to 32% of these patients.

Diagnosis Chest radiograph is relatively insensitive but may show widened mediastinum in up to 62% of cases. ECG may be normal in one-third of the cases. Negative D-dimer can rule out aortic dissection in low-risk patients, but if the suspicion is high, further investigation should be carried out. If the patient is stable, a CT scan with aortic dissection protocol or MRI is a good screening test in the ED. If unstable, patients need emergent transesophageal echocardiography (TEE).

Treatment Ascending dissections are managed surgically and descending dissections medically.

Pneumothorax

Pneumothoraces are classified as primary spontaneous pneumothorax (PSP) and secondary spontaneous pneumothorax (SSP). PSP occurs without underlying lung disease, and SSP is secondary to underlying lung disease. Pneumothorax most often occurs at rest.

Symptoms and signs Pneumothorax presents as an acute onset of pleuritic chest pain and dyspnea. Physical examination findings are decreased chest excursion on the side of pneumothorax, absent breath sounds, hyperresonance on percussion, and reduced tactile vocal fremitus. If the pneumothorax is large, patients may be in distress with labored breathing, tachycardia, and hypotension.

Diagnosis Chest radiograph is adequate to diagnose pneumothorax. The pneumothorax appears as a dark area with no vascular markings with a white pleural border. Point-of-care ultrasound (POCUS) has high sensitivity and specificity (90% and 98%, respectively); thus POCUS can rule out the diagnosis of pneumothorax rapidly and accurately.

Treatment Small pneumothoraces (<3 cm for PSP and <1 cm for SSP) are managed conservatively with supplemental oxygen and follow-up chest radiographs. If a patient presents with a tension pneumothorax with mediastinal tracheal shift and hemodynamic compromise, a quick bedside needle decompression (passing a long angiocatheter or spinal needle in the second or third intercostal space in the midclavicular line) improves mortality outcomes. If stable, a chest tube insertion followed by pleurodesis is the recommended treatment.

Esophageal rupture

Esophageal rupture (Boerhaave syndrome) is a potentially fatal condition that results from a full-thickness esophageal tear leading to mediastinitis and shock. It was first described by Boerhaave, who identified esophageal rupture following severe retching and vomiting. Risk factors for the rupture include recent endoscopic procedures, esophagitis from infections, medications or caustic ingestion, Barrett esophagus, and esophageal cancers.

Symptoms and signs Esophageal rupture presents with a sudden, severe, excruciating, retrosternal chest pain occurring after severe retching or vomiting. Patients may have dyspnea, odynophagia, or fever. Physical examination will likely be significant for tachycardia, tachypnea, diaphoresis, and possible subcutaneous emphysema. If patients present late in the course, they may have fever and shock due to mediastinitis.

Diagnosis Chest radiograph may show pneumomediastinum, mediastinal widening, and pleural effusion. Computed tomography provides more information, including an abscess or fluid collections. Gastrografin esophagogram usually establishes the diagnosis. Performing an esophagogastroduodenoscopy (EGD) is controversial, as it can worsen the perforation and introduce air into the mediastinum.

Treatment Medical management (NPO, antibiotics, total parenteral nutrition) is acceptable for stable patients with contained perforation. Urgent surgery should be performed within 24 hours in patients with free perforation or when medical management fails. Endoscopic therapy may be used in poor surgical candidates.

Other causes of chest pain

Other causes of chest pain are discussed in the following table with symptoms, signs, and further enquiry to understand the etiology of the chest pain (Table 7-3). Once we know that the cause of the chest pain is not life-threatening or one of the causes that require an inpatient workup, patients may be discharged with outpatient management and follow-up.

TIPS TO REMEMBER

- The most important step in the management of chest pain is an initial rapid assessment to rule out the causes that may lead to death (STEMI, PE, pneumothorax, aortic dissection, esophageal rupture).

- History and physical examination are crucial in the evaluation of chest pain, then followed by ECG and chest radiograph.

- Do not miss ST-segment elevation on the ECG.

- Risk factors for coronary artery disease predict long-term risk of ACS, but they have a limited role in identifying ACS with ongoing symptoms. The absence of risk factors will not exclude ACS.

- ECG is the easiest and simplest tool for diagnosis of ACS, but due to its low sensitivity, serial ECGs should be performed in a patient with ongoing chest pain. If there is ST deviation or T-wave inversion during the periods of symptoms, this suggests ischemia.

- All patients with suspected ACS should undergo serial cardiac biomarker sampling. If baseline data are negative, further sampling should be obtained 6 to 8 hours later depending on symptom onset.

- Early risk stratification is a crucial step in the management of ACS.

- A serial rise and fall in troponin associated with ACS may help distinguish ACS from non-ACS conditions.

- For STEMI, door to balloon time for primary PCI should be 90 minutes. If transferred from a non-PCI center, it is 120 minutes.

Table 7-3. Other Causes of Chest Pain

Condition	Symptom	Signs	Further Enquire
Musculoskeletal	Aching pain, worsened by movement, sometimes respirophasic. Tender to touch	May have chest wall erythema/ swelling. Light and deep palpation may reproduce the symptoms	Recent weight lifting, heavy exercise, trauma, slept in an abnormal posture/ new bed
Esophageal disorders	Esophageal spasm presents as tightness or burning or squeezing pain. Esophagitis may present similarly, but burning pain is the common complain	Pharyngeal erythema from reflux	New medications, caustic ingestion, and similar problems in the past
Reflux disease	Burning or tightness. Sensation of warmth/ discomfort traveling up the retrosternum with sour taste in the mouth and sometimes ends with coughing Worse on lying down and more symptomatic at night after a late or large meal at night	Pharyngeal erythema. Epigastric tenderness if associated with gastritis or peptic ulcer disease	New medications, eating patterns, positions worsening the symptoms
Peptic ulcer disease/gastritis	Epigastric pain and retrosternal pain described as burning sensation	Epigastric tenderness	New medications, smoking, alcohol history, and stress and feeding habits. Other family members being affected for infectious gastritis

(continued)

Table 7-3. Other Causes of Chest Pain (*Continued*)

Condition	Symptom	Signs	Further Enquire
Stable angina	Exertional central chest discomfort that is described as a pressure, heaviness, tightness, crushing, indigestion, or discomfort that radiates to neck, jaw, arms, or shoulders. Usually lasts 2 to 10 min. Relieved by rest or nitroglycerine	Ejection systolic murmur if the cause is aortic stenosis Pulmonic heave in pulmonary hypertension Pallor in anemia	Exacerbating factors such as bleeding, stress, and cold exposure. Other conditions such as aortic stenosis or pulmonary hypertension can present with angina
Pneumonia	Pleuritic chest pain with cough, fevers, and dyspnea	Pleural rub along with other signs of pneumonia	Ask to show the area of pain, as patients often develop musculoskeletal pain from recurrent coughing and the respirophasic pain may not be a pleuritic pain
Herpes zoster/ postherpetic neuralgia	Acute sharp pain in a dermatomal distribution	Acute infection can present with vesicular rash. Postherpetic neuralgia patients may have a faint healed rash	History of dermatomal zoster rash in the past if this was not due to active zoster
Stress/mental health issues	Fleeting pain lasting seconds or days	May have precordial tenderness	Palpate other areas of the body, as patients with neurotic disorders or fibromyalgia have tenderness in most other sites of the body

- Fibrinolytic therapy is recommended only if primary PCI is not immediately available and the delay from hospital presentation to a PCI capable facility is >120 minutes
- Thrombolysis for STEMI can be done for up to 12 hours after symptom onset. There is no benefit beyond that period.
- Aortic dissection is a difficult diagnosis to make, and high levels of vigilance are required. Chest radiograph may show a widened mediastinum, but the test is not very sensitive.
- Using clinical pretest probability scores such as Wells score can help categorize the patients as PE likely or PE unlikely. For the PE unlikely group, negative D-dimer rules out PE.
- If the clinical suspicion for PE is high, do not wait for the image confirmation; start therapeutic anticoagulation if there is no obvious contraindication.
- Pneumothorax is a clinical diagnosis supported by chest radiograph. Do not wait for chest tube insertion; if there is tension pneumothorax, proceed with needle decompression.
- Esophageal rupture in the hospital is often secondary to a recent procedure. Have a low index of suspicion for rupture if patients have had any upper GI procedures recently, or if they have known esophageal pathology.
- Gastroesophageal disorders and musculoskeletal problems are the most common causes of chest pain in the emergency department and the outpatient clinic.

COMPREHENSION QUESTION

1. A 38-year-old woman with no significant medical history presents to the emergency department with left-sided pleuritic chest pain, shortness of breath, and dizziness for a day. She became short of breath while watching television. When she tried to get up, she felt light-headed, so she went back to bed. She awakened this morning with severe chest pain that worsened with cough and deep breathing. She is physically active and runs 5 miles at least 4 times per week. There is no history of trauma, fever, chills, or rigors. She has had no similar episodes in the past. She does not smoke. She drinks a glass of wine occasionally. She is not married and has never been pregnant. She takes oral contraceptive pills but no other medications. She works for a pharmaceutical company and travels to most parts of the world. She just returned from Australia 2 days ago. Examination is significant for moderate distress, respiratory rate of 28/min, heart rate of 124/min, blood pressure 110/68 mm Hg, temperature of 100.3°F, and saturating 87% on room air. Routine labs are normal except a white cell count of 12,000 cells/mm^3 with a left shift. Troponin is mildly elevated at 0.104 ng/mL (normal high <0.034). ECG shows sinus tachycardia but is otherwise normal. Chest radiograph shows

left upper lobe infiltrate. Wells score is 4, and the D-dimer is elevated at 2.8 μg/mL. Pulmonary embolism is considered as the cause of her symptoms.

What do we do next?

A. Get lower-extremity Doppler to rule out DVT.

B. Get V/Q scan.

C. Get CT-PA.

D. Start weight-based enoxaparin 1 mg/kg and order a CT-PA.

E. Start antibiotics for community-acquired pneumonia and discharge home.

Answer

1. **D.** She has a pulmonary embolism until proven otherwise. CT angiogram is the next investigation of choice, but we should not waste time to confirm the diagnosis. The earlier the anticoagulation is started, the better the outcomes will be, since the anticoagulation will help prevent further clot extension. Troponins can be elevated in up to 50% of patients with a large thromboembolic clot burden. Troponin level normalizes within 40 hours in PE. This is compared with the troponin elevation after myocardial infarction, which may remain elevated for 5 to 14 days. Elevated troponins carry a poorer prognosis compared with negative troponins in patients with PE.

SUGGESTED READINGS

Bautz B, Schneider JI. High-risk chief complaints I: chest pain—the big three (an update). *Emerg Med Clin North Am*. 2020;38(2):453–498.

Bense L, Wiman LG, Hedenstierna G. Onset of symptoms in spontaneous pneumothorax: correlations to physical activity. *Eur J Respir Dis*. 1987;71(3):181–186.

Fruergaard P, Launbjerg J, Hesse B, et al. The diagnoses of patients admitted with acute chest pain but without myocardial infarction. *Eur Heart J*. 1996;17(7):1028–1034.

Gulati M, Levy PD, Mukherjee D, et al. 2021 AHA/ACC/ASE/CHEST/SAEM/SCCT/SCMR Guideline for the Evaluation and Diagnosis of Chest Pain: A Report of the American College of Cardiology/American Heart Association Joint Committee on Clinical Practice Guidelines. *Circulation*. 2021;144(22):e368–e454.

Hagan PG, Nienaber CA, Isselbacher EM, et al. The International Registry of Acute Aortic Dissection (IRAD): new insights into an old disease. *JAMA*. 2000;283(7):897–903.

Henrikson CA, Howell EE, Bush DE, et al. Chest pain relief by nitroglycerin does not predict active coronary artery disease. *Ann Intern Med*. 2003;139:979–986.

Klinkman MS, Stevens D, Gorenflo DW. Episodes of care for chest pain: a preliminary report from MIRNET. Michigan Research Network. *J Fam Pract*. 1994;38(4):345–352.

Kontos MC, Diercks DB, Kirk JD. Emergency department and office-based evaluation of patients with chest pain. *Mayo Clin Proc*. 2010;85(3):284–299.

Leise MD, Locke GR 3rd, Dierkhising RA, et al. Patients dismissed from the hospital with a diagnosis of noncardiac chest pain: cardiac outcomes and health care utilization. *Mayo Clin Proc*. 2010;85(4):323–330.

Lindenmann J, Matzi V, Neuboeck N, et al. Management of esophageal perforation in 120 consecutive patients: clinical impact of a structured treatment algorithm. *J Gastrointest Surg.* 2013;17:1036–1043.

Pasricha PJ, Fleischer DE, Kalloo AN. Endoscopic perforations of the upper digestive tract: a review of their pathogenesis, prevention, and management. *Gastroenterology.* 1994;106(3):787–802.

The PIOPED Investigators. Value of the ventilation/perfusion scan in acute pulmonary embolism. Results of the prospective investigation of pulmonary embolism diagnosis (PIOPED). *JAMA.* 1990;263(20):2753–2759.

van Belle A, Büller HR, Huisman MV, et al. Effectiveness of managing suspected pulmonary embolism using an algorithm combining clinical probability, D-dimer testing, and computed tomography. *JAMA.* 2006;295(2):172–179.

Wells PS, Anderson DR, Rodger M, et al. Derivation of a simple clinical model to categorize patients probability of pulmonary embolism: increasing the models utility with the SimpliRED D-dimer. *Thromb Haemost.* 2000;83(3):416–420.

Wright RS, Anderson JL, Adams CD, et al. 2011 ACCF/AHA focused update of the guidelines for the management of patients with unstable angina/non-ST-elevation myocardial infarction (updating the 2007 guideline): a report of the American College of Cardiology Foundation/American Heart Association Task Force on Practice Guidelines. *Circulation.* 2011;123(18):2022–2060.

A 50-year-old Patient With Worsening Dyspnea

Akshay Kohli, MD and Mingchen Song, MD, PhD

A 50-year-old man was admitted to the hospital with worsening dyspnea, fever, cough, and increased purulent sputum production. He states that he thought he had a cold for the past 3 days, which he tried to manage with acetaminophen.

The patient has been a smoker for 30 years and he still smokes 1 pack a day, having cut down from 3 packs a day before. One year ago, he was diagnosed with chronic obstructive pulmonary disease (COPD). Since being diagnosed, he has been taking an albuterol inhaler as needed and tiotropium bromide (Spiriva) daily. He has no other medical conditions and no known allergies.

The patient is alert but in mild respiratory distress. Temperature is 38.1°C (101.5°F), blood pressure is 130/84 mm Hg, pulse rate is 110/min, and respiration rate is 28/min. Oxygen saturation with the patient breathing ambient air is 87%. Breath sounds are diffusely decreased with bilateral expiratory wheezes; he is using accessory muscles to breathe. He does not have any peripheral edema or elevated jugular venous distension (JVD). With the patient breathing oxygen, 2 L/min by nasal cannula, arterial blood gases (ABGs) are pH 7.27, Pco_2 60 mm Hg, and Po_2 62 mm Hg; oxygen saturation is 91%. His CBC shows leukocytosis of 11,000, and chest x-ray does not show any new infiltrates or pneumothorax.

What is your differential diagnosis and evaluation?

Patients with a history of COPD who present to the hospital for acute-onset shortness of breath may have a disease or diagnosis other than acute exacerbation of COPD (AECOPD). These need to be carefully considered and ruled out. Diagnoses other than AECOPD include the following:

1. Pneumonia: This can be present as an independent entity or be present concomitant with AECOPD (pneumonia might be a cause of AECOPD). It might be difficult to differentiate it from a COPD exacerbation just based on clinical picture, as both may have fevers, chills, purulent sputum, and leukocytosis. Tests to order:
   a. Chest x-ray—look for infiltrates. However, the chest x-ray might be normal in a patient with developing pneumonia. In patients with high suspicion for pneumonia, CT scan might be needed.
   b. A bedside point-of-care ultrasound (POCUS) can be used to look for localized B-lines. B-lines are comet-tail artifacts that indicate subpleural interstitial edema. (Lung ultrasound has a high sensitivity and specificity for the diagnosis of pneumonia, but it is operator dependent.)
   c Sputum culture
   d. Procalcitonin (helpful if it is negative)

2. Pulmonary embolism (PE): The initial presentation of a PE can be shortness of breath only. Features of AECOPD might be missing, including increased sputum production or fever. Investigations to consider:
   a. D-Dimer and/or Doppler sonogram of lower extremities

   b. Chest computed tomography (CT) with pulmonary embolism protocol

3. Pneumothorax: Patients who have severe emphysema are at higher risk. Patients may have pleuritic chest pain and worsening hypoxemia; however, both these clinical findings are nonspecific.
   a. Chest x-ray—look at the chest x-ray yourself

   b. POCUS—loss of lung sliding and lung point sign

4. Pulmonary edema/congestive heart failure exacerbation: A proportion of patients with COPD may also have congestive heart failure and they may present with acute shortness of breath and wheezing, which is difficult to differentiate from AECOPD. Often, patients are treated for both a COPD exacerbation and a CHF exacerbation when the initial clinical picture is overlapping the two diagnoses.
   a. Chest x-ray with signs of vascular congestion (increased hilar markings, dilated blood vessels going to periphery)

   b. Diffuse bilateral B-lines on lung ultrasound

   c. JVD can help assess volume status

Basic diagnostic workup

- Obtain a detailed history and physical
- Chest x-ray (although not of diagnostic value in AECOPD, it is helpful to rule out other differentials of acute-onset dyspnea)
- Electrocardiogram (ECG)
- Basic labs (complete blood count, basic metabolic panel)
- Respiratory viral panel (such as COVID-19, respiratory syncytial virus and influenza, etc)
- ABG/VBG (helpful in somnolent patients to determine whether somnolence is caused by hypercapnia)

What is the most likely diagnosis?
Answer: Acute exacerbation of COPD (AECOPD). This patient has a known history of COPD and is on maintenance therapy. He has respiratory failure likely due to a COPD exacerbation precipitated by an upper respiratory tract infection.

How would you approach this patient?
Answer: Next step in therapy. The goal of oxygen therapy in a patient with COPD should be 88% to 92%. You should start the patient on a short-acting inhaled bronchodilator such as albuterol as well as an anticholinergic agent such as

ipratropium bromide. Additionally, you should begin IV corticosteroids and IV antibiotics. You should consider placing the patient on noninvasive positive-pressure ventilation (NPPV).

CASE REVIEW

Acute exacerbations of COPD are common. When a patient with known COPD presents with respiratory failure, the first step is to differentiate it from other causes that may present similarly. Exacerbations of COPD must be distinguished from pneumonia, pneumothorax, pulmonary embolism (PE), and congestive heart failure (CHF). Pneumonia and pneumothorax can usually be diagnosed by chest radiography. PE can be difficult to diagnose in patients with COPD, and spiral CT angiography should be used if embolic disease is suspected. Your suspicion of PE should be high in patients with risk factors such as prolonged immobilization, a history of cancer, recent trauma, or a history of clotting disorders. PE should also be suspected if the patient is in hypoxic respiratory failure rather than a hypercarbic respiratory failure and in those patients who do not respond to appropriate treatment for a COPD exacerbation. Patients with respiratory failure due to heart failure usually have a history of systolic or diastolic heart failure. On physical exam, these patients have bibasilar crackles, elevated JVD, and peripheral edema of their lower extremities. The CXR will show pulmonary vascular congestion and sometimes pulmonary edema. Elevated brain natriuretic peptide (BNP) will further support this diagnosis.

Now back to our patient, there are no signs of heart failure nor does the CXR show any pulmonary vascular congestion or pulmonary edema. Pneumonia and pneumothorax can be excluded based on findings on chest auscultation and CXR. The patient does not have any risk factors for PE, and the ABG is consistent with a COPD exacerbation. Although PE cannot be fully excluded without a spiral CT scan of the chest, we should see if the patient responds to initial treatment for a COPD exacerbation over the next few days.

What is COPD?

Answer: The Global Initiative for Chronic Obstructive Lung Disease (GOLD) defines COPD as "A common, preventable, and treatable disease that is characterized by persistent respiratory symptoms and airflow limitation that is due to airway and/or alveolar abnormalities usually caused by significant exposure to noxious particles or gases."

This definition has two important components: persistent respiratory symptoms, which are a clinical finding (eg, shortness of breath), and airflow limitation, which is assessed by pulmonary function testing.

What is chronic bronchitis?

Answer: Chronic bronchitis is defined as chronic productive cough for 3 months in each of 2 successive years.

What is emphysema?
Answer: Emphysema is an abnormal and permanent enlargement of the airspaces distal to the terminal bronchioles, accompanied by destruction of airspace walls.

What is the pathophysiology of COPD?
Answer: Inhalation of cigarette smoke or other noxious particles, such as smoke from biomass fuels, causes lung inflammation. In patients with COPD, this inflammatory response may induce parenchymal tissue destruction (resulting in emphysema) and disruption of normal repair and defense mechanisms (resulting in small airway fibrosis). This leads to gas trapping and progressive airflow limitation.

How is the severity of COPD defined?
Answer: The severity of airfl ow limitati on is defi nedusing the GOLD criteria as below
In patients with FEV_1/FVC ratio <0.70 the severity of COPD is defined as follows:

GOLD Stage	Severity	FEV_1
GOLD 1	Mild	FEV_1 ≥80% predicted
GOLD 2	Moderate	50% < FEV_1 <80% predicted
GOLD 3	Severe	30% < FEV_1 <50% predicted
GOLD 4	Very severe	FEV_1 <30% predicted

These values are based on postbronchodilator FEV_1.
    There is only a weak correlation between FEV_1, symptoms and impairment of a patient's health status. Therefore, formal symptomatic assessment is important.

What is acute exacerbation of COPD (AECOPD)?
Answer: An exacerbation is defined as an acute worsening of respiratory symptoms that results in additional therapy (ie, more than baseline).
    Key symptoms of exacerbations include increased dyspnea, increased sputum purulence and volume, increased cough, and wheezing. Exacerbations can be classified as mild, moderate, or severe based on the symptoms and management required to relieve those symptoms. Exacerbation is considered severe when a patient requires hospitalization or a visit to the emergency room. It may also be associated with acute respiratory failure.

What are the triggers of an acute exacerbation?
Answer:

- Respiratory viral infections: The most common virus isolated is human rhinovirus (cause of common cold)
- Bacterial infections
- Environmental factors such as pollution

When to hospitalize?

The first step in evaluation of a patient with AECOPD is to triage to outpatient treatment versus hospitalization.

Some indications for assessing the need hospitalization include the following:

- Severe symptoms such as sudden worsening of resting dyspnea, high respiratory rate, decreased oxygen saturation, confusion, or drowsiness
- Acute respiratory failure
- Onset of new physical signs (eg, cyanosis, peripheral edema)
- Failure to respond to initial medical management
- Presence of serious comorbidities (eg, heart failure, new arrhythmias)
- Insufficient support at home

Hospitalized patients can be classified based on clinical signs as follows:

1. No respiratory failure—respiratory rate (RR): 20 to 30 breaths per minute; no use of accessory respiratory muscles; no changes in mental status; hypoxemia improved with supplemental oxygen via Venturi mask 24% to 35% inspired oxygen (Fi_{O_2}); no increase in Pa_{CO_2}.

2. Acute respiratory failure—non-life-threatening: RR greater than 30 per minute; using accessory muscles of respiration; no change in mental status; oxygenation improved with supplemental oxygen with greater than 35% Fi_{O_2}; hypercarbia, ie, Pa_{CO_2} is increased compared with baseline or elevated to 50 to 60 mm Hg.

3. Acute respiratory failure—life-threatening: RR greater than 30 per minute; using accessory muscles of respiration; acute changes in mental status; hypoxemia not improved with supplemental oxygen or Fi_{O_2} greater than 40%; hypercarbia, ie, Pa_{CO_2} is increased compared with baseline or elevated above 60 mm Hg, or presence of acidosis (pH <7.25).

Imaging:

A chest x-ray is not useful in diagnosing COPD, but it is valuable in excluding alternative diagnoses and establishing the presence of significant comorbidities such as pulmonary fibrosis, bronchiectasis, pleural diseases, skeletal diseases (eg, kyphoscoliosis), and cardiac diseases (eg, cardiomegaly).

Radiologic changes associated with COPD usually include signs of lung hyperinflation (flattened diaphragm and an increase in the volume of retrosternal air space), hyperlucency of the lungs, and rapid tapering of vascular markings.

Chest CT scan is useful to diagnose pneumonia. A CT scan with PE protocol is helpful in patients who have high clinical suspicion for a pulmonary embolism.

Pharmacologic therapies

- Beta-adrenergic agonists: All patients with COPD exacerbation should receive prompt treatment with inhaled short-acting beta-adrenergic agonists (SABA) such as albuterol or levalbuterol. They have a rapid onset of action and have been shown to produce bronchodilation in COPD. They can be administered via a nebulizer, metered-dose inhaler (MDI) with a spacer, or dry powder inhaler (DPI). They are usually combined with a short-acting muscarinic antagonist (SAMA) such as ipratropium.

  We can use a nebulizer or MDI (both have equal efficacy), but some clinicians prefer a nebulizer because many patients have difficulty using proper MDI technique in the setting of an exacerbation.

  Dose: 2.5 mg (3 mL) via nebulizer or 1–2 inhalations of MDI (90 μg per inhalation) every 1 h for 2–3 h and then every 2–4 h depending on response to the therapy.

Continuous nebulization is not recommended.

- Muscarinic antagonist: In acute exacerbations, short-acting muscarinic antagonists (SAMA) are usually used in combination with SABA. Ipratropium 0.5 mg is mixed with albuterol 2.5 mg in a 3-mL nebulizer and is used every hour for 2–3 doses and then every 2–4 hours as described above. Although there has been no proven benefit of adding SAMA to SABA therapy in AECOPD, this practice is based on the benefit of SAMA and SABA in patients with stable COPD.

  GOLD strategy advises the continuation of long-acting beta agonists and or long-acting muscarinic antagonists.

- Systemic glucocorticoids: systemic glucocorticoids not only shorten recovery time in AECOPD, but also improve oxygenation, decrease risk of early relapse or treatment failure, and shorten the length of hospitalization.

Prednisone 40 mg per day for 5 days is recommended. However, depending on the severity of exacerbation, many clinicians use higher doses. Frequently used regimens range from prednisone 30–60 mg once daily to methylprednisolone 60–125 mg 2 to 4 times daily. Recent studies have failed to show an increased risk of treatment failure with lower doses of corticosteroids.

Oral therapy is equally efficacious when compared with IV therapy. However, IV steroids can be used in patients who cannot tolerate oral administration while in a severe exacerbation.

In patients with impending respiratory failure, many clinicians use IV high-dose steroids such as methylprednisolone 60 mg IV 1 to 4 times daily. However, there are limited data supporting this practice.

Duration of therapy is not clearly established, but GOLD guidelines suggest prednisone 40 mg/day for 5 days. The European Respiratory Society/American Thoracic Society guidelines suggest a longer course.

Even a short course of systemic glucocorticoids is associated with an increased risk of adverse events such as hyperglycemia, pneumonia, sepsis, venous thromboembolism, and fracture. Care needs to be taken while prescribing steroids in patients with a high risk of these side effects.

- Antibiotics: Most guidelines recommend antibiotics for patients with moderate to severe COPD exacerbation that requires hospitalization. GOLD recommends antibiotics in patients with any of the following:
  1. Increase in dyspnea, sputum volume, and sputum purulence
  2. Presence of 2 of the cardinal symptoms if increased purulence of sputum is 1 of the 2 symptoms
  3. Requirement for noninvasive or invasive mechanical ventilation

Choice of antibiotic is usually based on patient factors and local resistance patterns.

Patients admitted to the ICU due to COPD should receive antibiotics even if there is no infiltrate on the chest x-ray.

Usually empiric treatment with an aminopenicillin with clavulanic acid, macrolide, or tetracycline is sufficient.

Patients with frequent exacerbations, severe airflow limitation, and/or exacerbations requiring mechanical ventilation should get sputum and/or tracheal aspirate cultures, as gram-negative organisms such as *Pseudomonas* or other resistant organisms may be present.

The route of administration depends on the ability of the patient to tolerate oral intake, but if possible it is preferable to give antibiotics orally.

Recommended length of antibiotic therapy is 5 to 7 days.

Respiratory support

Oxygen therapy
Patients with hypoxemia need supplemental oxygen. Target saturations of 88% to 92% are recommended. Higher targets are associated with worsening hypercapnia and worse outcomes.

The following devices are available for delivery of supplemental oxygen:

1. Nasal cannula
2. Simple face mask
3. Non-rebreathing mask
4. High-flow nasal cannula

Usually a high fraction of inhaled oxygen (Fi_{O_2}) is not required to correct hypoxemia associated with COPD exacerbation. A patient with hypoxemia who is not correcting with relatively low Fi_{O_2} should prompt consideration of another concomitant cause, such as pulmonary embolism, acute respiratory distress syndrome, pulmonary edema, or severe pneumonia.

High-flow nasal cannula

High-flow nasal therapy (HFNT) delivers heated and humidified supplemental oxygen at rates up to 60 liters per minute. It has been associated with decreased respiratory effort, decreased work of breathing, and improved gas exchange. In patients with AECOPD, it has been reported to improve oxygenation and ventilation, decrease hypercarbia, and improve health-related quality of life. However, the current evidence is based on relatively smaller studies and limits the interpretation of the value of HFNT in COPD patient populations. Larger well-designed studies are needed to assess its effectiveness.

Ventilatory support

Noninvasive ventilation (NIV)

NIV has been found to reduce mortality and decrease intubation rate in patients with COPD exacerbation. COPD patients can develop acute respiratory acidosis (Pa_{CO_2} >45 mm Hg [6 kPa] or pH <7.35) due to hypoventilation and benefit from a noninvasive ventilation trial of bilevel positive airway pressure (BiPAP). The initial settings of BiPAP include an inspiratory positive airway pressure (IPAP) of 8 to 12 cm H_2O and expiratory pressure (EPAP) of 5 cm H_2O. For patients with AECOPD, NIV has been shown to have a success rate of 80% to 85%.

Relative contraindications include an uncooperative patient, decreased level of consciousness, hemodynamic instability, inadequate mask fit, severe respiratory acidosis, or patients at high risk of aspiration who are not able to protect their airways or clear secretions.

Once a patient is started on NIV, frequent reassessment for improvement in mental status (due to CO_2 washout and improvement in hypercapnia) is needed. Serial blood gasses can be done to document improvement. Arterial blood gas is not necessary as there is a good correlation between arterial and venous blood gas for pH and Pco_2.

Complications of NIV include local irritation or ulceration, air leaks, nasal dryness, gastric insufflation, and aspiration.

Invasive mechanical ventilation (IMV)

Patients with life-threatening respiratory failure are candidates for invasive mechanical ventilation. A bedside scoring system (BAP-65) has been found to predict the need for IMV in patients with acute COPD exacerbations. Failure of NIV and use of IMV as rescue therapy are associated with greater morbidity, hospital length of stay, and mortality.

In patients with very severe COPD, the decision to use IMV should be based on the likely reversibility of the precipitating event, the patient's wishes, and the availability of intensive care facilities. Early clarification of the patient's own treatment goals and wishes, such as an advance directive or "living will," makes these decisions easier in the acute setting.

Risks of IMV include ventilator-associated pneumonia, barotrauma, volutrauma, and the risk of prolonged ventilation and consequential need for tracheostomy.

Supportive care:
For patients hospitalized with AECOPD, supportive care is important and includes the following:

1. Thromboprophylaxis: Hospitalization for COPD exacerbation increases the risk for deep-vein thrombosis and pulmonary embolism. Appropriate pharmacologic and/or mechanical thromboprophylaxis should be used based on the patient's risk factors. Low-molecular-weight heparin is the preferred medication.

2. Smoking cessation: Hospitalization can provide an opportunity for patients to move toward smoking cessation. Counseling and resources can be provided to help start the process. Nicotine replacement therapy can help reduce symptoms of nicotine withdrawal during hospitalization.

Hospital discharge and follow-up
Older age, severity of underlying COPD, requirement for long-term oxygen at discharge, presence of comorbidities (eg, cardiovascular disease, lung cancer), and presence of *Pseudomonas aeruginosa* in the sputum are all known to negatively influence mortality after a hospital discharge. Many patients may never return to their baseline after an exacerbation.

Criteria for discharge
There are no fixed criteria for discharge. However, the decision should be based on sufficient improvement in the manifestations of COPD, patient stability, and decrease in frequency of nebulizer treatments. If the patient is near prehospital baseline, discharge is probably appropriate. Care must be taken to assess home environment and ability to manage activities of daily living (ADLs).

TIPS TO REMEMBER

- COPD is characterized by persistent respiratory symptoms and airflow limitation.

- Acute worsening of respiratory symptoms that result in additional therapy is defined as an acute exacerbation.

- Mainstay of treatment includes short-acting bronchodilator(s), systemic glucocorticoids, antibiotics, and oxygen supplementation.

- Noninvasive ventilation has been found to reduce mortality and decrease the need for intubation in COPD exacerbation. Frequent reassessment for response to therapy is of utmost importance. Be mindful of contraindications of NIV such as inability to protect airways.

- Invasive mechanical ventilation is reserved for patients with life-threatening respiratory failure and failed noninvasive ventilation.

COMPREHENSION QUESTIONS

A 65-year-old Caucasian man with history of hypertension, COPD, and heart failure with preserved ejection fraction was admitted with worsening dyspnea, cough, and increased purulent sputum production. He states that he had a mild fever and generalized fatigue for past 3 days, which he tried to manage with acetaminophen. His home medications include metoprolol succinate 50 mg daily, salbutamol inhaler PRN, and tiotropium bromide inhaler daily.

Vital signs:
- Blood pressure 110/76
- Respiratory rate 32/min
- Heart rate 118/min
- Oxygen saturation 87%
- Temperature 100.8°F

On physical examination, he is using accessory muscles to breathe. There are audible expiratory wheezing and inspiratory crackles, and diminished breath sounds in lower lobes upon auscultation.

CXR shows hyperinflation but no focal infiltrate. ABG results include pH 7.25, P_{CO_2} 75 mm Hg, and P_{O_2} 55 mm Hg.

1. What is the most likely diagnosis?
   A. COPD exacerbation
   B. Pneumonia
   C. Pulmonary embolism
   D. CHF exacerbation

Answer:

A. COPD exacerbation.

Rationale:

   A. COPD exacerbation: Most likely diagnosis, given the patient's history and examination findings such as expiratory wheezing, diminished breath sounds, and use of accessory muscles. Moreover, the patient is hypoxic and tachypneic, and ABG shows hypercapnia.
   B. Pneumonia: Patient's fever, tachycardia, hypoxia, and physical examination showing crackles can point toward pneumonia, but there is no focal infiltrate on chest x-ray so it is less likely.
   C. Pulmonary embolism: Patient's hypoxia, tachycardia, and relatively clear CXR without consolidation can point to PE, but hypercarbia makes it less likely. Patients with PE who have no other comorbidities will usually be tachypneic and hyperventilate, leading to low P_{CO_2} levels.

D. CHF exacerbation: Patient's hypoxia, tachycardia, hypoxia, and crackles on examination can point toward CHF exacerbation, but there is no pulmonary edema noted in chest x-ray so it is less likely.

2. What would you do next?
   A. Intubate and transfer to ICU
   B. Start non-breather
   C. Start high-flow nasal cannula
   D. Start noninvasive ventilation (BiPAP 10/5)
   E. Consult palliative care medicine for end-stage lung disease

Answer:

D. Start noninvasive ventilation (BiPAP 10/5)

Rationale:

Patient is noted to be in acute respiratory distress as noted by tachypnea and use of accessory muscles. Moreover, ABG shows CO_2 retention, which means that he is unable to ventilate well; this is common in COPD patients due to air trapping and airflow obstruction. The treatment for this is to bronchodilate so that there is better air flow to the alveoli and improved gas exchange. While the medications take time to bronchodilate, patients need support with ventilation. This can be achieved with noninvasive ventilation such as BiPAP or, if that fails, mechanical ventilation. Supplementation of oxygen with high-flow nasal cannula may improve the saturation, but it does not improve hypercapnia.

3. You start noninvasive ventilation. When you check on the patient 30 minutes later, he is less uncomfortable but rather lethargic.

Physical examination: less wheezing on auscultation, but still diminished breath sounds.

Repeat ABG: pH 7.20, P_{CO_2} 79 mm Hg, P_{O_2} 68 mm Hg (on 10 L)

What do you do next?
   A. Continue current noninvasive ventilation, repeat ABG in 30 minutes
   B. Change noninvasive ventilation setting, increase BiPAP from 10/5 to 12/5, repeat ABG in 30 minutes
   C. Intubate and transfer to ICU
   D. Consult pulmonology for urgent bronchoscopy for mucus plugging
   E. Start hypertonic saline nebulizer to facilitate mucus clearance

Answer:

C. Intubate and transfer to ICU

Rationale:

The patient has been on noninvasive ventilation for about 30 minutes and has not shown any improvement; in fact he looks worse. The next best step is to intubate rather than waiting more. Initial trial of NIV is necessary and has shown decrease in the rate of intubation, but if improvement is not seen, intubation should not be delayed. Giving more time on NIV has not been shown to improve outcomes and is rather detrimental.

SUGGESTING READINGS

Global Initiative for Chronic Obstructive Lung Disease. 2022 GOLD Reports. Accessed November 30, 2023. goldcopd.org/2022-gold-reports

Wedzicha JA, Miravitlles M, Hurst JR, et al. Management of COPD exacerbations: a European Respiratory Society/American Thoracic Society guideline. *Eur Respir J.* 2017;49(3):1600791.

A 40-year-old Woman With Shortness of Breath

Omar Siddiqui, MD and Youssef Chami, MD

A 40-year-old female smoker is admitted to the inpatient service with shortness of breath, progressive over the last 12 months. The shortness of breath is worse with exertion, is chronic in nature, and has progressed in severity over the last year. She reports a history of asthma but does not recall having any formal testing done for it in the past. At the time of admission, she is short of breath even with minimal activity. A chest x-ray shows bilateral opacities that are interpreted as possible pneumonia. Treatment for this admission is started with IV corticosteroid therapy, antibiotics, and frequent nebulization with bronchodilators to treat asthma exacerbation with pneumonia.

By the fourth hospital day, despite aggressive treatment, she does not appear to have had any clinical improvement in her symptoms. In fact, she feels as if she has become worse, not better. On examination, she is anxious in appearance and in clear respiratory distress. She is able to communicate in only a few words at a time, between her labored breaths. She is afebrile, with a heart rate of 95 beats/min and a blood pressure of 150/100 mm Hg. Her jugular venous pulse (JVP) is estimated at 16 cm. Lung examination is remarkable for very harsh breath sounds with coarse-sounding expiratory wheezes bilaterally, and decreased breath sounds at the bases. Cardiac examination reveals a systolic murmur prominent at the apex, and 2+ lower-extremity pitting edema up to the knees is found.

When questioned further, in addition to her history of shortness of breath with exertion, the patient notes frequent nighttime episodes of shortness of breath, requiring her to sit up in bed for extended periods before sleeping again to allow her to "catch her breath." A remote history of extended febrile illness is recalled from childhood, for which she does not recall getting specific treatment.

1. In light of this patient's reported symptoms by history, what is the most likely primary diagnosis?

2. What may be the significant underlying factor in this case?

3. What management decisions would you need to make at this time?

Answers

1. The combination of the patient's historic features, physical examination findings, and lack of response to usual asthma therapy supports a diagnosis of congestive heart failure (CHF), not asthma.

2. The patient's murmur and remote history of untreated childhood febrile illness suggest the diagnosis of rheumatic heart disease as the underlying factor.

3. If the patient has CHF, the IV corticosteroid therapy may be making her hypervolemia worse, and beta-agonist therapy may also be exacerbating her decreased cardiac function. Discontinuing these medications and initiating a trial of diuresis with a loop diuretic, while waiting on confirmatory testing for CHF, would be appropriate. The chest x-ray done at admission should be reviewed again for evidence of CHF. Additional testing may include an electrocardiogram (ECG), B-type natriuretic peptide (BNP), and an echocardiogram to definitively characterize cardiac function and the degree of structural heart disease that may be present.

CASE REVIEW

While asthma is typically episodic, this patient's history suggests she has had chronic and progressive symptoms. Additionally, her nighttime attacks appear more consistent with paroxysmal nocturnal dyspnea (PND), not asthma. On examination, her elevated JVP of 16 cm, harsh breath sounds with "cardiac wheezing," decreased breath sounds at her bases, and lower-extremity edema are all signs of a hypervolemic state. These features all suggest a diagnosis of CHF. Other physical examination findings that may be found include an S3 heart sound and a positive hepatojugular reflux. The patient's systolic heart murmur, possibly related to mitral regurgitation, and her remote history of an untreated childhood febrile illness, suggestive of rheumatic fever, make the diagnosis of rheumatic heart disease likely. Because she is demonstrating signs and symptoms of hypervolemia secondary to CHF, it would be reasonable to stop the asthma therapy and to start a trial of diuresis with a loop diuretic. Monitoring serum electrolytes is important in this situation. IV corticosteroid therapy has likely increased fluid retention and made her clinical status worse. Unnecessary beta-agonist therapy may also be putting more strain on her cardiac function if CHF is the primary etiology. These medications should be stopped. Because of the high prevalence of coronary artery disease (CAD) with any new diagnosis of CHF, it is also important to obtain an ECG. Depending on the clinical circumstances, an urgent cardiology consultation also may be appropriate. A CXR may be useful to assess for signs of CHF such as pulmonary edema, which may be confused with a pneumonic infiltrate outside of clinical context, and may help to estimate heart size. When the diagnosis of CHF is unclear, checking a BNP level can be supportive. An echocardiogram would provide more definitive information on structural heart disease, including wall thickness, left ventricular ejection fraction (EF), and degree of valvular involvement.

CONGESTIVE HEART FAILURE

Initial Diagnosis

Clinical presentation

The most common symptoms of congestive heart failure include dyspnea with activity or rest, orthopnea, paroxysmal nocturnal dyspnea, fatigue, and reduced exercise tolerance. If patients have a history of chronic heart failure, the symptoms of presentation during an acute exacerbation are usually similar to previous episodes of acute decompensation.

Clinical signs to look for include peripheral edema, pulmonary rales, jugular venous distention, hepatojugular reflux, and the presence of a third heart sound ("S3 gallop"). Consider acute coronary syndrome if the patient is having chest discomfort.

Heart failure symptoms can be divided into left-sided and right-sided symptoms. Symptoms of left-sided heart failure appear when there are increased filling pressures in the left ventricle, causing hydrostatic pressure in the pulmonary circulation. Patients will report orthopnea, paroxysmal nocturnal dyspnea, or exertional dyspnea that results from the pulmonary edema developing from left-sided heart failure. Right-sided heart failure is a result of increased filling pressures in the right ventricle; the most common etiology for right-sided heart failure is left-sided heart failure. Symptoms of right-sided heart failure include abdominal or peripheral edema, decreased appetite from gut edema, and a sensation of bloating.

Symptoms and signs related to peripheral hypoperfusion, such as cold and clammy skin, somnolence or altered mental status, and oliguria should raise concerns for possible cardiogenic shock. Hypoperfusion is difficult to assess clinically, so a low threshold should be maintained clinically. Hypoperfusion usually presents with low systolic blood pressure (BP <90 mm Hg), tachycardia (heart rate >100 bpm), respiratory distress (respiratory rate >25 bpm), and oxygen desaturation.

Triggering factors

Initial history on presentation should include an assessment for factors that commonly trigger acute decompensation of heart failure. The most common preventable reasons are dietary noncompliance and medication nonadherence. Otherwise, the natural history of heart failure involves progression of the disease causing recurrent acute decompensations.

Diagnostic workup

Cardiogenic shock, respiratory failure, myocardial infarction, and malignant arrhythmia should always be rapidly excluded during the initial evaluation. Although most heart failure patients will not present with these complicating

Table 9-1. Signs and Symptoms of HeartFailure

	Sensitivity	Specificity
Symptom		
Dyspnea	66%	52%
Orthopnea	21%	81%
Paroxysmal nocturnal dyspnea	33%	76%
Edema (by history)	23%	80%
Sign		
Resting heart rate >100 beats/min.	7%	99%
Rales	13%	91%
Edema (on examination)	10%	93%
Third heart sound	31%	95%
Neck vein distension	10%	2%

Reproduced with permission from Lüscher T. Diagnosis of CHF - often a trap in itself. *J Renin Angiotensin Aldosterone Syst.* 2000:1(1);2-36.

factors, the high mortality associated with them means that every patient should be screened for them on presentation.

- Cardiogenic shock can be evaluated based on physical exam and vital signs. If hypoperfusion is clinically suspected, then it is safer to admit the patient to a critical care bed and empirically start ionotropic therapy followed by invasive hemodynamics (Swann catheter placement).
- An initial ECG and telemetry (if required) will help evaluate for malignant arrhythmia. Consider malignant arrhythmia particularly if the patient endorses syncope or presyncope or has a history of arrhythmias. If the patient has a cardiac device such as a pacemaker or defibrillator, then device interrogations should be performed when arrythmia is suspected.
- Three serial troponins collected will help rule out an acute coronary syndrome.

History and physical exam should always be supplemented with basic lab work and imaging to confirm the diagnosis of decompensated heart failure.

- Complete metabolic panel → These labs will help establish renal function, which helps in dosing of diuretic therapy and when electrolyte abnormalities need to be addressed.

- BNP or NT pro-BNP → These labs have a high sensitivity for detecting cardiac disease in patients presenting with progressive dyspnea. Dyspnea in patients without normal or unchanged BNP is very likely to have non-cardiac etiology. Of note, patients taking sacubitril-valsartan will have a medication-induced elevation of BNP but not NT pro-BNP.
- Serial troponins → As mentioned above, three serial troponin draws should be ordered to assess for acute coronary syndrome presenting as decompensated heart failure. A chronic and mild troponin elevation can be due to subendocardial hypoperfusion from decompensated heart failure. An elevated left ventricular end-diastolic pressure (LVEDP) from decompensated heart failure can cause mild, chronic myocardial injury resulting in the abnormal troponin. The troponin trend in that case will be plateau-like without the typical dramatic peak and fall seen in acute coronary syndrome.
- Complete blood count → Anemia is an overlooked exacerbating factor in heart failure and should always be treated to improve overall cardiovascular function.
- Chest x-ray → Should be used to detect pulmonary congestion in patients presenting with acute dyspnea.
- Echocardiogram → An echo should be ordered only if this is the patient's first episode of decompensated heart failure or if a new cardiac pathology is suspected based on history, physical exam, and prior lab or imaging.

Many of the patients presenting with acute decompensated heart failure will have a history of prior cardiac evaluation. Make sure to scan their inpatient and outpatient chart briefly to determine any prior workup for etiology of heart failure, any device therapy the patient is currently using, and the patient's current home medications for heart failure.

It is also important to know the classifications of heart failure, as they affect long-term management and treatment. Patients should always get an echocardiogram on their first heart failure admission to determine left ventricular ejection fraction (LVEF). Based on LVEF, patients should be screened for comorbidities that contribute to HFrEF or HFpEF.

INPATIENT MANAGEMENT

Regardless of volume status, the patient's cardiopulmonary stability takes precedence. If hypoperfusion is evident, patient should be started on ionotropic and pressor therapy as needed with ICU admission. If mechanical ventilation is required for respiratory stability, then intubation should not be delayed due to ongoing workup.

During decompensated heart failure, the clinician should also focus on noncardiac acute conditions that can precipitate the decompensation; consider anemia, sepsis, acute pulmonary illness, or metabolic derangements.

Universal Definition and Classification of Heart Failure (HF)

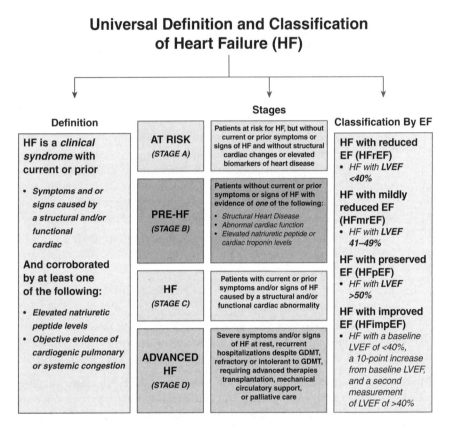

Figure 9-1. Universal definition and classification of heart failure (HF). (Reproduced with permission from Abramov D, Kittleson MM. The universal definition of heart failure: strengths and opportunities. *J Card Fail.* 2021;27(6):622–624.)

If the patient is stable from a hemodynamic and respiratory standpoint, then the next step is improving the volume status. Patients with acute decompensated heart failure present with similar vascular congestion regardless of their left ventricular function or etiology of heart failure. Decongestive treatment should be tailored according to the patient's prior exposure to diuretics and current renal function.

Patients who were previously on a loop diuretic as maintenance therapy should be given an IV dose of at least twice their maintenance dose. If renal function is acutely impaired, then consider a higher IV dose; a commonly used rule of thumb is 40 mg of furosemide for every 1 mg/dL of creatinine. Loop diuretics are preferred due to their rapid onset and short half-life. Intravenous diuretic therapy is preferred to overcome impaired enteral absorption, which can occur with vascular congestion in the gastrointestinal tract.

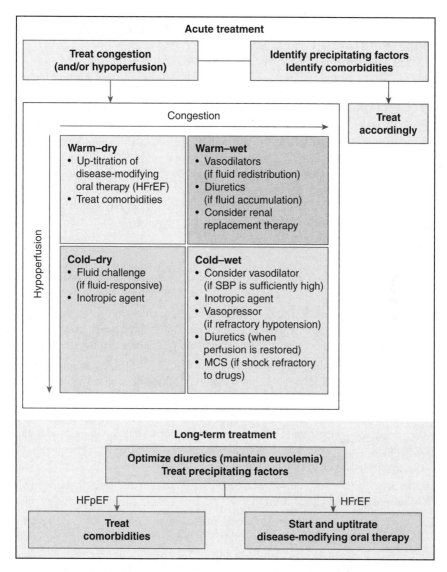

Figure 9-2. Inpatient Management of CHF. (Reproduced with permission from Jong, P, Vowinckel E, Liu PP, et al. Prognosis and determinants of survival in patients newly hospitalized for heart failure. *Arch Intern Med.* 2002;162:168.)

Loop diuretics are protein-bound and secreted in the proximal convoluted tubule. Impairment in renal function means that a higher diuretic dose is needed to achieve a plasma concentration sufficient to induce diuresis. The peak effect of IV loop diuretics occurs within the first 2 hours, and sodium excretion returns to baseline within 6 to 8 hours. To maintain decongestive therapy, IV loop diuretics should be redosed every 8 to 12 hours.

The target with decongestive therapy is to remove a net of 1.5 to 2 L of fluid over a 24-hour period. Diuretic dosing should be adjusted to aim for that target. If the patient is not achieving target fluid removal even with escalated doses of IV loop diuretics, then a combination of diuretics with different mechanisms of action can be used to create nephron blockade to induce diuresis. If a combination of diuretics is being tried, then the cardiology consult service should be working with the patient as well. The most commonly used diuretic for managing acute heart failure exacerbations is IV furosemide. Furosemide 40 to 80 mg can be used with metolazone 2.5 to 5 mg for a synergistic effect, with metolazone being given at least 30 minutes prior to furosemide. If multiple diuretics are unable to achieve desired volume control, then renal replacement therapy should be considered, facilitated by an inpatient nephrology consult.

Additional key points

- Consider stopping or decreasing other vasoactive medications while patients are on IV diuretic therapy to prevent hypotension.
- Do not initiate negative inotropes such as beta blockers or calcium channel blockers while the patient is in acute decompensated heart failure, as this can further deteriorate cardiac output and potentiate cardiogenic shock.
- Sinus tachycardia is a normal response to vascular congestion and decompensated heart failure, as it is a compensatory mechanism to increase cardiac output. Treating volume status by decongestion will resolve the sinus tachycardia.
- Atrial arrythmias such as atrial fibrillation or atrial flutter are triggered by vascular congestion; again, treating the volume status will help treat the arrythmia. Atrial arrythmias can be either the cause or consequence of heart failure decompensation.
- Strict intake and output measurements ("I&Os") are useful in assessing a patient's response to diuretic therapy and in maintaining volume control.
- Electrolytes should be monitored at least once daily and repleted aggressively while a patient is on IV diuretic therapy. Worsening renal function with inadequate urine output is a worrying sign and should raise concerns for refractory heart failure, right ventricular failure, pulmonary hypertension, or vascular shunting.
- Sodium restriction (2 g) and fluid restriction help familiarize patients with dietary restrictions for heart failure treatment and help resolve an acute exacerbation. Patients should have a consult with a dietitian at least once during their combined heart failure admissions.

Perform daily physical exams to assess the patient's volume status. Discuss symptomatic improvement with the patient daily as well. By the time patients are euvolemic, they should be able to comfortably lie down flat without dyspnea and ambulate per their baseline. Euvolemic patients should have returned to their baseline oxygen requirement and exercise tolerance.

LONG-TERM MANAGEMENT

Predischarge Management

Addressing vascular congestion is important for treating acute decompensated heart failure, but it has not shown to improve long-term survival. Any patient with a history of hospitalization for heart failure is at increased risk for another episode and has a disease-associated mortality similar to that of many malignancies.

Initiating guideline-directed medical therapy for heart failure while the patient is still admitted in the hospital has been shown to improve compliance and outpatient follow-up. Both of these factors are critical to increasing long-term survival and decreasing recurrent hospitalizations.

Medical therapy for heart failure with reduced ejection fraction (HFrEF) is different from treatment for heart failure with preserved ejection fraction (HFpEF). Long-term management for HFpEF is focused on treating comorbidities such as hypertension, obstructive sleep apnea, atrial arrhythmias, and obesity.

HFrEF has established data supporting specific medical therapies to improve survival and symptoms. The cornerstone of medical therapy is focused on "triple therapy," which includes the following:

- ACE/ARB/ARNI: lisinopril, ramipril, and enalapril are the most studied. Sacubitril/valsartan has recent data showing comparatively better outcomes, but be careful of hypotension when starting this drug.
- Beta blocker: Beta blockers should be initiated only once acute decompensation of heart failure has resolved, with a very slow titration of increased dosing.
- Metoprolol succinate, carvedilol, or bisoprolol are the three drugs studied for HFrEF patients. Nebivolol can be considered in elderly patients.
- Mineralocorticoid receptor antagonist: Spironolactone or eplerenone. These agents may cause hyperkalemia in combination with ACE/ARB/ARNI, and patients should have outpatient monitoring of electrolytes and renal function within a week of hospital discharge.

At the very least, a beta blocker and ACE/ARB/ARNI should be initiated prior to discharge and with close renal monitoring within 1 week of discharge. If renal function allows, aldosterone should be added during follow-up.

Recent data about the use of SGLT-2 inhibitors in HFrEF are very promising, regardless of the patient's diabetic status. Be mindful that initiating an SGLT-2 inhibitor can cause significant diuresis, so any existing maintenance diuretic a patient is on should be reduced in dose.

Diuretic therapy has not shown to improve mortality but does help control symptoms. Patients should be transitioned from IV diuretic therapy to the minimum required oral maintenance dose to maintain euvolemia.

If a diagnosis of HFrEF is made for the first time, then the cardiology consult service should be contacted to consider ischemic evaluation *prior to hospital discharge* to rule out an ischemic etiology.

Postdischarge Management

A follow-up visit in clinic within 7 to 10 days of hospital discharge is recommended by international guidelines and has been shown to improve medication adherence as well as to prevent rehospitalization. Close outpatient follow-up is essential for increasing medication doses and altering therapy to eventually get a patient on maximally tolerated guideline drive medical therapy for heartfailure. Higher doses of these critical medications have shown to have neurohormonal benefits in a dose-dependent fashion. Outpatient follow-up also allows for serial reevaluation of the patient's symptoms and potential need for device therapies such as chronic resynchronization therapy (CRT) or a defibrillator for primary prevention (ICD).

SUGGESTED READINGS

Arrigo M, Jessup M, Mullens W, et al. Acute heart failure. *Nat Rev Dis Primers.* 2020;6:16.

Metra M, Teerlink JR. Heart failure. *Lancet.* 2017;390(10106):1981–1995.

Murphy SP, Ibrahim NE, Januzzi JL. Heart failure with reduced ejection fraction: a review. *JAMA.* 2020;324(5):488–504.

Savarese G, Stolfo D, Sinagra G, et al. Heart failure with mid-range or mildly reduced ejection fraction. *Nat Rev Cardiol.* 2022;19:100–116.

Sharma A, Verma S, Bhatt D, et al. Optimizing foundational therapies in patients with HFrEF. *J Am Coll Cardiol Basic Trans Science.* 2021;7(5):504–517.

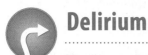

Delirium

Dorcas Adaramola, MD, MPH and Edgard
Cumpa, MD

A 75-year-old Woman With Mental Status Changes

A 75-year-old woman with a history of chronic obstructive pulmonary disease is evaluated in the intensive care unit (ICU) for altered mental status. Three days prior she had a repair of an aortic dissection and was extubated uneventfully. She is agitated, pulling at her lines, attempting to climb out of bed, and asking to leave the hospital. Her arterial blood gas values are normal. The patient has no history of alcohol abuse. Calm reassurance, orientation efforts, and having family members present have done little to reduce the patient's agitated behavior.

1. What is the diagnosis for the patient's altered mental status?

2. What is the most appropriate therapy for this patient's altered mental status?

Answers

1. This patient has an acute confusional state known as delirium.

2. The first focus of treatment in a patient with delirium is to ensure that the underlying condition, when identified, is being adequately treated. This is the most effective way of reversing the delirium. Antipsychotic agents should be used *only* in cases of severe agitation or psychosis with risk of harm to self or others. In this case a low dose of haloperidol may be used, such as 0.5 mg to 1 mg. This can be given orally or IM. Other agents that may be used include low-dose quetiapine (helpful when there is associated insomnia for its strong hypnotic properties), risperidone, or olanzapine. Ziprasidone should be used with caution due to its significant QTc-prolonging properties. There is no evidence that second-generation antipsychotics are superior to haloperidol for delirium. Haloperidol is not associated with significant respiratory suppression. All antipsychotic agents increase the risk of torsades de pointes, to varying degrees, as well as

extrapyramidal side effects and neuroleptic malignant syndrome. Patients with parkinsonism should be given atypical antipsychotics instead of haloperidol. The plan should be for short-term use only, with the drug being discontinued as soon as the risk for harm or psychotic symptomatology is eliminated. Benzodiazepines are not ideal as they may precipitate delirium. The risk of short-term and long-term mortality is increased with delirium.

A 79-year-old Woman With Agitation After Surgery

You have been called to evaluate a 79-year-old woman who underwent right hip replacement 3 days ago. She woke up from general anesthesia 12 hours after extubation. She has become increasingly agitated, yelling at the nurses and pulling at IV lines. Her medical comorbidities include a history of Alzheimer's dementia and chronic atrial fibrillation, for which she is on warfarin therapy. She has no other pertinent personal or family medical history. Current medications are donepezil, memantine, atenolol, and low-molecular-weight heparin.

On physical examination today, temperature is 37.2°C (99.0°F), blood pressure is 100/68 mm Hg, pulse rate is 100/min and irregular, respiration rate is 18/min, and BMI is 21. The patient can move all 4 extremities. She is inattentive and disoriented to time and place and exhibits combativeness alternating with hypersomnolence. The remainder of the neurologic examination is unremarkable, without evidence of focal findings or meningismus.

1. What is the most likely diagnosis?

Answer

1. Acute worsening of confusion in elderly patients with chronic dementia usually results from an acute medical problem. Patients with dementia are at greater risk for delirium after surgery with general anesthesia. This patient who recently had right hip surgery under general anesthesia most likely has postoperative delirium.

DELIRIUM

Diagnosis

Delirium is defined as changes in the level of consciousness with difficulty focusing, sustaining, or shifting attention. The changes develop and occur over a short period of time, usually hours to days, and fluctuate during the course of the day.

Delirium often involves other cognitive deficits, changes in level of arousal, and altered sleep-wake cycle, and it may include psychotic features such as hallucinations and/or delusions. It is a clinical syndrome often precipitated by an underlying medical condition or medical issue with or without a background of reduced cognitive reserve.

Key features of delirium include the following:

- Altered level of consciousness
- Change in cognition
- Onset over hours to days
- Fluctuating course
- Behavioral changes
- Sleep alterations

Common causes of delirium include certain commonly prescribed medications, including opioids, sedative-hypnotics, and polypharmacy. Medication withdrawal states and medication side effects (such as those associated with quinolones) also are common precipitants in the elderly. Other common causes include infections, metabolic abnormalities, and brain disorders. The infections that most commonly underlie delirium include sepsis, pneumonia, and urinary tract infections. Electrolyte abnormalities, hypercarbia, hypoxemia, hyperglycemia, and hypoglycemia also may precipitate delirium. CNS infections, seizures, and hypertensive emergencies can cause delirium. Lack of sleep and poor sleep are important contributing factors.

A mnemonic of some use to remember the possible etiologies of delirium is **I WATCH DEATH**:

Infectious: encephalitis, meningitis, syphilis, pneumonia, and urinary tract infection

Withdrawal: alcohol and sedative-hypnotics

Acute metabolic: acidosis, alkalosis, electrolyte disturbances, and hepatic or renal failure

Trauma: heat stroke, burns, and postoperative

CNS pathology: abscesses, hemorrhage, seizures, stroke, tumors, vasculitis, and normal pressure hydrocephalus

Hypoxia: due to anemia, carbon monoxide poisoning, hypotension, pulmonary embolus, and pulmonary or cardiac failure

Deficiencies: vitamin B_{12}, niacin, and thiamine

Endocrinopathies: hyperglycemia or hypoglycemia, hyperadrenocorticism or hypoadrenocorticism, hyperthyroidism or hypothyroidism, and hyperparathyroidism or hypoparathyroidism

Acute vascular: hypertensive encephalopathy and shock

Toxins: medications, drugs, pesticides, and solvents

Heavy metals: lead, manganese, and mercury

Management of a patient with delirium starts with anticipating and instituting effective measures to avoid the factors listed above, use of frequent orientation, use of sensory aids such as hearing aids and/or eyeglasses, ensuring supportive restorative sleep, and ensuring early mobilization of patients following surgery where possible.

The evaluation of a patient with delirium should always include a complete history. This may require obtaining collateral information from family members, friends, and/or nursing staff. A thorough review of the medical record may help to identify risk factors and uncover underlying conditions.

One important part of the history is to find out whether the patient has a prior diagnosis of dementia or sundowning or any notable symptoms of reduced cognitive reserve. Sometimes a formal diagnosis has not been made but the family has recognized lapses of memory, mood swings, or disturbances of behavior. A history of similar difficulty during prior hospitalizations may be a helpful clue. This is essential and often requires the clinician interview of a close relative. Although challenging for a busy resident on a call night, its importance cannot be minimized. Having a history of sundowning strongly predicts the presence of some underlying cognitive impairment.

It is important to understand the relationship between dementia and delirium. Having a diagnosis of dementia predisposes a patient to developing delirium while hospitalized, and vice versa. If a patient develops delirium while in the hospital, he or she is at increased risk for a later diagnosis of dementia.

Other elements of the history should focus on any symptoms of infections, exposures, or metabolic abnormalities. One needs to take a detailed medication history, as well as a good diet and social history, including a detailed alcohol and drug use history.

The physical examination should be head-to-toe. Many causes of delirium may be missed without a thorough physical examination. Vitals are essential to take and review, including a pulse oximetry. The lung examination may uncover pneumonia or CHF as the etiology. Cardiac examination may lead you to consider cardiac ischemia, CHF, or an arrhythmia. Abdominal examination may cause you to consider bowel impaction, gastrointestinal bleeding, or ischemia. Urinary retention is a common contributor to delirium. A complete neurologic examination, as possible, may help diagnose encephalitis, meningitis, seizure, or stroke. Don't forget to do a good skin examination so a pressure ulcer or an allergic reaction is not missed. Don't forget to check the patient's hearing and vision as these, too, often contribute to altered mental status and may be easily fixed with eyeglasses or hearing aids.

Delirium constitutes a medical emergency. Patients who present with acute delirium should be screened quickly for readily reversible causes such as hypoglycemia, hypoxia, and medication overdose. Further evaluation should be targeted based on the history and physical examination. Tests to consider include thyroid function tests, toxicology screen, drug levels, ammonia, cortisol, vitamin B_{12}, arterial blood gas, lumbar puncture, electroencephalography, neuroimaging, electrocardiography, and/or telemetry. Testing should be guided by clinical history rather than a shotgun approach. There is no evidence to support routine use of head CT scanning. Head CT/MRI should be done only if there is history of head trauma, suspicion of encephalitis, or new focal neurologic finding, or if no other identifiable cause can be found.

Treatment

Assess and ensure patient safety first. Treatment should focus on the underlying acute illness as well as preventing possible complications. Management of the underlying condition and removal of suspected medications are important. Patients with an acute delirium are at risk for complications, including respiratory failure, malnutrition, pressure ulcers, and venous thromboembolism. Airway protection, nutritional support, skin care, and venous thromboembolism prophylaxis should be started. Patient behavior that may place the patient at risk of harm should be actively managed, such as discouraging frequent getting up in an unsupervised, unsteady patient with a risk of falls, and removing feeding tubes and IV lines as possible. Physical restraints should be avoided. Restoring sensory input including the use of eyeglasses, hearing aids, and physical touch are helpful. Family involvement and use of sitters may be beneficial. Normal sleep-wake cycles should be encouraged; avoiding naps during the day and having patients sleep in a quiet room with low lighting are suggested. Supporting the normal sleep cycle with a sleep aid such as melatonin may be helpful.

Pharmacologic management is indicated in patients with severe agitation who are at a safety risk to themselves or staff. Start with the lowest dose possible and adjust to the patient's response. Low-dose haloperidol (0.5–1.0 mg orally or intramuscularly) may be used to control harmful agitation or psychotic symptoms. Benzodiazepines are indicated only in cases of sedative drug and alcohol withdrawal. Otherwise they should not be used in patients with delirium. Thiamine supplementation should be considered in all patients with delirium (Figure 10-1).

Approach to the Patient With Delirium

TIPS TO REMEMBER

- Delirium is an alteration of consciousness that develops over a short period of time.
- Recognizing that the disorder is present and uncovering the underlying etiology is essential.
- Delirium is a medical emergency.

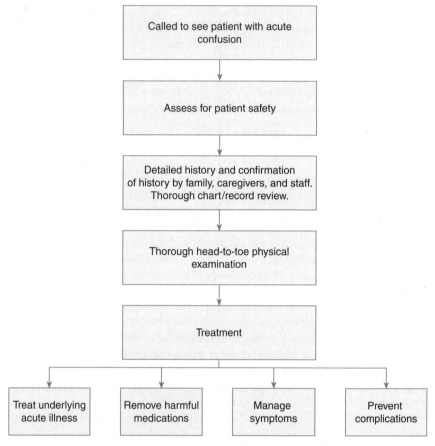

Figure 10-1. Approach to the patient with delirium.

● Pharmacologic management should be used only in patients with severe agitation and psychosis who pose a safety risk to themselves or staff or in patients who are at risk to impede essential medical care.

● Preventing complications of delirium is also a hallmark of treatment.

COMPREHENSION QUESTIONS

1. In the initial evaluation of a patient with acute confusion, what are the two most important things to do first?

Answer

First, assess and ensure patient safety. Second, information gathering is essential. This information should include a comprehensive history and physical examination, including confirming the history with a thorough chart review and discussions with family members, caregivers, and staff. A good medication and substance use inquiry may provide the key.

2. In the management of patients with agitated delirium, what essential elements of care should be considered?

Answer

Determining the underlying cause and targeting treatment are paramount. Supportive care, optimizing sensory input, and using orientation protocols are essential elements as well. Medications and physical restraints should be used only as a last resort and in cases of imminent harm.

SUGGESTED READINGS

Inouye SK. Delirium in older persons. *N Engl J Med.* 2006;354:1157–1165.
Marx JA, Hockberger RS, Walls RM, Rosen P. *Rosen's Emergency Medicine.* 7th ed. St. Louis: Mosby; 2009.
Schneider LS, Tariot PN, Dagerman KS, et al. Effectiveness of atypical antipsychotic drugs in patients with Alzheimer's disease. *N Engl J Med.* 2006;355:1525–1538.
Sink KM, Holden KF, Yaffe K. Pharmacological treatment of neuropsychiatric symptoms of dementia. *JAMA.* 2005;293:596–608.

Diabetes Emergencies

Sonaina Imtiaz, MD and Michael Jakoby, MD, MA

A 22-Year-Old Woman With Nausea, Vomiting, and Abdominal Pain

A 22-year-old woman presents to the emergency department for evaluation and management of progressively worsening nausea, vomiting, and abdominal pain for 2 days. She also reports increased urination and thirst. Examination is notable for resting tachycardia, mild tachypnea, dry mucous membranes, and modest, diffuse pain on palpation of the abdomen. Capillary blood glucose (CBG) is >600 mg/dL.

Initial electrolyte panel reveals sodium 130 mEq/L, potassium 4.5 mEq/L, chloride 92 mEq/L, bicarbonate 10 mEq/L, blood urea nitrogen (BUN) 20 mg/dL, creatinine (Cr) 1.3 mg/dL, and glucose 652 mg/dL. Anion gap is 28. Arterial blood gas is notable for pH 7.21, Pco_2 34 mm Hg, Po_2 80 mm Hg, and calculated bicarbonate 14 mEq/L. Large amounts of glucose and ketones are present on urinalysis, but nitrites and leukocyte esterase are undetectable. Complete blood count (CBC) shows modest leukocytosis and elevation of neutrophil count. Markers of liver function, amylase, lipase, ECG, and chest plain films are unremarkable.

Based on the clinical picture, this patient has diabetic ketoacidosis.

1. How is diabetic ketoacidosis (DKA) diagnosed?

2. How should DKA patients be evaluated?

3. What are the appropriate steps in DKA management?

Answers

1. DKA is diagnosed by the simultaneous occurrence of hyperglycemia, ketonemia and ketonuria, and anion gap acidemia. The differential diagnosis of ketosis is presented in Table 11-1, and the American Diabetes Association (ADA) diagnostic criteria for DKA are presented in Table 11-2.

2. Metabolic confirmation of the diagnosis includes timely measurements of glucose, urine or serum ketones (chiefly β-hydroxybutyrate), and electrolytes to allow computation of an anion gap (Na–Cl–HCO$_3$). The three leading causes of DKA are infection, medication noncompliance, and newly diagnosed type 1 diabetes mellitus. In a recent series of adults age ≥18 years with established type 1 diabetes and recurrent DKA, discontinuation of insulin was the precipitating cause for nearly 70% of patients. Infections occur frequently enough that all patients in DKA should be screened for respiratory and urinary tract infections. Other potential precipitants of DKA include major cardiovascular events, pancreatitis, sepsis, cocaine abuse, treatment with several medications including

Table 11-1. Etiologies of Ketosis

Etiology	Glucose
Fasting (infancy, pregnancy)	N, D
Prolonged exercise	N, occ D
Ketogenic diet	N, occ D
DKA	**I**
Adrenal insufficiency	D
GH insufficiency (children)	D
Ketotic hypoglycemia	D
Alcoholic ketoacidosis	Varies
Isopropyl alcohol poisoning	N
Salicylate poisoning	Varies

N, normal; D, decreased; I, increased; occ, occasionally.

Table 11-2. American Diabetes Association (ADA) Diagnostic Criteria for DKA

	Mild	Moderate	Severe
Glucose (mg/dL)	>250	>250	>250
pH	7.25–7.30	7.00–7.24	<7.00
HCO$_3^-$ (mM)	15–18	10–14	<10
Urine ketones	+	+	+
Serum ketones	+	+	+
Osmolality	Varies	Varies	Varies
Anion gap	>10	>12	>12
Sensorium	Alert	Drowsy	Stupor/coma

glucocorticoids, atypical antipsychotic agents, SGLT2 inhibitors and thiazide diuretics, and interruption of insulin delivery during management with an insulin pump.

3. Management of DKA requires prompt correction of fluid deficits and electrolyte abnormalities and treatment with IV insulin. Patients are initially hydrated with 0.9% (normal) saline until volume depletion is treated and then changed to 0.45% (half-normal) saline to correct hyperosmolarity. If serum potassium is <3.3 mEq/L, IV insulin is held and supplemental potassium delivered at 20–40 mEq/h until potassium level is >3.3 mEq/L. If serum potassium falls in the range of 3.3–5.2 mEq/L, 20–30 mEq of potassium is added to each liter of IV fluid. Supplemental potassium is held if serum potassium level exceeds 5.2 mEq/L, and potassium level is monitored every 2 hours. IV insulin is administered as a 0.1-U/kg bolus followed by a 0.1-U/h infusion. The rate is doubled if glucose level fails to fall by ≥50 mg/dL/h. When serum glucose is ~200 mg/dL, dextrose is added to IV fluid until resolution of DKA to prevent hypoglycemia. DKA is considered resolved if the patient's anion gap is <12 and serum bicarbonate ≥16 mEq/L.

CASE REVIEW

DKA is a life-threatening complication of type 1 diabetes mellitus and may also occur in patients with type 2 diabetes and significant insulinopenia. Absolute (type 1 diabetes) or severe relative (type 2 diabetes) deficiency of insulin activity, coupled with excess activity of counterregulatory hormones (glucagon, epinephrine, and cortisol) and unrestrained lipolysis in adipose tissue, leads to hyperglycemia and ketonemia. Dehydration and electrolyte abnormalities are due mainly to osmotic diuresis from glucosuria. There were more than 220,000 hospital admissions for DKA in 2017, with in-hospital mortality rates ranging from 0.1% for patients <45 years of age to 2.6% for patients ≥75 years of age. Hospital admissions for DKA are costly; in a recent study of DKA admissions to Hennepin County Medical Center in Illinois, January 2017 to January 2019, the median cost per admission was nearly $30,000.

Diagnosis

Common symptoms of DKA include nausea, vomiting, abdominal pain, polyuria, polydipsia, blurry vision, lethargy, and shortness of breath. Tachycardia, hypotension, dry mucous membranes, poor skin turgor, and diffuse abdominal pain to palpation are usually found on physical examination. Patients are also often tachypneic and may exhibit Kussmaul breathing, characteristic rapid and deep respirations. The breath of DKA patients may smell "fruity" of acetone.

The diagnosis of DKA is made by documenting anion gap acidemia in the setting of hyperglycemia. Diagnostic criteria for DKA are presented in Table 11-2. Although the patient's age may make type 1 diabetes seem unlikely, approximately 30% of type 1 diabetes cases are diagnosed in patients over age 18 years.

Workup of presumptive DKA should be directed at quickly confirming the diagnosis and identifying potential etiologies. Documenting hyperglycemia, an anion gap acidemia, and ketonemia confirms the diagnosis of DKA. The ADA recommends that all patients with DKA undergo an initial evaluation that includes arterial blood gas analysis, urine/serum ketones, measurements of plasma glucose, electrolytes, Cr and BUN, CBC, and blood and urine cultures. Corrected serum sodium for hyperglycemia can be calculated by adding 1.6 mEq/L for every 100 mg/dL that plasma glucose is greater than 100 mg/dL.

Treatment

Patients in DKA are significantly volume depleted (up to 0.1 L/kg) and require hydration with isotonic fluid (normal saline or Ringer's lactate) to correct hypovolemia. After administration of at least 3 to 4 L of isotonic fluid and documented improvement in heart rate and blood pressure, patients can be hydrated with hypotonic fluid, usually half-normal saline, at a rate ranging from 4 to 14 mg/kg/h (typical rates are 250–500 mL/h). Although serum potassium level may be elevated on presentation due to acidemia, patients with DKA have large total body potassium deficits (3–5 mEq/kg) and require potassium repletion. Potassium may be withheld from fluids at levels >5.2 mEq/L, but 20 to 40 mEq of potassium chloride should be added to IV fluids at levels <5.2 mEq/L. An electrolyte panel should be checked every 2 to 4 hours to closely monitor changes in potassium levels, bicarbonate, and anion gap.

Parenteral insulin is preferred due to the ability to quickly achieve high insulin levels and suppress ketogenesis, although there are protocols for frequent administration of SC insulin aspart (NovoLog) or insulin lispro (Humalog) to manage mild DKA. Unless circulating potassium level is significantly low (<3.3 mEq/L), IV insulin should be started as a 0.1-U/kg bolus followed by 0.1-U/kg/h infusion. CBG is measured hourly, and dextrose is added to fluids when CBG is <200 to 250 mg/dL. IV insulin should be continued until the anion gap has closed (<12) and serum bicarbonate is ≥16 mEq/L. Patients require basal insulin therapy with NPH, insulin glargine (Lantus), or insulin detemir (Levemir), and the insulin infusion must be overlapped by 1 hour with the initial dose of NPH or 2 hours with the initial dose of glargine or detemir before termination to avoid recurrence of ketoacidosis. A summary of recommendations for insulin dosing, hydration, and potassium repletion is presented in Table 11-3.

Sodium bicarbonate may be administered when DKA is severe (pH <7.0). The recommended dose is 100 mEq of bicarbonate with 20 mEq potassium chloride in 400 mL sterile water over 2 hours, with the dose repeated every 2 hours as necessary until pH improves to >7.0. Bicarbonate is coadministered with potassium to help avoid hypokalemia. Treatment with sodium bicarbonate does not substitute for therapy with adequate insulin and hydration, and the utility of adding bicarbonate to insulin is unclear. In a study comparing administration of insulin and bicarbonate with insulin alone in patients with severe DKA (pH 6.90–7.14), time to resolution of acidemia was no faster in the group of

Table 11-3. Recommendations for Insulin, Fluids, and Potassium Management

Intervention	
Insulin	0.1 U/kg bolus, and then 0.1 U/kg/h infusion
	0.14 U/kg/h infusion w/o bolus
	0.14 U/kg bolus if CBG fails to fall by ≥10% from baseline first hour
	Hold insulin until potassium ≥3.3 mEq/L
Fluids	Severe hypovolemia—several liters normal saline (NS) at 1 L/h
	Mild hypovolemia and low sodium level—250–500 mL/h NS
	Mild hypovolemia and normal or high sodium—250–500 mL/h half NS
	Add dextrose when CBG <200–250 mg/dL
	Switch to hypotonic fluid (half NS) when volume deficit corrected
Potassium	K^+ <3.3 mEq/L—hold insulin and administer KCl 40 mEq/h
	K^+ 3.3–5.2 mEq/L—administer KCl 20–40 mEq/h
	K^+ >5.2 mEq/L—monitor K^+ level every 2 h

patients who received bicarbonate in addition to parenteral insulin. Bicarbonate replacement may be considered if arterial pH is ≤6.9 and patients show signs of heart failure or refractory hypotension.

Hypophosphatemia is common in DKA, although administration of parenteral phosphate has not been shown to accelerate metabolic recovery. Serum phosphate levels fall significantly after stopping parenteral administration of supplemental phosphate, and the P_{50} curve for peripheral oxygen delivery is no different in treated or untreated patients. Treatment with supplemental phosphate should be considered only in patients with a phosphate level <1 mg/dL and evidence of cardiac dysfunction, respiratory depression, or hemolytic anemia. A 20- to 30-mEq dose of sodium or potassium phosphate can be administered in 1 L of IV fluid. Hypophosphatemia usually resolves quickly once patients resume eating.

An Elderly Patient With Hyperglycemic Hyperosmolar State

A 68-year-old male is brought from his nursing home to the emergency department for evaluation of confusion. Over the past 48 hours, the patient has grown progressively more confused and complained of increased thirst. History is notable for type 2 diabetes, hypertension, and dyslipidemia. Diabetes is managed with glyburide, which the patient has refused over the past few days. CBG from the nursing home is reported as > 400 mg/dL. Tachycardia and hypotension (BP 84/52 mm Hg) are noted. The patient is disoriented to place and time and does not follow commands.

Admission electrolyte panel is notable for serum sodium 124 mEq/L, chloride 92 mEq/L, bicarbonate 22 mEq/L, BUN 62 mg/dL, Cr 1.6 mg/dL, and glucose 850 mg/dL. Other serologies and CBC are unremarkable. Urinalysis is notable for large glucose and no ketones. No acute hemorrhages, ischemic changes, or masses are apparent on CT of the head. No infiltrates or effusions are visible on plain films of the chest, and ECG shows sinus tachycardia and nonspecific ST-segment changes.

1. What are the diagnostic criteria for hyperglycemic hyperosmolar state (HHS)?

2. What are important risk factors for HHS?

3. How should HHS patients be evaluated and managed?

Answers

1. HHS is diagnosed when patients present with altered mental status of some degree in the setting of severe hyperglycemia (plasma glucose ≥ 600 mg/dL) and hyperosmolarity (≥ 320 mOsm/L). Unlike DKA, there is no significant ketoacidosis.

2. Key risk factors for HHS are presented in Figure 11-1. Advanced age, residence in an institutional setting, infections, and cardiovascular events are all potential risk factors for HHS. Some patients may have undiagnosed type 2 diabetes at presentation. Occasionally, patients have been started on medications such as glucocorticoids that significantly exacerbate hyperglycemia.

3. Prompt fluid resuscitation, parenteral insulin, and potassium repletion are the most important factors in management. The approach to management is similar to patients with DKA presented in Table 11-3 except that insulin infusion rate is reduced by approximately half when glucose is <300 mg/dL to slow the fall in osmolarity and reduce the possibility of cerebral edema.

> • Age >70 years
> • Nursing home resident
> • Infection
> • Myocardial infarction
> • Stroke
> • Undiagnosed/untreated type 2 diabetes
> • Drugs (glucocorticoids, diuretics, beta-blockers)

Figure 11-1. Risk factors for HHS.

CASE REVIEW

Diagnosis

Hyperglycemic hyperosmolar state (HHS) occurs when severe elevation of plasma glucose leads to hyperosmolarity and altered mental status. Diagnostic criteria include plasma glucose ≥600 mg/dL, osmolarity ≥320 mOsm/L, and altered mental status, ranging from mild confusion to coma, in the absence of ketoacidosis (pH ≥7.30). Insulinopenia leads to impaired glucose uptake by skeletal muscle and inappropriate gluconeogenesis in liver, resulting in hyperglycemia that in turn induces osmotic diuresis and prerenal azotemia, further worsening hyperglycemia by limiting glucosuria. Attenuated thirst response, as a consequence of either aging or central nervous system injury, also plays a role. There is sufficient insulin activity to suppress lipolysis and ketogenesis, distinguishing HHS from DKA.

Risk factors for HHS are listed in Figure 11-1. HHS patients tend to be much older than DKA patients, as HHS typically occurs in patients with type 2 diabetes mellitus. Patients may live in institutional settings and not have free access to water. In addition to altered mental status, they may exhibit neurologic findings mimicking stroke that resolve with treatment of hyperosmolarity. Volume depletion is severe (0.1–0.2 L/kg), and signs such as tachycardia, hypotension, dry mucous membranes, and poor skin turgor are usually present on examination. Patients with poorly controlled hypertension may exhibit normotensive blood pressures that are an unusual change from baseline. Cardiopulmonary emergencies are well-known precipitants of HHS, and patients should be examined carefully for signs of coronary ischemia, heart failure, or chronic obstructive pulmonary disease (COPD) exacerbations. Infections also commonly trigger HHS, and patients require prompt evaluation for urinary tract infections and pneumonia. Glucocorticoids, thiazide diuretics, and beta blockers may worsen preexisting diabetes or hyperglycemia, and medications should be carefully reviewed.

Treatment

Initial evaluation of patients with presumptive HHS is similar to workup of patients with DKA. Key laboratories include electrolytes, markers of renal and hepatic function, CBC, and amylase or lipase. Urinalysis and cultures of blood and urine should be obtained. Given the high risk of cardiopulmonary disease, ECG, chest films, and cardiac enzymes also should be screened.

The incidence of HHS is less than 1% of hospitalizations for patients with diabetes, but the mortality rate for HHS is as high as 10% to 20% or more than 10-fold higher than DKA. In a large series of nearly 500 patients presenting with HHS, age, severity of altered mental status on presentation, degree of hyperosmolarity, and renal function were independent predictors of mortality risk. Goals of therapy are volume repletion and treatment of hyperglycemia with parenteral fluids and insulin, respectively, to correct hyperosmolarity. Electrolyte imbalances should be corrected, as patients are also total-body potassium depleted and require careful monitoring of potassium levels and therapy with supplemental potassium in IV fluids. Precipitating events (eg, infection, coronary ischemia) also need to be identified and treated promptly.

Fluids, insulin, and supplemental potassium are initiated and managed mostly as discussed in management of DKA and summarized in Table 11-3. However, when plasma glucose falls below 300 mg/dL, dextrose is added to IV fluids and insulin rate is reduced (eg, to 0.05 units/kg/h) to maintain plasma glucose in the range of 200 to 300 mg/dL until patients recover to baseline mental status as a protection against possible cerebral edema. Capillary glucose is monitored hourly and electrolytes every 2 hours while patients are managed with IV insulin. Patients require SC insulin to prevent recurrence of severe hyperglycemia, and IV insulin is overlapped by 1 to 2 hours with the first dose of SC basal insulin.

A Case of a Type 1 Diabetes Mellitus Patients With Severe Hypoglycemia

A 19-year-old female with type 1 diabetes of nearly 15 years' duration is admitted to the hospital for extreme alcohol consumption. After recovery to baseline mental status, a diet and basal/bolus insulin regimen are ordered. The patient is dosed with insulin lispro before her evening meal, but she vomits before starting to eat and skips the meal. Approximately 2 hours later, the patient is found unconscious. Capillary blood glucose is 48 mg/dL.

1. What are the diagnostic criteria for hypoglycemia?
2. What are key risk factors for hypoglycemia?
3. How is hypoglycemia treated?

Answers

1. For nonpregnant adults with diabetes, the ADA now defines hypoglycemia with 3 levels of severity. Level 1 hypoglycemia is defined as blood glucose <70 mg/dL but ≥54 mg/dL. Level 2 is a blood glucose <54 mg/dL, and level 3 is hypoglycemia complicated by altered mental status or physical state that requires treatment of the episode by a third party. Most patients experience neuroglycopenic symptoms ranging in severity from dizziness or weakness to overtly altered mental status and autonomic symptoms including palpitations, tremor, anxiety, sweating, and hunger.

2. Important risk factors for hypoglycemia in patients with diabetes are presented in Figure 11-1. Hypoglycemia is much more common in patients with type 1 diabetes than those with type 2 diabetes, although patients treated with insulin or

insulin secretagogues for type 2 diabetes are at risk of low blood sugars. Patients with type 1 diabetes report an average of 3 severe hypoglycemic events per year and male sex, adolescence, longstanding diabetes (>40 years' duration), history of severe hypoglycemia, and high glucose variability were found to be independent risk factors for severe hypoglycemia in the Type 1 Diabetes Exchange Clinical Registry. Randomized controlled trials of patients with type 1 and type 2 diabetes have demonstrated 2- to 3-fold increased risks of severe hypoglycemia in the tight glycemic control arms compared with the control arms.

3. Hypoglycemia should be treated with 15 to 20 g of fast-acting carbohydrates (eg, 4 oz of fruit juice or 4 glucose tablets) and blood glucose level rechecked 15 to 20 minutes after treatment. The process is repeated until blood glucose remains at least >70 mg/dL. Once glucose exceeds this threshold, the patient should eat a small snack to avoid recurrent hypoglycemia. Glucagon should be used to treat hypoglycemia in patients who are unable to consume carbohydrates by mouth (eg, due to altered mental status as in this patient's case). These patients should also be provided with a snack once they are safe to consume food. In hospital, patients with IV access can be administered 25 g of parenteral dextrose as half an ampule of D50 (50% dextrose solution) or 250 mL of 10% dextrose solution.

CASE REVIEW

Diagnosis

Hypoglycemia is the limiting factor for treatment of patients with diabetes, and the risk of hypoglycemia increases as treatment of hyperglycemia is intensified to reduce HbA1c. Symptoms of hypoglycemia typically occur at a plasma glucose threshold of 65 to 70 mg/dL, although patients with poorly controlled diabetes may have symptoms at significantly higher glucose thresholds (pseudohypoglycemia) while intensive management of hyperglycemia can reduce the threshold for symptoms of hypoglycemia and a significant counterregulatory response. Patients with frequent or recurrent severe hypoglycemia may develop a significantly reduced sympathoadrenal response and lack of symptoms during episodes of hypoglycemia, a condition called hypoglycemia unawareness.

Use of continuous glucose monitoring (CGM) in type 1 diabetes patients appears to show that clinically important (glucose <54 mg/dL) hypoglycemia is more common than previously known, with some patients experiencing 2 to 3 episodes daily. In patients with insulin-managed type 2 diabetes, there does not appear to be an increased rate of hypoglycemia detected by CGM compared with capillary blood glucose monitoring 4 times daily. However, insulin, sulfonylureas, and meglitinides pose a direct risk of hypoglycemia in patients with type 2 diabetes, while use of agents such as metformin, thiazolidinediones, glucagon-like peptide 1 (GLP-1) receptor agonists, dipeptidyl peptidase 4 (DPP-4) inhibitors, and sodium-glucose cotransporter 2 (SGLT2) inhibitors may increase the risk of hypoglycemia if used in combination with insulin or an insulin secretagogue.

Studies of the impacts of hypoglycemia on cognitive function have provided mixed results. In the Diabetes Control and Complications Trial and the long-term follow-up trial Epidemiology of Diabetes Interventions and Complications, patients randomized to tight glycemic control had equivalent performances on psychometric testing up to 18 years from randomization as patients in the control arms of the trials despite a much higher rate of hypoglycemia. However, older adults with diabetes who experience hypoglycemia have a significantly increased risk of dementia. Additionally, hypoglycemia increases fall risk in elderly patients and increases time off work among middle-aged adults.

Treatment

Acute management of hypoglycemia was discussed in the answer to question 3. Prevention of hypoglycemia requires healthcare providers to inquire about occurrence of low blood sugars at every office visit for patients managed with insulin or insulin secretagogues. Patients should be instructed to always bring their glucose meter or CGM device to appointments for download and review. All patients should receive education, preferably from a certified diabetes educator, on management of level 1 or level 2 hypoglycemia, and spouses, partners, family members, or friends should receive instruction on administration of glucagon to treat severe hypoglycemia. Education regarding meal plans, particularly carbohydrate consumption, and adjustment of diet and medications to avoid hypoglycemia in circumstances that increase risk of low blood glucose such as exercise, mitigates the risk of hypoglycemia and improves overall glycemic control.

Patients with frequent or severe hypoglycemia may need treatment to more conservative blood glucose and HbA1c targets than those considered optimal for reducing risk of microvascular complications in nonpregnant adults, to minimize frequency of low blood sugars and maximize safety. In patients with hypoglycemia unawareness, a sustained period of hypoglycemia avoidance may restore the sympathoadrenal and symptomatic response to low blood glucose. Management with sensor-augmented insulin pumps that have threshold-suspend or predictive low-glucose suspend capabilities reduce the frequency of hypoglycemia in patients with type 1 diabetes, particularly nocturnal hypoglycemia. When possible, patients with diabetes and frequent or severe hypoglycemia should be referred to an endocrinologist for glycemic management.

TIPS TO REMEMBER

- DKA and HHS are life-threatening emergencies of type 1 and type 2 diabetes, respectively. DKA occurs due to an absence of insulin activity that results in both hyperglycemia and ketogenesis. Relative insulinopenia and dehydration lead to severe hyperglycemia in HHS, but there is sufficient insulin activity to prevent ketogenesis.

- DKA is distinguished by the biochemical triad of hyperglycemia, ketonemia, and anion gap acidemia. Medical noncompliance, infection, and newly recognized type 1 diabetes mellitus are the three most common etiologies of DKA.

- Severe hyperglycemia, hyperosmolarity, and altered mental status without ketoacidosis are the defining manifestations of HHS. There are several risk factors for HHS including advanced age, residence in an institutional setting, cardiovascular disease, infection, and medications that exacerbate hyperglycemia such as glucocorticoids or thiazide diuretics.

- IV insulin, hydration, and supplemental potassium are the key interventions for successful management of both DKA and HHS. Patients require frequent monitoring of CBG and serum electrolytes during treatment.

- SC insulin is required to prevent recurrence of ketoacidosis in DKA and control hyperglycemia in both DKA and HHS after acute metabolic derangements have been successfully managed. Insulin infusion should overlap the first dose of SC insulin by 1 to 2 hours depending on the basal SC insulin chosen.

- Hypoglycemia should be promptly treated with 15 to 20 g of fast-acting carbohydrates in patients who can eat and with glucagon in patients who are unable to eat. In hospital, parenteral dextrose is also a treatment option. All patients should have a repeat blood glucose check in 15 to 20 min and be treated to a blood glucose at least >70 mg/dL. A small snack should be provided to prevent recurrence of hypoglycemia.

SUGGESTED READINGS

Action to Control Cardiovascular Risk in Diabetes Study Group, Gerstein HC, Miller ME, et al. Effects of intensive glucose lowering in type 2 diabetes. *N Engl J Med*. 2008;358:2545–2559.

Agesen RM, Kristensen PL, Beck-Nielsen H, et al. Effect of insulin analogs on frequency of non-severe hypoglycemia in patients with type 1 diabetes prone to severe hypoglycemia: much higher rates detected by continuous glucose monitoring than by self-monitoring of blood glucose—The Hypo-Ana Trial. *Diabetes Technol Ther*. 2018;20(3):247–256.

American Diabetes Association Professional Practice Committee. 17. Diabetes Advocacy: Standards of Medical Care in Diabetes—2022. *Diabetes Care*. 2022;45(Suppl 1):S254–S255.

American Diabetes Association. Standards of Medical Care in Diabetes—2006. *Diabetes Care*. 2006;29(suppl_1):s4–s42.

Amiel SA, Sherwin RS, Simonson DC, Tamborlane WV. Effect of intensive insulin therapy on glycemic thresholds for counterregulatory hormone release. *Diabetes*. 1988;37(7):901–907.

Andrade-Castellanos CA, Colunga-Lozano LE, Delgado-Figueroa N, Gonzalez-Padilla DA. Subcutaneous rapid-acting insulin analogues for diabetic ketoacidosis. *Cochrane Database Syst Rev*. 2016;2016(1):CD011281.

Arnaud M, Pariente A, Bezin J, et al. Risk of serious trauma with glucose-lowering drugs in older persons: a nested case-control study. *J Am Geriatr Soc*. 2018;66(11):2086–2091.

Beck RW, Riddlesworth TD, Ruedy K, et al. Continuous glucose monitoring versus usual care in patients with type 2 diabetes receiving multiple daily insulin injections: a randomized trial. *Ann Intern Med.* 2017;167(6):365–374.

Benoit SR, Zhang Y, Geiss LS, et al. Trends in diabetic ketoacidosis hospitalizations and in-hospital mortality—United States, 2000–2014. *MMWR Morb Mortal Wkly Rep.* 2018;67:362–365.

Cryer PE. Glycemic goals in diabetes: trade-off between glycemic control and iatrogenic hypoglycemia. *Diabetes.* 2014;63(7):2188–2195.

Diabetes Control and Complications Research Group. The effect of intensive treatment of diabetes on development and progression of long-term complications in insulin-dependent diabetes mellitus. *N Engl J Med.* 1993;329:977–986.

Diabetes Control and Complications Trial/Epidemiology of Diabetes Interventions and Complications Research Study Group, Jacobson AM, Musen G, et al. Long-term effect of diabetes and its treatment on cognitive function. *N Engl J Med.* 2007;356:1842–1852.

Fanelli CG, Epifano L, Rambotti AM, et al. Meticulous prevention of hypoglycemia normalizes the glycemic thresholds and magnitude of most neuroendocrine responses to, symptoms of, and cognitive function during hypoglycemia in intensively treated patients with short-term IDDM. *Diabetes.* 1993;42(11):1683–1689.

Fisher JN, Kitabchi AE. A randomized study of phosphate therapy in the treatment of diabetic ketoacidosis. *J Clin Endocrinol Metab.* 1983;57:177–180.

Fisher JN, Shahshahani MN, Kitabchi AE. Diabetic ketoacidosis: low-dose insulin therapy by various routes. *N Engl J Med.* 1977;297:238–247.

Geelhoed-Duijvestinjin PH, Pedersen-Bjergaard U, Weitgasser R, et al. Effects of patient-reported non-severe hypoglycemia on healthcare resource use, work-time loss, and wellbeing in insulin-treated patients with diabetes in seven European countries. *J Med Econ.* 2013;16(12):1453–1461.

Gubitosi-Klug RA, Braffett BH, White NH, et al. Risk of severe hypoglycemia in type 1 diabetes over 30 years of follow-up in the DCCT/EDIC Study. *Diabetes Care.* 2017;40(8):1010–1016.

Iqbal A, Heller SR. The role of structured education in the management of hypoglycemia. *Diabetologia.* 2018;61(4):751–760.

Kamel KS, Halperin ML. Acid-base problems in diabetic ketoacidosis. *N Engl J Med.* 2015;372(6):546–554.

Kitabchi AE, Murphy MB. Consequences of insulin deficiency. In: Skyler J, ed. *Atlas of Diabetes.* 4th ed. New York: Springer US; 2012.

Kitabchi AE, Umpierrez GE, Miles JM, Fisher JN. Hyperglycemic crises in adult patients with diabetes. *Diabetes Care.* 2009;32(7):1335–1343.

Kitabchi AE, Umpierrez GE, Murphy MB, et al. Management of hyperglycemic crises in patients with diabetes. *Diabetes Care.* 2001;24(1):131–153.

Kitabchi AE, Umpierrez GE, Murphy MB, Kreisberg RA. Hyperglycemic crises in adult patients with diabetes: a consensus statement from the American Diabetes Association. *Diabetes Care.* 2006;29(12):2739–2748.

Lyerla R, Johnson-Rabbett B, Shakally A, et al. Recurrent DKA results in high societal costs—a retrospective study identifying social predictors of recurrence for potential future intervention. *Clin Diabetes Endocrinol.* 2021;7:13.

Morris LR, Murphy MB, Kitabchi AE. Bicarbonate therapy in diabetic ketoacidosis. *Ann Intern Med.* 1986;105:836–840.

Newcomer JW. Second-generation (atypical) antipsychotics and metabolic effects: a comprehensive literature review. *CNS Drugs.* 2005;19(Suppl 1):1–93.

Pasquel FJ, Umpierrez GE. Hyperosmolar hyperglycemic state: a historic review of the clinical presentation, diagnosis, and treatment. *Diabetes Care.* 2014;37(11):3124–3131.

Peden NR, Braaten JT, McKendry JB. Diabetic ketoacidosis during long-term treatment with continuous subcutaneous insulin infusion. *Diabetes Care.* 1984;7(1):1–5.

Randall L, Begovic J, Hudson M, et al. Recurrent diabetic ketoacidosis in inner-city minority patients: behavioral, socioeconomic, and psychosocial factors. *Diabetes Care.* 2011;34(9):1891–1896.

Seaquist ER, Anderson J, Childs B, et al. Hypoglycemia and diabetes: a report of the workgroup of the American Diabetes Association and Endocrine Society. *J Clin Endocrinol Metab.* 2013;98(5):1845–1859.

Steineck I, Ranjan A, Norgaard K, Schmidt S. Sensor-augmented insulin pumps and hypoglycemia prevention in type 1 diabetes. *J Diabetes Sci Tech.* 2017;11(1):50–58.

Tannenbaum H, Dreyer N. Ketotic hyperosmolar coma. *Lancet.* 1973;2(7830):635–639.

Taylor SI, Blau JE, Rother KI. SGLT2 inhibitors may predispose to ketoacidosis. *J Clin Endocrinol Metab.* 2015;100(8):2849–2852.

Umpierrez GE, Khajavi M, Kitabchi AE. Review: diabetic ketoacidosis and hyperglycemic hyperosmolar syndrome. *Am J Med Sci.* 1996;311(5):225–233.

Umpierrez GE, Latif K, Stoever J, et al. Efficacy of subcutaneous insulin lispro versus continuous intravenous regular insulin for the treatment of patients with diabetic ketoacidosis. *Am J Med.* 2004;117(5):291–296.

Weinstock RS, Xing D, Maahs DM, et al. Severe hypoglycemia and diabetic ketoacidosis in adults with type 1 diabetes: results from the T1D Exchange clinic registry. *J Clin Endocrinol Metab.* 2013;98(8):3411–3419.

Yaffe K, Falvey CM, Hamilton N, et al. Association between hypoglycemia and dementia in a biracial cohort of older adults with diabetes mellitus. *JAMA Intern Med.* 2013;173(14):1300–1306.

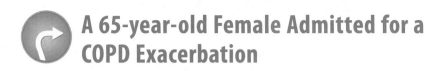

A 65-year-old Female Admitted for a COPD Exacerbation

Vanessa Williams, MD and Michael Jakoby, MD, MA

A 65-year-old female is admitted to the hospital to manage a chronic obstructive pulmonary disease (COPD) exacerbation. History is notable for type 2 diabetes mellitus diagnosed 2 years ago and currently managed with metformin. She reports no missed doses of metformin at home. She denies any microvascular complications. Hemoglobin A1c (HbA1c) checked on admission to the hospital was 8.5%.

Initial evaluation reveals the patient to be in mild respiratory distress but capable of eating. Weight and height are recorded as 100 kg and 162 cm, respectively (BMI 38.1). Admission plasma glucose (glc) is 262 mg/dL, and serum creatinine is 0.9 mg/dL. The admitting service writes orders for insulin lispro (LP) with meals and insulin glargine (Glarg) at bedtime as presented in Figure 12-1. The night nurse calls the on-call intern to report bedtime capillary blood glucose (CBG) is 326 mg/dL (see Figure 12-1).

The patient responds well to therapy with methylprednisolone, levofloxacin, and ipratropium-albuterol. Her CBG pattern (mg/dL) by the morning of hospital day 2 is shown in Table 12-1.

Glycemic control improves after advancing LP doses. However, on hospital day 4, the patient feels sweaty and tremulous in the morning, and CBG before breakfast is measured at 58 mg/dL. At bedtime on hospital day 3, CBG was 104 mg/dL.

1. What is the best approach to manage the patient's type 2 diabetes mellitus?

2. How can the patient's unanticipated exacerbation of hyperglycemia on the night of admission be corrected?

3. How should insulin be adjusted on hospital day 2 to improve glycemic control?

4. How should hypoglycemia occurring the morning of hospital day 4 be addressed?

Answers

1. A basal/bolus insulin regimen is the preferred approach to diabetes management on non–critical care hospital services. Typically, a basal insulin analog such as insulin glargine is combined with a prandial insulin analog such as insulin lispro.

2. Correction factor (CF) insulin should be dosed as presented in Figure 12-2. Rapid-acting insulin analogs, such as insulin lispro or insulin aspart, are

Since BMI is greater than 25, estimate daily calories with the Mifflin–St. Jeor equation:

$(9.99 \times 100 \text{ kg}) + (6.25 \times 162 \text{ cm}) - (4.92 \times 65) - 161 = 1530 \text{ kcal/day}$

Carbohydrates (g/meal) = 1530/24 = 64 g/meal

Total daily insulin (TDI) = 0.6 units/kg × 100 kg = 60 units

Basal insulin (units/day) = TDI × 1/2 = 60/2 = 30 units

Prandial insulin (units/meal) = TDI × 1/6 = 60/6 = 10 units

Figure 12-1. Initial diet and insulin orders.

preferred for CF insulin. Capillary blood glucose (CBG) correction target is usually 140 or 150 mg/dL (see Figure 12-2).

3. Persistently elevated CBG measurements during the day but stable CBG measurements from night to morning indicate a need to increase prandial insulin doses. See Figure 12-3 for instructions regarding adjustments of prandial insulin dosing. In this case, insulin lispro should be increased by 20% at each meal to 12 units (see Figure 12-3).

4. Fall in CBG from night to morning indicates that the patient's basal insulin requirement needs to be reduced by approximately 20%. Reducing the basal insulin dose to 24 units at bedtime is likely to avoid additional morning hypoglycemia.

CASE REVIEW

Overview

Diabetes mellitus is a common comorbidity of patients admitted to the hospital and has a significant impact on clinical outcomes. In the 20-year period from 1995 to 2014, the number of hospital discharges listing diabetes mellitus with or without complications as one of the diagnoses increased about 2-fold to almost 8.3 million in 2014. A study of 2030 consecutive admissions to Georgia Baptist Medical Center in Atlanta, Georgia, in 1998 found a 26% prevalence of preexisting diabetes

Table 12-1. Capillary Blood Glucose Measurements

Day	0300	Breakfast	Lunch	Dinner	Bedtime
Admission					254
Day 1	185	173	158	174	162
Day 2	—	155			

ISF = 1500/TDI = 1500/54 = 28

CF insulin = (measured CBG − 140)/ISF = (254 − 140)/28 = 4 U of lispro

Figure 12-2. Correction factor insulin dosing.

and 12% prevalence of newly recognized hyperglycemia. Diabetes mellitus and hyperglycemia have been linked to poor clinical outcomes in both the critical care and non–critical care settings and for multiple clinical presentations including myocardial infarction, stroke, pneumonia, and heart failure.

A growing body of evidence indicates that basal/bolus insulin is the superior approach to managing diabetes on non–critical care hospital services. In the RABBIT-2 trial, patients with type 2 diabetes mellitus admitted to general medicine services were randomized to a basal/bolus insulin protocol with insulin glulisine dosed at meals with insulin glargine administered daily for basal insulin or a sliding scale insulin protocol (regular insulin dosed depending on capillary blood glucose [CBG] measurements). Glycemic control was significantly better for basal/bolus insulin–managed patients than for sliding scale insulin–managed patients. A basal/bolus insulin protocol study at Carle Foundation Hospital in Urbana, Illinois, documented significant improvements in both glycemic control and hospital length of stay for patients on general medicine. Basal/bolus insulin was compared with sliding scale regular insulin for general surgery patients in the RABBIT-2 Surgery trial, and basal/bolus insulin–managed patients had better blood glucose control, fewer surgical morbidities, and shorter stay in the surgical intensive care unit than patients managed with sliding scale insulin.

Diet Management

Diet orders are important in effective hospital diabetes management. Caloric requirements for height/weight proportionate patients can be estimated as 20 to 25 kcal/kg per day, with 50% of calories provided as carbohydrate. Caloric requirements for overweight or obese patients (BMI >25) can be estimated using the Mifflin-St. Jeor equation. Orders should be written so that equal amounts of carbohydrate are provided at each meal (consistent carbohydrate diet). An example of diet and initial insulin orders for the patient under consideration is presented in Figure 12-1.

CBG stable from bedtime to morning, no basal insulin adjustment

CBG 141 to 179 mg/dL throughout the day, increase prandial insulin by 20%

New lispro dose = 9 × 1.2 = 11 U

Figure 12-3. Insulin dosing adjustments.

Initial Management of Basal and Prandial Insulin

Most basal/bolus insulin protocols stop outpatient diabetes medications and make estimates of the patient's total daily insulin (TDI) requirements based on weight in kilograms. TDI is usually divided equally between prandial and basal insulin. However, patients receiving glucocorticoids have a disproportionate need for prandial insulin and may have better glycemic control if TDI is divided as two-thirds for prandial insulin and one-third for basal insulin. Renal impairment may lower TDI requirements, as exogenous insulin is mainly cleared by the kidney. Therefore, TDI should be reduced by 25% when glomerular filtration rate (GFR) is below 50 mL/min/1.73 m^2 and by 50% when GFR is below 10 mL/min/1.73 m^2 or if the patient requires dialysis.

Protocols often include orders for supplemental insulin to correct elevated CBG. If no protocol is available, correction factor insulin can be estimated using the "rule of 1500" as discussed later in the chapter. American Diabetes Association glycemic targets are CBG 140–180 mg/dL before meals, with tighter glycemic control (CBG 110–140 mg/dL) as an option if it can be achieved without frequent hypoglycemia.

Correction Factor (CF) Insulin

When an unanticipated high CBG occurs, potential causal factors should be investigated and corrected, if possible. A CBG may be increased above target due to a delayed or omitted insulin dose, a delayed meal with measurement of a CBG within 4 hours after the meal, inadequate standing insulin doses, unplanned carbohydrate consumption between meals or before bedtime, dextrose-containing fluids or parenteral medications, initiation of peritoneal dialysis, and initiation of glucocorticoid therapy.

Most formulas for estimating insulin sensitivity factor (ISF) and determining CF insulin dose have been developed for patients with type 1 diabetes mellitus. The SIU Hospital Diabetes Team typically uses the "rule of 1500" to estimate ISF when CBG is elevated and CF insulin is required. A target-corrected CBG of 140 to 150 mg/dL is typically chosen, and the difference between measured and target CBG is then divided by ISF to determine the dose of CF insulin as illustrated in Figure 12-2. When administered at meals, it is important to clarify with nursing staff that CF insulin is administered in addition to scheduled prandial insulin. If CF insulin is administered at bedtime, CBG should be rechecked 3 to 4 hours later to determine CF insulin dose efficacy and screen for possible hypoglycemia due to overcorrection.

Adjustments to Insulin Orders

While the patient is admitted to the hospital, it is important to adjust standing insulin orders to achieve the CBG targets discussed above. Stable CBG from bedtime to morning indicates that basal insulin is dosed appropriately and does not need to be adjusted. When CBG increases from bedtime to morning, basal insulin should be increased. If CBG falls significantly from night to morning without the use of CF insulin, basal insulin dose is excessive and should be reduced.

Persistent elevation of CBG values during the day implies that prandial insulin doses (LP) should be increased. The CBG after a dose of mealtime insulin is a measure of how well the dose covered carbohydrate at that meal; for example, lunch CBG is a measure of the efficacy of breakfast prandial insulin. The SIU Pocket Insulin Dosing Card shown in Figure 12-4 gives guidance for adjusting prandial and basal insulin doses. Insulin dosing adjustments for this clinical vignette are presented in Figure 12-3.

Hypoglycemia

A CBG <70 mg/dL is considered mild hypoglycemia, and a CBG <40 mg/dL or an episode of a low blood glucose requiring third-party intervention for resolution is considered severe hypoglycemia. Hypoglycemia should be treated immediately to avoid potential complications such as confusion, loss of consciousness, or seizures. In addition, assessment and adjustment of the current insulin regimen should be performed with every episode of hypoglycemia to decrease the risk of future hypoglycemia.

Mild hypoglycemia should be managed according to the "rule of 15's": 15 g of oral glucose followed by repeat CBG monitoring in 15 minutes. Appropriate sources of supplemental glucose include 4 oz of fruit juice, 6 oz of regular soda, 1 to 2 teaspoons of honey, 3 to 4 glucose tablets, or a tube of glucose gel. The goal of treatment is to raise CBG above 80 mg/dL without causing rebound hyperglycemia. A small snack, which should include a source of protein, may be required after initial treatment to avoid recurrent hypoglycemia, especially if the next meal will be delayed by at least 1 hour.

When patients are too impaired to consume an oral source of glucose safely, either parenteral glucose or glucagon should be administered. A half or full ampule of 50% dextrose (12.5–25 g dextrose) or 125–250 mL of 10% dextrose (12.5–25 g dextrose) can be administered as an IV bolus, or glucagon 0.5–1.0 mg can be given by SC, IM, or IV administration.

Most patients experience a combination of autonomic (palpitations, tremor, anxiety, perspiration, or hunger) and neuroglycopenic (weakness, dizziness, drowsiness, or confusion) symptoms during an episode of hypoglycemia. Patients who do have symptoms of hypoglycemia when CBG is <70 mg/dL usually have an artifactually low CBG. There are multiple causes of artifactually low CBGs in the hospital setting, including residual isopropyl alcohol, poor perfusion, edema, anemia, and supplemental oxygen therapy. In this setting, it is important to repeat the CBG and ensuring that the isopropyl alcohol fully dries before testing. The earlobe is an optional site for CBG testing as it is usually unaffected by poor

Stop all outpatient diabetes medications.

Diabetic diet with 20 to 25 kcal/kg total calories.

Oral medications/new hyperglycemia:

Admit glc <200 mg/dL: 0.5 U/kg per day TDI; admit glc ≥200 mg/dL: 0.6 U/kg per day TDI

Basal insulin + oral medications as outpatient:

Admit glc <200 mg/dL: 0.6 U/kg per day TDI; admit glc ≥200 mg/dL: 0.7 U/kg per day TDI

Basal and prandial insulin as outpatient:

Admit glc <200 mg/dL: greater of TDI = 0.7 U/kg per day or outpatient TDI × 1.2

Admit glc ≥200 mg/dL: greater of TDI = 0.8 U/kg per day or outpatient TDI × 1.3

Standard dosing:

Lantus (Glarg) dose = TDI/2; Humalog (LP) dose (each meal) = TDI/6

Steroid treated:

Lantus (Glarg) dose = TDI/3; Humalog (LP) dose (each meal) = (TDI × 2)/9

Adjustments if glc high:

AM glc >QHS glc	Increase Glarg
AM glc >QHS glc	Increase supper LP
Lunch glc high	Increase breakfast LP
Supper glc high	Increase lunch LP
QHS glc high	Increase supper LP

If glc 141 to 179 mg/dL, increase by 20%.

If glc 180 to 219 mg/dL, increase by 25%.

If glc ≥220 mg/dL, increase by 35%.

Daily adjustments if glc <70 mg/dL:

Use guide for glc high to determine insulin dose to adjust.

If glc <70 mg/dL, decrease by 20%.

If glc <50 mg/dL, decrease by 35%.

Figure 12-4. SIU Pocket Insulin Dosing Guide.

perfusion and edema. However, some patients have hypoglycemia unawareness, although this usually occurs in the setting of longstanding diabetes treated with insulin and complicated by frequent hypoglycemia.

TIPS TO REMEMBER

- Prevalence of diabetes mellitus and hyperglycemia in the hospital is high, and management of hyperglycemia has a significant impact on outcomes, such as hospital length of stay and risk of hospital readmission.

- Ambulatory medications should be stopped and basal/bolus insulin should be substituted for patients admitted to general medicine who are able to eat. Many hospitals have basal/bolus insulin protocols, and there are protocols published in the peer-reviewed literature.

- Correction factor insulin should be administered to treat unanticipated high blood glucoses. If a supplemental insulin dosing protocol is unavailable, the "rule of 1500" can be used to estimate the insulin sensitivity factor and determine correction factor insulin dose.

- Insulin should be adjusted to achieve pre-meal blood glucoses <140 mg/dL and random glucoses <180 mg/dL.

- Mild hypoglycemia should be treated according to the "rule of 15's" (15 g of glucose and repeat capillary blood glucose measurement in 15 minutes). Severe hypoglycemia should be managed with parenteral glucose or glucagon.

SUGGESTED READINGS

American Diabetes Association Professional Practice Committee. 16. Diabetes care in the hospital: standards of medical care in diabetes—2022. *Diabetes Care.* 2022;45(suppl 1):S244–S253.

Capes SE, Hunt D, Malmberg K, et al. Stress hyperglycemia and prognosis of stroke in nondiabetic and diabetic patients: a systematic overview. *Stroke.* 2001;32:2426–2432.

Davidson PC, Hebblewhite HR, Steed RD, Bode BW. Analysis of guidelines for basal-bolus insulin dosing: basal insulin, correction factor, and carbohydrate to insulin ratio. *Endocr Pract.* 2008;14:1095–1101.

Gebreegziabher Y, McCullough PA, Bubb C, et al. Admission hyperglycemia and length of hospital stay in patients with diabetes and heart failure: a prospective cohort study. *Congest Heart Fail.* 2008;14:117–120.

Goyal A, Mehta SR, Diaz R, et al. Differential clinical outcomes associated with hypoglycemia and hyperglycemia in acute myocardial infarction. *Circulation.* 2009;120:2429–2437.

Jakoby M, Alnijoumi M, Soriano S, et al. Impact of a pocket insulin dosing guide on utilization of basal/bolus insulin by internal medicine resident physicians. *Diabetes.* 2012;61(suppl 1):A21–A22.

Jakoby M, Kumar J, Six B, Hall M. Basal/bolus insulin is superior to prevalent methods of diabetes management on the general medicine service at a regional medical center. *Carle Selected Papers.* 2007;50:1–7.

Krinsley JS. Association between hyperglycemia and increased hospital mortality in a heterogeneous population of critically ill patients. *Mayo Clin Proc.* 2003;78:1471–1478.

McAlister FA, Majumdar SR, Blitz S, et al. The relation between hyperglycemia and outcomes in 2,471 patients admitted to the hospital with community acquired pneumonia. *Diabetes Care.* 2005;28:810–815.

Mifflin MD, St. Jeor ST, Hill LA, et al. A new predictive equation for resting energy expenditure in health individuals. *Am J Clin Nutr.* 1990;51:241–247.

Moghissi ES, Korytkowski MT, Dinardo M, et al. American Association of Clinical Endocrinologists and American Diabetes Association consensus statement on inpatient glycemic control. *Diabetes Care.* 2009;32:1119–1131.

Snyder RW, Berns JS. Use of insulin and oral hypoglycemic medications in patients with diabetes mellitus and advanced kidney disease. *Semin Dial.* 2004;17:365–370.

Umpierrez G, Smiley D, Zisman A, et al. Randomized study of basal-bolus insulin therapy in the inpatient management of patients with type 2 diabetes (RABBIT 2 Trial). *Diabetes Care.* 2007;30:2181–2186.

Umpierrez GE, Isaacs SD, Bazargan N, et al. Hyperglycemia: an independent marker of in-hospital mortality in patients with undiagnosed diabetes. *J Clin Endocrinol Metab.* 2002;87:978–982.

Umpierrez GE, Smiley D, Jacobs S, et al. Randomized study of basal–bolus insulin therapy in the inpatient management of patients with type 2 diabetes undergoing general surgery (RABBIT 2 Surgery). *Diabetes Care.* 2011;34:256–261.

Diarrhea in Hospitalized Patients

Ramprasad Jegadeesan, MD and
Sayeeda Azra Jabeen, MD, FACP

A 72-year-old Man With Diarrhea

A 72-year-old man was admitted to the hospital 7 days ago with a fall resulting in a left hip fracture. He underwent successful surgery to repair the hip fracture with an open reduction internal fixation procedure. He has been progressing well with physical therapy. His pain is well controlled with hydrocodone. Other medications include metoprolol, hydrochlorothiazide, simvastatin, docusate, ranitidine, and enoxaparin. He received antibiotics (ceftriaxone) intraoperatively. He has no known drug allergies. He is a nonsmoker and does not drink alcohol. You were called by the nurse today because the patient has developed diarrhea that is described as loose, nonbloody stools. He had 3 episodes yesterday and 1 episode today. His vital signs are normal. His abdominal examination is unremarkable. Rectal examination reveals brown liquid stool in the vault that is Hemoccult negative.

1. What is the most likely etiology of his diarrhea? How would you treat his diarrhea?

Answer

1. This patient's diarrhea is likely medication induced. It is unlikely to be antibiotic-related given that he only received the ceftriaxone intraoperatively and the surgery was a week ago. The most likely offending medications include docusate as well as metoprolol and ranitidine. Non-antibiotic-associated diarrhea (non-AAD) generally improves with removal of the offending medication(s). No additional treatment is usually needed. It is unlikely to be *Clostridium difficile*-induced diarrhea given its mild nature. If patient fails to improve with discontinuation of the offending medications or the diarrhea significantly worsens, one should then consider testing for *Clostridium difficile*.

A 78-year-old Woman With Profuse Diarrhea

A 78-year-old woman was admitted to the hospital 2 weeks ago with community-acquired pneumonia. She was initially started on levofloxacin IV. Despite antibiotics, her condition deteriorated, and she required intubation and mechanical ventilation. In the ICU, her antibiotics were changed to piperacillin, tazobactam, and cefuroxime. Tube feeds were initiated while she was on the ventilator. She improved clinically and was extubated 3 days ago. Since transfer to the general medical floor, she developed profuse, watery, nonbloody diarrhea that is foul smelling. Episodes occur 6 to 8 times per day. She has no fever or chills. Her white blood cell count is elevated to 14,000.

1. What is the most likely etiology of her diarrhea? How would you treat her diarrhea?

Answer

1. *Clostridum difficile*–induced diarrhea is the most likely etiology given her antibiotic usage. The description of the diarrhea is also consistent with *C difficile*–induced diarrhea. Although she was on tube feeds, the clinical course and the elevated white blood cell count make tube feed–induced diarrhea unlikely. She should undergo stool testing for *C difficile* infection with glutamate dehydrogenase enzyme immunoassay (GDH EIA) as the initial step, and then confirming positive results with either nucleic acid amplification testing alone (such as polymerase chain reaction [PCR] or toxin EIA), followed by nucleic acid amplification testing if the toxin EIA is negative. If she tests positive for *C difficile* then she should be treated with a standard regimen of vancomycin (125 mg orally 4 times daily for 10 days).

HOSPITAL-ACQUIRED DIARRHEA

Hospital-acquired diarrhea is defined as 3 or more loose bowel movements per day, for at least 1 day, or a significant increase in stool frequency above baseline and occurring 72 hours after admission.

Diarrhea acquired in the hospital can be broadly classified into 2 major categories:

A. Non-antibiotic-associated diarrhea (non-AAD)
B. Antibiotic-associated diarrhea (AAD)

Non-antibiotic-associated Diarrhea

This diarrhea is caused by agents, other than antibiotics, started during hospitalization. The classic presentation is diarrhea that is benign and self-limited. It

Table 13-1. Medications That Cause Diarrhea

Common Medications Causing Diarrhea Through Nonosmotic Effect	Magnesium-containing Medications	Medications Containing Osmotic Agents	Others Agents Causing Diarrhea
• Colchicine	• Nutritional supplements	• Ingestion of elixir containing sorbitol or mannitol (such as acetaminophen or theophylline)	• Tube feeds (occur in 30% of patients on general medical and surgical floors)
• Chemotherapeutic agents	• Antacids		
• Cholinergic agents	• Laxatives		• Bowel preparation
• Digoxin			
• H_2 blockers			• Contrast agents
• Metformin			
• Metoclopramide			• Fecal impaction/ overflow incontinence
• Misoprostol			
• NSAIDs			
• Olsalazine			
• Propranolol			
• Quinidine			
• Serotonin receptor uptake inhibitors			

is recognized by a lack of constitutional symptoms such as fever, large-volume diarrhea, dehydration, abdominal pain, or leukocytosis. Diarrhea resolves once the offending agent is discontinued.

The pathogenesis of non-AAD is due to nonosmotic means or as a result of recognized side effects of medications. Many drugs contain inert carriers for the active compound. These inert carriers, however, are osmotically active. Inert carriers, such as sorbitol, magnesium, and docusate sodium, may cause diarrhea. Table 13-1 shows the most commonly used medications and agents that cause diarrhea.

Diagnosis

Most episodes of non-AAD do not require any investigation or imaging. A good history, a thorough physical examination, including rectal examination (to assess for fecal impaction), and a thorough chart review to look for any offending agents should be performed. Non-AAD is noninfectious and self-limited, and investigations should be performed only if the results will influence management and outcome. Routine stool examination for enteric pathogens, ova, and parasites is usually unrewarding and not cost-effective. One does not need to and should not order stool studies for ova and parasites in patients with hospital-acquired diarrhea, especially in immunocompetent patients. Fecal white blood cell testing should not be ordered, as it is neither sensitive nor specific. Immunocompromised patients (such as those with organ transplants or late-stage HIV infection) occasionally contract diarrhea due to causes other than *C difficile*, and consultation with a gastroenterologist or an infectious disease physician could be considered if diarrhea persists and no cause is apparent. In the rare situation when a patient is hospitalized after very recent overseas travel and then contracts diarrhea, causes of traveler's diarrhea should be considered. In an outbreak of norovirus, especially if vomiting is present, norovirus testing by reverse transcriptase PCR could be considered.

Treatment

Stable patients with mild symptoms may respond to withdrawal of the offending agent (if any), while patients with moderate or severe symptoms (including those with fever, hypotension, leukocytosis, acute kidney injury, or a decreased serum bicarbonate level) should be tested for *C difficile* infection. Identify and remove the offending agent. Most patients do not require specific therapy, as the diarrhea is self-limiting. Therapy should mainly be directed at preventing dehydration.

Antibiotic-associated Diarrhea

AAD is the most common cause of diarrhea in hospitalized patients, representing an important source of morbidity, mortality, and cost. It is estimated that 10% to 15% of all hospitalized patients treated with antibiotics will develop AAD.

The pathogenesis is due to prolonged use of multiple antibiotics, especially broad-spectrum agents with poor intestinal absorption or high biliary excretion. These antibiotics induce a change in the composition and function of the intestinal flora and therefore result in a higher incidence of AAD. A decrease in the colonic anaerobic flora interferes with carbohydrate and bile acid metabolism. Osmotic or secretory diarrhea may occur. Overgrowth of opportunistic pathogens takes place as a result of microbiologic and metabolic alterations.

AAD can be classified into 2 distinct categories:

I. Diarrhea related to the direct effects of antibiotics

II. Diarrhea related to an enteric pathogen (primarily *C difficile*)

Diarrhea related to the direct effects of antibiotics

Diagnosis: This diarrhea often presents as an annoyance, presenting with frequent loose and watery stools without fever, leukocytosis, or severe abdominal cramps. Diarrhea occurs due to a change in the composition and function of intestinal flora.

Additionally, nonantimicrobial effects of antibiotics can occur. Erythromycin can act as a motilin receptor agonist and accelerate the rate of gastric emptying, thus causing diarrhea. The clavulanate in amoxicillin–clavulanate appears to stimulate small bowel motility, thus causing diarrhea. In rare instances, penicillins may cause segmental colitis, resulting in diarrhea. Some antibiotics, such as clindamycin, cephalosporins, ampicillin, amoxicillin, and amoxicillin–clavulanate, can cause both types of diarrhea.

Typically, no pathogens are identified. There is no diagnostic test specific for benign, self-limiting AAD. One should not order routine stool culture for ova and parasites in patients with hospital-acquired diarrhea, especially in immunocompetent patients with a benign presentation.

Treatment: Effective treatment is generally limited to discontinuation of the implicated agent, with or without therapy with antiperistaltic agents. Probiotics such as those in live-culture yogurt may be helpful. See Table 13-2.

Diarrhea related to enteric pathogens (primarily due to *C difficile* infection)

Enteric pathogen-related diarrhea accounts for 15% to 20% of all AAD cases. The cardinal symptom of the disease is diarrhea, which can range from a mild illness to life-threatening pseudomembranous colitis. *C difficile* infection (CDI) manifests with a profuse, mucous, foul-smelling diarrhea associated with cramps and tenesmus. Frank bleeding is rare, although fecal occult blood and leukocytes are frequently detected. Constitutional symptoms are common and include nausea, vomiting, dehydration, and low-grade fever. Mild leukocytosis is frequently present and may occur even in the absence of diarrhea. An occasional leukemoid reaction can be seen. Diarrhea commonly develops during treatment but may appear as late as 8 weeks after discontinuation of antibiotics. CDI should be highly suspected in patients with leukocytosis of unknown etiology even in the absence of diarrhea, especially in the severely ill elderly, hospitalized patient on antimicrobials, or those who have recently completed a course of antimicrobials, including antifungal agents.

Table 13-2. Antimicrobial Agents That May Induce *Clostridium difficile* Diarrhea or Colitis

Frequently Associated	Occasionally Associated	Rarely Associated
Fluoroquinolones, clindamycin, penicillins (broad spectrum), cephalosporins (broad spectrum)	Macrolides Trimethoprim Sulfonamides	Aminoglycosides, tetracyclines, chloramphenicol, metronidazole, vancomycin (drugs used to treat *C difficile* can rarely cause *C difficile* diarrhea)

C difficile causes diarrhea via toxin-mediated effects on the large bowel. Both *C difficile* toxins A and B exhibit potent enterotoxic and cytotoxic effects that are responsible for the clinical manifestations. Toxic megacolon and subsequent perforation are possible complications if the CDI goes untreated. A dramatic clinical picture of marked colonic distention, peritoneal irritation, fever, and elevated white blood count may occur. Hypoalbuminemia, hypovolemia, and ascites are common features.

Diagnosis: Cytotoxin assay or tissue culture assays are considered to be the gold standard with 94% to 100% sensitivity and 99% specificity, but cell culture tests are expensive and time-consuming, limiting their clinical utility and resulting in delay in both diagnosis and implementation of infection control measures. Enzyme immunoassays (EIAs) are faster. EIAs are available to detect glutamate dehydrogenase (GDH) and toxins A and B, all produced by *C difficile*. The GDH EIA is 92% sensitive and 93% specific but should not be used alone, as it does not distinguish between toxigenic and nontoxigenic strains of *C difficile*. The toxin A/B EIA is 97% specific, but since its sensitivity may be as low as 73%, it too should not be used alone. Nucleic acid amplification tests such as PCR and loop-mediated isothermal amplification (LAMP) identify toxigenic *C difficile* by detecting tcdA, tcdB, or tcdC genes, which regulate toxin production. These tests have sensitivities and specificities well over 90%.

In light of the limited sensitivity of some toxin EIAs and the increased identification of asymptomatic colonization with nucleic acid amplification testing, the optimal approach may be to combine rapid testing methods. Algorithms that include nucleic acid amplification testing have the best sensitivity (68% to 100%) and specificity (92% to 100%). Clinical guidelines suggest using a GDH EIA as the initial step, and then confirming positive results with either nucleic acid amplification testing alone, or toxin EIA followed by nucleic acid amplification testing if the toxin EIA is negative. However, the best diagnostic approach remains controversial, and multistep algorithms may be impractical in some laboratories. Imaging is usually not required in mild cases. Abdominal CT scan in patients with pseudomembranous colitis demonstrates pronounced colonic wall thickening. If suspecting toxic megacolon, a plain abdominal x-ray may show marked colonic distention (>7 cm) or thumbprinting, with or without pneumatosis intestinalis. CT often reveals colonic wall thickening, lumen obliteration, pericolonic fat stranding, and ascites with toxic megacolon.

Treatment: Indication for treatment:

1. Patients with typical CDI manifestations and a positive diagnostic assay.
2. Empiric therapy is indicated when a substantial delay in laboratory confirmation is expected, or for fulminant CDI.

Treatment is *not* indicated in patients who have a positive diagnostic assay but are asymptomatic.

The initial step in the treatment of CDI is tapering the antibiotic regimen and cessation of the inciting antibiotic as soon as possible, as this may influence the risk of CDI recurrence. Infection control practices must be implemented, including contact precautions and hand hygiene. Hand hygiene should include washing using soap and water, as this is more effective than alcohol-based agents in removing *C difficile* spores.

Treatment of initial episode of nonsevere *C difficile* infection

Either vancomycin or fidaxomicin is recommended over metronidazole for an initial episode of CDI. The dosage is vancomycin 125 mg orally 4 times per day or fidaxomicin 200 mg twice daily for 10 days. In settings where access to vancomycin or fidaxomicin is limited, we suggest using metronidazole for an initial episode of nonsevere CDI only. The suggested dosage is metronidazole 500 mg orally 3 times per day for 10 days.

Treatment of Fulminant *C difficile* infection

Fulminant CDI, previously referred to as severe, complicated CDI, may be characterized by hypotension or shock, ileus, or megacolon. For fulminant CDI, vancomycin administered orally is the regimen of choice. If ileus is present, vancomycin can also be administered per rectum. The vancomycin dosage is 500 mg orally 4 times per day and 500 mg in approximately 100 mL normal saline per rectum every 6 hours as a retention enema. Intravenously administered metronidazole should be administered together with oral or rectal vancomycin, particularly if ileus is present. The metronidazole dosage is 500 mg IV every 8 hours. Use of high doses of vancomycin is safe, but elevated serum concentrations have been noted with high doses, prolonged exposure, renal failure, and disrupted intestinal epithelial integrity. Hence, it may be appropriate to monitor trough serum concentration in such circumstances to rule out drug accumulation.

A rising WBC count ($\geq$25,000) or a rising lactate level ($\geq$5 mmol/L) is associated with high mortality and may be helpful in identifying patients whose best hope for survival lies with early surgery. Subtotal colectomy with preservation of the rectum is an established surgical procedure. Diverting loop ileostomy with colonic lavage followed by antegrade vancomycin flushes is an alternative approach that may lead to improved outcomes.

Treatment of Recurrent *C difficile* infection

Relapse is defined as complete resolution of symptoms while a patient is on CDI treatment and reappearance of diarrhea and other symptoms after completion of CDI treatment. Approximately 25% of patients treated for CDI with vancomycin can be expected to experience at least 1 additional episode. Recurrence rates are significantly lower following treatment of an initial CDI episode with fidaxomicin compared with vancomycin.

1. Treat a first recurrence of CDI with oral vancomycin as a tapered and pulsed regimen rather than a second standard 10-day course of vancomycin. After

the usual dosage of 125 mg 4 times per day for 10–14 days, vancomycin is administered at 125 mg 2 times per day for a week, 125 mg once per day for a week, and then 125 mg every 2 or 3 days for 2–8 weeks, in the hope that *C difficile* vegetative forms will be kept in check while allowing restoration of the normal microbiota. Alternatively, 10-day course of fidaxomicin can be used and is preferred over oral vancomycin if available.

2. Antibiotic treatment options for patients with >1 recurrence of CDI include oral fidaxomicin, oral vancomycin therapy using a tapered and pulsed regimen, or a standard course of oral vancomycin followed by rifaximin.

3. Fecal microbiota transplantation is recommended for patients with multiple recurrences of CDI who have failed appropriate antibiotic treatments.

TIPS TO REMEMBER

- Diarrhea acquired in the hospital can be broadly classified into 2 major categories: non-AAD and AAD.

- Laboratory evaluation should only include assessment for *C difficile* and only in patients at risk. Additional stool studies are not needed.

- Oral vancomycin should be the initial treatment of nonsevere CDI. Treatment is not indicated in patients who have a positive *C difficile* diagnostic assay but are asymptomatic.

- In patients with recurrent CDI episodes, we suggest fidaxomicin as the initial treatment regimen rather than oral vancomycin.

SUGGESTED READINGS

Aranda-Michel J, Giannella RA. Acute diarrhea: a practical review. *Am J Med.* 1999;106(6):670–676.

Bagdasarian N, Rao K, Malani PN. Diagnosis and treatment of *Clostridium difficile* in adults: a systematic review. JAMA 2015;313:398–408.

Bartlett JG. Clinical practice. Antibiotic-associated diarrhea. *N Engl J Med.* 2002;346(5):334–339.

Gilligan PH. Diarrheal disease in the hospitalized patient. *Infect Control.* 1986;7(12):607–609.

Johnson S, Lavergne V, Skinner AM, et al. Clinical Practice Guideline by the Infectious Diseases Society of America (IDSA) and Society for Healthcare Epidemiology of America (SHEA): 2021 Focused Update Guidelines on Management of *Clostridioides difficile* Infection in Adults. *Clin Infect Dis.* 2021;73(5)1:e1029–e1044.

Kelly C, Lamont T. Treatment of *Clostridium difficile* infection in adults. In: Calderwood S, Baron E, eds. *UpToDate.* 2012.

Kyne L, Moran A, Keane C, O'Neill D. Hospital-acquired diarrhea in elderly patients: epidemiology and staff awareness. *Age Ageing.* 1998;27(3):339–343.

Lamont T. Clinical manifestations and diagnosis of *Clostridium difficile* infection in adults. In: Calderwood S, Baron E, eds. *UpToDate.* 2012.

Lamont T. Epidemiology, microbiology, and pathophysiology of *Clostridium difficile* infection in adults. In: Calderwood S, Baron E, eds. *UpToDate.* 2012.

McDonald LC, et al. Clinical practice guidelines for *Clostridium difficile* infection in adults and children: 2017 update by the Infectious Diseases Society of America (IDSA) and Society for Healthcare Epidemiology of America (SHEA). *Clin Infect Dis.* 2018;66:e1.

Mullish BH, Williams HR.Clin Med (Lond). *Clostridium difficile* infection and antibiotic-associated diarrhoea. 2018 Jun;18(3):237–241. doi: 10.7861/clinmedicine.18-3-237.PMID: 29858434

Polage CR, Gyorke CE, Kennedy MA, et al. Overdiagnosis of *Clostridium difficile* infection in the molecular test era. *JAMA Intern Med.* 2015;175:1792–1801.

Stern S, Cifu A, Altkorn D. Diarrhea, acute. In: Benoit J, Stein S, eds. *Symptom to Diagnosis: An Evidence Based Guide.* 2nd ed. New York: McGraw-Hill (Lange Clinical Medicine); 2010.

Surawica CM, Brandt LJ, Binion DG, et al. Guidelines for diagnosis, treatment, and prevention of *Clostridium difficile* infections. *Am J Gastroenterol.* 2013;108:478–498.

Thielman NM, Guerrant RL. Clinical practice. Acute infectious diarrhea. *N Engl J Med.* 2004;350(1):38–47.

Yamada T. Approach to the patient with diarrhea. In: Yamada T, ed. *Handbook of Gastroenterology.* Philadelphia: Lippincott Williams & Wilkins; 1998:84–96.

An 86-year-old Woman With Fever and Chills

Zainab Alnafoosi, MD, Muhammad Farooq Asghar, MD and Vidya Sundareshan, MD, MPH

An 86-year-old female with a history of hypertension, COPD, coronary artery disease, and CHF with an ejection fraction (EF) of 40% was admitted to the hospital 4 days ago with respiratory failure secondary to decompensated systolic heart failure. She was intubated in the ED and was transferred to the ICU for further management. In the ICU, she required a central line due to poor IV access. A Foley catheter was placed for urine output monitoring. IV furosemide was given for diuresis, and after 48 hours in the hospital she was successfully extubated. She maintained her oxygen saturation of more than 90% on 4 liters of oxygen. Patient was then transferred to a regular floor. Her medication list includes furosemide 80 mg IV twice daily, lisinopril 40 mg daily, amlodipine 10 mg daily, metoprolol 50 mg twice daily, aspirin 325 mg daily, tiotropium bromide inhaler daily, and enoxaparin 40 mg SC injection daily. Now, 4 days after admission, the patient is complaining of fever and chills since last night. She has no cough, sputum production, postnasal drip, diarrhea, abdominal pain, suprapubic tenderness, or flank pain.

Her vital signs are as follows: temperature 39.2°C, BP 135/85 mm Hg, pulse 110/min, and respiratory rate 18/min. She is awake, alert, and oriented; central line in the internal jugular vein is without evidence of any discharge or surrounding erythema. There is pedal edema bilaterally. Cardiac examination shows a normal S1 and S2 without any gallops or murmur; respiratory examination shows vesicular breathing with bibasilar crackles (which have improved since admission). Abdomen is soft and nontender, and bowel sounds are normal. Neurologic examination is nonfocal. Skin examination does not reveal any abnormalities. The patient still has a Foley catheter in place.

1. What is the diagnosis?

2. What is your next step in evaluation?

Answers

1. The patient has a nosocomial fever at present, which is defined as a fever of at least 38.3°C occurring in a hospitalized patient 48 hours or more after admission in whom neither fever nor infection was present on admission.

2. Once we have confirmed the fever, the next step is figuring out its source. The patient has had a thorough history and physical examination, which failed to reveal any etiology of fever, so we will start our evaluation with CBC, CMP, 2 sets of blood cultures, urinalysis, and a chest x-ray.

Fever is a sign of inflammation, not infection. It is not a specific response to infection, but rather is a response to any form of tissue injury that is sufficient to trigger an inflammatory response. Proinflammatory cytokines, the hypothalamus, and cellular and end-organ systems may be triggered by microorganisms, exogenous pyrogens, tissue inflammation, ischemia, or injury. This might explain why some hospitalized patients with fever have no apparent infection. Studies indicate that among patients with nosocomial fever, 40% to 70% of cases are caused by infectious etiologies, including hospital-associated infections with antimicrobial-resistant organisms, while 15% to 50% of the cases originate from noninfectious etiologies such as malignancies, postprocedure or postsurgical conditions, or organ ischemia. In 10% to 30% of cases, the etiology is unclear. The distinction between inflammation and infection is an important one, not only for the evaluation of fever but also for curtailing the use of antibiotics to treat fever. The degree of fever is not an indication of the presence or severity of infection. High-grade fevers can be associated with noninfectious processes (eg, drug fever), while fever can sometimes be mild or absent in patients with life-threatening infections.

FEVER IN HOSPITALIZED PATIENTS

For several reasons, fever that develops in hospitalized patients warrants a thoughtful evaluation. First, hospitalized patients are usually severely ill and often have complex underlying illnesses. Second, organisms commonly found in nosocomial infections in seriously ill patients include *Staphylococcus aureus*, *Enterococcus*, gram-negative bacilli, and fungi. Infections due to these organisms are characterized by necrotizing destruction of tissue and high rates of associated bloodstream invasion. Third, hospital-acquired organisms are likely to exhibit broad resistance to antimicrobials, making appropriate selection of antibiotic therapy more challenging. Additionally, infections with multidrug-resistant organisms (MDROs) lead to longer lengths of stay and increased health care costs. Finally, fever may herald exacerbation or progression of the disease that prompted hospitalization.

Diagnosis

If the patient is able to communicate, he or she should be interviewed to take a detailed history and identify localizing complaints. The patient's verbal history and the hospital chart should be reviewed thoroughly for history of relevant antecedent problems (eg, prior postoperative infections with MDROs, renal disease, adverse reactions to drugs). If the patient is unable to communicate, the chart and medical personnel can provide helpful information concerning duration of intravascular accesses, catheters, amount and purulence of sputum or wound drainage, changes in skin condition, apparent abdominal or musculoskeletal pain or tenderness, difficulty in handling respiratory secretions and feeding, consistency of bowel movements, and changes in requirements for supplemental oxygen.

A thorough physical examination is invaluable:

- Skin examination may demonstrate findings suggestive of drug reaction, vasculitis, endocarditis, or soft tissue necrosis.

- All IV and intra-arterial line sites should be inspected; a tender IV access site, with or without purulence, can indicate septic thrombophlebitis. Spreading erythema, warmth, and tenderness that appear to indicate cellulitis of an extremity also can be the hallmarks of deep venous thrombophlebitis, pyarthrosis, or gout.

- After the first 24 hours postoperatively, wounds should be examined; this may require fenestrating or changing a cast to allow examination of a fractured extremity if no other source of fever is found.

- Head and neck examination can provide important signs of systemic and localized infection.

- Purulent sinusitis can occur in nasally or orally intubated patients and may have a paucity of associated symptoms.

- Cardiac examination may demonstrate a pericardial friction rub due to Dressler syndrome in a patient with an acute myocardial infarction; a new or changing murmur might be due to endocarditis.

- Abdominal findings can be misleadingly unremarkable in the elderly, in patients with an obtunded sensorium, and in patients receiving sedatives. They may be confounding in the patient with recent abdominal or thoracic surgery. Abdominal pain and tenderness may be localized (cholecystitis, intra-abdominal abscess, diverticulitis) or generalized (diffuse peritonitis, ischemic bowel, antibiotic-associated colitis). Examination of the genitalia and rectum may demonstrate epididymitis, prostatitis, prostatic abscess, or perirectal abscess. Blood cultures are the only mandatory diagnostic test in patients with a new fever; the rationale is that clinical findings cannot reliably exclude bacteremia and mortality is high without appropriate treatment. Remember to obtain at least 2 sets of blood cultures from separate venipuncture sites prior to initiation of antimicrobial therapy. Each set of blood cultures should include 2 bottles (both aerobic and anaerobic). This practice increases the yield of blood cultures and helps in distinguishing true bacteremia from contamination. Further investigations may be indicated depending on the clinical assessment.

- Sputum: Sputum Gram stain and culture are indicated for febrile patients with any of the following findings—new sputum production; a change in the color, amount, or thickness of their sputum; a new or progressive pulmonary infiltrate; an increased respiratory rate; or increased oxygenation requirements.

- Urine: Urinalysis and urine culture are indicated for febrile patients with urinary symptoms, a urethral catheter, urinary obstruction, renal calculi, recent genitourinary surgery, or neutropenia.

- Chest imaging: A chest radiograph is easily obtainable in the hospital and worthwhile in many patients with respiratory symptoms or signs. It may detect a new or progressive pulmonary infiltrate and identify a respiratory source of fever other than pneumonia or tracheobronchitis that would otherwise be missed because it may not be associated with sputum production.

- Laboratory studies: Transaminases, bilirubin, alkaline phosphatase, amylase, lipase, and lactate measurements are indicated for patients with abdominal pain or whose abdominal examination cannot be reliably assessed. Serum sodium, potassium, glucose, and cortisol levels should be drawn if adrenal insufficiency is in the differential. Thyroid-stimulating hormone (TSH), T3, and T4 levels should be drawn if thyroid storm is expected. Blood should be drawn for measurement of direct antiglobulin, plasma free hemoglobin, and haptoglobin, as well as a repeat blood type and crossmatch if an acute hemolytic transfusion reaction is suspected.

- Abdominal imaging: Abdominal imaging is indicated for patients with symptoms or signs of an intra-abdominal process but for whom laboratory testing has not identified the cause of the symptoms or signs. It is also indicated for patients who have a reason to have an intra-abdominal infection and no alternative source of the fever has been identified, even if there are no symptoms or signs of an abdominal process.

- Sinus evaluation: Evaluation for sinusitis is appropriate for patients with purulent nasal drainage and recent mechanical ventilation or whose evaluation has otherwise been completely negative. The evaluation begins with a radiographic evaluation looking for sinus opacification. CT is the preferred modality. Culture of sinus fluid obtained by endoscopic-guided middle meatus aspiration is indicated for patients with sinus opacification and persistent fevers in absence of other obvious causes for fever.

- It is imperative to keep a broad differential diagnosis when investigating a nosocomial fever. Clinicians should remain mindful that hospitalized patients may have more than 1 infection. Also, signs of infection and inflammation (eg, leukocytosis) may be altered in immunocompromised patients. Keep in mind that previously acquired infections may be unmasked during hospitalization especially in immunocompromised patients with prolonged hospitalization and critical illness (eg, some cases of invasive aspergillosis).

Treatment

Treatment of fever should be directed at its underlying causes, some of which are discussed in separate chapters in this book.

Perhaps the 2 most important clinical questions that need to be answered when a patient develops a new fever in the hospital are as follows:

1) Is empiric or presumptive antibiotic therapy warranted?

2) Do we need to remove the patient's intravascular catheter?

- Hospitalized patients who develop a new fever should be treated with empiric antibiotics if they are deteriorating, in shock, or neutropenic, or if they have a ventricular assist device. Empiric therapy should also be started for patients who have a temperature ≥38.9°C because most fevers in this range will be infectious. For other patients, further diagnostic workup with ongoing clinical assessment prior to the initiation of antibiotic therapy is reasonable.

- Whether to routinely remove an intravascular catheter (or other devices) in a febrile patient is a controversial and evolving issue. In general, factors to take into consideration are the severity of illness, age of the catheter, and probability that the catheter is the source of fever.

- Fever itself does not generally require treatment with antipyretics (eg, acetaminophen) or external cooling (eg, cooling blanket, ice packs). Exceptions to this are when the fever may be detrimental to the outcome (eg, increased intracranial pressure) or is ≥41.0°C. If body temperature exceeds the "critical thermal maximum," which is thought to be 41.6°C, life-threatening complications can ensue (eg, rhabdomyolysis, organ failure).

Fever in hospitalized patients can be categorized into infectious and noninfectious causes.

Common causes of fever in hospitalized patients include the following:

A. *Infections*
  1. Pneumonia
  2. UTI
  3. Catheter-related bloodstream infections (CRBSIs)
  4. Surgical site infection
  5. *Clostridium difficile* colitis
  6. Sinusitis
  7. Abdominal abscess
  8. Other infections

B. *Noninfectious causes*
  1. Drug-induced fever
  2. Reaction to blood products
  3. Deep venous thrombosis

4. Pulmonary embolism (PE)

5. Infarctions

6. Acute pancreatitis

7. Acalculous cholecystitis

8. Adrenal insufficiency

9. Malignant hyperthermia

10. Neuroleptic malignant syndrome (NMS)

11. Serotonin syndrome (SS)

12. Postoperative fever

13. Fever related to procedures

Infections in hospitalized patients

Hospital-acquired pneumonia Hospital-acquired (or nosocomial) pneumonia (HAP) is pneumonia that occurs 48 hours or more after admission and did not appear to be incubating at the time of admission.

The most common organisms responsible for HAP are *Pseudomonas aeruginosa, Staphylococcus aureus including methicillin-resistant S aureus (MRSA), Enterobacter, Klebsiella pneumoniae, Escherichia coli, Proteus, Serratia marcescens, Haemophilus influenzae,* and streptococci. Additional information can be found in Chapter 22. The symptoms and signs associated with HAP include fever, cough, increasing oxygen requirements, purulent sputum, and abnormal breath sounds.

UTI in hospitalized patients Nosocomial urinary tract infections are a common complication in hospitalized patients. The use of urinary catheters is the major risk factor for the development of these infections. Urinary tract infection should be suspected as a cause of nosocomial fever in any patient who has had an indwelling bladder catheter for more than a few days. The diagnosis of urinary tract infection is difficult in chronically catheterized patients because these catheters tend to be colonized with bacteria. Therefore, a positive urine culture does not always reflect infection in a chronically instrumented patient. Additional information can be found in Chapter 42.

Catheter-related bloodstream infection (CRBSI) Infections caused by indwelling vascular catheters should be suspected in any case of unexplained fever when a catheter has been in place for more than 48 hours, or when purulence is found at the catheter insertion site. Other clinical manifestations include hemodynamic instability, altered mental status, catheter dysfunction (as occurs with intraluminal clot), and clinical signs of sepsis that start abruptly after catheter infusion. Complications related to a bloodstream infection (eg, suppurative thrombophlebitis, endocarditis, osteomyelitis, metastatic infection) also may be observed.

Microbiologic confirmation of CRBSI may be made based on blood cultures obtained prior to initiation of antibiotic therapy, and with exclusion of alternative sources for blood stream infection. Ideally, at least 2 sets of blood cultures should be obtained from peripheral veins via separate venipuncture sites. When this is not feasible, 1 blood culture set from set may be drawn peripherally and the other blood culture set may be drawn from the catheter hub. Do not draw blood cultures solely from the catheter hub since this site is commonly colonized with skin flora.

In general, the first step for treatment of systemic IV catheter-related infection requires a determination regarding catheter management.

Catheter removal is warranted in the following circumstances:

- Severe sepsis
- Hemodynamic instability
- Endocarditis or evidence of metastatic infection
- Erythema or exudate due to suppurative thrombophlebitis
- Persistent bacteremia after 72 hours of antimicrobial therapy to which the organism is susceptible
- Bloodstream infections such as *Candida* spp, *S aureus*, or *P aeruginosa*

Catheters that have been left in place should be removed if cultures confirm the presence of catheter-related septicemia. There are 2 situations in which catheters can be left in place if the patient shows a favorable response to antimicrobial therapy:

A. When catheter removal is not easily accomplished (eg, tunneled catheters)

B. When the responsible organism is *Staphylococcus epidermidis*

However, relapse after systemic antimicrobial therapy is higher when catheters have been left in place, and this relapse is less likely when antibiotic lock therapy is used.

Empiric antibiotic therapy for CRBSI in health care settings should include agents with activity against MRSA; vancomycin is a reasonable agent. Patients with neutropenia or sepsis should also receive empiric antibiotic therapy for gram-negative organisms (including *Pseudomonas*). Patients known to be colonized with drug-resistant organisms should receive empiric antibiotic therapy selected in view of their pertinent previous cultures; therapy should be tailored based on subsequent culture data. Following initiation of empiric treatment, antibiotic therapy should be tailored in light of culture and susceptibility results once data are available.

Transesophageal echocardiogram (TEE) should be pursued in the setting of *S aureus* bacteremia to rule out infective endocarditis (IE). Possible exceptions include patients whose fever and bacteremia resolve within 72 hours following catheter removal and who have no underlying cardiac predisposing conditions or clinical signs of endocarditis.

In general, for uncomplicated CRBSI with negative blood cultures following catheter removal and institution of appropriate antibiotic therapy, the duration of therapy is 10 to 14 days (day 1 being the first day on which negative blood cultures are obtained). Patients with persistent bacteremia >72 hours following catheter removal should receive treatment for at least 4 to 6 weeks. For patients with complications related to bacteremia (such as suppurative thrombophlebitis, endocarditis, osteomyelitis, or metastatic infection), the duration of therapy should be tailored accordingly depending on the nature of infection. Patients with CRBSI must be monitored closely during and following therapy to detect relapses or signs of metastatic infection. Blood cultures should be drawn after treatment has been initiated to demonstrate clearance of bacteremia. Repeatedly positive blood cultures and/or persistent symptoms 72 hours after catheter removal with appropriate antibiotic therapy should prompt evaluation for sequelae of CRBSI such as those listed above.

Surgical site infection In hospitalized patients who have undergone surgical procedures, fever may develop due to surgical site infection. Wound infections typically appear at 5 to 7 days after surgery. Most infections do not extend beyond the skin and subcutaneous tissues and can be managed with debridement and antimicrobial therapy to cover *Streptococcus*, *Staphylococcus*, and anaerobes.

Necrotizing wound infections are produced by clostridia or β-hemolytic streptococci. Unlike other wound infections, which appear 5 to 7 days after surgery, necrotizing infections are evident in the first few postoperative days. There is often marked edema around the incision, and the skin may have crepitus and fluid-filled bullae. Spread to deeper structures is rapid and produces progressive rhabdomyolysis and myoglobinuric renal failure. Treatment involves extensive debridement and IV antibiotics. The mortality is high (above 60%) when treatment is delayed.

Clostridium difficile colitis Enterocolitis from *C difficile* should be suspected in cases of nosocomial fever accompanied by watery diarrhea especially in patients who have received antibiotics or chemotherapy within 2 weeks. The diagnosis requires documentation of *C difficile* toxin in stool samples or evidence of pseudomembranes on proctosigmoidoscopy.

Empiric antibiotics should not be necessary unless the diarrhea is severe or the patient appears toxic. Therapy can include oral vancomycin or fidaxomicin for 10 to 14 days with the first episode. Although rarely necessary, surgical intervention is required when *C difficile* colitis is associated with progressive sepsis, ileus, toxic megacolon, or signs of peritonitis despite antibiotic therapy. The procedure of choice is subtotal colectomy. Additional information can be found in Chapter 13.

Sinusitis Fever due to sinusitis should be considered in patients who were recently intubated or have indwelling nasogastric or nasotracheal tubes. Evaluation for sinusitis is appropriate for patients with purulent nasal drainage or whose evaluation has otherwise been completely negative. The evaluation begins with a radiograph looking for sinus opacification. CT is the preferred modality. Culture of sinus fluid obtained by endoscopic-guided middle meatus aspiration is indicated for patients with sinus opacification and no other cause for fever. Additional information can be found in Chapter 41.

Abdominal abscess An abdominal abscess may present with fever. Patients who undergo abdominal surgeries are at risk. Abdominal abscesses typically become symptomatic 1 to 2 weeks after laparotomy. Septicemia occurs in approximately 50% of cases. CT of the abdomen will reveal the localized collection in more than 95% of cases. Initial antimicrobial therapy should be directed at gram-negative enteric pathogens, including anaerobes (eg, *Bacteroides fragilis*), but definitive treatment requires surgical or percutaneous drainage.

Other infections Other infections that should be considered in selected patient populations are endocarditis (in patients with prosthetic valves), meningitis (in neurosurgical patients and those with HIV infection), and spontaneous bacterial peritonitis (in patients with cirrhosis and ascites).

Noninfectious causes

Drug-induced fever Drug-induced fever can be the result of a hypersensitivity reaction, an idiosyncratic reaction, or an infusion-related phlebitis. The therapeutic agents most often implicated in drug fever are amphotericin, cephalosporins, penicillin, phenytoin, procainamide, quinidine, vancomycin, cimetidine, carbamazepine, hydralazine, and rifampin. The onset of the fever varies from a few hours to a few weeks after the initiation of drug therapy. The fever can appear as an isolated finding or can be accompanied by other manifestations such as rigors, myalgias, leukocytosis, eosinophilia, rash, and hypotension. Approximately half of patients have rigors, and about 20% develop hypotension, indicating that patients with drug fever can appear to be seriously ill which further complicates the clinical picture.

Drug fever is a diagnosis of exclusion. In most patients, the only way to know if a patient has a drug fever is by stopping the offending drug(s). The usual approach is to discontinue the most probable offending drug first, followed sequentially by cessation of other drugs if fever persists. Discontinuing all medications at once may eliminate the fever but may also put the patient at risk from the underlying disease and prevent identification of the causative drug. In most cases, resolution of drug fever will occur within 72 to 96 hours of discontinuing the offending drug.

Reaction to blood products Hospitalized patients who receive blood products can develop fever either due to acute hemolytic or nonhemolytic febrile reactions, or sometimes due to bloodborne transmission of infections. Additional information can be found in Chapter 28.

Deep venous thrombosis DVT can present with fever, although more common manifestations of DVT include asymmetric extremity edema, pain, or erythema.

In a hospitalized febrile patient, if no other etiology for fever is identified, the patient should be evaluated with venous Doppler of both lower extremities. Additional information can be found in Chapter 29.

Pulmonary embolism Fever in hospitalized patients can be associated with PE. The most common symptoms of acute PE are dyspnea (at rest or with exertion), pleuritic pain, cough, calf pain, or swelling. The most common signs are tachypnea, tachycardia, rales, decreased breath sounds, an accentuated pulmonic component of the second heart sound, and jugular venous distension. Additional information can be found in Chapter 29.

Infarctions Ischemic injury in any organ will trigger a local inflammatory response, and this can produce a fever. Myocardial and cerebrovascular infarctions are usually heralded by other symptoms, but bowel infarction can be clinically silent in elderly, debilitated patients, or patients with depressed consciousness. The only sign of a bowel infarction may be an unexplained fever or metabolic (lactic) acidosis. Additional information can be found in Chapters 1, 3, and 26.

Acute pancreatitis Fever can be a prominent symptom in acute pancreatitis. Additional information can be found in Chapter 1.

Acalculous cholecystitis Acalculous cholecystitis is an uncommon but serious disorder reported in up to 1.5% of critically ill patients. The clinical manifestations of acalculous cholecystitis include fever, nausea, vomiting, abdominal pain, and right upper quadrant tenderness. Abdominal findings can be minimal or absent, and fever may be the only presenting manifestation. Elevations in serum bilirubin, alkaline phosphatase, and amylase can occur but are variable. Additional information can be found in Chapter 1.

Adrenal insufficiency An adrenal crisis usually occurs in patients with previously undiagnosed adrenal insufficiency when subjected to a serious infection or other major stress, patients with known adrenal insufficiency who do not take stress-dose glucocorticoid during a serious infection or other major stress, patients with acute bilateral adrenal infarction or hemorrhage, or patients whose chronic glucocorticoid therapy is abruptly withdrawn. Distributive shock is the predominant manifestation of an adrenal crisis, but fever, nausea, vomiting, abdominal pain, weakness, fatigue, lethargy, hypoglycemia, confusion, or coma also may be present. Acute adrenal crisis is more commonly seen in primary adrenal insufficiency (Addison disease) than in disorders of the pituitary gland causing secondary adrenocortical hypofunction.

An early morning low serum cortisol concentration (<3 μg/dL [<80 nmol/L]) is strongly suggestive of adrenal insufficiency. The diagnosis is made by cosyntropin stimulation test, which tests the ability of ACTH to increase cortisol production. Failure of an appropriate rise in cortisol levels in response to ACTH indicates primary adrenal insufficiency. If the diagnosis is suspected acutely, draw a blood sample for cortisol determination and treat with IV hydrocortisone.

Malignant hyperthermia   A rare but important cause of elevated body temperatures in the immediate postoperative period is malignant hyperthermia. It is an inherited disorder with an autosomal dominant pattern, and it is characterized by excessive release of calcium from the sarcoplasmic reticulum in skeletal muscle in response to halogenated inhaled anesthetic agents (eg, halothane, isoflurane, desflurane) and depolarizing neuromuscular blockers (eg, succinylcholine). The calcium influx into the cell cytoplasm somehow leads to an uncoupling of oxidative phosphorylation and a marked rise in metabolic rate.

The clinical manifestations of malignant hyperthermia include hypercapnia, muscle rigidity, increased body temperature, depressed consciousness, and autonomic instability. The generalized muscle rigidity can progress rapidly to widespread myonecrosis (rhabdomyolysis) and subsequent myoglobinuric renal failure. The heat generated by the muscle rigidity is responsible for the marked rise in body temperature (often above 40°C) in malignant hyperthermia. The altered mental status in malignant hyperthermia can range from confusion and agitation to obtundation and coma. Autonomic instability can lead to cardiac arrhythmias, fluctuating blood pressure, or persistent hypotension.

The first suspicion of malignant hyperthermia should prompt immediate discontinuation of the offending anesthetic agent. Specific treatment for muscle rigidity is with dantrolene sodium, a muscle relaxant that blocks the release of calcium from the sarcoplasmic reticulum. When given early in the course of malignant hyperthermia, dantrolene can reduce the mortality rate from 70% or higher (in untreated cases) to 10% or less. Treatment is extended to 3 days to prevent recurrences. Patients should be aggressively hydrated to keep adequate urine output, and cooling blankets should be used to keep body temperature below 38.5°C. Electrolytes and renal functions as well as blood counts should be monitored closely because patients can develop electrolyte imbalance and renal failure due to rhabdomyolysis. They are also prone to develop DIC.

Neuroleptic malignant syndrome   NMS is strikingly similar to malignant hyperthermia in that it is a drug-induced disorder characterized by four clinical features: increased body temperature, muscle rigidity, altered mental status, and autonomic instability. As the name implies, NMS is caused by neuroleptic agents (antipsychotic medications). Note that drugs other than neuroleptic agents can trigger NMS, so the name of this syndrome may be misleading.

Most cases of NMS begin to appear 24 to 72 hours after the initiation of drug therapy, and almost all cases are apparent in the first 2 weeks of drug therapy. The onset is usually gradual and can take days to fully develop. In 80% of cases, the initial manifestation is muscle rigidity or altered mental status. The change in mental status can range from confusion and agitation to obtundation and coma. Hyperthermia is a defining symptom, with temperatures of more than 38°C in most patients. Autonomic instability can produce cardiac tachyarrhythmias, labile blood pressure, and tachypnea.

The serum CK level is typically more than 1000 U/L in NMS. Leukocytosis with left shift may be present, with WBC counts up to 40,000/μL. The clinical presentation of NMS can be easily confused with sepsis. The serum CK level will distinguish NMS from sepsis, however.

The single most important measure in the management of NMS is immediate removal of the offending drug. If NMS is caused by discontinuation of dopaminergic therapy, it should be restarted immediately with plans for a gradual reduction in dosage at a later time. General measures, including volume resuscitation and evaluation for multiorgan involvement (eg, rhabdomyolysis), are the same as described for malignant hyperthermia.

Dantrolene sodium can be given intravenously for severe cases of muscle rigidity. Bromocriptine is a dopamine agonist that has been used successfully in treating NMS when given orally at a dose of 2.5 to 10 mg 3 times daily. Some improvement in muscle rigidity can be seen within hours after the start of therapy, but the full response often takes days to develop. Hypotension is a troublesome side effect. There is no advantage of bromocriptine over dantrolene, except in patients with advanced liver disease (where dantrolene is not advised). Benzodiazepines can be used as adjunctive therapy in moderate to severe cases. Treatment of NMS should continue for about 10 days after clinical resolution because of delayed clearance of many neuroleptics (2–3 weeks of treatment if depot preparations are implicated).

Serotonin syndrome Another important cause of fever in hospitalized patients is serotonin syndrome (SS). Overstimulation of serotonin receptors in the central nervous system produces a combination of mental status changes, autonomic hyperactivity, and neuromuscular abnormalities. The severity of illness can vary widely, and the most severe cases can be confused with any of the other hyperthermia syndromes.

There are several serotonergic drugs that are capable of producing serotonin syndrome. These include the following:

- Drugs that decrease serotonin breakdown such as MAOIs (including linezolid)
- Drugs that increase serotonin release such as amphetamines, MDMA ("ecstasy"), cocaine, and fenfluramine
- Drugs that decrease serotonin reuptake such as SSRIs, TCAs, dextromethorphan, meperidine, fentanyl, and tramadol
- Serotonin receptor agonists such as lithium, sumatriptan, buspirone, and LSD

The onset of serotonin syndrome is usually abrupt (in contrast to NMS, where the full syndrome can take days to develop), and more than half of the cases are evident within 6 hours after ingestion of the responsible drug(s). The clinical findings include mental status changes (eg, confusion, delirium, coma), autonomic hyperactivity (eg, mydriasis, tachycardia, hypertension, hyperthermia, diaphoresis), and neuromuscular abnormalities (eg, hyperkinesis, hyperactive deep tendon reflexes, clonus, muscle rigidity). The clinical presentation can vary markedly. Mild cases may include only hyperkinesis, hyperreflexia, tachycardia, diaphoresis, and mydriasis. Moderate cases often have additional findings of hyperthermia (temperature >38°C), clonus, and agitation. The clonus is most obvious in the patellar deep tendon reflexes, and horizontal ocular clonus also may be present. Severe cases of SS often present with delirium, hyperpyrexia (temperature >40°C), widespread muscle rigidity, and spontaneous clonus. Life-threatening cases are marked by rhabdomyolysis, renal failure, metabolic acidosis, and hypotension.

The first step in the diagnostic evaluation is to establish recent ingestion of 1 or more serotonergic drugs. Hyperthermia and muscle rigidity can be absent in mild cases of the illness. The features that most distinguish SS from other hyperthermia syndromes are hyperkinesis, hyperreflexia, and clonus. However, in severe cases of SS, muscle rigidity can mask these clinical findings. Severe cases of SS can be difficult to distinguish from malignant hyperthermia and neuromuscular malignant syndrome, and the history of drug ingestion is important in these cases too (note that some drugs can be implicated in both NMS and SS).

As is the case with all drug-induced hyperthermia syndromes, removal of the precipitating drug(s) is the single most important element in the management. The remainder of the management includes measures to control agitation and hyperthermia, and the use of serotonin antagonists. Many cases of SS resolve within 24 hours after initiation of therapy, but serotonergic drugs with longer half-lives can produce more prolonged symptomatology.

Benzodiazepines are considered essential for the control of agitation and hyperkinesis in SS. Physical restraints should be avoided because they encourage isometric muscle contractions, and this can aggravate skeletal muscle injury and promote lactic acidosis.

Cyproheptadine is a serotonin antagonist that can be given in severe cases of SS. Neuromuscular paralysis may be required in severe cases of SS to control muscle rigidity and extreme elevations of body temperature (41°C). Nondepolarizing agents (eg, vecuronium) should be used for muscle paralysis because succinylcholine can aggravate the hyperkalemia that accompanies rhabdomyolysis. Dantrolene is not effective in reducing the muscle rigidity and hyperthermia in SS.

Postoperative fever Surgery always involves some degree of tissue injury, and major surgery can involve considerable tissue injury. Because inflammation and fever are the normal response to tissue injury, fever is a likely consequence of major surgery. Fever in the first day following a major surgery is reported in 15% to 40% of patients, and in most of these cases, there is no associated infection. These fevers are short-lived and usually resolve within 24 to 48 hours. If the fever is very high, the patient has other systemic symptoms, or fever lasts beyond 48 hours, a thorough evaluation looking for an infectious process should be done.

Fever related to procedures The following procedures or interventions can be accompanied by noninfectious fever:

A. Hemodialysis: Febrile reactions during hemodialysis can be attributed to endotoxin contamination of the dialysis equipment, but endovascular infections including access-related infection remain on the differential. Blood cultures are recommended for all patients who develop fever during hemodialysis, but the dialysis does not have to be terminated unless the patient shows signs of sepsis (eg, mental status changes or hypotension). Empiric antibiotics are recommended for patients who appear septic. Vancomycin and ceftazidime are appropriate empiric antibiotics to be used pending culture results.

B. Bronchoscopy: Fiber-optic bronchoscopy is followed by fever in 5% of cases. The fever usually appears 8 to 10 hours after the procedure, and it subsides spontaneously in 24 hours. The probable cause is release of endogenous pyrogens from the lung during the procedure. The fever is often associated with leukocytosis, but pneumonia and bacteremia are rare. There is no need for blood cultures or empiric antimicrobial therapy unless the fever does not subside or the patient shows signs of sepsis (eg, mental status changes, hypotension).

TIPS TO REMEMBER

● History and physical examination are the most important parts of your evaluation of a hospitalized patient with fever.

● Etiologies include infectious and noninfectious causes.

● Blood cultures are the only mandatory test in hospitalized patients with new-onset fever.

● Additional workup should be targeted based on the clinical scenario and clues obtained from your history and physical examination.

COMPREHENSION QUESTIONS

Refer back to the 86-year-old patient with fever described at the beginning of the chapter.

The patient has several risk factors for the development of nosocomial infections. These include Foley catheter, central venous catheter, recent intubation, and mechanical ventilation. The patient's laboratory studies show a WBC count of 16,000 with a neutrophilia of 85%. Renal function, AST, ALT, and alkaline phosphatase are all within normal range. Her urine is positive for high leukocyte esterase and has WBCs of 42 per high-power field and many bacteria. Her chest x-ray shows improving pulmonary edema and infiltrates. Blood cultures showed no growth.

1. What is your next step?
2. When should a catheter-related bacteriuria be treated?
3. If a patient has a vascular catheter and develops fever, under which circumstances should the catheter be removed?

Answers

1. Once it is established that the patient has a UTI, urine cultures should be sent, Foley catheter removed (or exchanged if ongoing catheterization is still indicated), and antibiotics started empirically. The antibiotics can be modified once culture results are available. This patient was started on vancomycin and cefepime and her urine cultures later grew >100,000 cfu/mL of enterococci that were sensitive to ampicillin, vancomycin, and nitrofurantoin. Her blood cultures remained negative for 5 days. The patient completed a 5-day course of ampicillin. Her fever subsided after 48 hours of starting the antibiotics. Foley catheter was removed after evaluating the patient and determining no further need for ongoing catheterization.

2. Symptomatic catheter-related bacteriuria should be treated. It is usually referred to as catheter-associated UTI. It is defined as the presence of fever >38°C, suprapubic tenderness, costovertebral angle tenderness, or otherwise unexplained systemic symptoms such as altered mental status, hypotension, or sepsis, together with urine culture that shows significant growth of bacteria (typically >100,000 cfu/mL). Patients who are no longer catheterized but had indwelling urinary catheters within the past 48 hours also are considered to have catheter-associated UTI if they meet these criteria.

Note that patients with indwelling urinary catheters have high rates of bacteriuria. This does not always infer urinary tract infection. Results of urinalysis and urine culture should be interpreted carefully in conjunction with clinical correlation.

3. Endovascular catheter removal is warranted in the following circumstances:
- Severe sepsis
- Hemodynamic instability
- Endocarditis or evidence of metastatic infection
- Erythema or exudate due to suppurative thrombophlebitis
- Persistent bacteremia after 72 hours of antimicrobial therapy to which the organism is susceptible
  - Subcutaneously tunneled central venous catheter tunnel tract infection or subcutaneous port reservoir infection
  - Infection with highly virulent organisms such as *S aureus, P aeruginosa,* and *Candida* species.

In the absence of the above-mentioned criteria, catheter salvage is reasonable if the infection was due to coagulase-negative Staphylococci or drug-susceptible Enterobacterales. In this case it is recommended to treat with systemic antibiotic therapy in conjunction with antibiotic lock therapy.

SUGGESTED READINGS

Dankul P, Karaketklang K, Jitmuang A. Nosocomial fever in general medical wards: a prospective cohort study of clinical characteristics and outcomes. *Infect Drug Resist.* 2021;14:3873–3881.

Irwin RS, Rippe JM, eds. *Irwin and Rippe's Intensive Care Medicine.* 6th ed. Philadelphia: Lippincott Williams and Wilkins; 2007:1015–1022.

Marino PL, Sutin KM. *The ICU Book.* 3rd ed. Philadelphia: Lippincott Williams and Wilkins; 2006:713–733.

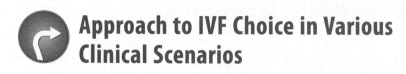

Approach to IVF Choice in Various Clinical Scenarios

Mohammed Al Hosaini, MD and Bemi (Oritsegbubemi) Adekola, MD

IV FLUID MANAGEMENT

Case 1

A 55-year-old female had a right total knee replacement done 1 day ago. She was started on lactated Ringer's at 120 mL/h. The patient has a history of hypertension, diastolic heart failure, and CKD stage III. Her current medications are morphine, atenolol, and ondansetron. The patient has been doing fine except for the pain at her surgery site. Her appetite is still poor due to her morphine-induced nausea. Her vitals are within normal limits, and the physical examination is not significant. Her labs show the following:

     Sodium: 138
     Potassium: 5.8
     Chloride: 100
     Bicarbonate: 24
     Blood urea nitrogen: 20
     Creatinine: 2.2 (baseline is 2.3)
     Glucose: 98
     Calcium: 8.9

Which of the following is the most appropriate regarding this patient's fluid management?
     A. Continue the same management.
     B. Stop lactated Ringer's.
     C. Stop lactated Ringer's and start normal saline.
     D. Stop lactated Ringer's and start dextrose 5% half-normal saline.

Case 2

A 63-year-old male patient was admitted by vascular surgery for evaluation of worsening peripheral vascular disease in his right leg. The patient is prepared to have arterial angiography the next day. He has a history of DM, hypertension, CKD stage IV, congestive heart failure, and left below-the-knee amputation 3 years ago for advanced peripheral vascular disease. The patient complains of right foot pain on walking for 2 blocks that has worsened over the last 2 months. He noted that his torsemide dose was increased 2 weeks ago because of worsening dyspnea on exertion. Since that time his dyspnea has been controlled. The patient is not in acute distress, and his vital signs are within normal limits. Physical examination is significant for 3-plus edema in the right leg and a cold hairless shin. His right dorsalis pedis and posterior tibial pulses are weak.

Which of the following is the most appropriate for this patient?
    A. Stop diuretics prior to angiography.
    B. Give bicarbonate sodium fluid prior to angiography.
    C. Continue diuretics.
    D. Give half-normal saline fluid prior to angiography.

FLUID MANAGEMENT

IV fluids are "medications" that have side effects. Using them in inappropriate settings can cause serious complications and prolong hospitalization stays. For example, patients with acute respiratory distress syndrome (ARDS) do better when they are on conservative fluid management. Loading patients with a high volume of fluids can cause pulmonary edema even in patients with no history of heart failure.

The most important indications for IV fluids are summarized in Table 15-1, and the suggested type of fluids to use for each of them will be suggested. Table 15-2 summarizes the compositions of different IV fluids.

Maintenance Fluids

Hospitalized patients are frequently placed on nothing by mouth for various reasons (surgeries, imaging, etc). During that time they must be provided with ongoing requirements of water, sodium, and potassium.

Water requirements can be calculated by the 4/2/1 rule. Four milliliters of water is needed per hour for each kilogram of the first 10 kg, 2 mL/kg for the second 10 kg, and 1 mL/kg for the rest of the weight. Daily sodium and potassium

Table 15-1. Indications for Intravenous Fluids

1. Maintenance fluid
2. Volume resuscitation
3. Hyponatremia
4. Hypernatremia
5. Hypercalcemia/tumor lysis syndrome/rhabdomyolysis
6. Contrast-induced nephropathy prophylaxis
7. Persistent hypoglycemia
8. Spontaneous bacterial peritonitis management
9. After large-volume paracentesis in cirrhosis patients

Table 15-2. Intravenous Fluids Composition

Parameter	Human Serum	D5W	0.45 NS	0.9 NS	Lactated Ringer's	Albumin	Hypertonic Saline
Na (mmol/L)	135–150	0	75	154	131	140	513
Cl (mmol/L)	95–105	0	75	154	111	128	513
K (mmol/L)	3.5–5.0	0	0	0	5	0	0
Ca (mmol/L)	2.2–2.6	0	0	0	2	0	0
HCO_3 (mmol/L)	24–28	0	0	0	29	0	0
Glucose (mg/dL)	70–100	5000	0	0	0	0	0
Albumin (g/L)	30–50	0	0	0	0	50	0
pH	7.3–7.4		5.4	6.0			
Osmolality	270–290	0	150	308	276	265	900

requirements are 1 to 2 and 0.5 to 1 mmol/kg, respectively. All the above are rough estimates, and one must use judgment when dealing with different patients. For example, patients with heart failure should get minimum fluids or perhaps none at all, and patients with chronic kidney disease (CKD) should not be placed on potassium.

The best maintenance fluid is half-normal saline. If the patient does not have diabetes, D5 half-normal saline is the best choice as it provides some calories to prevent starvation-induced ketoacidosis. Do not forget to add potassium to the fluid order.

Basic maintenance fluids with potassium are not enough for patients on fasting states for prolonged periods of time (more than 48–72 h). Other minerals, vitamins, amino acids, and fatty acids should be given to these patients by tube feedings or by total parenteral nutrition.

Volume Resuscitation

Patients who have lost volume or have become dehydrated need fluids that expand the extracellular space to support blood pressure. Isotonic fluids do not cross cell membranes and thus stay in the extracellular space. They will support blood pressure and increase organ perfusion in shock patients.

Isotonic fluids include normal saline, lactated Ringer's, and albumin. Albumin provides high oncotic pressure and brings fluids to the intravascular space. Theoretically, albumin should therefore support blood pressure more than the other 2 fluids; however, there is no evidence that shows albumin does better than normal saline, and it is much more expensive. Both lactated Ringer's and normal saline are inexpensive and effective fluids. Be aware, however, that using large volumes of lactated Ringer's may cause hyperkalemia, and so normal saline may often be the best choice of the two.

When giving volume to resuscitate patients, start with boluses of 500 milliliters to 1 liter over 30 minutes. If patients have end-stage renal disease or advanced heart failure, boluses of 250 milliliters may be used to avoid precipitating acute pulmonary edema. Boluses should be repeated until the central venous pressure (if internal jugular vein central line monitoring is available) and the mean arterial blood pressure improve. After blood pressure is stabilized, isotonic fluid rates can be lowered to a fixed rate per hour. Follow up the heart rate and the urine output to adjust the rate. Patients should make at least 0.5 mL/kg/h of urine.

Treatment of hypercalcemia/prevention of AKI in tumor lysis syndrome/prevention of AKI in rhabdomyolysis

High serum calcium, uric acid, and myoglobin have significant toxicities. Hypercalcemia causes mental status changes, kidney salt wasting with dehydration, vomiting, and serious arrhythmia. High uric acid can precipitate in the tubules and cause anuric acute kidney injury. Myoglobin has significant kidney toxicity as well. IV hydration is a major part of the prevention and treatment of these three disorders. Aggressive hydration increases the glomerular filtration rate and thus increases the urinary excretion of these substances. Isotonic saline is the fluid that is most commonly used for this purpose.

Patients with hypercalcemia should be placed on 200 to 300 mL/h of NS. The urine output should be at least 100 to 150 mL/h. Hydration alone will not decrease the calcium level, and therefore bisphosphonate with or without calcitonin should be used as well. Tumor lysis syndrome is seen in patients with high cell burden tumors who are on chemotherapy. Tumor cell death will lead to the release of potassium, phosphate, and nucleic acids. The metabolism of such a high load of purines will cause hyperuricemia. Patients at risk for tumor lysis syndrome are usually those with aggressive lymphomas and leukemia. Before starting chemotherapy these patients should be started on isotonic saline at 2 to 3 $L/m^2/24$ h. Urine output should be at least 100 mL/h. Furosemide may be added to increase the urine output. Allopurinol or rasburicase is used to decrease uric acid production. Uric acid, kidney function, and electrolytes should be monitored closely.

Trauma, immobility, and drugs are the most common etiologies of rhabdomyolysis. The myoglobin released from myocytes can precipitate acute kidney injury. Patients with serum creatinine kinases (CK) of more than 5000 and those with rapidly increasing CK from baselines lower than 5000 are at high risk for AKI. Aggressive hydration with NS to keep urine output to at least 200 to 300 mL/h is recommended. Hydration may be stopped when CK stops rising.

Alkalinization of the urine is thought to increase uric acid solubility and thus decrease its precipitation in the tubules. Alkalinization may also decrease free ion release from myoglobin (which in turn decreases its toxicity to the kidney). However, there is no clear clinical evidence to support the use of alkalinization. Some clinicians still recommend using sodium bicarbonate in the fluids to achieve a urine pH of at least 6.5 in these patients. If this is done, closely monitor the serum bicarbonate and the arterial pH (serum bicarbonate of 30 or arterial pH of 7.5 indicates the need to stop this process).

Hydration in these disorders is aggressive, and the risk of pulmonary edema should always be kept in mind. Serial lung and lower extremity examinations are recommended to watch for signs of fluid overload. The hydration rate should be adjusted downward for patients with baseline cardiac dysfunction.

Contrast-induced nephropathy prevention

Contrast material used for CT imaging and in arterial angiography procedures has the potential to cause acute kidney injury. Contrast-induced nephropathy has a significant effect on morbidity and mortality; therefore, prevention of contrast-induced AKI should be a goal. There are conflicting data regarding who should get prophylaxis and what the best prophylaxis procedures are. However, patients with estimated glomerular filtration rates of less than 60 mL/1.73 m^2 are at high risk, and IV fluids (especially normal saline or sodium bicarbonate) definitely decrease the risk of contrast nephropathy. It is probably wise to give prophylactic fluids to patients with CKD stage III or more. Isotonic sodium bicarbonate fluid can be made by adding 3 ampules of $NaHCO_3$ (a total of 150 mL) to 850 mL of D5W. Give 3 mL/kg/h of sodium bicarbonate fluid 1 hour before contrast administration and continue for 6 hours after. An alternate protocol is to give 1 mL/kg of NS 6 hours prior to the contrast and to continue that for 6 to 12 hours after.

Persistent Hypoglycemia

Sometimes patients get too much insulin. Most of the time orange juice or half an ampule of dextrose 50% will take care of the hypoglycemia. If the patient has renal dysfunction, sometimes the hypoglycemia will persist for hours. This is also true if an elderly patient or a patient with CKD takes too much sulfonylurea and does not eat enough. Hypoglycemia in these cases can last for a few days. In cases like these, it becomes impractical to give dextrose ampules alone. A better approach is to start the patient on continuous IV dextrose 5% or 10% and follow the blood sugar levels.

Spontaneous Bacterial Peritonitis

Cirrhosis patients with spontaneous bacterial peritonitis (SBP) are at high risk for acute kidney injury. This is because of the decreased effective arterial circulation that results in decreased kidney perfusion. Albumin infusion has been shown to decrease this risk and in turn decrease the mortality in these patients.

Once SBP is diagnosed, start the patient on a 1-time dose of 1.5 g/kg IV albumin. Give another 1 g/kg on day 3.

Post–large-volume Paracentesis

Patients with diuretic-resistant cirrhotic ascites need frequent paracenteses. Sometimes, a large volume of ascites fluid needs to be removed. Following removal of a large volume of fluid, patients will be at risk for circulatory collapse and renal failure. Infusion of albumin may decrease this risk. When paracentesis of more than 5 liters is performed, it is reasonable to give 6 to 8 grams of IV albumin for each liter removed.

TIPS TO REMEMBER

- IV fluids should be used only when indicated. The "liberal" use of IV fluids can have adverse reactions.
- Half-normal saline with dextrose and potassium supplements is probably the best maintenance fluid to use for patients fasting for short periods of time.
- Normal saline and lactated Ringer's are the fluids of choice for shock patients.
- Isotonic fluids are used in patients with hypercalcemia to keep the urine output to at least 100 cm^3/h.
- Patients at risk for tumor lysis syndrome should be on isotonic fluids to prevent uric acid–induced AKI. Urine output should be at least 100 cm^3/h.
- Patients at risk for myoglobin-induced AKI should be on isotonic fluids to keep the urine output to at least 200 cm^3/h.
- Sodium bicarbonate or normal saline should be used in patients with CKD stage III or more to prevent contrast nephropathy.
- IV albumin use is currently indicated only in patients with SBP or after paracentesis of at least 5 L of ascites fluid.

Answers

1. **D**. Lactated Ringer's is the most likely cause of the hyperkalemia in this patient with a history of CKD. Thus, it should be stopped. The patient is nauseated and her oral intake is still poor, so she needs maintenance fluid. The best maintenance fluid in this patient would be D5 1/2 NS. There is no evidence of hypovolemia on examination, so NS is better to be avoided, especially given this history of heart failure in this patient.

2. C. This patient is at high risk for contrast nephropathy because of his advanced CKD. Sodium bicarbonate decreases the risk of contrast nephropathy. However, this patient has evidence of hypervolemia (edema in his right leg) and his diuretic dose was recently increased. Starting fluids, whether hypotonic or isotonic, or discontinuing the diuretics will put him at risk for acute exacerbation of his congestive heart failure. This risk most likely outweighs the benefit of giving isotonic fluid. Diuretics will help make this patient euvolemic and improve the stroke volume; this in turn will increase the kidney perfusion and help decrease the risk of contrast nephropathy in this patient.

SUGGESTED READINGS

Dale D, Federman D. *ACP Medicine*. Vol. 2. 3rd ed. New York: WebMD; 2007:1976–1979.

McPhee S, Papadakis M. *Current Medial Diagnosis and Treatment*. 50th ed. New York: McGraw-Hill; 2011:867–868.

Gastrointestinal Bleeding

Zafar Quader, MD, FASGE and Zak
Gurnsey, MD, FACP

A 65-year-old Man With Melena and Hematemesis

A 65-year-old man presents to the ED with a 3- to 4-day history of melena with episodes of hematemesis. He is nauseous and light headed when he stands up and appears a little confused.

Medical history is significant for HTN and chronic back pain. He is a construction worker lifting heavy loads. After work every day for the past 30-plus years he consumes 6 to 8 beers. He smokes about a pack of cigarettes daily. His medications include lisinopril 20 mg qd, as well as Tums for heartburn and several ibuprofen 200-mg tablets almost daily for chronic aches and pains.

The patient's vital signs are as follows: temperature 37.2°C; respiratory rate 16; blood pressure 100/70 and heart rate 100 (supine); blood pressure 80/55 and heart rate 125 (upright). On physical exam you encounter a middle-aged male in mild distress.

HEENT shows pallor, with mildly icteric sclera. Cardiovascular exam shows regular rhythm with postural changes. Lungs are clear. Abdomen is mildly distended with mild epigastric tenderness. No hepatosplenomegaly is appreciated. Bowel sounds are normal and active. Stool for occult blood is positive. CNS exam is nonfocal, but patient is lethargic. Nasogastric tube inserted in the ED returns a clear colorless fluid.

ED labs show the following: hemoglobin 6.6, hematocrit 18%, platelets 94,000, MCV 104. CMP shows BUN 64, Cr 1.2, AST 66, ALT 30, total bilirubin 2.8, and INR 2.3.

What do you do first in evaluating and managing this patient?

This patient's vitals, physical examination, and laboratory data suggest volume loss and hemodynamic instability. In any case of GI bleeding, ABCs (airway, breathing, circulation) always come first. The patient requires rapid evaluation and treatment, including volume resuscitation and then workup for the cause of his bleeding.

In the ED this patient was noted to have postural changes as well as some obtundation indicating a volume loss of 15% to 30%. Immediate volume resuscitation with fluids and blood products is necessary. IV saline or LR should be immediately started. Two wide-bore IVs (14–18 gauge) should be inserted for rapid infusion if needed. Blood and platelets should be transfused, and any underlying coagulopathy needs to be corrected with vitamin K or FFP if needed. If a decision for admission is made, the patient needs to be sent to a monitored bed in, at the least, an IMC or CCU unit. After the ABCs are managed, further evaluation can progress.

What is your most likely diagnosis and what is the differential diagnosis?

This is a 65-year-old man with what appears to be a UGI bleed. He has significant risk factors for GI bleeding (age, alcohol abuse, and NSAID usage) and presents with several episodes of melena and hematemesis. At this point the cause is unclear and could be multifactorial. A clear return on NG tube lavage does not rule out UGI bleed. Definitive diagnosis will require an esophagogastroduodenoscopy. The differential diagnosis in this patient includes the following:

1. PUD, gastritis, esophagitis (remember age, NSAID use, alcohol abuse)
2. Variceal bleed or portal hypertensive gastropathy (alcohol, jaundice, and thrombocytopenia)
3. Mallory-Weiss tear (emesis with possible retching)

Analysis: This case represents the approach to a patient with an upper GI bleed with a focus on initial assessment and resuscitation, as well as a discussion of the differential diagnoses.

Acute gastrointestinal bleeding is a very common clinical problem associated with significant morbidity and mortality. The annual rate of hospitalizations in the United States is around 30 to 100 patients per 100,000, with about 400,000 hospital admissions annually.

UPPER GASTROINTESTINAL BLEEDING

Etiology of severe UGI bleed in 1000 consecutive admissions (UCLA-Cure research Group) diagnosed by endoscopy:

1. PUD 35.3%
2. Esophageal or gastric varices 22.6%

3. UGI angiomas 4%

4. Mallory-Weiss tears 3.1%

5. Gastric or duodenal erosions 1.2%

6. Esophagitis 4.6%

7. Dieulafoy lesion 3.0%

8. Portal hypertensive gastropathy or post-banding ulcers 5.4%

9. Epistaxis 2.3%

10. Other causes or no etiology 15.4%

UGI bleeding may present with the following:

1. Hematemesis 30%

2. Melena 20%

3. Both 50%

4. Hematochezia alone 5% to 10%

History

A focused history should revolve around such questions as length of time and progression of bleeding, associated symptoms (nausea, retching, abdominal pain), prior history of GI bleeding, and medication usage.

Physical

Vital signs revealing hypotension, tachycardia, tachypnea, and hypoxia can help determine the degree of blood loss. Postural changes are associated with about a 15% loss in blood volume, and baseline hypotension/mental status changes indicate about a 30% loss of blood volume. Historic trending also will give an idea of volume loss. Other physical examination findings to look for include dry mucus membranes, poor skin turgor, and evidence of chronic liver disease (jaundice, ascites, hepatomegaly, spider angiomas, and caput medusae).

Labs

The laboratory evaluation should focus on blood and volume status as well. The hemoglobin and hematocrit should be assessed for degree of anemia. Keep in mind, though, that an acute bleeding episode will not have an immediate impact on the hemoglobin level due to lack of equilibrizing. Low platelet levels may indicate underlying liver disease. BUN and creatinine should be assessed for renal complications due to volume loss. An exceedingly high BUN:creatinine ratio (>20) may indicate GI bleeding. This is because the blood is digested in the GI tract, with byproducts being reabsorbed and causing the BUN to rise. PT/INR and PTT should be assessed to look for any underlying coagulopathies, which may impact the ability to reverse the bleeding. Liver enzymes should be assessed to determine underlying acute and/or chronic liver disease.

Initial assessment

Resuscitation should commence immediately and concurrently with the initial evaluation. As noted above, in all urgent/emergent situations, the first approach revolves around the ABCs (airway, breathing, circulation). Patients with upper GI bleeding may develop the inability to protect their airways. This may be due to persistent vomiting and/or associated lethargy due to blood loss with inadequate perfusion of vital organs. If this occurs, the patient needs to be intubated for airway protection.

MANAGEMENT

Volume resuscitation

As in all cases of sudden volume loss, patients with GI bleeding need adequate vascular access. This is ideally accomplished with two large-bore (18 gauge or larger) peripheral IV sites. This will allow rapid infusion of volume (such as normal saline or Ringer lactate) and blood products (such as packed red blood cells, fresh frozen plasma, and platelets).

Patients should be kept NPO.

Blood products

Packed red blood cells should be considered for transfusion based on degree of reported or witnessed blood loss, degree of anemia, and degree of hemodynamic instability. Transfusion of other blood products, such as fresh frozen plasma and platelets, should be considered based on the laboratory evaluation and/or underlying coagulopathies. Hemoglobin should be maintained above 7 to 8 g/dL and platelet count above 50,000. INR should be below 2. A restrictive transfusion strategy is used in stable patients (not hypotensive or with cardiovascular disease). RBC transfusions given only at Hb <7 g/dL with a posttransfusion target of 7 to 9 g/dL are better than a liberal transfusion strategy, decreasing 45-day mortality and further bleeding in patients with UGI hemorrhage.

Other medications

Besides IV fluids and blood products, other medications should be considered. Home medications should be discontinued (in line with the patient's NPO status). Proton-pump inhibitors should be ordered for all patients with active GI bleeding, in either continuous or bolus IV routes. Octreotide infusion should be used for upper GI bleeding cases with a suspected cause of esophageal varices. Octreotide is a somatostatin analog that reduces the portal venous pressure.

Bed status
Patients with upper GI bleeding should be monitored in an ICU or IMC setting with frequent evaluations of hemodynamic status.

Consults
A gastroenterology consult should be obtained in all cases of upper GI bleeding. For those patients with hemodynamic instability, this consult needs to be obtained emergently.

Diagnostic approach
Upper endoscopy is the mainstay of definitive diagnosis in cases of upper GI bleeding. Imaging like CT or angiography may also help localize an area of bleeding depending upon the amount of bleeding.

Treatments for Upper GI Bleeding (Depends on Diagnosis)

Esophageal varices
Esophageal varices are dilated veins in the submucosa of the esophagus caused by portal hypertension. They are asymptomatic until they present as an upper GI bleed. Diagnosis is made via endoscopy. Treatment options include banding, sclerotherapy, transjugular intrahepatic portosystemic shunt (TIPS), and liver transplantation. Nonselective beta blockers are used to prevent bleeding or rebleeding in patients with esophageal varices. They are not, however, used for primary prophylaxis of esophageal varices.

Gastric varices
Gastric varices are dilated veins in the submucosa of the stomach caused by portal hypertension. They are asymptomatic until they present as an upper GI bleed. Diagnosis is made via endoscopy. Gastric varices are extremely difficult to treat or eradicate. They often rebleed and have a high mortality rate. Treatment options include gastric variceal obliteration with cyanoacrylate (which is not approved by the US FDA), balloon-occluded retrograde transvenous obliteration intragastric balloon tamponade (BRTO), TIPS, and liver transplantation.

Peptic ulcer disease
Peptic ulcer disease most commonly occurs in the duodenum but may also occur in the esophagus or stomach. Abdominal pain is usually an associated symptom. Causes generally include *Helicobacter pylori* infection, NSAID usage (most common), and antiplatelet medication usage (eg, aspirin, clopidogrel). Malignancy also is a potential cause. Diagnosis may be considered on clinical suspicion but is confirmed with endoscopy. Treatment focuses on the underlying cause. Any offending medications are discontinued. *H pylori* infections are treated with a combination of antibiotics and a proton-pump inhibitor. Multiple biopsies should be taken to help rule out malignancy.

Esophagitis

Esophagitis is inflammation of the lining of the esophagus. Common causes include GERD (acid reflux), chemical ingestions, alcohol, and infections (*Candida*, HSV, CMV). Diagnosis may be considered on clinical suspicion but is confirmed with endoscopy. Treatment focuses on the underlying cause. Any offending medications are discontinued. Proton-pump inhibitors are generally prescribed regardless of the cause. Mucosal coating agents like sucralfate act as a barrier to avoid acid injury.

Gastritis

Gastritis is inflammation of the lining of the stomach. Common causes include alcohol, NSAID usage, severe illness (stress, burns, trauma, sepsis), and *H pylori* infection. Diagnosis may be considered on clinical suspicion but is confirmed with endoscopy. Treatment focuses on the underlying cause. Any offending medications are discontinued. Histamine receptor blockers or proton-pump inhibitors are generally prescribed regardless of the cause. Other potential medications to use include sucralfate, bismuth, and misoprostol.

Mallory-Weiss tear

Mallory-Weiss tears occur in the mucosa at the gastroesophageal junction after episodes of severe retching and vomiting. The bleeding may stop on its own, or endoscopic treatment via cauterization or epinephrine injection can be used.

Portal Hypertensive Gastropathy

PHG or gastric antral vascular ectasia (GAVE) occurs as a result of portal hypertension and subsequent engorgement of the gastric mucosa vasculature. The mucosa becomes quite friable, lending itself to bleeding from underlying vessels. Treatment is geared toward reducing portal venous pressure with the use of nonselective beta blockers. Endoscopic treatment with thermal coagulation or mechanical clips of individual bleeding vessels also can be used.

Angiodysplasias

Angiodysplasias are small vascular malformations seen in the lining of the GI tract during endoscopy. They are a common cause of unexplained or recurrent GI bleeding. They are usually multiple and may occur throughout the upper and lower GI tracts. Treatment is usually via thermal coagulation during endoscopy.

Aortoenteric fistula

Aortoenteric fistulas usually occur as a result of erosion of an abdominal aortic aneurysm into the duodenum. Prior aortic vascular surgery and graft infection also increases the risk. This situation requires emergent surgical intervention. These patients have a high mortality rate.

Dieulafoy lesions

Dieulafoy lesions are caused by caliber-persistent arterioles in the submucosa. The larger size and pulsatile nature of the arteriole cause the small layer of overlying submucosa to erode, leading to bleeding into the stomach or GI lumen. Even with endoscopy, they are difficult to diagnose because of an intermittent bleeding pattern. Endoscopic treatment options include epinephrine injection, electrocoagulation, photocoagulation, endoscopic clipping, and banding.

Cameron lesions

Cameron lesions are small, linear erosions or ulcers seen at the gastroesophageal junction. They are associated with hiatal hernias. They are usually asymptomatic. They may lead to iron-deficiency anemia due to continuous and chronic bleeding in small amounts.

A 62-year-old Woman With Bright Red Blood per Rectum

Patient is a 62-year-old female who presents to the ED after developing bright red blood per rectum (BRBPR) that started last night. She has had a total of 8 episodes of BRBPR. She denies any abdominal pain, rectal pain, weight loss, or fevers. She does complain of fecal incontinence with these episodes. She has never had any previous episodes of GI bleeding. She has a history of diabetes mellitus type 2 and hyperlipidemia. Her home medications include metformin and simvastatin. She denies any tobacco or alcohol use. She had a colonoscopy 3 years ago that revealed diverticulosis without any other significant findings. On examination, she is awake and pleasant with a blood pressure of 136/74 mm Hg, heart rate of 84 bpm, respiratory rate of 16 breaths/min, and oxygen saturation of 98% on room air. She is afebrile. Her HEENT, cardiovascular, and respiratory examinations are all normal. Her abdomen is soft without any tenderness or distention. Bowel sounds are normal. Rectal examination reveals some red blood on the examination finger.

Laboratory data show hemoglobin 12.5, hematocrit 37, and platelets 215,000. BUN is 15 and creatinine is 1.1. INR is 0.9. AST is 34 and ALT is 30.

1. What is the most likely diagnosis?

2. What is the initial goal of evaluation and patient care?

3. What else is on the differential diagnosis?

Answers

This is a 62-year-old female with sudden onset of BRBPR that began last night. She has no other symptoms. A previous colonoscopy was negative for polyps or malignancy. Her vitals and physical examination show that she is hemodynamically stable. She has mild anemia. She requires further workup for these episodes of lower GI bleeding.

1. The most likely diagnosis is diverticular bleeding.

2. The initial goals of her care revolve around monitoring volume status and anemia levels. She will require a nonurgent GI consult.

3. The differential diagnosis includes malignancy, inflammatory bowel disease (IBD), ischemic colitis, hemorrhoids, and angiodysplasias. Do not forget that up to 10% of UGI bleeds present as hematochezia only.

HEMATOCHEZIA AKA LOWER GI BLEED

Acute LGI bleeding, defined as bleeding distal to the duodenum but most commonly the colon, has an annual hospitalization rate of 20 per 100,000 adults. In most patients with hematochezia, the bleeding stops spontaneously, allowing elective diagnostic evaluation. However, 10% to 40% of patients with a colonic source of bleeding will have a recurrent bleed within 48 hours of the initial event. Mortality is reported between 3% and 5% because the incidence of LGI bleeding increases markedly in patients older than 65 years. The strongest predictors of mortality are advanced age, intestinal ischemia, and comorbid illnesses. In patients with severe hematochezia after resuscitation and ruling out UGI bleeding, urgent colonoscopy is recommended so as to provide an accurate diagnosis and opportunity for hemostasis during the exam.

Common Causes of Severe Hematochezia (706 Cases)

1. Diverticulosis	32.6%
2. Ischemic colitis	12.2%
3. Internal hemorrhoids	10.8%
4. Rectal ulcers	8.5%
5. Ulcerative, Crohn, other colitis	7.5%
6. Colon angiomas or radiation telangiectasias	7.2%
7. Postpolypectomy bleeds	7.1%
8. Colon cancer or polyps	6.1%

History
A focused history should revolve around such questions as history of length of time and progression of bleeding, associated symptoms (such as abdominal pain, rectal pain, and weight loss), prior history of GI bleeding, and medication usage.

Physical
Vital signs revealing hypotension, tachycardia, tachypnea, and hypoxia can help determine the degree of blood loss. Other physical examination findings to look

for include dry mucus membranes, poor skin turgor, and evidence of hemorrhoids or rectal masses.

Laboratory

The laboratory evaluation should focus on blood and volume status as well. The hemoglobin and hematocrit should be assessed for degree of anemia. Keep in mind, though, that an acute bleeding episode will not have an immediate impact on the hemoglobin level due to lack of equilibrizing. BUN and creatinine should be assessed for renal complications due to volume loss. PT/INR and PTT should be assessed to look for any underlying coagulopathies, which may impact the ability to reverse the bleeding.

Volume resuscitation

As in all cases of sudden volume loss, patients with GI bleeding need adequate vascular access. This is ideally accomplished with two large-bore (18 gauge or larger) peripheral IV sites. This will allow rapid infusion of volume (such as normal saline or Ringer lactate) and blood products (such as packed red blood cells, fresh frozen plasma, and platelets). Patients should be kept NPO.

Blood products

Packed red blood cells should be considered for transfusion based on the degree of reported or witnessed blood loss, degree of anemia, and degree of hemodynamic instability. Transfusion of other blood products, such as fresh frozen plasma and platelets, should be considered based on the laboratory evaluation and/or underlying coagulopathies.

Medications

Besides IV fluids and blood products, other medications should be considered. Home medications should be discontinued (in line with the patient's NPO status). This is especially true for such medication classes as NSAIDs, anticoagulants, and antiplatelet drugs.

Consults

A gastroenterology consult should be obtained.

Diagnostic approach

Colonoscopy will help visualize and localize an area of bleeding. It also allows for direct intervention. Radionuclide scanning may help localize bleeding to a particular quadrant of the abdomen. It is performed by tagging red blood cells with a radionuclide tracer. It has drawbacks in that it requires a bleeding rate of approximately 0.1 mL/min and does not allow for therapeutic intervention. Angiography is another option. It does not require bowel preparation and does allow for intervention via embolization. Drawbacks include a bleeding rate requirement of approximately 1.0 mL/min and the use of IV contrast, which may be contraindicated in cases of chronic kidney disease.

Treatments for Lower GI Bleeding (Depending on Diagnosis)

Diverticulosis

Diverticula may develop along the colonic wall. These small outpouches occur through weaknesses in the colonic wall musculature. They are most common in the sigmoid colon. They are usually asymptomatic. If stretched too far, the blood vessels within the outpouches may bleed. Treatment is generally supportive, with fluid resuscitation and, at times, blood transfusions. If diverticular bleeding is a recurrent problem, the ultimate treatment may be surgical removal of the section of colon with predominant diverticular disease.

Colonic angiodysplasias

Angiodysplasias are small vascular malformations seen in the lining of the GI tract during endoscopy. They are a common cause of unexplained chronic or recurrent GI bleeding. They are usually multiple and may occur throughout the upper and lower GI tracts. Treatment is usually thermal therapy during colonoscopy.

Colorectal malignancy

Colon cancer may present as rectal bleeding or anemia. Associated symptoms of weight loss and change in bowel habits should be investigated. Colon cancer usually occurs later in life. The US Preventive Services Task Force and various specialty societies recommend age 45 as the starting point for screening colonoscopy. Diagnosis requires histopathologic samples from endoscopic biopsies. Treatment depends on the stage and may include endoscopic therapy, surgery, chemotherapy, and/or radiation therapy.

Inflammatory bowel disease

IBD has two main forms: Crohn disease and ulcerative colitis. It should be suspected in younger patients with lower GI bleeding with associated symptoms of fever, malaise, and abdominal pain. Diagnosis is made via autoimmune and genetic serum markers and via endoscopic biopsies. Treatment typically involves anti-inflammatory and other immunosuppressive agents.

Ischemic colitis

Ischemic colitis occurs due to lack of blood flow to an area of the colon. This is usually due to decreased blood pressure (ie, volume loss or septic shock) or a stoppage in blood flow (ie, atherosclerotic disease or thromboembolic disease). Treatment starts with supportive care, including fluid resuscitation and pain management. Surgical excision of the ischemic area may be needed if the area develops gangrene or perforation. Most of the time, however, bleeding secondary to ischemic colitis resolves without any treatment.

Hemorrhoids

Hemorrhoids can occur internally or externally in relation to the dentate line. Bleeding typically occurs with a bowel movement. External hemorrhoids will be painful as well. Diagnosis is via digital rectal examination or endoscopy.

Treatment begins with supportive care but may ultimately include rubber band ligation or surgical excision.

Rectal ulcers

These may be solitary or multiple, and they may be found especially in elderly or debilitated patients with constipation or in hospitalized patients with fecal management systems. Treatment is correcting the underlying cause and endoscopic therapy.

Upper GI bleeding

Cases of upper GI bleeding that exhibit very rapid transit of the blood through the GI tract may present as BRBPR. These patients are likely to have significant hemodynamic instability. If upper GI bleeding is suspected as the cause of BRBPR, the approaches outlined in the first half of this chapter should be employed. The much more common appearance of stool in relation to upper GI bleeding is that of melena, or black tarry stools.

TIPS TO REMEMBER

- ABCs first. Adequate vascular access and sufficient volume resuscitation are necessary in all cases of GI bleeding. Prudent use of PRBCs, platelets, and FFP is advisable.
- PUD is the most common cause of UGI bleeding.
- Proton-pump inhibitors should be empirically started in all cases of upper GI bleeding.
- Endoscopy is the standard for diagnosis in cases of upper GI bleeding.
- Most cases of lower GI bleeding will resolve spontaneously.
- Rule out UGI bleed as the cause in all cases of severe hematochezia.

COMPREHENSION QUESTIONS

1. A 54-year-old male with a history of alcoholism presents to the ED after experiencing hematemesis of 200 mL bright red blood at home. He complains of fatigue and is pale in appearance. His blood pressure is 98/46 and heart rate is 112. What is the next step in this patient's management?
    A. Nasogastric tube placement
    B. Gastroenterology consult
    C. Transfusion of 2 U of packed red blood cells
    D. Placement of two large-bore peripheral IV sites and initiation of IV fluid boluses

2. An 80-year-old female with a history of atrial fibrillation, hypertension, and coronary artery disease presents with a 1-day history of abdominal pain and rectal

bleeding with bright red blood. The pain is dull and vague, is located in the left lower quadrant, and has been getting worse over time. Her warfarin therapy was stopped several months ago due to concerns regarding frequent falls. Her blood pressure is 136/78 and heart rate is 64. On examination, she has severe tenderness on palpation of the left lower quadrant with some associated guarding. What is the most likely diagnosis?
    A. Hemorrhoids
    B. Peptic ulcer disease
    C. Diverticulosis
    D. Ischemic colitis

3. A 26-year-old male with no prior medical history complains of a 3-day history of nausea with vomiting and diarrhea. He has several episodes of each per day. His fiancé had similar symptoms that resolved spontaneously 2 days ago. Earlier today, he developed hematemesis of bright red blood during his episodes of nausea with vomiting. His vital signs and physical examination are essentially normal. What is the most likely diagnosis?
    A. Esophageal varices
    B. Peptic ulcer disease
    C. Esophagitis
    D. Mallory-Weiss tear

Answers

1. **D**. This patient has several indicators of volume loss, including the amount of hematemesis, pale appearance, and hypotension with compensatory tachycardia. The other options are all likely to occur in the urgent management of this patient, but appropriate vascular access and aggressive volume resuscitation are the initial concerns in an attempt to stabilize this patient so that further interventions (ie, blood transfusions, endoscopy) may occur.

2. **D**. This elderly female most likely has ischemic colitis. Her history of atrial fibrillation without current anticoagulation treatment places her at an increased risk of developing thromboembolic disease. Her abdominal pain is also characteristic of ischemic colitis, as it is worse on physical examination than reported during the history and it is located in a typical area for ischemic colitis. Abdominal pain would not be expected with hemorrhoids or diverticulosis. Peptic ulcer disease should present with upper GI bleeding or melena, but not typically with bright red lower GI bleeding.

3. **D**. This patient has likely developed a Mallory-Weiss tear due to recurrent vomiting and retching. He has no noted history of alcohol abuse or liver disease, acid reflux, or abdominal pain that would make the other choices more likely.

SUGGESTED READINGS

Barkun AN, Bardou M, Kuipers EJ, et al. International consensus: recommendations on the management of patients with non-variceal gastrointestinal bleeding. *Ann Intern Med.* 2010;152:101–113.

Cappell MS, Friedel D. Initial management of acute upper gastrointestinal bleeding: from initial evaluation up to gastrointestinal endoscopy. *Med Clin North Am.* 2008;92:491–509.

Gralnek IM, Barkun AN, Bardou M. Current concepts: management of acute bleeding from a peptic ulcer. *N Engl J Med.* 2008;359:928–937.

Jensen DM. The ins and outs of diverticular bleeding. *Gastrointest Endosc.* 2012;75:389–391.

Laine L, Jensen DM. Management of patients with ulcer bleeding. *Am J Gastroenterol.* 2012;107:345–360.

Longo DL, Fauci AS, Kasper DL, et al, eds. *Harrison's Principles of Internal Medicine.* 18th ed. New York: McGraw-Hill; 2012.

Manning-Dimmitt LL, Dimmitt SG, Wilson GR. Diagnosis of gastrointestinal bleeding in adults. *Am Fam Physician.* 2005;71(7):1339–1346.

McQuaid KR. Gastrointestinal disorders. In: McPhee SJ, Papadakis MA, eds. *Current Medical Diagnosis & Treatment.* New York: McGraw-Hill; 2012.

Sepe PS, Yachimski PS, Friedman LS. Gastroenterology. In: Sabatine M, ed. *Pocket Medicine: The Massachusetts General Hospital Handbook of Internal Medicine.* 2nd ed. Philadelphia: Lippincott Williams & Wilkins; 2004:1–26.

Strate LL, Naumann CR. The role of colonoscopy and radiological procedures in the management of acute lower intestinal bleeding. *Clin Gastroenterol Hepatol.* 2010;8:333–343.

Washington University School of Medicine, Cooper DH, Krainik AJ, et al. *The Washington Manual of Medical Therapeutics.* 32nd ed. Philadelphia: Lippincott Williams & Wilkins; 2007.

Hypertension Management in the Emergency Department and Hospital

John M. Flack, MD, MPH, Asad Cheema, MD, Ashley Hill, DNP and Priyanka Bhandari, MD

A 64-year-old Woman With Severe BP Elevation and Shortness of Breath

A 64-year-old woman presents to the emergency department with complaints of increasing shortness of breath with progressively lesser physical exertion to the point that she is SOB at rest. For the last 3 days, she has slept on 4 pillows. Established medical conditions are long-standing hypertension, diabetes, and osteoarthritis. Home BP usually ranges from 160 to 174 systolic, 76 to 88 diastolic. The last 4 clinic BP readings over the past 6 months have been approximately similar. Over the past 5 years she has been prescribed lisinopril 20 mg/d, which she takes each morning. She estimates that she misses 1 or 2 doses per year. BP today is 218/102 mm Hg without orthostatic change, pulse is 100 beats per minute, lungs show loud popping rales in the lower to mid posterior areas, an S3 gallop is audible, and extremities are cool and edematous. The chest x-ray shows cardiac enlargement and bilateral fluffy infiltrates. A subsequent echocardiogram showed a reduced ejection fraction of 38% but no segmental wall motion abnormalities or valvular dysfunction. Her kidney function is normal.

Case commentary

This patient has long been undertreated with a single drug despite persistent BP elevations. The undertreatment of this patient originated, in all likelihood, by initiating antihypertensive drug therapy with a single drug, then cemented in place by repeated episodes of therapeutic inertia—ie, documenting BP elevations in clinical settings without intensification of the antihypertensive drug regimen. Unequivocally this patient has a hypertensive emergency. Her BP is definitely high enough to be the cause of the cardiopulmonary dysfunction observed: pulmonary edema and acute heart failure. Urgent admission to a critical care setting with immediate treatment with IV medications (eg, nitro-glycerin) is indicated.

Hypertension management in the clinic is also relevant to hypertension man-agement in the emergency department and hospital because, not infrequently, patients seen in clinic are referred to this location for evaluation and treatment. It is critically important to understand key information in the history, physical, and laboratory data that guides clinical decision-making. We will define extreme hypertension treatment failure phenotypes—hypertensive urgency, hypertensive emergency—as well as the clinical presentation of abrupt withdrawal from beta blockers or other sympatholytic drugs. Many of the aforementioned patient types will present with severe BP elevations (≥180/110 mm Hg), but not invariably; patients with true hypertensive emergencies may present with BP elevations near but lower than this threshold, while a hypertensive urgency can present with BP much higher than this threshold.

CLINICAL DEFINITIONS OF SEVERE BP ELEVATIONS

Poorly controlled BP

Poorly controlled BP or hypertension is commonly encountered in ambulatory clinics and emergency departments. In fact, patients seen in in ambulatory clinical settings with poorly controlled BP are not infrequently referred to the emergency department for evaluation, where they may receive IV or oral medication, such as clonidine, to abruptly lower BP. There is, however, no proven clinical indication for this potentially dangerous clinical intervention.

We operationalize the definition of poorly controlled BP to overlap nearly entirely with the accepted definition of hypertensive urgency. That is, when BP is 180/110 mm Hg or higher instead of labeling the patient as having a hypertensive urgency, we prefer to label them in almost all instances as having poorly controlled BP or hypertension. The rationale for this is that making the diagnosis of hypertensive urgency strongly implies the need for acute BP lowering over the next few hours to prevent target-organ injury. However, the perceived immediate need for BP lowering is based on a medical judgement of impending target-organ dysfunction/failure. What is typically underweighted is the risk for precipitating target-organ ischemia when BP is abruptly low-ered with either IV or oral antihypertensive medications such as clonidine while the perceived risk of target-organ dysfunction/failure is strikingly exag-gerated. Our position is consistent with a recent published statement by the European Society of Cardiology that discourages the use of the term *hyperten-sive urgency*, as they recognize that the treatment of such patients is no differ-ent than that of other patients with uncontrolled BP. When patients with BP above this threshold are labelled with *poorly controlled BP*, there is no implied urgency regarding the need for BP lowering. Accordingly, in patients with poorly controlled BP our focus is on maximizing adherence to the prescribed antihypertensive drug regimen, reinforcing diet and lifestyle modifications (especially dietary sodium restriction), and optimizing the prescribed antihypertensive drug regimen.

Hypertensive Urgency

Hypertensive urgency has been defined as BP elevations ≥180/110 mm Hg without evidence of new or worsening target-organ injury. Table 17-1 displays the varied clinical presentations of target-organ injury. Again, this terminology should be used infrequently, if ever, in the clinical care of patients with severe BP elevations without new or worsening target-organ injury.

Rebound Hypertension

Rebound hypertension occurs when beta blockers or select other central adrenergic inhibitors (eg, clonidine) are abruptly discontinued. These patients will present with evidence of sympathetic nervous system hyperactivity (tachycardia and BP elevations above pretreatment levels) because of the rapid uncovering of beta-adrenergic receptors with upregulated sensitivity that are exposed to high levels of catecholamines. These patients will present for care in both ambulatory clinics and emergency departments. Clinicians should have a high degree of suspicion for rebound hypertension in patients with acute BP elevations and signs of sympathetic nervous system overactivity. In this situation, it is reasonable to use IV labetalol to pharmacologically block both alpha- and beta-adrenergic receptors to interrupt this cycle of sympathetic discharge. Alternatively, selected patients may be managed by simply restarting their beta blocker or central adrenergic inhibitor (eg, clonidine). In patients with known intermittent nonadherence to prescribed antihypertensive medications, beta blockers and central adrenergic inhibitors should be avoided if at all possible.

Hypertensive Emergency

Hypertensive emergency is diagnosed typically with BP greater than 180/110 mm Hg in persons with new or worsening target-organ injury (Table 17-1). A general rule of thumb is that the diagnosis of hypertensive emergency should be made when the BP elevation is, in your clinical judgement, likely high enough or has occurred rapidly enough to be the cause of the observed new or worsening target-organ injury. In other words, if the BP is 170/98 mmm Hg in a patient presenting with pulmonary edema and heart failure, they should be considered to have a hypertensive emergency. Another patient with no prior history of hypertension may present with signs of hypertensive encephalopathy if their BP rapidly rises to ~160/100 mm Hg during an episode of acute glomerulonephritis.

The initial evaluation of these critically ill patients should be focused on a targeted history, physical exam, and diagnostic testing to gain insight into the

Table 17-1. Blood Pressure–Related Target-Organ Injury

Retinal
- Papilledema
- Hemorrhage
- Exudates
- Cotton wool spots

Brain
- Hypertensive encephalopathy
- Transient ischemic attack (TIA)
- Stroke (atherothrombotic or hemorrhagic)

Vascular
- Microangiopathic hemolysis
- Aortic dissection

Heart/Lungs
- Acute coronary syndrome/myocardial infarction
- Acute heart failure
- Pulmonary edema

Kidney
- New or worsening azotemia
- Hematuria

Table 17-2. Clinically Available Clues Indicative of Prior Poorly Controlled BP

1. Retinopathy
    - Arteriolar narrowing, A-V nicking
    - Focal/general arteriolar narrowing, prominent arteriolar silver wiring
    - Hemorrhages, exudates, cotton wool spots, papilledema
2. Cardiac examination
    - Laterally displaced and/or enlarged PMI
    - S4 gallop
3. Electrocardiogram
    - Inverted or biphasic P-wave in lead V1
    - Voltage criteria for LVH

A-V, arteriovenous; LVH, left ventricular hypertrophy; PMI, point of maximal impulse.

reason(s) for the severe BP elevation as well as to determine the extent of the target-organ injury. Table 17-2 lists potential clues to the presence of long-standing uncontrolled hypertension. Garnering diagnostic clues is important because it is not uncommon for patients with severe BP elevations to present for care with minimal to no documented history of prior BP control.

Treatment of such patients should take place in a closely monitored, critical setting with the use of IV antihypertensive medications to lower BP. However, the specific treatment approaches to the various types of hypertensive emergencies are beyond the scope of this chapter.

Hazards of Overzealous BP Lowering

Long-standing hypertension, especially if uncontrolled, leads to remodeling of resistance arterioles. Resistance arterioles importantly mediate autoregulation in pressure-sensitive organs such as the brain and kidney. That is, when BP falls they dilate and when BP rises they constrict to keep blood flow and therefore oxygen delivery constant. Resistance arterioles that have remodeled can no longer maximally vasodilate, and, to the degree they can, vasodilation happens rather sluggishly. Thus, acutely dropping BP with oral or IV drugs risks precipitating target-organ ischemia—especially in patients with poorly controlled hypertension over the long term.

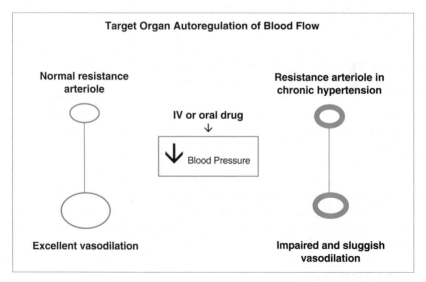

Figure 17-1. Why rapid blood pressure lowering can cause target-organ ischemia in chronic hypertension. The remodeling of resistance arterioles is proportional to the duration and severity of the BP elevation.

In this situation, practitioners routinely overestimate the risk from the current severe BP elevations while dramatically underestimating the risk from abruptly lowering BP. In most instances, severe BP elevations without new or worsening target-organ injury should not be targeted for immediate reduction by pharmacologic means. Overzealous BP lowering can occur in either hypertensive urgency or emergency as a consequence of oral or intravenously administered antihypertensive agents.

Managing Hypertension in the Emergency Department

The emergency department presents a tremendous challenge with regard to obtaining accurate BP measurements because, in no small part, of the hurried and chaotic environment and the absence of time-consuming standard BP measurement protocols. It is, however, common for BP measurements to trend significantly lower when repeated in this setting. There is no proven clinical benefit in patients with hypertensive urgencies for hospitalizing them compared with sending them home from the emergency department. In these patients it is prudent to ascertain their adherence to their prescribed regimen as well as to scrutinize their regimen, optimize it, and arrange for early follow-up in an ambulatory clinic. We have previously shown efficacious BP lowering and safety in patients presenting to an urban emergency department who were prescribed 1 or more prescriptions for antihypertensive drug therapy.

Hospital Management of Hypertension

Therapeutic goals

Inpatient management of BP can be challenging given the myriad reasons leading to hospital admissions. The goal of treatment during hospitalization is not BP normalization but rather to keep the BP below an imminent danger zone (<220/120 mm Hg). Consideration should be given to identifying reversible causes of BP elevations such as pain, hypoxia, hypercarbia, or IV saline-containing fluid infusions. When considering different treatment modalities, a targeted patient evaluation should take place while paying close attention to focused history-taking and a targeted physical examination. You should focus on hypertension duration, treatment history, clinical complications, adherence to BP medications, and identifying the clinical manifestations of target-organ injury by focusing on pressure-sensitive organs, the heart, lungs, nervous system, and eyes. Therapeutic modifications should focus on intensification of the prescribed oral drug regimen and coordination of subsequent follow-up with ambulatory care providers.

Therapeutic principles

It is important to remember the absence of any persuasive unconfounded evidence of any kind that even suggests the abrupt normalization of BP confers clinical benefit over the short term in any setting. That said, an important guiding principle is for inpatient hypertension management to set the stage for good postdischarge outcomes. That is, educate patients and their families about hypertension and diet/lifestyle modifications and spend time either constructing an effective drug regimen or deconstructing and rebuilding a suboptimal drug regimen. Also, antihypertensive drug therapy should never be prescribed to an inpatient for abrupt BP lowering without examining the patient. This will prevent the common clinical practice of writing as-needed administration of IV (or oral) antihypertensive drugs based on BP levels exceeding prespecified levels that are often only modestly elevated and even below the diagnostic threshold for hypertensive urgency. Importantly, understand and treat the patient—don't just treat the BP number.

Uncontrolled BP

Uncontrolled hypertension is commonly encountered in hospital settings. Long-acting antihypertensive drugs are the staple of antihypertensive drug therapy. However, their maximal effect of BP lowering takes ~4 weeks to become mostly or fully manifest. Thus, within the time frame of a typical hospitalization, even the most appropriate and effective antihypertensive drug regimen that has been uptitrated or initiated during the hospitalization simply will not have had enough time to maximally lower BP. Accordingly, it is irrational to try and normalize BP while hospitalized. Importantly, unnecessary exposure to IV saline or sodium by any route, oral or IV, will raise BP in most hypertensives and should therefore be avoided. Also, take time to scrutinize the prescribed antihypertensive drug regimen and take steps to optimize it as adapted from the American College of Cardiology/American Heart Association (ACC/AHA) hypertension guideline outlined in Table 17-3.

Perioperative Hypertension Management

Many patients scheduled for surgery have established hypertension and take antihypertensive drugs. During the induction phase of general anesthesia, BP and pulse rate can rise significantly, especially among those with poorly controlled BP (>210/105 mm Hg). With continued anesthesia, there is a risk of hypotension because of loss of baroreceptor integrity and inhibition of sympathetic nervous system activity. Perioperative BP lability increases the risk for coronary ischemia, stroke, bleeding, and neurologic dysfunction. Elective surgery scheduled for patients with BP >180/110 mm Hg might be delayed until better BP control is attained. Regarding specific drugs, chronic beta-blocker therapy should be continued up until the time of surgery and reinstituted during the postoperative period when feasible; however, beta-blocker therapy should not be initiated on the day of surgery in beta blocker–naïve patients, as it may be associated with clinical harm. Postoperatively it may, though, be necessary to utilize IV beta blockers and other

Table 17-3. Three-step Approach to Constructing Effective Hypertension Drug Regimens

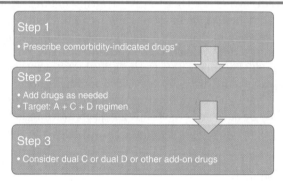

A, ACE inhibitor or ARB; C, calcium antagonist; D, thiazide-like or thiazide diuretic.

*Comorbidities	
Atrial fibrillation	ARB or ACE
Aortic disease	Beta blocker
Chronic kidney disease	ACE or ARB
-Post kidney transplant	Calcium antagonist
Heart failure	
-Reduced EF	GDMT beta blockers
	Aldosterone antagonists
	ARNI (ACE or ARB if ARNI not available)
-Preserved EF	ARNI
Secondary stroke prevention	Thiazide or thiazide-like diuretic
	ACE
	ARB
Stable ischemic heart disease	GDMT beta blockers
	ACE or ARB
-Angina	GDMT beta blockers
-Post-MI or ACS	GDMT beta blockers
-Aortic insufficiency	Avoid drugs that drugs that slow the HR (beta blockers, non-DHP calcium antagonists)

ACE, angiotensin-converting enzyme inhibitor; ACS, acute coronary syndrome; ARB, angiotensin receptor blocker; ARNI, angiotensin receptor/neprilysin inhibitor; DHP, dihydropyridine; EF, ejection fraction; GDMT, guideline-directed medical therapy (carvedilol, metoprolol succinate, bisoprolol); HR, heart rate; MI, myocardial infarction.

antihypertensive drugs in patients who are NPO or have impaired gut absorption. Angiotensin-converting enzyme (ACE) inhibitors, angiotensin receptor blockers (ARBs), and probably sacubitril/valsartan should be discontinued the day before surgery to avoid intraoperative hypotension.

During the postoperative period when BP is elevated, reversible causes of a pressor response should be sought including pain, tracheal suction, infusions of saline-containing fluids, hypoxia, and hypercarbia. When pharmacologic BP control is needed, clevidipine, a very short-acting dihydropyridine calcium antagonist, is a preferred agent; its metabolism is unaffected by kidney and hepatic function as it is metabolized by red blood cell esterases. In comparison to nicardipine, a longer-acting dihydropyridine calcium antagonist, clevidipine appears more effective at keeping BP within a narrow prespecified range.

Preparing the Patient for Discharge

Since complete hypertension control is not the goal during an acute hospitalization, once the drug regimen has been optimized, arrange for post-hospital follow-up within 1 to 2 weeks of discharge. There is rarely a good reason for prolonging the inpatient stay to normalize or nearly normalize the BP. Make use of the acute hospitalization to teach and/or reinforce how to minimize dietary sodium intake as well as the important reason for doing this. Most of the antihypertensive drugs lower BP more effectively when the dietary intake of sodium is reduced. High levels of dietary sodium intake can cause marked resistance to BP-lowering drugs.

The patient in our case study should have an antihypertensive drug regimen that starts with comorbidity-indicated drugs. The ARNI drug sacubitril/valsartan has proven clinical benefit in heart failure with reduced and preserved ejection fraction and should replace lisinopril—although some patients may not be able to access this drug because of cost and insurance coverage. The ACE inhibitor should be discontinued at least 36 hours before initiating sacubitril/valsartan. Beta blockers and aldosterone antagonists also should be included in the drug regimen with the caveat that the beta blocker should not be started in the setting of decompensated left ventricular function and could therefore be started post-discharge. Ultimately if a fourth drug is needed for BP control, given the normal kidney function, opt for chlorthalidone rather than a loop diuretic.

Screening for Secondary Forms of Hypertension

Table 17-4 displays the types of patients with established hypertension who should be screened for secondary causes of hypertension. It must be recognized that in many confirmed cases of secondary hypertension, especially in middle-aged and older patients, the secondary cause is superimposed on primary hypertension. This guidance is important because all patients with established hypertension should not be screened for secondary causes.

Table 17-4. When to Support Secondary Forms of Hypertension

Resistant or refractory hypertension

Hypertensive emergency

Abrupt onset of hypertension

Hypertension onset prior to 30 years of age

Diastolic hypertension in patients ≥65 years of age

Unprovoked[1] or excessive[2] hypokalemia

Incidentaloma

Hypertension and depressed kidney function—especially in current or prior smokers with evidence of vascular atherosclerosis

[1]Not taking a diuretic.
[2]Hypokalemia persisting >1 month after discontinuation of a diuretic *or* potassium <3.0 mEq/L while taking a diuretic.

Table 17-5 displays common and/or important causes of secondary hypertension and the approach to screen for these conditions. Although diagnostic testing is discussed, in most instances you will likely refer the patient to the appropriate subspecialist for confirmatory testing.

Obstructive Sleep Apnea

This is perhaps the most commonly encountered form of secondary hypertension. One of the screening questionnaires listed in Table 17-5 is typically administered and scored to qualify the patient for a definitive sleep study. There is a known epidemiologic association between primary aldosteronism and sleep apnea.

Primary Aldosteronism

This form of secondary hypertension is infrequently diagnosed relative to its clinical prevalence. Even 10% of normotensives appear to have primary aldosteronism (PA). Just over 50% of patients with resistant hypertension and suppressed renin levels have PA. We usually undertake multiday salt loading in patients with plasma aldosterone 10 ng/dL or higher with suppressed (or near suppressed) renin <1 ng/mL/h. The diagnosis of PA is made when the 24-hour urinary excretion of aldosterone does not suppress to <12 μg per 24 hours after 3 days of oral salt loading (need at least 200 mmol of sodium in the 24-hour collection). Adrenal vein sampling is the test of choice to determine whether aldosterone hypersecretion lateralizes and is amenable to adrenalectomy. Bilateral aldosterone hypersecretion is identified in the majority of PA cases.

Table 17-5. Screening and Diagnostic Testing for Secondary Hypertension

	Screen Test	**Diagnostic Test**
Sleep apnea	STOP-BANG, Berlin Questionnaire, Epworth Sleepiness Scale	Home or overnight sleep study
Primary aldosteronism	Early AM plasma aldosterone and renin	Oral salt-loading test
Renovascular	Renal artery duplex scan	Angiography – Traditional – CT – MRA with gadolinium enhancement – Carbon dioxide
Cushing syndrome	Late-night salivary cortisol or 1-mg overnight dexamethasone suppression test	24-hour urinary free cortisol
Pheochromocytoma	Plasma free metanephrines	24-hour urinary fractionated metanephrines

Renovascular

The ACC/AHA guideline recommends medical therapy for most patients with critical renal artery stenosis but notes that hypertensive patients with azotemia (ischemic nephropathy), heart failure/flash pulmonary edema, or refractory hypertension can be considered medical treatment failures and therefore potentially candidates for revascularization. Accordingly, it is only in these patient types that we undertake an evaluation for critical renal artery stenosis. The overwhelming majority of patients with atherosclerotic renal artery obstruction either smoke currently or previously smoked. Our renal artery imaging modality of choice is carbon dioxide angiography because it is devoid of nephrotoxicity and many of the patients in whom we pursue this diagnosis have depressed kidney function. Some patients, mostly women, may alternatively have fibromuscular dysplasia, so if this is suspected then the appropriate screening should be done.

Cushing Syndrome

Screen for this condition in hypertensive patients with incidentalomas and/ or signs of cortisol excess, pigmented abdominal striae, acne, hirsutism, round facies, cervical buffalo hump, rapid weight gain, osteoporosis, etc. This condition is, however, significantly less common than either sleep apnea or PA. An AM cortisol of <50 nmol/L after 1 mg of dexamethasone the prior evening essential rules out this diagnosis in all but a few percent of cases.

Pheochromocytoma

This is a distinctly uncommon cause of secondary hypertension, but missing this diagnosis can have devastating consequences. Most patients have a cluster of symptoms such as headache, palpitations, tachycardia, and paroxysm of sweating; even when patients have suggestive symptoms, pheochromocytoma is almost never the cause. Given the very low prevalence of this condition, the overwhelming majority of positive screening tests are false positives. Normetanephrine or metanephrine elevations more than 3-fold greater than the upper range of normal or elevations of both metanephrine and normetanephrine fractions are more likely to be true than false positives.

Summary

Much restraint should be shown when treating elevated BP in the emergency department and inpatient settings. Rarely will a patient with severely elevated BP in the absence of new or worsening target-organ injury need abrupt lowering of their BP with either oral or IV medications. Nevertheless, it is commonly done in both settings. In both ambulatory and emergency department clinical settings, the focus should be on optimizing the currently prescribed antihypertensive drug regimen and arranging for timely follow-up in an ambulatory clinical setting. True hypertensive emergencies should be admitted to closely monitored critical care settings and treated with IV antihypertensive agents. Most patients hospitalized primarily for severe BP elevations and/or target-organ injury should be evaluated for secondary causes of hypertension.

SUGGESTED READINGS

Anker SD, Butler J, Filippatos G, et al. Empagliflozin in heart failure with preserved ejection fraction. *N Engl J Med.* 2021;385(16):1451–1461.

Aronson S, Dyke CM, Stierer KA, et al. The ECLIPSE trials: comparative studies of clevidipine to nitroglycerin, sodium nitroprusside, and nicardipine for acute hypertension treatment in cardiac surgery patient. *Anesth Analg.* 2008;107:1110–1121.

Brody A, Rahman T, Red B, et al. Safety and efficacy of antihypertensive prescription at emergency department discharge. *Acad Emerg Med.* 2015;22(5):632–635.

Brown JM, Siddiqui M, Calhoun D, et al. The unrecognized prevalence of primary aldosteronism: a cross-sectional study. *Ann Intern Med.* 2020;173(1):10–20.

Ceccato F, Boscaro M. Cushing's syndrome: screening and diagnosis. *High Blood Press Cardiovasc Prev.* 2016;23(3):209–215.

Cherney D, Straus S. Management of patients with hypertensive urgencies and emergencies: a systematic review of the literature. *J Gen Intern Med.* 2002;17(12):937–945.

Chiu HY, Chen PY, Chuang LP, et al. Diagnostic accuracy of the Berlin questionnaire, STOP-BANG, STOP, and Epworth sleepiness scale in detecting obstructive sleep apnea: a bivariate meta-analysis. *Sleep Med Rev.* 2017;36:57–70.

Funder JW, Carey RM, Mantero F, et al. The management of primary aldosteronism: case detection, diagnosis, and treatment: an Endocrine Society clinical practice guideline. *J Clin Endocrinol Metab.* 2016;101:1889–1916.

Kirk LF Jr, Jash RB, Katner HP, Jones T. Cushing's disease: clinical manifestations and diagnostic evaluation. *Am Fam Physician.* 2000;62(5):1119–1127, 1133–1134.

Lenders JWM, Duh QY, Eisenhofer G, et al. Pheochromocytoma and paraganglioma: an endocrine society clinical practice guideline. *J Clin Endocrinol Metab.* 2014;99(6):1915–1942.

Lipari M, Moser LR, Petrovitch EA, et al. As-needed intravenous antihypertensive therapy and blood pressure control. *J Hosp Med.* 2016;11(3):193–198.

Patel KK, Young L, Howell EH, et al. Characteristics and outcomes of patients presenting with hypertensive urgency in the office setting. *JAMA Intern Med.* 2016;176(7):981–988.

Travieso-Gonzalez A, Nunez-Gil IJ, Riha H, et al. Management of arterial hypertension: 2018 ACC/AHA versus ESC guidelines and perioperative implications. *J Cardiothorac Vasc Anesth.* 2019;33:3496–3503.

Van den Born BH, Lip GYH, Brguljan-Hitij J, et al. ESC council on hypertension position document on the management of hypertensive emergencies. *Eur Heart J Cardiovasc Pharmacother.* 2019;5(1):37–46.

Varon J, Marik PE. Perioperative hypertension management. *Vasc Health Risk Manag.* 2008;4(3):615–627.

Whelton PK, Carey RM, Aronow WS, et al. 2017 ACC/AHA/APA/ABC/ACPM/AGS/APhA/ASH/ASPC/NMA/PCNA guideline for the prevention, detection, evaluation and management of high blood pressure in adults. *Hypertension.* 2018;71:e13–e115.

Zannad F, Ferreira JP, Pocock SJ, et al. SGLT2 inhibitors in patients with heart failure with reduced ejection fraction: a meta-analysis of the EMPEROR-Reduced and DAPA-HF trials. *Lancet.* 2020;396(10254):819–829.

An 89-year-old Man With Acute Respiratory Failure Requiring Intubation

Zak Gurnsey, MD, FACP

Mr. Daniels is an 89-year-old male with a history of COPD, hypertension, and coronary artery disease. He is admitted to the ICU for acute respiratory failure due to exacerbation of his COPD. He requires intubation and mechanical ventilation. The day after admission, his wife presents evidence of a universal DNR order form. After discussing this with the health care team, it is decided to maintain the current treatment plan of intubation and mechanical ventilation. The patient's son, who was previously appointed the patient's health care power of attorney, disagrees with this decision. He would like the patient to be extubated, removed from mechanical ventilation, and allowed to pass away from natural causes. Before a treatment plan decision is ultimately reached, the patient suffers cardiac arrest and is unable to be revived. The patient is pronounced dead by his attending physician.

1. Was the code status clearly determined?

2. Who is allowed to make health care decisions for this patient?

3. Who may pronounce this patient dead?

Answers

1. This case is an example of common scenarios that arise when taking care of critically ill patients and dealing with end-of-life decisions. The patient's previous wishes were stated by the universal DNR order form. This should have been verified at admission before the patient was initially intubated.

2. Because the patient's son is designated as the health acre power of attorney, he has the right to make medical decisions.

3. The attending physician is allowed to pronounce this patient deceased.

CODE STATUS AND DEATH

This chapter will discuss areas of health care that are tied to laws and regulations. These may differ from state to state. It is important to understand the rules of the state in which one practices medicine. Unless otherwise stated, general comments in this chapter will be based on reference to Illinois law.

Code Status

All patients interacting with the health care system should ideally have their code status determined. It is important to determine this prior to a cardiopulmonary arrest situation so that the patient's wishes may be fulfilled during a catastrophic event. Performing CPR and life-sustaining measures on a patient who has previously decided against these may be grounds for criminal consequences.

One should approach code status determination as "all or none." It is not generally recommended to provide the different treatment options during a code situation as individual decision points. Certain patient scenarios will make the "all or none" stance more difficult. For instance, a patient with COPD who has previously been intubated may feel very strongly about never being intubated again. On the other hand, the patient may elect for full cardiac resuscitation during a potentially fatal heart attack. It is extremely important to have candid and upfront conversations with all patients regarding code situations.

DNR stands for do not resuscitate. DNI stands for do not intubate. The view of vasopressor medications as life-prolonging measures will differ among physicians and health care institutions.

If a patient elects for DNR code status, a universal DNR order form should be filled out. Copies should be kept with the patient, with that patient's physicians, and at relevant health care institutions.

Advance Directives

Advance directives will vary in their form and their power. The original advance directive developed was a living will (Figure 18-1). This simply states that the patient does not want life prolonged when death is imminent. It is rather vague and does not give any decisional direction prior to a possibly deadly event.

The universal DNR order form is also considered an advance directive (Figure 18-2).

Having a previously determined advance directive is one part of the process. The other important step is determining who will carry out those decisions or help make new decisions. To this end, governments have developed acts that regulate who may make decisions. In Illinois, it is called the Healthcare Surrogacy Act (Figure 18-3). This spells out the steps to use to determine a decision maker based on that person's relationship with the patient. The surrogate must agree to be the decision maker in order for the act to be completed.

A predetermined decision maker is commonly revealed through health care power of attorney paperwork. This allows a preselected person to make health care–related decisions for the patient any time that the patient is not able to do so. This form takes precedence over the surrogate form. Thus, a patient's best friend may be allowed to make decisions over the patient's spouse or child.

Pronouncing Death

In general, death is determined by means of cardiac or brain death. There are specific protocols for determining brain death. They are beyond the scope of the discussion here. Any licensed physician is allowed to determine cardiac death.

❧Living Will❧
DECLARATION

This declaration is made this _____ day of_____ (month, year).

I,_____, born on _____, being of sound mind, willfully and voluntarily make known my desires that my moment of death shall not be artificially postponed.

If at any time I should have an incurable and irreversible injury, disease, or illness judged to be a terminal condition by my attending physician who has personally examined me and has determined that my death is imminent except for death delaying procedures, I direct that such procedures which would only prolong the dying process be withheld or withdrawn, and that I be permitted to die naturally with only the administration of medication, sustenance, or the performance of any medical procedure deemed necessary by my attending physician to provide me with comfort care.

In the absence of my ability to give directions regarding the use of such death delaying procedures, it is my intention that this declaration shall be honored by my family and physician as the final expression of my legal right to refuse medical or surgical treatment and accept the consequences from such refusal.

Signed_____

City, County and State of Residence_____

The declarant is personally known to me and I believe him or her to be of sound mind. I saw the declarant sign the declaration in my presence (or the declarant acknowledged in my presence that he or she had signed the declaration) and I signed the declaration as a witness in the presence of the declarant. I did not sign the declarant's signature above for or at the direction of the declarant. At the date of this instrument, I am not entitled to any portion of the estate of the declarant according to the laws of intestate succession or, to the best of my knowledge and belief, under any will of declarant or other instrument taking effect at declarant's death, or directly financially responsible for declarant's medical care.

Witness _____

Witness _____

History
(Source: P.A. 85-1209.)
Annotations
Note. This section was Ill.Rev.Stat., Ch. 110 1/2, Para. 703.

Rev 5/2012

Figure 18-1. Sample living will declaration.

• DO-NOT-RESUSCITATE • DNR • DO-NOT-RESUSCITATE • DNR • DO-NOT-RESUSCITATE • DNR •

(Page 1 of 2)

Illinois Department of Public Health

UNIFORM DO-NOT-RESUSCITATE (DNR) ADVANCE DIRECTIVE

Patient Directive

I, ______________________________, born on ____________, hereby direct the following in the event of:
(print full name) (birth date)

1. **FULL CARDIOPULMONARY ARREST (When both breathing and heartbeat stop):**

☒ **Do Not Attempt Cardiopulmonary Resuscitation (CPR)**
(Measures to promote patient comfort and dignity will be provided.)

2. **PRE-ARREST EMERGENCY (When breathing is labored or stopped, and heart is still beating):**

SELECT ONE

❑ **Do Attempt Cardiopulmonary Resuscitation (CPR) -OR-**

❑ **Do Not Attempt Cardiopulmonary Resuscitation (CPR)**
(Measures to promote patient comfort and dignity will be provided.)

Other Instructions ____

Patient Directive Authorization and Consent to DNR Order (Required to be a valid DNR Order)

I understand and authorize the above Patient Directive, and consent to a physician DNR Order implementing this Patient Directive.

Printed name of individual | Signature of individual | Date

-OR-

Printed name of (circle appropriate title):
legal guardian
OR agent under health care power of attorney
OR healthcare surrogate decision maker
| Signature of legal representative | Date

Witness to Consent (Required to have a witness to be a valid DNR Order)

I am 18 years of age or older and acknowledge the above person has had an opportunity to read this form and have witnessed the giving of consent by the above person or the above person has acknowledged his/her signature or mark on this form in my presence.

Printed name of witness | Signature of witness | Date

Physician Signature (Required to be a valid DNR Order)

I hereby execute this DNR Order on ________________.
Today's date

Signature of attending physician | Printed Name of attending physician | Physician's telephone number

◆ *Send this form or a copy of both sides with the individual upon transfer or discharge.* ◆

• DNR • DO-NOT-RESUSCITATE • DNR • DO-NOT-RESUSCITATE • DNR • DO-NOT-RESUSCITATE •

Figure 18-2. Uniform do-not-resuscitate (DNR) advance directive form.

DO-NOT-RESUSCITATE • DNR • DO-NOT-RESUSCITATE • DNR • DO-NOT-RESUSCITATE • DNR

(Page 2 of 2)

Illinois Department of Public Health
UNIFORM DO-NOT-RESUSCITATE (DNR) ADVANCE DIRECTIVE

Patient's name _____

Summarize medical condition:

When This Form Should Be Reviewed

This DNR order, in effect until revoked, should be reviewed periodically, particularly if –

- The patient/resident is transferred from one care setting or care level to another, or
- There is a substantial change in patient/resident health status, or
- The patient/resident treatment preferences change.

How to Complete the Form Review

1. Review the other side of this form.
2. Complete the following section.
   If this form is to be voided, write "VOID" in large letters on the other side of the form.
   After voiding the form, a new form may be completed.

Date   **Reviewer**   **Location of review**   **Outcome of Review**
❏ No change
❏ FORM VOIDED; new form completed
❏ FORM VOIDED; **no** new form completed

Date   **Reviewer**   **Location of review**   **Outcome of Review**
❏ No change
❏ FORM VOIDED; new form completed
❏ FORM VOIDED; **no** new form completed

Date   **Reviewer**   **Location of review**   **Outcome of Review**
❏ No change
❏ FORM VOIDED; new form completed
❏ FORM VOIDED; **no** new form completed

Advance Directives

I also have the following advance directives: **Contact person** (name and phone number)

❏ Health Care Power of Attorney   _____

❏ Living Will   _____

❏ Mental Health Treatment   _____
   Preference Declaration

◆ *Send this form or a copy of both sides with the individual upon transfer or discharge.* ◆

IOCI 0741-10

DNR • DO-NOT-RESUSCITATE • DNR • DO-NOT-RESUSCITATE • DNR • DO-NOT-RESUSCITATE

Figure 18-2. (*Continued*)

755 ILCS 40/25. Surrogate decision making:

Sec. 25. Surrogate decision making. (a) When a patient lacks decisional capacity, the health care provider must make a reasonable inquiry as to the availability and authority of a health care agent under the Powers of Attorney for Health Care Law [755 ILCS 45/4-1 et seq.]. When no health care agent is authorized and available, the health care provider must make a reasonable inquiry as to the availability of possible surrogates listed in items (1) to (4) of this subsection. The surrogate decision makers, as identified by the attending physician, are then authorized to make decisions as follows: (i) for patients who lack decisional capacity and do not have a qualifying condition, medical treatment decisions may be made in accordance with subsection (b-5) of Section 20 [755 ILCS 40/20]; and (ii) for patients who lack decisional capacity and have a qualifying condition, medical treatment decisions including whether to forgo life-sustaining treatment on behalf of the patient may be made without court order or judicial involvement in the following order of priority:

(1) the patient's guardian of the person

(2) the patient's spouse

(3) any adult son or daughter of the patient

(4) either parent of the patient

(5) any adult brother or sister of the patient

(6) any adult grandchild of the patient

(7) a close friend of the patient

(8) the patient's guardian of the estate

The health care provider shall have the right to rely on any of the above surrogates if the provider believes after reasonable inquiry that neither a health care agent under the Powers of Attorney for Health Care Law [755 ILCS 45/4-1 et seq.] nor a surrogate of higher priority is available.

Where there are multiple surrogate decision makers at the same priority level in the hierarchy, it shall be the responsibility of those surrogates to make reasonable efforts to reach a consensus as to their decision on behalf of the patient regarding the forgoing of life-sustaining treatment. If 2 or more surrogates who are in the same category and have equal priority indicate to the attending physician that they disagree about the health care matter at issue, a majority of the available persons in that category (or the parent with custodial rights) shall control, unless the minority (or the parent without custodial rights) initiates guardianship proceedings in accordance with the Probate Act of 1975 [755 ILCS 5/1-1 et seq.]. No health care provider or other person is required to seek appointment of a guardian.

(b) After a surrogate has been identified, the name, address, telephone number, and relationship of that person to the patient shall be recorded in the patient's medical record.

(c) Any surrogate who becomes unavailable for any reason may be replaced by applying the provisions of Section 25 [755 ILCS 40/25] in the same manner as for the initial choice of surrogate.

(d) In the event an individual of a higher priority to an identified surrogate becomes available and willing to be the surrogate, the individual with higher priority may be identified as the surrogate. In the event an individual in a higher, a lower, or the same priority level or a health care provider seeks to challenge the priority of or the life-sustaining treatment decision of the recognized surrogate decision maker, the challenging party may initiate guardianship proceedings in accordance with the Probate Act of 1975 [755 ILCS 5/1-1 et seq.].

(e) The surrogate decision maker shall have the same right as the patient to receive medical information and medical records and to consent to disclosure.

Figure 18-3. Excerpt from Illinois Healthcare Surrogacy Act.

Health care institutions will usually have a policy that allows nonphysicians to pronounce death as well. For instance, two licensed registered nurses (RNs) may be allowed to pronounce death.

Death Summary

The death summary should have the same format as the discharge summary. Listed items should include admission and death dates, admission diagnosis, presumed cause of death, physicians/consultants on the case, important procedures and imaging, important lab and test results, a summary of the hospital course, and the events ultimately leading to the patient's death.

Other items to consider may include code status, details of prior discussions with the patient and/or family, autopsy request, and organ donor status.

TIPS TO REMEMBER

● Code status should be determined for all patients, especially the elderly and those with chronic medical conditions. This should be reviewed at regular intervals.

● Using advance directives will help determine decision makers when patients are unable to make decisions themselves.

COMPREHENSION QUESTIONS

1. A patient is admitted to the hospital with pneumonia. He has a history of COPD. The patient gives his nurse a copy of a universal DNR order form that he filled out with his primary care physician 6 months ago. His wishes for DNR code status are confirmed at this time. The patient becomes lethargic and minimally arousable. His respiratory status worsens, and the health care team determines that intubation and mechanical ventilation may be helpful. What should they do?
    A. Intubate the patient. He has a treatable condition and he may fully recover.
    B. Intubate the patient. The physician should always do something. Allowing a patient to die is unacceptable.
    C. Do not intubate the patient. The patient has clearly stated his wishes.

2. A comatose patient in the ICU cannot make his own decisions. A decision maker needs to be determined. A health care power of attorney has not been previously determined. The patient's wife, mother, and two sons are all willing to be the decision maker. Who is the decision maker?
    A. Wife
    B. Mother
    C. Oldest son
    D. Youngest son

3. A patient who was admitted yesterday after an acute myocardial infarction suffers ventricular fibrillation and is unable to be resuscitated. Which of these individuals is *not* allowed to pronounce the patient as dead?
    A. The attending physician
    B. The ICU resident
    C. The patient's daughter, who is an attorney
    D. Two ICU nurses

Answers

1. **C.** This patient should not be intubated. The universal DNR order form indicates how to treat this patient in this situation. Do not confuse DNR with "do not treat." This patient's pneumonia, COPD, and respiratory failure should be aggressively treated with any indicated medications and treatments, including noninvasive positive pressure ventilation. The treatment plan must stop, though, before it reaches intubation and mechanical ventilation.

2. **A.** Following the steps in the surrogate act, the patient's wife is appointed his decision maker. If the wife was not willing or able to be the decision maker, the next person in line would be the patient's mother.

3. **C.** The patient's daughter, regardless of her advanced degree, is not allowed to pronounce someone dead. The other listed individuals all have the authority to do so.

SUGGESTED READINGS

Illinois Department of Public Health. IDPH Online. Accessed December 5, 2023. dph.illinois.gov

Illinois General Assembly. Illinois General Assembly Home Page. Accessed December 5, 2023. www.ilga.gov

Illinois Guardianship & Advocacy Commission. Welcome to the Illinois Guardianship & Advocacy Commission. Accessed December 5, 2023. gac.illinois.gov

Living Will ID. Living Will Forms by State. Accessed December 5, 2023. https://www.caringinfo.org/planning/advance-directives/by-state/

Longo DL, Fauci AS, Kasper DL, et al, eds. *Harrison's Principles of Internal Medicine.* 18th ed. New York: McGraw-Hill; 2012.

Rabow MW, Pantilat SZ. Palliative care and pain management. In: McPhee SJ, Papadakis MA, eds. *Current Medical Diagnosis & Treatment 2012.* New York: McGraw-Hill; 2012.

Washington University School of Medicine, Krainik AJ, Lubner SJ, Reno HEL. *The Washington Manual of Medical Therapeutics.* 32nd ed. Philadelphia: Lippincott Williams & Wilkins; 2007.

Airway Management

Raj Sreedhar, MD

An 82-year-old man is brought to the ED after becoming acutely dyspneic. He has a past history of stroke, hypertension, and emphysema. On exam, his vital signs are BP 150/90, heart rate 110/min, respiratory rate 30/min, and oxygen saturation 88% on 6 liters of oxygen via nasal cannula. He appears to be in distress. On neurologic exam he is lethargic, with weakness in his right arm and leg. He has flaring of his nostrils and accessory muscle use. He is tachypneic, and bilateral rhonchi are present on auscultation. He has no wheeze. The patient has tachycardia with regular rhythm and no murmurs. The rest of the exam was unremarkable. Labs show a creatinine of 2.4 and potassium of 5.4. ABG results are pH 7.2, P_{CO_2} 53, P_{O_2} 62, and HCO_3 18. Chest x-ray shows bilateral basal infiltrates.

What is the next step in management of this patient?
- A. Noninvasive ventilation
- B. Intubation and mechanical ventilation
- C. Oxygen at 100% via non-rebreather mask
- D. High-flow nasal cannula

It was decided to intubate this patient and place him on mechanical ventilation.

What Is Intubation?

Intubation is the process of introducing an artificial tube into the trachea for the purpose of assisting in ventilation.

What Precautions Are Needed Prior to Intubation?

Airway, breathing, and circulation (the ABCs) are core concepts in the management of a critically ill patient.

When intubating a patient, it is important to remember the 6 Ps:

1. Preparation and preoxygenation
2. Pretreatment
3. Putting the patient to sleep (sedation with/without paralysis)
4. Positioning the patient
5. Placement of tube
6. Postintubation management

You decide to intubate this patient. What is the ideal method to preoxygenate the patient?

A. High-flow oxygen at Fi_{O_2} of 100%

B. Bag-valve mask ventilation

C. No need to preoxygenate, as this is an emergency

D. Non-rebreather mask at Fi_{O_2} of 100%

Preoxygenation

Bag-valve mask ventilation is the preferred method to achieve optimal artificial breaths prior to sedating the patient for intubation. It involves using a full face mask with a bag and a steady supply of high-flow oxygen. Compression and decompression of this bag not only helps in increasing oxygen reserve for the patient while they are apneic but also assists in removal of carbon dioxide (ventilation).

Preparation for intubation entails gathering and testing the supplies needed (endotracheal tubes, stylet, blades, handles, medications, alternate airway methods) as well as planning for a surgical airway if orotracheal intubation fails.

For airway managers, it is important to achieve and maintain competency and proficiency in this procedure.

Stratifying the difficulty of a patient's airway is vital before attempting intubation. A simplified acronym for this assessment is LEMON:

- **Look**: Observe for obvious anatomic variations
- **Evaluate**: 3, 3, 2 rule for an easier intubation
  - o Fitting 3 fingers in an open mouth between upper and lower incisors
  - o Fitting 3 fingers between the edge of the chin and the hyoid bone
  - o Fitting 2 fingers between the hyoid bone and the notch of the thyroid cartilage
- **Mallampati score**: The more of the posterior pharynx you can see, the easier it will be
- **Obstruction**: Possible foreign body, airway edema, vomitus, etc
- **Neck mobility**: Anything that prevents ideal positioning or movement of the neck will make intubation more difficult

Pretreatment

This is done in some patients to account for the physiologic response of the body to the intubation, as a catecholamine surge can result in increased sympathetic activity (elevated heart rate and blood pressure), increased intracranial pressure, and bronchospasm. It is necessary to anticipate postintubation hypotension due to sedative agents or vasodilation. Having vasopressors on standby is important.

Positioning

For intubation, it is important to place and position the patient appropriately so as to achieve optimal view of the vocal cords. The operator stands cephalad while the patient is supine and maneuvered to a "sniffing position" where the oral-pharyngeal-laryngeal axes are closely aligned.

What medications would you use to sedate this patient for intubation?

A. Etomidate and succinylcholine

B. Ketamine and fentanyl

C. Propofol and rocuronium

Sedation and Paralysis for Intubation

Sedation helps in relaxing the patient, decreasing the gag reflex, mitigating the catecholamine surge, and relaxing the airway muscles to obtain optimal view.

Paralysis after deep sedation aids in preventing the gag reflex and emesis during intubation and in obtaining optimal views of the larynx.

Given together, the sedative and paralytic agent helps in achieving rapid induction of anesthesia so as to place endotracheal tube into trachea.

The sedation induction agents are as follows:

1. Etomidate: 0.3 mg/kg IV, quick onset, lasts 3–12 min. This is a common "go-to" choice. There is some concern that it may cause adrenal suppression in septic patients.

2. Ketamine: 1.5 mg/kg IV, onset in <1 min, lasts 10–20 min. It acts as an anesthetic, amnestic, and analgesic. It causes bronchodilation and a catecholamine surge resulting in increased blood pressures and heart rate. ketamine works well in unstable sepsis patients and those with reactive airway disease. Avoid in cardiovascular disease.

3. Propofol: 1.5–2.5 mg/kg IV, onset in 45 s, lasts 5–10 min. Typically used in hemodynamically stable patients, status epilepticus, and reactive airway disease. It has a higher chance for causing hypotension and myocardial depression.

The common paralytic drugs are depolarizing and nondepolarizing agents. The only depolarizing agent is succinylcholine, which mimics acetylcholine at the postsynaptic receptor and depolarizes the muscles fasciculations. There are more nondepolarizing agents, and the commonly used ones are rocuronium and vecuronium.

4. Succinylcholine: 1.5 mg/kg IV, onset in 45 s, lasts 5–10 min. Widely used but has many contraindications: hyperkalemia, recent trauma or burn injury, and malignant hyperthermia.

5. Rocuronium: 1.2 mg/kg IV, onset in 60 s, lasts 15–40 min. Frequently used in children.

This patient was intubated using propofol and rocuronium. Succinylcholine should be avoided, as the patient's potassium level is elevated.

Ketamine is typically not used in patients where elevated intracranial pressure is suspected. This patient was lethargic and not moving the right side of his body.

Placement of the tube

Optimal visualization of the vocal cords is vital before insertion of the endotracheal tube. Visualization can be by direct laryngoscopy or via a video-laryngoscope.

Once vocal cords are visualized, the operator asks to be handed the endotracheal tube without taking eyes off the vocal cords and watches for passage of the tube through the vocal cords.

The cuff of the endotracheal tube is inflated.

Postintubation Management

How would you confirm proper tube placement?

Physical examination methods such as auscultation of chest and epigastrium, visualization of thoracic movement, fogging in the tube, and capnography (end-tidal CO_2) can be used to ensure the tube is in the airway.

Additional methods such as chest x-ray or point-of-care ultrasound also can be used to ensure proper placement.

Securing the tube in place, placing the patient on the ventilator, elevating the head of the bed to prevent ventilator-associated infections, determining a postintubation sedation plan, and daily ventilator wean assessment are all necessary steps in management of the intubated patient.

SUGGESTED READINGS

Myatra SN, Dhawan I, D'Souza SA, et al. Recent advances in airway management. *Indian J Anaesth.* 2023;67(1):48–55.

Shetty SM, Ashwini N. Airway management guidelines: an overview. In: Ubaradka RS, Gupta N, Bidkar PU, et al, eds. *The Airway Manual.* Singapore: Springer; 2023.

Patient in Need of Nutritional Support

Cheryl Burns, RDN, CDCES and Michael Jakoby, MD, MA

A 77-year-old man is admitted to the coronary care unit (CCU) after a massive anterior myocardial infarction and cardiopulmonary arrest. The patient is mechanically ventilated and supported with an aortic balloon pump. His health history is notable for hypertension and hyperlipidemia, although he has never been diagnosed with diabetes mellitus, chronic kidney disease, or stroke. Prior to admission, the patient lived with his wife and performed his activities of daily living without difficulty.

Examination reveals a 70-in, 67-kg (body mass index [BMI] 21) male patient intubated, mechanically ventilated, and sedated with propofol. The patient's wife reports a ~10% weight loss in the year prior to admission. He opens his eyes to verbal commands and nods appropriately to yes/no questions. Bowel sounds are easily audible, and nursing staff reports a large bowel movement yesterday. Laboratories are notable for random glucose 97 mg/dL, creatinine 0.7 mg/dL, albumin 2.8 g/dL, hemoglobin 9.6 mg/dL, and total cholesterol 115 mg/dL (patient was prescribed atorvastatin 40 mg daily prior to admission). It is hospital day 4, and the CCU team and the patient's family are concerned about his nutritional status. The patient has done poorly on attempts at weaning mechanical ventilation.

1. How would you approach nutritional screening and assessment in this patient?

2. What are the indications and options for nutritional support in this patient?

3. What are the chief considerations for starting and continuing nutrition support?

Answers

1. Given the high prevalence of malnutrition or risk of developing malnutrition among hospitalized patients, nutritional screening should be performed on admission for all patients. There are several nutritional screening tools that have been validated to identify patients with malnutrition on admission or at high risk for developing malnutrition during a hospital stay as well as complications (eg, increased hospital length of stay) as a consequence of poor nutritional status. Three commonly used screening tools are presented in Table 20-1, and patients at high risk of malnutrition at time of admission are described in Table 20-2. Providers should be familiar with the nutritional screening policies and screening tools at their hospitals.

Table 20-1. Nutritional Risk Screening Tools for Hospitalized Patients

Screening Tool	Parameters
NRS-2002	BMI <20.5, weight loss within 3 months, reduced caloric intake in the past week, ICU status
MUST	Current weight, current height, weight 3–6 months ago, "acute disease effect" (patient likely to have no nutritional intake for >5 d)
MNA	Food intake past 3 months, weight loss past 3 months, mobility, psychological distress or acute illness, neuropsychological problems, BMI

MNA, Mini Nutritional Assessment; MUST, Malnutrition Universal Screening Tool; NRS, Nutritional Risk Screening; SGA, Subjective Global Assessment.

From Reber E, Gomes F, Vasiloglou MF, et al. Nutritional risk screening and assessment. *J Clin Med.* 2019;8(7):1065.

Table 20-2. Patients at High Risk for Malnutrition.

- Underweight (BMI <18.5)
- Recent loss of ≥10% of usual body weight
- Food insecurity
- Alcoholism
- Nothing to eat in the past 5 d
- History of eating disorder, cognitive dysfunction, or depression
- Malabsorptive disorder, enteric fistulas, or draining wounds
- Hypermetabolic states (trauma, sepsis, burns)
- Treatment with catabolic drugs (glucocorticoids, immunosuppressants, chemotherapeutic agents)

   Nutritional assessments should be performed for all patients identified with malnutrition or at high risk of malnutrition on initial screening. There are multiple components to a formal nutritional assessment, including a thorough dietary history, anthropometric measurements (ie, weight, height, computation of BMI), physical examination, and review of selected biochemistries (eg, pre-albumin level). Interpretation of BMI is presented in Table 20-3. A nutritional assessment should be performed by a registered dietitian with the training and time to conduct it appropriately. The Subjective Global Assessment (SGA) is the most widely utilized nutritional assessment tool at this time. It classifies patients as well nourished (SGA A), moderately malnourished (SGA B), or severely malnourished (SGA C).

2. Inadequate oral caloric intake resulting in manifest or impending malnutrition is the indication for artificial nutrition. In the critical care setting, it is common for patients to be unable to meet their caloric requirements and require artificial nutrition. The two options for providing nutrition support are enteral nutrition (EN) and parenteral nutrition (PN). EN requires the ability to provide supplements to the patient's gastrointestinal (GI) tract through feeding tubes (ie, nasogastric, gastric, or jejunal), and PN requires placement of a central venous catheter. EN is preferred over PN unless there is a contraindication to using the GI tract for nutrition support (eg, ileus, enterocutaneous fistula). A decision tree to provide guidance choosing EN or PN is presented in Figure 20-1.

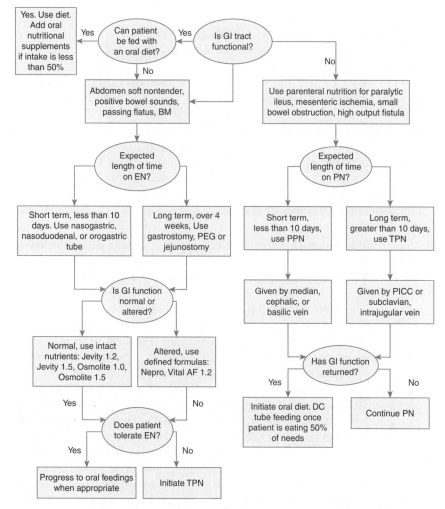

Figure 20-1. Decision tree for use of enteral nutrition (EN) or parenteral nutrition (PN).

Table 20-3. Classification of Body Mass Index (BMI, kg/m^2).

BMI	Category
<18.5	Underweight
≥18.5–24.9	Normal weight
≥25–29.9	Overweight
30–34.9	Class 1 obesity
35–39.9	Class 2 obesity
≥40	Class 3 obesity

Although limited, the best available data support starting critically ill patients on EN within 48 hours of mechanical ventilation whenever possible. A large, multicenter, randomized, controlled trial found best clinical outcomes for patients when PN was delayed to hospital day 8. Data on timing of artificial nutrition for noncritically ill patients are fragmentary. For example, noncritically ill patients who underwent emergency GI surgery and started EN within 48 hours of the procedure had reduced hospital mortality and length of stay (LOS) compared with delaying start of EN to hospital days 3–6. On noncritical medicine services, a stepwise approach of food fortification, oral nutritional supplements, and then EN is generally followed in patients failing to meet caloric targets, although definitive recommendations on the timing for each step is lacking. Inadequate nutritional intake in the context of acute illness is defined as consuming less than 50% of daily energy and protein needs over 5 days.

3. Initial considerations in starting artificial nutrition include determination of total daily caloric requirement, optimal distribution of calories between macronutrients (carbohydrates, protein, and lipids), total daily fluid requirement (including free water), and special electrolyte or micronutrient requirements (eg, potassium restrictions in patients with renal failure). Whenever possible, decisions regarding the optimal choice of EN supplement or composition of PN should be made by a qualified registered dietitian. Formulas to estimate daily caloric requirements in critically and noncritically ill patients are presented in Table 20-4. The composition of selected enteral supplements is presented in Table 20-5, and guidelines for biochemical evaluation of patients before and during support with artificial nutrition are presented in Table 20-6. Triglycerides should be checked at baseline and then periodically as needed if the level is elevated. Radiographic confirmation that any blindly placed tube (small-bore or large-bore) is properly positioned in the GI tract should be obtained prior to use. For patients in a prolonged supine posture, the head of the bed should be raised to ≥30 degrees to minimize risk of reflux. Gastric residual volume, occurrence of emesis, and frequency of bowel movements require regular monitoring

Table 20-4. Formulas for Estimating Daily Caloric Requirements.

Patients	Formulas
Noncritically ill	Mifflin-St. Jeor (MSJ) equations
	(Resting energy needs are calculated with an adjustment for injury factor; weight [W] is in kilograms, height [H] is in centimeters, and age [A] is in years.)
	Men: $(9.99 \times W) + (6.25 \times W) - (4.92 \times W) + 5$
	Women: $(9.99 \times W) + (6.25 \times W) - (4.92 \times W) - 161$
	Adjustment: MSJ $\times 1.2$ for minor injury or surgery
	MSJ $\times 1.3 - 1.5$ for major surgery, infected wounds, burns
Critically ill	Harris-Benedict equation (HBE)
	Men: $66.4730 + (13.7516 \times W) + (5.0033 \times H) - (6.7550 \times A)$
	Women: $655.0955 + (9.5634 \times W) + (1.8496 \times H) - (4.6756 \times A)$
	Ireton-Jones equation
	$(5 \times W) - (11 \times A) + (244 \text{ if male}) + (239 \text{ if trauma present}) + (840 \text{ if burns present}) + 1784$
Ventilated	Original Penn State equation
	(T_{max} is maximum temperature [°C] in past 24 h and V_E is minute ventilation in L/min.)
	$(1.1 \times HBE) + (140 \times T_{max}) + (32 \times V_E) - 5340$
	Modified Penn State equation
	$(0.85 \times HBE) + (175 \times T_{max}) + (33 \times V_E) - 6433$

in patients receiving EN. Capillary blood glucose should be monitored regularly for patients supported with either EN or PN.

CASE REVIEW: NUTRITIONAL SUPPORT IN THE HOSPITALIZED PATIENT

Diagnosis

Malnutrition among hospitalized patients is common and consequential. In a recent study using the SGA to assess patients admitted to ward medicine services, the prevalence of stage B/C malnutrition was 31% at time of admission. Nutritional status did not improve or worsened for some patients during the course of hospitalization; at time of discharge, 36% were found to have SGA stage B/C

Table 20-5. Macronutrient Composition of Selected Enteral Supplements.

Product	Cal/mL	Protein (g/L)	Carbohydrates (g/L)	Fat (g/L)
Jevity 1.2	1.2	56	169	39
Jevity 1.5	1.5	64	216	50
Osmolite 1 Cal	1.0	44	144	35
Osmolite 1.5 Cal	1.5	63	204	49
TwoCal HN	2.0	84	219	91
Nepro	1.8	81	161	96
Vital AF 1.2	1.2	75	111	54

Table 20-6. Laboratory Monitoring for Patients Receiving Artificial Nutrition.

Parameter	Frequency	Rationale
Sodium, potassium, blood urea nitrogen, creatinine	Baseline Daily until stable 1–2 weekly when stable	Monitor renal function and key electrolytes
Glucose	Baseline At least twice daily until stable Weekly if no hyperglycemia	Facilitate glycemic management in patients with hyperglycemia
Magnesium, phosphate	Baseline Daily until stable Weekly when stable	Depletion is common and could be exacerbated by refeeding syndrome
Calcium, albumin	Baseline Daily until stable Weekly when stable	Monitor for hyper- or hypocalcemia; albumin level required to interpret total calcium measurements
Liver function and INR	Baseline Twice weekly until stable Weekly when stable	Changes in liver function may occur with overfeeding; elevated INR may indicate vitamin K and fat-soluble vitamin deficiencies
Complete blood count	Baseline 1–2 times weekly until stable Weekly when stable	Anemia is common in malnutrition and may indicate iron, folate, or vitamin B_{12} deficiencies

malnutrition. Another recent study that evaluated the malnutrition among surgical patients but utilized the NRS-2002 found a prevalence of approximately 20%. Malnutrition increases rates of decubitus ulcers and infections, impairs functional status, and increases hospital LOS, readmission rates, and mortality. Given the frequency and clinical implications of malnutrition in the hospital, universal screening within the first 24 to 48 hours of admission is indicated. Table 20-1 presents the parameters used in three common hospital nutrition screening tools.

Patients whose screening or clinical condition indicate malnutrition or high risk for malnutrition should undergo a formal nutritional assessment. In this patient's case, prolonged admission to a critical care unit with mechanical ventilation and inability to meet daily caloric requirements make a nutritional assessment and plan for nutrition support mandatory. Major components of a nutritional assessment include careful dietary history, anthropometric measures, physical examination, and assessment of selected laboratory results. Dietitians obtain manual dietary assessments from patients or family members if the patient is unable to provide history as in this case. Semiquantitative food records of nursing staff also are reviewed when available. Weight loss prior to hospital admission is also determined. In a recent study conducted in Germany, low food intake prior to hospital admission was documented in slightly more than 20% of patients, and low food intake has also been identified as an independent risk factor for mortality among hospitalized patients.

Height and weight are the anthropometric measurements most readily obtained in hospitalized patients. Although measures of body composition such as skinfold measurements, bioelectrical impedance, and imaging studies (eg, computed tomography and dual-energy x-ray absorptiometry) provide better assessments of lean body mass and nutritional status, they are not practical to obtain. BMI <18.5 is an indicator of malnutrition, although BMI does not reflect potential recent weight loss or low caloric intake. For example, a study using the NRS-2002 found evidence of malnutrition or significant risk of malnutrition in nearly 25% of obese patients admitted to hospital. Targeted physical examination to identify potential signs of malnutrition supplements, computation of BMI, and examination findings indicative of malnutrition are summarized in Table 20-7.

Several laboratory parameters have been investigated as markers of nutritional status, although all have significant limitations and some are not readily available in clinical practice. Potential serologic markers of nutritional status are presented in Table 20-8. All the potential markers are affected by factors independent of energy status such as inflammation, hepatic function, and renal function, although prealbumin (formerly transthyretin) and retinol-binding protein are the most reliable. A diagnosis of malnutrition cannot be made with biochemical markers alone, although results may help confirm a suspicion of malnutrition or high risk for malnutrition based on findings from screening tools, dietary history, and examination.

Table 20-7. Clinical Signs of Malnutrition.

Region	Finding	Potential Deficiencies
Scalp	Sparse, dry, dull hair, scaly skin	Protein, essential fatty acids, zinc
Eyes	Loose skin around orbits, conjunctival pall or	Protein, calorie deficit, iron, folate, or B_{12} (as cause of anemia)
Face	Bitemporal wasting	Protein, fat, calorie deficit
Oral cavity and lips	Cheilitis, stomatitis, gingivitis, pale tongue, atrophied papillae	B-complex vitamins, vitamin C, niacin, and iron
Neck	Prominent clavicles	Protein, fat, calorie deficit
Hands	Interosseous wasting	Protein, calorie deficit
Nails	Pallor, clubbing, ridging, dark, curled at ends	Protein, iron, B_{12}
Torso	Prominent bones/skeletal features	Protein, fat, calorie deficit
Skin	Petechiae/purpura, pallor, hyperpigmentation, decubitus ulcers or poorly healing wounds	Vitamins A, C, and K, B-complex vitamins, biotin, zinc, essential fatty acids, protein
Extremities	Edema	Protein, thiamine

Management

Metabolic rate is increased during periods of acute illness and injury. In a study that included a subset of patients who had basal metabolic rate (BMR) measured by indirect calorimetry during noncritical care admissions and 6 weeks after hospital discharge, BMR was approximately 20% higher during the hospital admission. Energy expenditures are even higher during critical illness and may be as much as 2-fold increased in the setting of major burns. When caloric intake is inadequate for energy expenditure, glycogenolysis, gluconeogenesis, proteolysis, and lipolysis are all significantly increased. In particular, mobilization of protein to provide amino acid precursors (eg, glutamine) for gluconeogenesis can result in a significant reduction in lean muscle mass. Losses of more than 10% of lean body mass in an acutely ill patient may be associated with rapid deterioration in clinical status.

Table 20-8. Potential Laboratory Markers of Malnutrition.

Parameter	Confounders	Utility
Prealbumin	Liver function, renal function, hyperthyroidism, inflammation	Best individual test
Retinol binding protein	Liver function, renal function, hyperthyroidism, vitamin A deficiency	As reliable as prealbumin if results available in a timely manner
Albumin	Liver function, renal function, inflammation	Poor specificity as levels fall commonly following acute illness or trauma independent of nutritional status
Transferrin	Inflammation, infection, liver function, renal function, hemochromatosis	Poor sensitivity and specificity due to many factors that make levels independent of energy intake
IGF-1	Liver function, infection, age	Falls rapidly during fasting but results may take days to become available
Lymphocyte count	Infection, hematologic disorders, immunosuppressant medications, steroids	Very poor specificity

Validated equations to estimate energy requirements in noncritically ill and critically ill patients are presented in Table 20-4. In general, the preferred contribution of macronutrients to total daily energy requirement is 45% to 55% from carbohydrates, 25% to 35% from lipids (fat), and 15% to 25% from protein. For patients who require EN, selected options and their macronutrient compositions are presented in Table 20-5. Special considerations in determining optimal protein-calorie support are presented in Table 20-9. Protein catabolism increases in proportion to severity of illness, with typical levels reaching 30 to 60 grams per day after elective surgery, 60to 90 grams per day in the setting of infection, 100 to 130 grams per day with sepsis or trauma, and >175 grams per day with major burns. These losses are reflected by an increase in the excretion of urea nitrogen, the major byproduct of protein breakdown. When possible, recommendations for total daily calories and macronutrient distribution should be obtained from a qualified registered dietitian. Utilization of nutrition support teams, when

Table 20-9. Daily Protein Requirements for Selected Clinical Conditions.

Condition	Daily Protein Requirement (g/kg)
Adult maintenance	0.8–1.0
Minor surgery	1.0–1.2
Major surgery	1.25–1.75
Surgery with trauma or sepsis	1.50–1.75
Obesity, critical care (based on ideal body weight)	
BMI 30.0–39.9	2.0
BMI >40	2.5
Pressure ulcers	
Stage I	1.1–1.2
Stage II	1.25–1.40
Stage III/IV (small or nondraining)	1.5
Stage III/IV (large or draining)	1.5–2.0
Sepsis	1.5–2.0
Renal failure (based on dry weight)	
Predialysis	0.8
Hemodialysis	1.2–1.3
Peritoneal dialysis	1.5–1.8
Continuous renal replacement therapy	2.0–2.5
Liver disease (based on dry weight)	
Hepatitis (acute or chronic)	1.5–2.0
Cirrhosis	1.0–1.5
Encephalopathy (grade 1 or 2)	0.5–1.0
Encephalopathy (grade 3 or 4)	0.5

available, has been demonstrated to improve appropriate use of artificial nutrition options and reduce LOS for ICU patients.

Carbohydrate requirements are increased in critical and noncritical acute illnesses, and too little carbohydrate in artificial nutrition may result in increased protein catabolism to provide glucogenic amino acids (primarily alanine) as a substrate for gluconeogenesis. A minimum of 2 g/kg/d carbohydrate in artificial nutrition is recommended, although estimates of the maximum rates of glucose oxidation in critically ill patients yield maximum daily glucose requirements in the range of 400 to 700 grams. In practice, 250 to 400 grams of dextrose or carbohydrate per 24 hours is provided in most artificial nutrition regimens to avoid stress-induced hyperglycemia or overfeeding. Even with appropriate carbohydrate as a proportion of total calories, hyperglycemia during the course of artificial nutrition is common. In a recent series of nondiabetes patients receiving PN, nearly 30% of patients experienced at least 1 blood glucose measurement >180 mg/dL during treatment, and the rate of hyperglycemia was approximately 20% at a glucose threshold >150 mg/dL in a population of EN-dependent stroke patients. PN- and EN-associated hyperglycemia is associated with increased morbidity and mortality. Fortunately, there are protocols for managing PN- and EN-associated hyperglycemia that are superior to approaches based on "sliding-scale insulin."

Fatty acids are required in artificial nutrition regimens to provide a source of calories and because numerous fatty acid derivatives (eg, phospholipids) are required for physiologic cellular processes. While the liver has an extensive capacity for de novo lipogenesis, linoleic acid (omega-6) and linolenic acid (omega-3) are not synthesized and must be provided from dietary sources. Current artificial nutrition guidelines recommend approximately 30% of total daily calories from fat, or about 1 g/kg/d.

Data on the prevalence of micronutrient (MN) deficiencies are usually published in the context of specific predisposing diseases or conditions. Alcoholism, chronic gastritis, inflammatory bowel diseases, chronic liver diseases, chronic renal failure, bariatric surgery, and critical illness are key conditions in which deficiencies of fat-soluble vitamins (A, D, E, and K), B-complex vitamins, ascorbic acid (vitamin C), and key minerals (iron, zinc, copper, and selenium) are well documented. Treatment with medications that reduce gastric acidity (iron, folate, and vitamin B_{12}), broad-spectrum antibiotics (vitamin K), diuretics (potassium, copper, zinc, and vitamin B_6), phenytoin (vitamin D and folate), salicylates (vitamin C and folate), and laxatives (fat-soluble vitamins, vitamin B_{12}, and calcium) can lead to vitamin or mineral deficiencies. Commercial trace element and multivitamin preparations can be added to PN, and most EN preparations are designed to provide dietary reference intakes of MNs for feedings that provide 1500 to 2500 kcal/d nutrition support. A registered dietitian or nutrition support team should be consulted if there is uncertainty whether MN requirements are being provided by standard multivitamin and trace element supplements for PN or standard EN preparations.

Refeeding syndrome (RS) may occur when nutrition is provided to a chronically malnourished patient. According to the latest American Society of Parenteral and Enteral Nutrition (ASPEN) consensus recommendations, diagnostic criteria for RS include a decrease in any or all of potassium, magnesium, and phosphorus levels by 10% to 20% (mild), 20% to 30% (moderate), or >30% (severe) from baseline, thiamine deficiency, or organ dysfunction occurring within 5 days of resuming calories. Serious complications of RS include congestive heart failure, hemolysis, rhabdomyolysis, seizures, and respiratory failure. Risk factors for refeeding syndrome include severe weight loss (BMI <14 or below 70% of ideal body weight), little or no caloric intake in the previous 5 to 10 days, history of an eating disorder or chronic alcoholism, and low levels of potassium, magnesium, or phosphorus prior to reintroduction of calories. RS appears to occur due to a rapid shift from protein and fat catabolism back to carbohydrate as the chief source of adenosine triphosphate (ATP), leading to rising insulin levels that result in substantial shifts in glucose, potassium, magnesium, and phosphorus into the intracellular space as well as sodium and fluid retention.

RS can be avoided by scrupulously correcting potassium, magnesium, and phosphorus deficits prior to initiating refeeding or start of artificial nutrition, keeping initial total daily calories conservative (eg, 10 kcal/kg/d), and slowly increasing caloric intake or support at a rate of 200 to 250 kcal/d until the patient's caloric target is reached. Patients at high risk for RS should be evaluated by a registered dietitian or nutrition support team prior to reintroduction of calories.

TIPS TO REMEMBER

- The prevalence of malnutrition on hospital medicine and surgery services is high, and all patients admitted to hospital should undergo nutritional **screening**. Patients identified on screening should undergo nutritional **assessment** by a registered dietitian.

- Malnutrition is consequential for both noncritical and critically ill patients and results in increased morbidity, hospital length of stay, and mortality.

- Patients unable to meet caloric targets for a sustained period require artificial nutrition, with enteral nutrition preferred to parenteral nutrition when possible.

- Refeeding syndrome is a potential complication during reintroduction of calories to severely malnourished patients. Correction of electrolyte (potassium, magnesium, and phosphorus) deficits and slow, conservative resumption of nutrition support can avoid refeeding syndrome.

COMPREHENSION QUESTIONS

1. In the case of the patient at the beginning of this chapter, what are the indications to start artificial nutrition?
   A. Mechanical ventilation
   B. Weight loss prior to admission
   C. Inability to eat

D. All of the above

E. None of the above

2. What laboratory information is most important before potentially starting artificial nutrition in this patient's case?

A. Prealbumin level

B. Albumin level

C. Phosphorus, potassium, and magnesium levels

D. Sodium, blood urea nitrogen (BUN), and creatinine levels

E. None of the above

3. What is the preferred mode of nutrition support for this patient?

A. Enteral nutrition (EN)

B. Parenteral nutrition (PN)

C. Partial caloric support from both EN and PN

Answers

1. **D**. Inability to consume enough calories to meet daily requirements, prolonged mechanical ventilation, and weight loss prior to admission are all indications to start artificial nutrition. In particular, nutrition support is usually started within 48 hours when patients in critical care units require intubation and mechanical ventilation.

2. **C**. Phosphorus, magnesium, and potassium levels are required to help determine the patient's risk for refeeding syndrome. Although the patient has only been in critical care 4 days without caloric intake, he is elderly and has documented weight loss prior to admission. Replacing deficits of phosphorus, magnesium, and potassium is important in preventing refeeding syndrome. Since the patient already meets criteria for nutrition support, a prealbumin level is unnecessary. Albumin level is a lower-quality marker of nutritional status than prealbumin. Although monitoring sodium, BUN, and creatinine levels is important during the course of artificial nutrition support, they do not risk-stratify patients for refeeding syndrome.

3. **A**. EN is preferred to PN when the GI tract can be used to delivery nutrition without complications, and there are no obvious contraindications for EN in this patient's case. Risks of complications such as infections and thrombosis are higher with PN than EN due to the requirement for a central venous catheter to start PN. Use of both modalities to deliver nutrition is occasionally indicated when a patient can tolerate a significant partial but inadequate rate of EN to meet nutritional requirements.

SUGGESTED READINGS

Agarwal E, Ferguson M, Banks M, et al. Malnutrition and poor food intake are associated with pro-longed hospital stay, frequent readmissions, and greater in-hospital mortality: results from the Nutrition Care Day Survey 2010. *Clin Nutr.* 2010;32:737–745.

Alchaer M, Khasawneh R, Heuberger R, Hewlings S. Prevalence and risk factors of total parenteral nutrition induced hyperglycemia at a single institution: retrospective study. *Metab Syndr Relat Disord.* 2020;18(5):267–273.

Banks M, Bauer J, Graves N, Ash S. Malnutrition and pressure ulcer risk in adults in Australian health care facilities. *Nutrition.* 2010;26:896–901.

Bier DM, Brosnan JT, Flatt JP, et al. Report of the IDECG Working Group on lower and upper limits of carbohydrate and fat intake. *Eur J Clin Nutr.* 1999;53:s177–s178.

Böhne SEJ, Hiesmayr M, Sulz I, et al. Recent and current low food intake—prevalence and associated factors in hospital patients from different medical specialties. *Eur J Clin Nutr.* 2022;76(10):1440–1448.

Casaer MP, Mesotten D, Hermans G, et al. Early versus late parenteral nutrition in critically ill adults. *N Engl J Med.* 2011;365:506–517.

Cheung NW, Napier B, Zaccaria C, Fletcher JP. Hyperglycemia is associated with adverse outcomes in patients receiving total parenteral nutrition. *Diabetes Care.* 2005;28(10):2367–2371.

da Silva JSV, Seres DS, Sabino K et al. ASPEN Consensus Recommendations for Refeeding Syndrome. *Nutr Clin Pract.* 2020;35(2):178–195.

Davidson P, Kwiatkowski CA, Wien M. Management of hyperglycemia and enteral nutrition in the hospitalized patient. *Nutr Clin Pract.* 2015;30(5):652–659.

Frankenfeld D, Smith JS, Cooney RN. Validation of 2 approaches to predicting resting metabolic rate in critically ill patients. *JPEN J Parenter Enteral Nutr.* 2004;28:259–264.

Frankenfeld DC. Energy dynamics. In: Matarese LE, Gottschlich MM, eds. *Contemporary Nutrition Support Practice: A Clinical Guide.* Philadelphia: WB Saunders; 1998:79–98.

Freemont RD, Rice TW. How soon should we start interventional feeding in the ICU? *Curr Opin Gastroenterol.* 2014;30(2):178–181.

Furhman MP, Charney P, Mueller CM. Hepatic proteins and nutrition assessment. *J Am Diet Assoc.* 2004;104:1258–1264.

Gariballa S, Forster S. Energy expenditure of acutely hospitalized patients. *Nutr J.* 2006;5:9.

Harris JA, Benedict FG. A biometric study of human basal metabolism. *Proc Natl Acad Sci USA.* 1918;4:370–373.

Hiesmayr M, Schindler K, Pernicka E et al. Decreased food intake is a risk factor for mortality in hospitalized patients: the NutritionDay survey 2006. *Clin Nutr.* 2009;28:484–491.

Inoue T, Misu S, Tanaka T, et al. Pre-fracture nutritional status is predictive of functional status at discharge during the acute phase with hip fracture patients: a multicenter prospective cohort study. *Clin Nutr.* 2017;36:1320–1325.

Ireton-Jones C, Jones JD. Why use predictive equations for energy expenditure assessment? *J Acad Nutr Diet.* 1997;97(Suppl):A44.

Jakoby MG, Nannapaneni N. An insulin protocol for management of hyperglycemia in patients receiving parenteral nutrition is superior to ad hoc management. *JPEN J Parenter Enteral Nutr.* 2012;36(2):183–188.

Lee SH, Jang JY, Kim HW, et al. Effects of early enteral nutrition on patients after emergency gastrointestinal surgery. *Medicine.* 2014;93(28):e323.

Leibovitz E, Giryes S, Makhline R, et al. Malnutrition risk in newly hospitalized overweight and obese patients: Mr NOI. *Eur J Clin Nutr.* 2013;67:620–624.

López-Gómez JJ, Delgado-García E, Coto-García C, et al. Influence of hyperglycemia associated with enteral nutrition on mortality in patients with stroke. *Nutrients.* 2019;11:996.

Mifflin MD, St. Jeor ST, Hill LA, et al. A new predictive equation for resting energy expenditure in healthy individuals. *Am J Clin Nutr.* 1990;51(2):241–247.

Mo YH, Rhee J, Lee E-K. Effects of nutrition support services on outcomes in ICU patients. *Yakugaku Zasshi*. 2011;131(12):1827–1833.

Park YE, Park SJ, Park Y, et al. Impact and outcomes of nutritional support team intervention in patients with gastrointestinal disease in the intensive care unit. *Medicine*. 2017;96:49.

Reber E, Gomes F, Vasiloglou MF, et al. Nutritional risk screening and assessment. *J Clin Med*. 2019;8(7):1065.

Schneider SM, Veyres P, Pivot X et al. Malnutrition is an independent actor associated with nosocomial infections. *Br J Nutr*. 2004;92:105–111.

Schuetz P. "Eat your lunch!" controversies in the nutrition of the acutely, noncritically ill medical inpatient. *Swiss Med Wkly*. 2015;145:w14132.

Shenkin A. Biochemical monitoring of nutrition support. *Ann Clin Biochem*. 2006;43:269–272.

Singer P, Berger MM, Van den Berghe G, et al. ESPEN Guidelines on parenteral nutrition: intensive care. *Clin Nutr*. 2009;28:387–400.

Skeie E, Sygnestveit K, Nilsen RM, et al. Prevalence of patients "at risk of malnutrition" and nutritional routines among surgical and non-surgical patients at a large university hospital during the years 2008–2018. *Clin Nutr*. 2021;40:4738–4744.

van Vliet IMY, Gomes-Neto AW, de Jong MFC, et al. High prevalence of malnutrition on both hospital admission and predischarge. *Nutrition*. 2020;77:110814.

An 80-year-old Woman With Pain After a Fracture Repair

Jacob Varney, MD and Alan J. Deckard, MD

An 80-year-old female is admitted to the hospital following a fall on an icy sidewalk. She suffered a left intertrochanteric hip fracture. There was no loss of consciousness or other injury. She was promptly transported to the ED for evaluation. Her primary physician admits her, completes a preoperative risk assessment, and consults the orthopedic surgery service after finding her to be suitable to undergo the risk of an orthopedic procedure. She has a history of well-controlled hypertension. She has no history of diabetes mellitus, coronary artery disease, kidney disease, congestive heart failure, or stroke. She is a nonsmoker, does not consume alcohol, and has no allergies. She takes hydrochlorothiazide 25 mg daily and lisinopril 20 mg daily. She had an appendectomy 40 years ago without complication. She is widowed, lives independently, and completes her activities of daily living, including light housework and climbing 1 flight of stairs, independently. She drives and manages her own finances.

The orthopedic surgery service surgically repaired the fracture with an open reduction and internal fixation. She tolerated the procedure well with spinal anesthesia. She is now on the medical-surgical floor. You are called by the orthopedic surgery resident, who asks that you manage her pain and hypertension. She is otherwise following routine postoperative orthopedic protocol for venous thromboembolism (VTE) prophylaxis, activity, diet, physical and occupational therapy, and wound care. The patient states her pain is rated at 8 out of 10 in severity during your evaluation.

Physical examination reveals a 5-ft 2-in, 52-kg (BMI 21) elderly Caucasian female in moderate distress from pain. Her pulse is 100 bpm and regular, BP is 150/90 mm Hg, RR is 20/min, and temperature is 37°C. Her skin is warm and dry with good capillary refill. Chest is clear to auscultation bilaterally with good inspiratory effort. Cardiac examination reveals tachycardia with a regular rhythm. S1 and S2 are noted without murmurs. Abdomen has normal bowel sounds and is nontender to palpation. Extremities show good pulses in all extremities with no edema. The left hip surgical dressing is intact and dry. The patient is oriented to person, place, and time. She has intact sensation and spontaneously moves all extremities, with significant pain noted in the left hip following any movement. Her pulse oximeter is 95% on room air. Postoperative hemoglobin is 9.8 g/dL.

1. **How would you describe the type of pain this patient is experiencing?**

2. **How would you approach the ongoing assessment and management of the patient's pain?**

3. **What are potential adverse effects of her pain treatment?**

Answers

Summary: A healthy 80-year-old female in the immediate orthopedic postoperative period needs a pain management approach to safely and effectively provide analgesia for her musculoskeletal pain. Control of the pain will lessen physical stress and allow more rapid rehabilitation. Safety concerns are especially noteworthy in patients with advanced age or comorbid conditions that affect analgesic metabolism and increase the likelihood of adverse effects.

1. Type of pain this patient is experiencing: acute somatic.
2. Pain assessment and control may be accomplished by the use of any of several patient pain-reporting scales and physical findings. A multimodal analgesic approach of NSAIDs, opioids, and local ice compresses would serve as an effective initial strategy.
3. Potential side effects include constipation, ileus, nausea, delirium, somnolence, allergic reactions, respiratory depression, hypotension, increased bleeding risk, gastritis, acute renal failure, and others, depending on the agent.

CASE REVIEW

The elderly patient in this clinical scenario has fracture-related and postoperative tissue injury pain consistent with acute somatic (nociceptive) pain. Pain scales, pulse rate, blood pressure, and observation of general comfort can be used to assess the severity of the pain and adequacy of treatment. While tachycardia and elevated blood pressure may be seen as a sympathetic response to acute pain, these findings are often absent and may be less significant than expected.

When patients with acute surgical pain are prescribed opioids alone for acute pain, 5% to 6% of patients continue opioid use chronically. In addition, higher inpatient opioid use is associated with higher discharge use of opioids. In light of the risks of chronic opioid use, it is important to minimize opioids perioperatively.

For surgical patients, "Enhanced Recovery After Surgery" (ERAS) protocols apply a multimodal approach with consideration for preoperative, intraoperative, and postoperative phases. One focus of ERAS protocols is to apply multimodal treatments to minimize postoperative opioid use. Multimodal analgesia is an essential approach to optimize analgesia, minimize opioids, and reduce side effects. Use of regional anesthesia preoperatively, postoperative intra-and periarticular injections, and neurostimulation employed by the surgical and anesthesia teams can significantly reduce opioid needs and accelerate functional recovery postoperatively.

It is critical for the internist to continue this multimodal approach in the perioperative period.

Many medications have been studied as components of a multimodal analgesic approach, including acetaminophen, nonsteroidal anti-inflammatory drugs (NSAIDs), gabapentin, ketamine, magnesium, dexamethasone, and lidocaine.

Scheduled acetaminophen at maximum recommended doses is often the foundation of inpatient analgesia. Nonsteroidal anti-inflammatory drugs or COX-2 inhibitors are effective for acute musculoskeletal pain and inflammation. Nonpharmacologic therapy such as local cold therapy can be applied to the postoperative site. Short-acting opioids can be prescribed if needed, with emphasis on utilizing the lowest tolerated doses and using oral opioids instead of IV if possible. Rarely, a short-term patient-controlled IV opioid delivery system is needed to deliver relief rapidly and safely. With improvement of pain in the subsequent postoperative days, opioids may be changed to oral form and titrated off.

See Figure 21-1 for a summary of the ERAS approach.

Acute adverse reactions to opioid analgesic agents include allergic reactions, sedation, increased risk for delirium, hypotension, respiratory depression, and nausea. It is important to note that sedation always precedes respiratory depression. Constipation is the only opioid side effect that persists with chronic use, for which management depends on stimulant-based laxatives such as senna or bisacodyl in addition to osmotic agents such as polyethylene glycol. NSAIDs may cause GI upset, peptic ulcer disease, or acute renal failure.

PAIN MANAGEMENT IN THE HOSPITAL

Diagnosis

Pain, specifically acute pain, is one of the most common symptoms encountered in the inpatient setting. It is a source of patient suffering, anxiety, physical stress, and metabolic demand. It is an important diagnostic clue in many disease processes and conditions. The etiology of pain should be evaluated as it is treated, so that its underlying cause can be appropriately addressed. The emotional and physical well-being of the patient requires that pain be effectively treated.

Nociceptive pain is a response to strong mechanical, thermal, or chemical stimuli generated by nociceptors. These stimuli are transmitted as nerve impulses that are interpreted as pain. Tissue injury induces inflammatory mediators that contribute to this response. Nociceptive pain can be categorized as either somatic (related to skin, muscles, bone, and other tissue of somatic embryologic origin) or visceral (related to internal organs). Neuropathic pain refers to peripheral or central nerve injury or dysfunction. Nociceptive pain responds favorably to local therapy, acetaminophen, NSAIDs, and opioid analgesics, while neuropathic pain is more responsive to selective serotonin and norepinephrine reuptake inhibitors, anticonvulsants such as gabapentin and pregabalin, and lidocaine.

Pain is always subjective, and the patient's report of pain should be respected. Pain is defined by the International Association for the Study of Pain as an unpleasant sensory and emotional experience associated with, or resembling that associated with, actual or potential tissue damage. There is no test to verify or quantify the severity of the pain except for the patient's word and behavioral

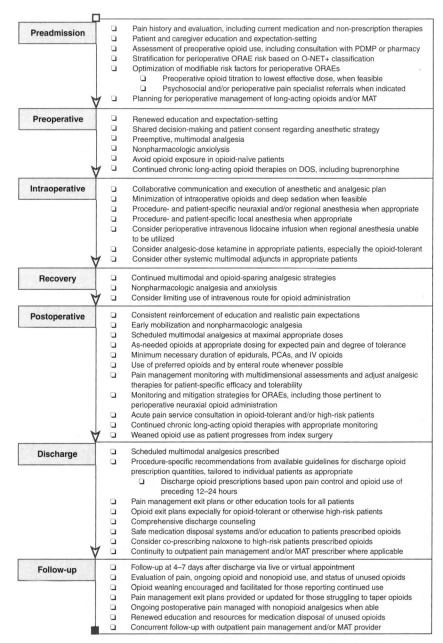

Preadmission	❏	Pain history and evaluation, including current medication and non-prescription therapies
	❏	Patient and caregiver education and expectation-setting
	❏	Assessment of preoperative opioid use, including consultation with PDMP or pharmacy
	❏	Stratification for perioperative ORAE risk based on O-NET+ classification
	❏	Optimization of modifiable risk factors for perioperative ORAEs
	❏	Preoperative opioid titration to lowest effective dose, when feasible
	❏	Psychosocial and/or perioperative pain specialist referrals when indicated
	❏	Planning for perioperative management of long-acting opioids and/or MAT

Preoperative	❏	Renewed education and expectation-setting
	❏	Shared decision-making and patient consent regarding anesthetic strategy
	❏	Preemptive, multimodal analgesia
	❏	Nonpharmacologic anxiolysis
	❏	Avoid opioid exposure in opioid-naïve patients
	❏	Continued chronic long-acting opioid therapies on DOS, including buprenorphine

Intraoperative	❏	Collaborative communication and execution of anesthetic and analgesic plan
	❏	Minimization of intraoperative opioids and deep sedation when feasible
	❏	Procedure- and patient-specific neuraxial and/or regional anesthesia when appropriate
	❏	Procedure- and patient-specific local anesthesia when appropriate
	❏	Consider perioperative intravenous lidocaine infusion when regional anesthesia unable to be utilized
	❏	Consider analgesic-dose ketamine in appropriate patients, especially the opioid-tolerant
	❏	Consider other systemic multimodal adjuncts in appropriate patients

Recovery	❏	Continued multimodal and opioid-sparing analgesic strategies
	❏	Nonpharmacologic analgesia and anxiolysis
	❏	Consider limiting use of intravenous route for opioid administration

Postoperative	❏	Consistent reinforcement of education and realistic pain expectations
	❏	Early mobilization and nonpharmacologic analgesia
	❏	Scheduled multimodal analgesics at maximal appropriate doses
	❏	As-needed opioids at appropriate dosing for expected pain and degree of tolerance
	❏	Minimum necessary duration of epidurals, PCAs, and IV opioids
	❏	Use of preferred opioids and by enteral route whenever possible
	❏	Pain management monitoring with multidimensional assessments and adjust analgesic therapies for patient-specific efficacy and tolerability
	❏	Monitoring and mitigation strategies for ORAEs, including those pertinent to perioperative neuraxial opioid administration
	❏	Acute pain service consultation in opioid-tolerant and/or high-risk patients
	❏	Continued chronic long-acting opioid therapies with appropriate monitoring
	❏	Weaned opioid use as patient progresses from index surgery

Discharge	❏	Scheduled multimodal analgesics prescribed
	❏	Procedure-specific recommendations from available guidelines for discharge opioid prescription quantities, tailored to individual patients as appropriate
	❏	Discharge opioid prescriptions based upon pain control and opioid use of preceding 12–24 hours
	❏	Pain management exit plans or other education tools for all patients
	❏	Opioid exit plans expecially for opioid-tolerant or otherwise high-risk patients
	❏	Comprehensive discharge counseling
	❏	Safe medication disposal systems and/or education to patients prescribed opioids
	❏	Consider co-prescribing naloxone to high-risk patients prescribed opioids
	❏	Continuity to outpatient pain management and/or MAT prescriber where applicable

Follow-up	❏	Follow-up at 4–7 days after discharge via live or virtual appointment
	❏	Evaluation of pain, ongoing opioid and nonopioid use, and status of unused opioids
	❏	Opioid weaning encouraged and facilitated for those reporting continued use
	❏	Pain management exit plans provided or updated for those struggling to taper opioids
	❏	Ongoing postoperative pain managed with nonopioid analgesics when able
	❏	Renewed education and resources for medication disposal of unused opioids
	❏	Concurrent follow-up with outpatient pain management and/or MAT provider

Figure 21-1. ERAS approach summary. (Reproduced from Hyland SJ, Brockhaus KK, Vincent WR, Spence NZ, Lucki MM, Howkins MJ, Cleary RK. Perioperative Pain Management and Opioid Stewardship: A Practical Guide. *Healthcare (Basel).* 2021 Mar 16;9(3):333)

response to the pain. Each patient's perception of pain is influenced by social, psychological, and biological factors. An individual's response to pain is as unique as is the response to analgesics. A thorough pain history should be performed for all patients, including severity assessment, localization, temporal features, aggravating and alleviating factors, previous use of analgesics, and previous alcohol or drug dependence. Physical examination should localize the pain and note the patient's response to pain. Clues to etiology can also be determined by the examination, such as costovertebral angle tenderness, rebound tenderness, reproducible chest pain, and others. Specialized physical exam maneuvers and techniques can help to diagnose or elicit specific etiologies of pain.

Pain scales should be used to quantify pain initially and to measure ongoing analgesic effectiveness. Scales may be self-assessment tools used by the patient to report to caregivers, or pain observation scales that target patients with cognitive impairments or communication challenges. The simplest self-assessment scales have the patient rate the pain on a 0 to 10 scale, with 10 being the most severe pain, or a 0 to 9 face scale, with a neutral face indicating no pain to a crying face meaning severe pain. Any scale may be used as long as it is patient appropriate and used consistently. A reasonable goal for a conscious patient is a pain rating of 3 or less out of 10 (Figure 21-2). It is appropriate to ask a patient what pain level is tolerable for him or her.

Wong-Baker FACES pain rating scale
See Figure 21-3.

Brief word instructions Point to each face using the words to describe the pain intensity. Ask the child to choose face that best describes own pain and record the appropriate number.

Original instructions Explain to the person that each face is for a person who feels happy because he has no pain (hurt) or sad because he has some or a lot of pain. *Face 0* is very happy because he doesn't hurt at all. *Face 1* hurts just a little bit. *Face*

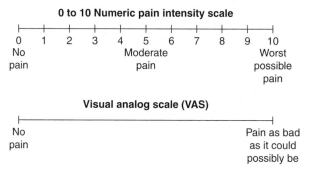

Figure 21-2. Examples of visual pain intensity assessment scales. (Reproduced with permission from Hockenberry MJ, Wilson D. *Wong's Essentials of Pediatric Nursing.* 8th ed. St. Louis: Mosby; 2009.)

Wong-Baker faces pain rating scale

	0	1	2	3	4	5
	No hurt	Hurts little bit	Hurts little more	Hurts even more	Hurts whole lot	Hurts worst
Alternate coding	0	2	4	6	8	10

Figure 21-3. Wong-Baker FACES pain rating scale. (Reproduced with permission from Hockenberry MJ, Wilson D. *Wong's Essentials of Pediatric Nursing.* 8th ed. St. Louis: Mosby; 2009.)

2 hurts a little more. *Face 3* hurts even more. *Face 4* hurts a whole lot. *Face 5* hurts as much as you can imagine, although you don't have to be crying to feel this bad. Ask the person to choose the face that best describes how he is feeling.

Rating scale is recommended for persons age 3 years and older.

Nonverbal patients and those with impaired cognition should be evaluated for pain despite an inability to communicate. Multiple tools exist, such as the Pain in Advanced Dementia (PAIN AD) (Figure 21-4) and Doloplus-2 tools for those with severe cognitive impairment and the Critical Care Pain Observation Tool (CPOT) or Behavioral Pain Scale (BPS) for patients in a critical care setting who are unable to verbalize.

Pain Assessment in Advanced Dementia: PAINAD

Items	0	1	2	Score
Breathing independent of vocalization	Normal	Occasional labored breathing. Short period of hyperventilation	Noisy labored breathing. Long period of hyperventilation. Cheyne-Stokes respirations.	(0–2)
Negative vocalization	None	Occasional moan or groan. Low-level of speech with a negative or disapproving quality	Repeated troubled calling out. Loud moaning or groaning. Crying	(0–2)
Facial expression	Smiling or inexpressive	Sad, frightened, frown	Facial grimacing	(0–2)
Body language	Relaxed	Tense. Distressed pacing. Fidgeting	Rigid. Fists clenched. Knees pulled up. Pulling or pushing away. Striking out	(0–2)
Consolability	No need to console	Distracted or reassured by voice or touch	Unable to console, distract or reassure	(0–2)
				TOTAL (0–10)

Instructions: Observe the patient for 3–5 minutes before scoring his or her behaviors. Score each item based on the patient's behavior (0, 1, 2). Add scores for each item to achieve a total score. Monitor changes over time and in response to treatment.

Figure 21-4. The Pain Assessment in Advanced Dementia (PAINAD) scale. (Reproduced with permission from Warden V, Hurley AC, Volicer L. Development and psychometric evaluation of the Pain Assessment in Advanced Dementia (PAINAD) scale. *J Am Med* Dir Assoc. 2003;4(1):9-15.)

Assessing the degree to which a patient's pain impacts their daily function is an underappreciated method of monitoring pain severity and efficacy of management.

Treatment

Nonpharmacologic methods of treating acute pain include relaxation techniques, hypnosis, acupuncture, transcutaneous electrical neural stimulation (TENS), massage therapy, and heat and cold topical treatments. Pharmaceutical agents include acetaminophen, NSAIDs, corticosteroids, opioids, lidocaine, ketamine, clonidine, and topical anesthetic agents. They may be administered locally, such as in intra-articular or regional blockade, orally, parenterally, or via epidural route. This discussion will focus on oral and parenteral agents used by most internal medicine residents. It is worthwhile to be aware of other modalities and the other medical professionals available to help with challenging patients. Depending on local availability and practice, consultation with pharmacy, pain medicine, anesthesia, interventional radiology, or palliative care can provide additional expertise and treatment options.

Analgesics reduce the sensation of pain by altering perception of pain in the CNS, inhibiting local pain and inflammatory mediator production, or interrupting the neural impulse in the spinal cord, such as with a neuraxial block. One should target the lowest effective dose of analgesic agent, taking into account metabolic pathways, comorbid illnesses, medication interactions, and potential side effects. Always have dosing references for specific agents available that include opioid equivalent dosing information.

Acetaminophen and NSAIDs, including COX-2 inhibitors, are step 1 agents in the WHO analgesic ladder. They are for pain on the low end of the severity scale. Acetaminophen may be used at 325 to 1000 mg per dose up to 4 g daily. It has antipyretic and analgesic properties. It can potentiate warfarin at higher dosing and may cause acute liver failure in overdoses. It does not have antiplatelet effects. Aspirin and NSAIDs, including COX-2 inhibitors, have anti-inflammatory, antipyretic, and analgesic effects. They have a variable effect on platelet function, may induce gastrointestinal bleeding, should be used with caution in patients with hepatic and renal disease, and should be avoided in patients with an aspirin allergy. Both acetaminophen and NSAIDs may be used in conjunction with opioid agents.

Step 2 agents include tramadol and the opioids codeine, hydrocodone, and meperidine. Meperidine is not recommended due to the potential for accumulation of metabolites and risk of seizures. These agents reach a dose-response plateau unlike step 3 agents. Tramadol is a unique medication with opiate and with serotonin norepinephrine reuptake inhibiting properties. It binds to opioid receptors. Tramadol is dosed at 50 to 100 mg every 6 hours prn. Dosing reduction is recommended for the elderly and those with renal or liver dysfunction. See Table 21-1 for other dosing comparisons of step 2 agents.

Table 21-1. Equianalgesic Doses of Opioid Analgesics

Medication	Onset	Duration	Parenteral Dosing (mg)	Enteral Dosing	Comments
Fentanyl	Rapid (<10 min)	Short (1–2 h)	0.1 mg IM/ IV/SC	Not available orally	Also available in patch form
Hydromorphone	Quick (15–30 min)	Moderate (4–5 h)	1.0–2.0 mg IM/IV/SC	7.5 mg	
Methadone	Slow (45–60 min)	Long (6–8 h)	10 mg IM/ IV/SC	20 mg	Commonly used for chronic pain
Morphine	Quick (15–30 min)	Moderate (4–6 h)	10 mg IM/ IV/SC	60 mg	
Oxycodone	Quick (15–30 min)	Moderate (4–6 h)	Not available parenterally	30 mg	
Meperidine	Variable (10–45 min)	Short (2–4 h)	75 mg IM/ IV/SC	300 mg	Typically not recommended due to efficacy studies
Codeine	Quick (15–30 min)	Moderate (4–6 h)	120 mg IM/ IV/SC	200 mg	Most commonly given orally

Note: For comparative reference only. Consult therapeutic sources for individual patient dosing.

Step 3 agents are morphine, hydromorphone, oxycodone, fentanyl, and methadone (see Table 21-1). Morphine is the standard to which the other agents are compared. Opioid-naïve patients should be started with lower doses than opioid-tolerant patients. There is no ceiling to the analgesic effect of these agents. The onset and duration of the agent help to determine the appropriate dosing interval and route of administration. Transdermal preparations of fentanyl should only be given for chronic pain of moderate or severe intensity. Some opioids are used in patient-controlled analgesia (PCA) regimens. Most institutions will have order sets that specify a patient-controlled dose, a lockout interval between doses, and a maximum dose per specific period of time. A basal rate of constant infusion may be given along with the patient-triggered doses. All the opioid agents may cause nausea, constipation, and neurologic or respiratory suppression. Bowel regimens including a mild stimulant agent (eg, senna) are strongly recommended on a scheduled basis, titrated to 1 bowel movement daily, with additional osmotic agents as needed. If constipation persists despite maximal initial therapies, specific treatment for opioid induced constipation can be implemented. Fiber supplementation in the context of opioid use is not advised, as this does not overcome the slowed peristalsis of opioid-induced constipation. Of note, there is no evidence for the benefit of docusate.

Antiemetics may be used as needed. Dosages should be adjusted with renal and hepatic impairment and used cautiously with lung disease, malnutrition, endocrine disease, and other psychotropic or sedative agents. Urinary retention due to opioids may be caused by increased bladder, ureteral, and urethral sphincter tone.

Intraspinal administration of opioids may be given with the assistance of the anesthesiology clinicians. Coordination of dosing after acute intraspinal analgesia requires timely and clear communication.

Naloxone may be given to reverse the effect of opioids. It should be used with caution in chronic opioid users. It can precipitate agitation, anxiety, nausea, and seizures.

TIPS TO REMEMBER

- The cause of acute pain should be determined prior to, or in conjunction with, treatment of the pain.
- Pain scales should be used to determine severity of pain and effectiveness of treatment.
- Multimodal analgesic therapy should be used whenever possible.
- Concurrent medications, comorbid medical conditions, age, and previous exposure to opioid agents should be considered in opioid dosing decisions.
- Bowel regimens should be standard anticipatory therapy on all patients taking opioids.

COMPREHENSION QUESTIONS

1. A 24-year-old female is hospitalized with a kidney stone and pyelonephritis. She is started on appropriate IV antibiotics and fluid therapy. She has no allergies and has never had opioids in the past. Her weight is 48 kg. Her colicky pain is rated at 7 to 8 out of 10 in severity at admission, with significant nausea and occasional vomiting. She has not passed the stone. What is/are reasonable analgesic option(s)?

    A. Fentanyl transdermal 12-µg/h patch every 3 days

    B. Acetaminophen 1000 mg orally every 8 hours as needed

    C. Naloxone 0.4 mg IV every 8 hours as needed

    D. Hydromorphone 0.6 mg IV every 3 hours as needed

2. A 65-year-old man is on his third postoperative day following a knee replacement. He is progressing as expected but is limited in physical therapy due to pain. He is only on IV morphine as needed every 3 hours. He is allergic to aspirin that caused hives and dyspnea. What agent should be avoided?
  A. Naproxen
  B. Acetaminophen/hydrocodone
  C. Oxycodone
  D. Clonidine

3. Which of the following agents is not commonly administered via PCA?
  A. Fentanyl
  B. Morphine
  C. Oxycodone
  D. Hydromorphone

Answers

1. **D.** Transdermal fentanyl should be used only with opioid-tolerant patients with moderate to severe chronic pain requiring continuous analgesic dosing. Acetaminophen is likely not potent enough to control this moderate to severe pain, and it may not be absorbed well orally due to the potential for vomiting. Naloxone is used to reverse the effects of opioids. Hydromorphone at this dose is appropriate for an opioid-naïve patient.

2. **A.** Naproxen should be avoided with a known allergy to aspirin. There is a potential for similar reactions. The others have no cross-reactivity to aspirin or other NSAIDs.

3. **C.** Oxycodone has no IV preparation available in the United States at the time of this writing, so it cannot be used in PCA systems.

SUGGESTED READINGS

Dayoub EJ, Jena AB. Does pain lead to tachycardia? Revisiting the association between self-reported pain and heart rate in a national sample of urgent emergency department visits. *Mayo Clin Proc.* 2015;90(8):1165–1166.

Helfand M, Freeman M. *Assessment and Management of Acute Pain in Adult Medical Inpatients: A Systematic Review.* Washington, DC: US Department of Veterans Affairs; 2008.

Hockenberry MJ, Wilson D. *Wong's Essentials of Pediatric Nursing.* 8th ed. St. Louis: Mosby; 2009.

Hyland SJ, Brockhaus KK, Vincent WR, et al. Perioperative pain management and opioid stewardship: a practical guide. *Healthcare (Basel).* 2021;9(3):333.

Mitchell SL. Advanced dementia. *N Engl J Med.* 2015;373(13):1276–1277.

Olmos AV, Steen S, Boscardin CK, et al. Increasing the use of multimodal analgesia during adult surgery in a tertiary academic anaesthesia department. *BMJ Open Qual.* 2021;10(3):e001320.

Small C, Laycock H. Acute postoperative pain management. *Br J Surg.* 2020;107(2):e70–e80.

Smith TW Jr, Wang X, Singer MA, et al. Enhanced recovery after surgery: a clinical review of implementation across multiple surgical subspecialties. *Am J Surg.* 2020;219(3):530–534.

Wachter RM, Goldman L, Hollander H. *Hospital Medicine.* Philadelphia: Lippincott Williams &
Wilkins; 2000.

Washington University School of Medicine Department of Medicine, Green GB, Harris IA, et al. *The
Washington Manual of Medical Therapeutics.* 31st ed. Philadelphia: Lippincott Williams & Wilkins;
2004.

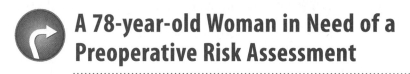

A 78-year-old Woman in Need of a Preoperative Risk Assessment

Robert Robinson, MD, MS, FACP

You are asked to perform a preoperative risk assessment on a 78-year-old woman with a traumatic femur fracture after slipping on ice. The patient takes no medications, has no known medical problems, has no cardiac symptoms, has no problems with easy bruising or prolonged bleeding, and is usually able to climb several flights of stairs. The patient has a 50-pack-year smoking history but quit about 10 years ago.

Physical examination is unremarkable except for evidence of the femur fracture.

Tests done in the ED show a normal sinus rhythm on ECG, hyperinflation of the lungs on chest x-ray, and unremarkable electrolytes and CBC. The surgical resident indicates that the surgery will take about 1 hour and will be done with regional anesthesia.

1. **What additional tests are needed to assess this patient's risk of perioperative cardiac complications?**

2. **Is it possible to quantify the patient's risk of perioperative cardiac complications?**

3. **What are this patient's risk factors for postoperative pulmonary complications?**

4. **What actions should be taken postoperatively to reduce the patient's risk of complications?**

Answers

1. The patient does not appear to have any active cardiac issues and has good exercise tolerance. The *ACC/AHA Guidelines on Perioperative Evaluation and Care for Noncardiac Surgery* indicate that it is reasonable to proceed to surgery under these circumstances without additional testing. The risk of a major adverse cardiac event (MACE) of death or myocardial infarction (MI) in this patient is low based on the type of surgery (nonvascular extremity) and the patient's cardiovascular history.

2. The *ACC/AHA Guidelines on Perioperative Evaluation and Care for Noncardiac Surgery* recommends the use of a validated risk assessment tool such as the Revised Cardiac Risk Index (RCRI) or American College of Surgeons National Surgical Quality Improvement Program (NSQIP) calculation to quantify the risk of MACE in surgical patients.

3. Postoperative pulmonary complications such as atelectasis, hypoxia, bronchospasm, and pneumonia are relatively common. Age (>60 years) and possible

COPD are known risk factors for postoperative pulmonary complications. Cigarette smoking is not a risk factor because the patient quit smoking about 10 years ago. The NSQIP has developed and validated a calculation to quantify the risk of postoperative pulmonary complications.

4. This patient would benefit from DVT prophylaxis, early mobilization, and incentive spirometry in the postoperative time frame. Due to the nature of the injury and surgery, the patient is at increased risk of DVT. Monitoring for evidence of bleeding, wound dehiscence, and infection should be routine after a surgical procedure.

CASE REVIEW

The medical history is the most effective and efficient perioperative risk assessment tool.

This patient has no known medical problems, good functional status (>4 METS), and no active cardiac issues. Using the *ACC/AHA Guidelines on Perioperative Evaluation and Care for Noncardiac Surgery* criteria, this patient can go to surgery without further cardiac testing or other intervention. Cardiac risk assessment tools can be used to quantify the risk of perioperative MACE and pulmonary complications. Additional testing, such as a cardiac stress test or echocardiography, will not enhance risk stratification and does not add value to patient care.

Part of a preoperative examination is to identify potential postoperative risks. This patient is at increased risk of pulmonary and thrombotic complications. Recommending DVT prophylaxis and incentive spirometry is appropriate.

PERIOPERATIVE MEDICINE

Cardiac Risk Assessment

The *ACC/AHA Guidelines on Perioperative Evaluation* encourage the use of a validated cardiac risk assessment tool to improve the accuracy and objectivity of the assessment.

The RCRI is straightforward and easy to calculate, but it was derived from a relatively small population at a single medical center. The utility of the RCRI has been confirmed in multiple settings and is noteworthy for excellent negative predictive value.

The NSQIP risk assessment tool was derived from a dataset of hundreds of thousands of patients at more than 1000 different hospitals in the United States. This tool requires complex calculations, so it is done with purpose-built calculators on computers or mobile devices. This increased complexity provides greater precision in the risk assessment and includes surgery-specific cardiovascular risks.

Table 22-1. Padua Prediction Score

Condition	Points
Active cancer	3
History of VTE	
Reduced mobility	
Known thrombophilic condition	
Surgery or trauma in the last month	2
Age ≥70 years	1
Cardiac failure or acute myocardial infarction	
Acute stroke	
Respiratory failure	
Active infection	
Rheumatologic disorder	
BMI ≥30	
A score of 4 or more is an indication for VTE prophylaxis	

Cardiac Risk Reduction

Cardiac risk reduction for noncardiac surgery is an area of active research. Recent studies have called into question the utility of strategies using revascularization and medications for this purpose.

VTE Prevention

DVT and PE can be prevented with several strategies including heparin, low-molecular-weight heparin, direct oral anticoagulants (DOACs), warfarin, aspirin, and mechanical devices. A VTE prevention strategy should be implemented in all hospitalized patients assessed to be a moderate risk or higher for VTE using the Padua Prediction Score (Table 22-1) or other validated VTE risk scoring system.

HIGH-RISK MEDICATIONS

There are medications that should be adjusted prior to surgery in order to help to minimize complications.

High-risk Medications in the Perioperative Timeframe

See Table 22-2.

Table 22-2. High-risk Medications in the Perioperative Timeframe

Medication	Risk	Potential Action	Guidelines
Anticoagulants	Bleeding	Discontinue	Yes
Aspirin	Bleeding	Discontinue	Yes
P2Y$_{12}$ inhibitors	Bleeding	Discontinue	Yes
Insulin and other diabetes drugs	Hypoglycemia	Modify dose Monitor glucose	
Narcotics	Sedation	Modify dose Monitor	
Narcotic antagonists	Exaggerated response to narcotics	Discontinue	
Seizure medications	Seizures	Ensure adequate dose administered	
ACE-I/ARBs	Hypotension	Modify dose	
Beta blockers	Hypotension	Modify dose	
Diuretics	Volume depletion Hypotension		

TIPS TO REMEMBER

- Use a validated cardiac risk assessment tool to quantitate the risk of MACE for the proposed surgery.
- Extensive testing does not add value to perioperative clinical care.
- High-risk medications (antiplatelets, anticoagulants, hypoglycemic agents, and steroids) require careful attention in the perioperative period.
- Surgical patients should be started on therapy to prevent DVTs.

COMPREHENSION QUESTIONS

1. You are evaluating the cardiac risk for a right total knee replacement in a 59-year-old male with diabetes (treated with insulin) and diabetic nephropathy (serum creatinine 1.5 mg/dL). The patient has difficulty walking due to severe osteoarthritis and is scheduled for surgery in 1 week. The patient denies cardiac symptoms and is able to climb 2 flights of stairs. His only limitation on mobility is knee pain at this time.

What additional information is needed to assess this patient's risk of surgical complications?

A. A cardiac stress test due to the presence of 2 risk factors (diabetes treated with insulin and renal disease)

B. An echocardiogram

C. A CBC, BMP, chest x-ray, and 12-lead ECG

D. None of the above

2. You are evaluating the cardiac risk for a right total knee replacement in a 59-year-old male with diabetes (treated with insulin), diabetic nephropathy (serum creatinine 1.5 mg/dL), and a history of myocardial infarction 6 months ago. The patient had left main coronary artery disease and underwent CABG.

The patient has difficulty walking due to severe osteoarthritis and is scheduled for surgery in 1 week. The patient denies cardiac symptoms and is able to climb two flights of stairs. His only limitation on mobility is knee pain at this time. The patient is taking a beta blocker for his CAD and has a resting pulse rate of 70 beats/min.

What additional information is needed to assess this patient's risk of surgical complications?

A. A cardiac stress test

B. An echocardiogram

C. A CBC, BMP, chest x-ray, and 12-lead ECG

D. None of the above

3. You are evaluating the cardiac risk for a right total knee replacement in a 77-year-old female with hypertension and a history of myocardial infarction 6 months ago. The patient underwent PCI at that time but is unsure if a stent was placed. The patient is on clopidogrel and a beta blocker.

The patient has difficulty walking due to severe osteoarthritis and is scheduled for surgery in 1 week. She denies cardiac symptoms and is able to climb 2 flights of stairs. Her only limitation on mobility is knee pain at this time.

What additional information is needed to assess this patient's risk of surgical complications?

A. A cardiac stress test

B. An echocardiogram

C. A CBC, BMP, chest x-ray, and 12-lead ECG

D. Information regarding the patient's PCI 6 months ago

E. None of the above

4. The case in Question 3 continues: Review of records from the patient's cardiologist shows that a drug-eluting stent was placed 7 months ago. How should this patient be managed?

A. Discontinue clopidogrel 3 to 7 days before surgery.

B. Delay surgery for 12 months.

C. Delay surgery for 6 months.

D. Discontinue clopidogrel 3 to 7 days before surgery; start patient on IV heparin for full anticoagulation before surgery.

Answers

1. **D.** The patient has no active cardiac issues and exercise tolerance >4 METS, so it is reasonable to proceed with surgery without additional testing. The patient has just 1 risk factor: diabetes treated with insulin. The patient's renal insufficiency is not severe enough to qualify as a risk factor.

2. **D.** No additional testing is indicated at this time. He has had a recent CABG and has no active cardiovascular symptoms. This patient is low risk for cardiovascular complications from surgery.

3. **D.** It is essential to know if the patient had a stent placed at the time of PCI, and also to know what type of stent was placed.

4. **A.** The patient has been on DAPT for more than 6 months since the DES was placed. It is reasonable to discontinue the clopidogrel for a short time to allow for this elective surgery. The clopidogrel should be restarted as soon as possible after the surgery.

SUGGESTED READINGS

Fleisher LA, Fleischmann KE, Auerbach AD, et al. 2014 ACC/AHA guideline on perioperative cardiovascular evaluation and management of patients undergoing noncardiac surgery: a report of the American College of Cardiology/American Heart Association Task Force on Practice Guidelines. *Circulation.* 2014;130(24):e278–e333.

Ford MK, Beattie WS, Wijeysundera DN. Systematic review: prediction of perioperative cardiac complications and mortality by the revised cardiac risk index. *Ann Intern Med.* 2010;152(1):26–35.

Gupta PK, Gupta H, Sundaram A, et al. Development and validation of a risk calculator for prediction of cardiac risk after surgery. *Circulation.* 2011;124(4):381–387.

Gupta H, Gupta PK, Fang X, et al. Development and validation of a risk calculator predicting postoperative respiratory failure. *Chest.* 2011;140(5):1207–1215.

Levine GN, Bates ER, Bittl JA, et al. 2016 ACC/AHA Guideline Focused Update on Duration of Dual Antiplatelet Therapy in Patients With Coronary Artery Disease: A Report of the American College of Cardiology/American Heart Association Task Force on Clinical Practice Guidelines: An Update of the 2011 ACCF/AHA/SCAI Guideline for Percutaneous Coronary Intervention, 2011 ACCF/AHA Guideline for Coronary Artery Bypass Graft Surgery, 2012 ACC/AHA/ACP/AATS/PCNA/SCAI/STS Guideline for the Diagnosis and Management of Patients With Stable Ischemic Heart Disease, 2013 ACCF/AHA Guideline for the Management of ST-Elevation Myocardial Infarction, 2014 AHA/ACC Guideline for the Management of Patients With Non-ST-Elevation Acute Coronary Syndromes, and 2014 ACC/AHA Guideline on Perioperative Cardiovascular Evaluation and Management of Patients Undergoing Noncardiac Surgery [published correction appears in Circulation. 2016;134(10):e192–e194]. *Circulation.* 2016;134(10):e123–e155.

A 72-year-old Man With Pneumonia

Robert Robinson, MD, MS, FACP

You are called by the ED and told of a 72-year-old male nonsmoker with a history of diabetes, coronary artery disease, and hypertension who presents with pneumonia and needs to be admitted to the hospital. The patient is febrile and tachypneic, has a blood pressure of 145/65, and has an oxygen saturation of 95% on room air. Physical examination is significant for rhonchi in the right lower lung fields, and a chest x-ray showing a right lower lobe infiltrate. Laboratory studies show a white blood cell count of 14,000 and no evidence of acute renal failure. COVID and influenza testing is negative, blood cultures have been obtained, and an unknown antibiotic has been started in the ED.

1. Should this patient be admitted to the hospital?
2. What historic information is needed to make a treatment decision for this patient?
3. What is the best initial treatment if this patient has no antibiotic allergies and no significant contact with the health care system?
4. What would be the best initial treatment if this patient has no antibiotic allergies and is a resident of a long-term care facility?

Answers

1. Yes, to a non-ICU setting. This patient is hemodynamically stable and has a CURB-65 score (an easy-to-use risk assessment method for community-acquired pneumonia [CAP] described below) of 2 (age, tachypnea), so it is reasonable to manage the patient out of the ICU.

2. A history of medication allergies, particularly antibiotic allergies, is essential for the development of a safe treatment plan. Additionally, because initial antimicrobial therapy is selected primarily based on the type of pneumonia a patient has, risk factors for other respiratory infections should be considered. A vaccination history (pneumonia, influenza, and COVID) may be helpful.

3. Combined therapy with ceftriaxone, cefotaxime, ceftaroline, ertapenem, or ampicillin/sulbactam *plus* a macrolide or doxycycline is first-line therapy. For patients who are unable to take beta-lactam/macrolide therapy, a respiratory fluoroquinolone is an alternative for a hospitalized patient with CAP. The use of respiratory fluoroquinolones is associated with a higher risk of *Clostridioides difficile* than with the beta-lactam/macrolide combination therapy.

4. Initial antibiotic choices for a CAP do not differ based on residence in a long-term care facility. The pneumonia category of health care–associated pneumonia (HCAP) was removed from the evidence-based 2016 ATS/IDS guidelines because of changing epidemiology and concerns regarding overtreatment with broad-spectrum antibiotics.

CASE REVIEW

This patient appears to have a CAP that requires hospital admission based on his CURB-65 score. Hemodynamic stability and a low CURB-65 score indicate that the patient is appropriate for admission to a non-ICU level of care. The patient does not meet the criteria for hospital-acquired pneumonia (HAP). COVID and influenza pneumonia should be considered in all patients. Additional history is needed to better assess risk factors for other pneumonias. A history of recent travel should raise concern for avian influenza, SARS, parasites, lung flukes, fungi, etc. Exposure to others who are symptomatic for a respiratory illness should raise concern for *Bordetella*, mycobacteria, *Legionella*, etc. A history of high-risk sexual behavior, injectable drug use, long-term steroid use, or a history of malignancy should raise concern for an immunocompromised status, and the differential diagnosis should include viral infections (ie, HIV, cytomegalovirus, varicella, and herpes), mycobacterial infections, fungal infections (including *Pneumocystis*), and atypical bacterial infections (eg, *Nocardia*, *Actinomyces*).

PNEUMONIA

Diagnosis

Pneumonia is suggested by a history that contains 1 or more symptoms of pneumonia such as cough, fever, pleuritic chest pain, dyspnea, and/or sputum production. The history is insensitive for the diagnosis of pneumonia but is essential for eliciting risk factors for immunocompetent status, as well as the likely type of pneumonia.

Physical examination may reveal fever, tachycardia, tachypnea, rales, and evidence of pulmonary consolidation (egophony and dullness to percussion). However, physical examination has not been shown to be sensitive for the diagnosis of pneumonia either.

A CBC, BMP, and blood cultures should be obtained on all patients with suspected pneumonia. The value of sputum cultures is controversial. Urine antigen testing (*Legionella* and *Streptococcus pneumoniae*) and viral testing (influenza, COVID and others) also may be helpful.

Chest radiography showing a new infiltrate with a compatible history and examination is considered the gold standard for the diagnosis of pneumonia. A chest x-ray should be ordered on all patients with suspected pneumonia. Comparison with prior radiographs (if available) should be made (Table 23-1).

Risk stratification with CURB-65

The CURB-65 criteria are an easy-to-use risk assessment method for CAP, and they are useful for determining which patients can be managed as outpatients (Table 23-2).

Table 23-1. Differential Diagnosis for Pulmonary Infiltrates

Acute Infiltrate	Chronic or Nonresolving Infiltrate
Pneumonia	Nonresolving infection
Pulmonary edema	ARDS
Aspiration pneumonitis	Lung abscess
Hemorrhage	Mycobacterial infection
Contusion	*Pneumocystis jiroveci*
Pulmonary infarction	Fungal infection
Postobstructive pneumonia	Chronic aspiration
Inhalation injury	Hypersensitivity pneumonitis
Radiation pneumonitis	Lipoid pneumonia
ARDS	Eosinophilic lung disease
	Malignancy
	Sarcoidosis
	Rheumatologic conditions
	Vasculitis
	Radiation pneumonitis
	Fibrosis
	Pulmonary alveolar proteinosis
	Parasites
	Pneumoconiosis
	Inhalation injury
	Cryptogenic organizing pneumonia

Table 23-2. CURB-65 Criteria

Criteria	Treatment Location
Confusion	0–1 criteria → outpatient
Uremia	2 criteria → inpatient
Respiratory rate >30	3 or more criteria → ICU
Systolic blood pressure ≤90	
Age ≥65	

Table 23-3. Common Bacterial Causes of Community-acquired Pneumonia

Typical Bacteria	Atypical Bacteria
Streptococcus pneumoniae	Mycoplasma pneumoniae
Haemophilus influenzae	Chlamydophila pneumoniae
Moraxella catarrhalis	Legionella pneumophila

Table 23-4. Nonbacterial Causes of Community-acquired Pneumonia

Viruses	Fungal
Influenza	Cryptococcus
Coronavirus	Histoplasma
Rhinovirus	Coccidioides
Varicella	Blastomyces

Microbiology of community-acquired pneumonia

CAP can be caused by so-called typical or atypical bacterial organisms. More than 100 organisms (bacteria, viruses, fungi, and parasites) have been identified as causative agents for CAP, but the vast majority of cases are caused by a short list of microbes (Tables 23-3 and 23-4).

Treatment

The initial treatment of patients with pneumonia is driven by patient allergies and drug availability. Duration of antibiotic therapy remains controversial. Duration ranges from 5 to 14 days (Table 23-5).

Consider de-escalation of antibiotic therapy 48 to 72 hours after initiation of antibiotics, depending on culture results and the clinical status of the patient.

Fungal pneumonia

Fungi causing respiratory infections are ubiquitous, and symptoms are often mild and nonspecific. Risk factors for severe fungal pneumonia include immunosuppression, abnormal pulmonary parenchyma (bronchiectasis, emphysema, and pulmonary fibrosis), and chronic lung disease. It is important to remember that exposures to large fungal loads can overwhelm an immunocompetent person's ability to adequately respond as well (Table 23-6).

Viral pneumonia

Viral respiratory tract infections are extremely common and have been a frequent cause of hospital admission during the COVID-19 pandemic. The vast majority of

Table 23-5. Treatment Recommendations From 2007 IDSA Guidelines

CAP (non-ICU status)	Respiratory fluoroquinolone alone
	or
	One of the following:
	    Third- or fourth-generation
	    cephalosporin
	    Ertapenem
	    Ampicillin/sulbactam
	    Macrolide or doxycycline

CAP (ICU status)	Antipneumococcal beta-lactam *and* Respiratory fluoroquinolone *or* a macrolide Add antipseudomonal coverage for patients with risk factors for *Pseudomonas* infection

HAP/VAP/HCAP (initial therapy)	One of the following:
	    Antipseudomonal cephalosporin
	    Antipseudomonal carbapenem
	    Piperacillin/tazobactam
	    Respiratory fluoroquinolone *or*
	    aminoglycoside
	    Linezolid *or* vancomycin

patients with viral pneumonias do not require hospitalization for these infections. Serious cases of viral pneumonia do require hospital admission and supportive care. Some viral respiratory tract infections have antiviral treatment options (Table 23-7). Treatment options for serious COVID infections are rapidly evolving. Consulting current evidence-based treatment protocols is essential for the management of COVID patients.

Health care costs

Antibiotic selection is one of the largest costs associated with the treatment of a patient with pneumonia. When possible, select a less expensive drug. Antipseudomonal carbapenems (meropenem, doripenem) and other newer antibiotics are quite expensive, often costing hundreds of dollars per dose.

Table 23-6. Fungal Causes of Pneumonia, Diagnostic Methods, and Treatment Options

Fungus	Diagnostic Tests	Initial Treatment
Aspergillus	CT of chest Bronchoscopy Culture Fungal antigen testing (1-3)-β-ᴅ-Glucan assay	Voriconazole or amphotericin B
Cryptococcus	Culture Fungal antigen testing PCR Bronchoscopy	Amphotericin B (until CNS disease is excluded)
Histoplasma	Urine antigen Culture	Amphotericin B
Blastomyces	Culture	Amphotericin B
Coccidioides	Antibody titers Culture	Amphotericin B or ketoconazole or fluconazole or itraconazole

Table 23-7. Selected Treatable Causes of Viral Pneumonia

Virus	Diagnosis	Treatment
Influenza	Rapid antigen test Culture	Zanamivir or oseltamivir plus rimantadine
Varicella	Culture	Acyclovir

Table 23-8. Selected Bioterrorism Agents

Bioterrorism Agent	Diagnosis	Treatment
Anthrax	Widened mediastinum and/or pleural effusions on CXR Culture, Gram stain	Ciprofloxacin or doxycycline
Pneumonic plague	Culture	Streptomycin or doxycycline or ciprofloxacin Respiratory isolation
Tularemia	Culture	Doxycycline or ciprofloxacin

Table 23-9. Cost-effective Treatments

Drug	Less Expensive Alternatives
Antipseudomonal carbapenem	Antipseudomonal cephalosporin or piperacillin/tazobactam
Linezolid	Vancomycin
Third-generation cephalosporin + macrolide	Respiratory fluoroquinolone
Ertapenem + macrolide	Respiratory fluoroquinolone

TIPS TO REMEMBER

- A detailed history is essential for determining appropriate treatment, focusing on risk factors for multidrug-resistant bacterial infection.

- HAP occurs 48 hours or more after hospital admission. Pneumonia diagnosed on hospital day 2 may be CAP, aspiration pneumonia, or an alternative diagnosis.

- Deterioration or slow clinical improvement warrants further investigation. Causes may include inadequate antibiotics, an alternative diagnosis, or a complication of pneumonia.

- Counseling smokers about smoking cessation and respiratory pathogen vaccination (COVID, influenza, or bacterial pneumonia) before discharge may have long-term benefits for patients.

COMPREHENSION QUESTIONS

1. While on night call, you are called to urgently evaluate a cross-cover patient. The patient is an 81-year-old female admitted 3 days prior for CAP. She was started on levofloxacin and low-molecular-weight heparin for DVT prophylaxis. The respiratory viral panel and blood and sputum cultures are thus far negative. The patient reports the sudden onset of dyspnea. She has no other chronic medical problems and is unable to recall any triggering events. The patient has a respiratory rate of 30, and her oxygen saturation is 85% on room air. Her examination is significant for rales in all lung fields, and she has no lower extremity edema, calf tenderness, or JVD.
    a) What is your differential diagnosis for the patient's dyspnea and hypoxia?
    b) What should be done to evaluate the cause or causes of the patient's dyspnea and hypoxia?
    c) What initial management is appropriate for this patient?

2. You are consulted by the orthopedic service to evaluate a patient with post-operative confusion. The patient is a 57-year-old male who underwent elective right knee replacement 5 days ago. The patient has no chronic medical problems and has been on DVT prophylaxis during the postoperative period. The patient is unable to provide a useful history, and physical examination is unrevealing. The patient is afebrile and his vital signs are stable.

Diagnostic studies reveal an elevated white blood cell count of 18,000, a hemoglobin of 8.5, and a right upper lobe infiltrate on chest x-ray that was not present in his preoperative chest x-ray.

  a) What is your differential diagnosis for the right upper lobe infiltrate?

  b) What is the most appropriate treatment for this patient?

3. You are called by the ED to admit a patient with pneumonia. The patient is a 61-year-old male smoker with no significant past medical history or contact with the health care system. He presented to the ED with a 4-day history of worsening cough, dyspnea, and fever. The ED physician has ordered blood and sputum cultures, obtained a chest x-ray, CBC, and BMP, and started IV levofloxacin. The hospital pneumonia order set has also been activated.

Examination of the patient reveals rhonchi and moderate respiratory distress. The patient has an elevated white blood cell count. No other laboratory studies are abnormal.

Chest x-ray shows a cavitary lung lesion.

  a) What other orders should be written for this patient?

Answers

1. a) The differential diagnosis for this patient is broad.

  a. Treatment failure of pneumonia due to antibiotic choice:

  - MRSA
  - *Pseudomonas*
  - Viral pneumonia
  - Fungal pneumonia
  - Mycobacteria

  b. A complication of pneumonia:

  - ARDS
  - Pleural effusions
  - Myocardial ischemia/infarction
  - CHF
  - Acute renal failure with volume overload
  - Acute exacerbation of COPD

    c. Aspiration event

    d. Pulmonary embolus

    e. Mucus plug

    f. Allergic response to the antibiotics

1.b) Consider ordering a chest x-ray, ECG, blood cultures, CBC, BMP, BNP, and cardiac enzymes urgently. An arterial blood gas may be needed if the patient's respiratory status does not rapidly improve with supplemental oxygen. A repeat upper respiratory viral panel also may be useful.

1.c) Remember your ABCs (airway, breathing, circulation). Provide adequate supplemental oxygen to increase the patient's oxygen saturation to 90% or better, order diagnostic studies, establish resuscitation status of the patient, and notify the attending. If the patient deteriorates, or does not improve rapidly, transfer to the ICU may be appropriate for management of the patient's acute respiratory failure. Further management will depend on the results of the initial diagnostic studies.

2.a) The differential diagnosis for this patient includes HAP, aspiration pneumonia, mucus plugging, and acute mitral regurgitation causing focal pulmonary edema.

2.b) After excluding acute mitral regurgitation, initiate antibiotic therapy for HAP. Postoperative patients receiving pain medications are at increased risk of aspiration pneumonia and mucus plugging secondary to low tidal volumes. Ensure that the head of the bed is elevated $\geq 45°$, sedating medications are minimized, and an appropriate respiratory hygiene protocol is initiated. If aspiration pneumonia is suspected, a speech therapy evaluation can determine if the patient has swallowing defects, such as poor muscle tone or vocal cord dysfunction.

3.a) This patient should be placed in respiratory isolation until tuberculosis can be excluded. Sputum should be sent for Gram stain, AFB, and fungal culture. An interferon-gamma release assay and/or a tuberculin skin test should be placed as well. A CT scan of the chest will assist in better characterization of the cavitary lung lesion noted on the CXR.

SUGGESTED READINGS

Bhimraj A, Morgan RL, Shumaker AH, et al. Infectious Diseases Society of America Guidelines on the Treatment and Management of Patients with COVID-19. *Clin Infect Dis.* 2020;ciaa478.

IDSA Guidelines on the Treatment and Management of Patients with COVID-19. Accessed December 9, 2023. www.idsociety.org/practice-guideline/covid-19-guideline-treatment-and-management/#

Kalil AC, Metersky ML, Klompas M, et al. Management of Adults With Hospital-acquired and Ventilator-associated Pneumonia: 2016 Clinical Practice Guidelines by the Infectious Diseases Society of America and the American Thoracic Society [published correction appears in *Clin Infect Dis.* 2017;64(9):1298] [published correction appears in *Clin Infect Dis.* 2017;65(8):1435] [published correction appears in *Clin Infect Dis.* 2017;65(12):2161]. *Clin Infect Dis.* 2016;63(5):e61–e111.

Metlay JP, Kapoor WN, Fine MJ. Does this patient have community-acquired pneumonia? Diagnosing pneumonia by history and physical examination. *JAMA.* 1997;278(17):1440.

Metlay JP, Waterer GW, Long AC, et al. Diagnosis and Treatment of Adults with Community-acquired Pneumonia. An Official Clinical Practice Guideline of the American Thoracic Society and Infectious Diseases Society of America. *Am J Respir Crit Care Med.* 2019;200(7):e45–e67.

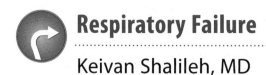

Respiratory Failure

Keivan Shalileh, MD

A 47-year-old Man With Severe Shortness of Breath

- A 47-year-old male presents to the ED with onset of severe shortness of breath 2 days ago, which has been progressively worsening. He also complains of cough productive of small amount of "clear" sputum, as well as mild wheezing.

- He is a current smoker (90 pack-years) and has history of severe COPD with emphysema.

- Vital signs: Blood pressure 124/78, pulse 76, respiratory rate 18, oxygen saturation 90% on 100% oxygen via non-rebreather mask, BMI 18.

- On physical exam: He opens eyes with repetitive verbal and tactile stimuli but does not follow commands and falls back to sleep immediately. Breath sounds are significantly decreased throughout both lungs, with no wheezes, rhonchi, or crackles. Cardiovascular exam reveals regular rate and rhythm, normal S1 and S2, and no murmurs or gallops. There is no JVD or peripheral edema.

- Venous blood gas: pH 7.22, $Pvco_2$ 95, Pvo_2 52, HCO_3^- 38. CO_2 from chemistry: 36

- Portable chest x-ray is shown in Figure 24-1.

1. What is the most likely etiology of this patient's presentation?

2. What type of respiratory failure does he have?

3. What are your next steps (in order of priority) in the management of this patient?

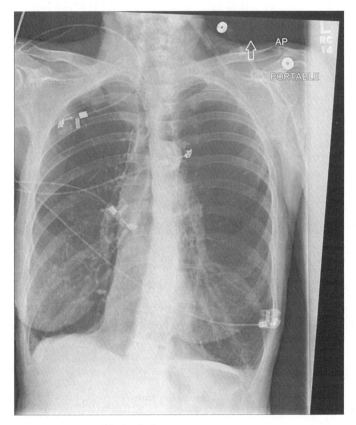

Figure 24-1. Portable (AP) chest x ray.

DEFINITIONS, PATHOPHYSIOLOGY, AND CLASSIFICATION

Acute respiratory failure (ARF)

- Respiratory (ventilatory) failure exists when the respiratory system cannot maintain gas exchange, causing dysfunction in other organs or threatening life.
- Numerically, it is defined as follows:

Pa_{O_2} <60 mm Hg (~Sp_{O_2} or Sa_{O_2}<88%–89%): hypoxemic (hypoxic) ARF
or
Pa_{CO_2} >50 mm Hg: hypercapnic (hypercarbic) ARF

- Can be mixed hypoxemic-hypercapnic.
- Traditionally: <1 month: acute respiratory failure (ARF), ≥1 month: chronic respiratory failure.

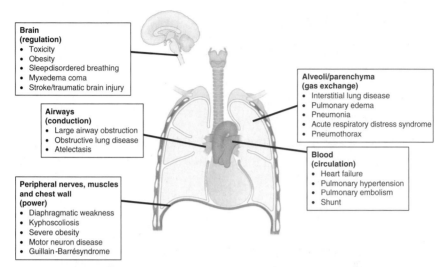

Figure 24-2. Causes of acute respiratory failure by anatomic site. Chapter 2 Functional Design of the Human Lung for Gas Exchange, Grippi MA, Antin-Ozerkis DE, Dela Cruz CS, Kotloff RM, Kotton C, Pack AI. *Fishman's Pulmonary Diseases and Disorders, 6e;* 2023. Available at: https://accessmedicine.mhmedical.com/content.aspx?bookid=3242&sectionid=270507440 Accessed: March 07, 2024, Copyright © 2024 McGraw-Hill Education. All rights reserved; Chapter 1 Fundamental Organizati on of the Nervous System, Waxman SG. *Clinical Neuroanatomy, 30e;* 2024. Available at: https://accessmedicine.mhmedical.com/content.aspx?bookid=3408&sectionid=283598767 Accessed: March 07, 2024.Copyright © 2024 McGraw-Hill Educati on. All rights reserved.

Causes of ARF

Can be classified by anatomic site or physiologic mechanism.
Causes of ARF By Anatomic Site (Figure 24-2)

- CNS ("won't breathe")
  - Reduced respiratory drive
  - Nondyspneic, bradypneic
- Other causes ("can't breathe")
  - Inability to ventilate despite effort
  - Generally symptomatic with dyspnea and respiratory distress

Causes of ARF by physiologic mechanism

1. Hypoventilation (causes hypoxemia or hypercapnia)
   Hypoxemia due to hypoventilation is easily corrected with supplemental O_2
   Causes of hypoventilation:
   - Reduced drive (regulation)
     - Obesity

- Brain injury
- Toxicity
- Central sleep apnea
- Central airways (conduction)
  - Obstructive sleep apnea
  - Subglottic stenosis
- Increased dead space/tidal volume (VD/VT) (conduction, gas exchange)
  - COPD
  - Atelectasis
  - Heart failure
  - PNA
- Problems with chest wall expansion (power)
  - Severe chest wall abnormality (kyphoscoliosis, flail chest)
  - Severe neuromuscular weakness (diaphragmatic paralysis, ALS)

2. Shunt (hypoxemia): mixing of oxygenated blood with non-oxygenated blood

Types of shunt:

- Anatomic
  - Intracardiac (PFO, VSD)
  - Extracardiac: extrapulmonary (PDA), intrapulmonary (AVM, hepatopulmonary syndrome)
- Physiologic
  - PE

Hypoxemia due to anatomic shunt cannot be fully corrected with any amount of supplemental O_2

Dx of anatomic shunt: agitated saline (bubble) echo

3. Ventilation-perfusion (V-Q) mismatch (O_2 or CO_2): Most common mechanism of hypoxemia

4. Diffusion limitation (O_2)

Relatively correctable with supplemental O_2: S_{PO2} or Pa_{O2} increase is usually proportional to the amount of O_2 supplied

Myriad of causes:

- PNA
- Atelectasis

- Pulmonary embolism
- Heart failure (with or without pulmonary edema)
- Hemodynamic collapse

Dx based on the constellation of Hx, exam, labs, and imaging findings

Bedside Approach to Evaluation and Treatment

1. Do your ABCDEFG

Airway

Breathing

Circulation

Drugs

Exposure

Food

Glucose

- Pulse oximetry with a good waveform is usually enough to determine presence of hypoxemia (do not waste time waiting for ABG):
  - If <89%: unlikely to have Pa_{O_2} >60
  - If >95%: unlikely to have Pa_{O_2} <60

Correct hypoxemia and treat shock immediately!

2. Assess for respiratory "distress" (ie, "distressful" breathing)
  - General appearance
  - Ability to speak
  - Respiratory rate
  - It is not always 18/min!
  - Accessory muscle use
  - Paradoxical breathing (thoracoabdominal movements)

3. Pay attention to disease progression
  - Do not waste time trying to convince yourself that the patient is fine!
  - Almost everyone in respiratory distress will eventually tire out.

4. Airway protection
  - Mental status: Awake, talking versus unresponsive, comatose
  - Audible gurgling or visible drooling
  - Cough matters, gag doesn't!
  - Some suggest palatal reflex instead of gag

5. Identify immediately correctable causes
   - Examine
   - Vital signs
   - POCUS, CXR, blood gas, lactate
   - Pneumothorax
   - Mucus plugging
   - Hypercapnia
   - $Pa_{CO_2} \approx Pv_{CO_2}$
   - pH (matters more than CO_2 level itself)
   - Upper airway obstruction
   - Heart failure, MI
   - Unstable (massive) pulmonary embolism
   - Don't assume anxiety!

6. Determine need for ventilatory support
   - O_2 for anyone with hypoxemia:
     Regular nasal cannula: up to 5 Lpm
     High-flow nasal cannula: up to 15 Lpm
     Venturi mask: adjustable, up to 50% O_2
     Non-rebreather mask: can provide 100% O_2
     Heated-humidified high-flow O_2 (eg, Opti-Flow, AirVo): separately adjustable flow and percentage: up to 100% O_2 and 60 Lpm of flow
   - Noninvasive positive pressure ventilation (NPPV):
     - Good evidence in COPD and cardiogenic pulmonary edema
     - Modest evidence in other situations
     - Pay attention to contraindications
   - Invasive mechanical ventilation

Contraindication to NPPV (items in bold are absolute contraindications):
- **At-risk airway**: inability to protect airways or clear secretions, vomiting, severe upper GI bleeding, massive hemoptysis, upper airway obstruction (eg, angioedema)
- Respiratory: **undrained pneumothorax**, aspiration PNA
- **Severe respiratory failure/distress**
- Neurologic: **severe CNS disturbance not due to hypercapnia** (seizure, toxic-metabolic encephalopathy, post–cardiac arrest), agitated or uncooperative patient

- Cardiovascular: hemodynamic instability, significant arrhythmias, acute MI
- Surgical: recent gastroesophageal surgery
- **Interface issues**: recent facial/head surgery, facial/head trauma or burn, deformity (unless helmet interface is available)
- **Lack of expertise, equipment, or appropriate monitoring setting**

7. Medications and other therapeutic measures

Directed at cause

- Inhaled beta-agonists (albuterol, levalbuterol):
  - Help with small airway obstruction
  - Immediate effect (unlike other meds)
  - Side effects: tachyarrhythmia, anxiety, tremors, lactic acidosis, hypoglycemia
  - Major relative contraindication: tachyarrhythmia, anxiety
- No proven clinical difference between albuterol and levalbuterol in terms of β_2 specificity
- Diuretics for pulmonary edema
  - Dry lung = happy lung
- Steroids
- Secretion clearance assistance: chest physical therapy, pulmonary toilet, mucolytics

8. Escalation of care/consult

- Does the patient need continuous hemodynamic or respiratory monitoring?
- Does the patient need treatments that cannot be provided at the current level of care?
- Is the patient worsening or at risk of immediate worsening?
- Do you need help?

TIPS TO REMEMBER

- Acute respiratory failure is an emergency.
- Don't forget ABCDEFG!
- Stabilize first, but don't forget that the condition may progress.

SUGGESTED READINGS

- Ancha S, Auberle C, Cash D, et al. *The Washington Manual of Medical Therapeutics.* 37th ed. Philadelphia: Lippincott Williams & Wilkins; 2022.
- Broaddus VC, Ernst JD, King TE Jr, et al. *Murray & Nadel's Textbook of Respiratory Medicine.* Philadelphia: Elsevier; 2022.
- Landsberg JW. *Manual for Pulmonary and Critical Care Medicine.* Philadelphia: Elsevier; 2018.
- West JB, Luks AM. West's *Respiratory Physiology: The Essentials.* Philadelphia: Lippincott Williams & Wilkins; 2020.
- West's Respiratory Physiology (Lippincott Connect) Eleventh, North American Edition by John B. West MD PhD DSc (Author), Andrew M. Luks MD (Author)

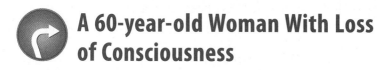

A 60-year-old Woman With Loss of Consciousness

Martha Hlafka, MD

A 60-year-old woman is admitted to the hospital after a loss of consciousness. She had a "strange feeling" before losing consciousness. Her husband stated that she fell to the ground and had generalized stiffening and then shaking. She was unresponsive for approximately 1 minute, had urinary incontinence, and was confused for a few minutes after regaining consciousness. She had a similar episode 2 months ago; evaluation at that time, which included electrocardiography, stress electrocardiography, and a continuous-loop event electrocardiographic recorder, revealed no abnormal findings. The patient takes no medications.

Physical examination including a full neurologic examination is normal.

MRI of the brain and electroencephalogram (EEG) during waking and sleeping also are normal.

1. What is the most likely diagnosis?

Answer

1. The patient likely had a seizure. Seizure is classified according to the history and physical examination. Diagnostic testing is used to confirm or clarify the suspected cause. When a patient has loss of consciousness with urinary incontinence and stiffening and shaking lasting 1 to 2 minutes, seizure should always be considered as the cause until proven otherwise. Even when there is a high clinical suspicion of epilepsy, normal MRI of the brain and EEG do not rule out that diagnosis.

SEIZURES

A seizure is defined as an abnormally excessive or synchronous discharge of electrical activity in the brain that results in a sudden change in behavior. Most seizures are precipitated by an inciting event. About 5% to 10% of the population will have at least 1 seizure in their lifetime, with the most common incidences in childhood and late adulthood. Epilepsy is defined as 2 or more seizures due to an underlying chronic process. Approximately 6 to 8 in every 1000 persons have epilepsy in the United States.

The most common causes of seizures are cerebrovascular disease, developmental brain disorders, remote head trauma, brain tumors, and neurodegenerative conditions. In epilepsy, seizure triggers include sleep deprivation, alcohol, flashing lights, and menstruation. Medications, including antibiotics, antipsychotic agents, and antidepressants, may lower seizure threshold, thus precipitating a seizure.

There are many conditions that may mimic seizures, including cardiac syncope, arrhythmias, transient ischemic attack (TIA), migraine, metabolic problems, intoxication, and vertigo. Psychogenic nonepileptic spells (PNES) are seizure-like episodes that are seen in patients with a conversion disorder. They mimic an epileptic seizure but do not have the EEG findings associated with seizures. Features commonly seen in PNES are biting the tip of the tongue, seizures lasting more than 2 minutes, seizures having a gradual onset, eyes being closed during a seizure, and side-to-side head movements. Features that are unusual in PNES are severe tongue biting, biting the inside of the mouth, and urinary and/or fecal incontinence.

Seizures are classified into 2 main types: generalized and focal (previously known as partial). Focal seizures may also progress to a full, generalized tonic-clonic seizure. The determination of whether a seizure is generalized or focal often depends on the description of behaviors that occurred before, during, and after the seizure. The International League against Epilepsy Commission on Classification and Terminology has developed a classification system for seizures based on clinical features of a seizure. These features include the presence or absence of motor behaviors, the type of motor behaviors if they occur, and whether the patient experiences impaired awareness of his/her behavior.

Generalized Seizures

Generalized seizures affect both cerebral hemispheres, usually with impaired awareness (consciousness). Generalized seizures may or may not exhibit motor behaviors.

Generalized nonmotor seizures, previously known as absence seizures or petit mal seizures, typically present as a sudden lapse of awareness without loss of postural control, lasting only about 5 to 10 seconds. Consciousness immediately returns, and there is no postictal confusion. There may be subtle motor signs with blinking or chewing movements of the jaw. These seizures usually start in childhood, and most patients have a spontaneous remission before adulthood.

Generalized motor tonic-clonic seizures, once known as grand mal seizures, are the most common type of seizure from conditions of a reversible cause, such as infections, metabolic derangements, withdrawal, and toxic ingestions. About 10% of patients with epilepsy experience generalized motor tonic-clonic seizures as their primary seizure type. Generalized motor seizures often begin without warning, and patients can exhibit an "ictal cry." The body stiffens in an initial tonic phase, and the patient falls to the ground. The tonic phase affects muscles of respiration as well as postural tone, resulting in cyanosis. After approximately 10 to 20 seconds, the extremities begin clonic movements, which generally last no more than 1 to 2 minutes. There is typically a postictal period during which the patient appears to be asleep or sleepy. There may be bladder or bowel incontinence and tongue-biting during the seizure. The patient wakes up gradually over the course of minutes to hours, often with associated confusion.

Focal Seizures

Focal seizures arise from a discrete area of the cerebral cortex then spread to neighboring regions, remaining localized to one cerebral hemisphere. The area of hyperexcitability may have developed secondary to injury, infection, genetic predisposition, or a developmental abnormality. If it is secondary to a CNS insult, it may be months or years after that injury before a patient develops seizures. Focal seizures may present with impaired awareness (previously called complex partial seizures) or without impaired awareness (previously called simple partial seizures).

In focal seizures with retained awareness, the person remains aware of their surroundings and remembers the events of the seizure. Symptoms may be localized motor, sensory, psychic, or autonomic in nature. Motor symptoms usually occur contralaterally to the cerebral hemisphere affected, with involuntary movements of the hand and can also include muscles of the face in a clonic fashion. The "Jacksonian march" is a progression of symptoms that starts in a small region, such as the fingers, and progresses to include more of the extremity. "Todd paralysis" is a temporary weakness in the affected area after the seizure that can last for minutes to hours. Sensory symptoms can include hallucinations, paresthesias, vertigo, smells, flushing, and sweats, among others.

Focal seizures with impaired awareness are the most common type of seizures in adults with epilepsy. They typically begin with a stereotypical aura that may be sensory, motor, autonomic, or psychic in quality. Impaired awareness begins soon afterwards, and the individual may first exhibit a motionless stare followed by involuntary behaviors. These behaviors can be simple, repetitive automatisms, such as lip smacking, or more complex such as running or eating. The seizures usually last less than 3 minutes, after which patients generally are confused or somnolent for up to an hour.

APPROACH TO NEW-ONSET SEIZURES

The first step in evaluating a patient with a suspected seizure is to rule out other conditions, such as syncope or TIA. As is most often the case, a complete history and physical examination are essential. The history should explore the patient's symptoms before, during, and after the episode. If the patient loses consciousness, witnesses to the event should be interviewed. The history should include questions about potential conditions that predispose to seizure: prior personal or family history of seizures, prior CNS infections or tumors, and history of stroke or TIA. The physical examination should include evaluation for signs of systemic illness, infection, and chronic illnesses or conditions that may be contributors to seizures. These include liver disease, kidney disease, developmental disorders, and neurocutaneous disorders such as neurofibromatosis. Based on the results of those examinations, one pursues appropriate diagnostic testing. Acute symptomatic seizures are usually secondary to an acute neurologic event or to a metabolic problem.

Diagnostic testing may be needed to confirm or clarify the underlying cause or precipitant of the seizure. Evaluation for metabolic problems, cardiac disease, cerebrovascular disorders, or vestibular dysfunction may be needed based on your history and physical examination. Laboratory investigations may include a complete blood count, serum electrolytes, kidney function, liver function, plasma glucose levels, and a toxicology screen.

A lumbar puncture is usually indicated if there are signs or symptoms suggesting an underlying infection of the brain or if the patient is immunocompromised. Electroencephalography (EEG) is the standard of the diagnostic workup. EEGs are done not only to formally diagnose seizures but also to classify the seizure type. However, it is important to note that a normal routine EEG does not rule out the possibility of a seizure. When a routine EEG is negative and seizure is still suspected, ambulatory EEG monitoring or inpatient continuous video EEG monitoring may be considered.

All patients with new-onset seizures should have neuroimaging to evaluate for structural conditions, such as stroke, intracerebral hemorrhage, or malignancy. In emergent situations such as acute intracerebral bleeding, infection, or tumor, CT is appropriate. However, MRI is superior to CT for detection of epileptogenic lesions and is preferred in non-emergent situations.

If a seizure has been provoked by a reversible cause, appropriate management should be aimed at correcting the underlying cause. Patients who have only had 1 seizure and have no risk factors for recurrence, such as an abnormal EEG or a known cause such as stroke, may not require further treatment.

In approximately 62% of patients with epilepsy, no cause of the seizures is found. Elderly patients more commonly have an identified etiology. Cerebrovascular disease is responsible for approximately 30% of seizures in older patients.

Antiepileptic drugs (AEDs) are used for patients with recurrent seizures and epilepsy. AEDs can be classified by efficacy into narrow spectrum (effective for focal seizures) and broad spectrum (effective for both focal and generalized seizures). AEDs have several drug interactions, potential for adverse events, and various side effects such that the choice of AED is a highly individualized one. A patient's age, sex, and comorbidities must be considered. Several AEDs are potential teratogens, particularly valproic acid, and others can interact with oral contraceptives, so care must be taken with women of child-bearing age. Phenobarbital, phenytoin, carbamazepine, and oxcarbazepine all induce hepatic cytochrome P450 enzymes, and valproic acid inhibits them. In patients with suspected drug interactions or underlying liver disease, gabapentin, pregabalin, and levetiracetam should be considered. Chronic use of first-generation antiepileptic drugs has been linked with an increased risk of osteoporosis and vitamin D deficiency; therefore, calcium and vitamin D should be started.

Patients diagnosed with epilepsy should be treated with single-agent pharmacotherapy. Monotherapy is better tolerated, less expensive, and associated with better medication adherence. If seizures persist, the monotherapy regimen should be changed to a different drug, again choosing a single-drug regimen. Second or third drugs may be added as needed if monotherapy is not sufficient.

Status Epilepticus

Status epilepticus is a medical emergency in which a patient experiences a continuous generalized seizure for more than 5 minutes, or more than 1 seizure within 5 minutes without a return to a normal level of consciousness. The 30-day mortality rate for status epilepticus is approximately 20%. Patients can experience short-term effects such as hyperthermia, pulmonary edema, and cardiac arrhythmias, as well as long-term consequences including cognitive dysfunction and epilepsy. Patients in status epilepticus are managed in an intensive care setting, and first-line treatment is IV benzodiazepines.

TIPS TO REMEMBER

- The first step in evaluating a patient with a suspected seizure is to rule out other conditions, such as syncope or transient ischemic attack, by taking a complete history and physical examination, and obtaining appropriate diagnostic testing.

- Focal seizures arise from a localized area and may indicate the possibility of an underlying lesion.

- Depending on the history, evaluation for metabolic problems, cardiac disease, cerebrovascular disorders, or vestibular dysfunction may be appropriate.

- A lumbar puncture is generally indicated only if there are signs or symptoms suggesting an underlying infection of the brain or if the patient is immunocompromised.

- All patients with a seizure should have a brain imaging, preferably MRI.

- Newly diagnosed epilepsy should be treated with single-agent pharmacotherapy. Monotherapy is better tolerated, less expensive, and associated with better adherence.

COMPREHENSION QUESTIONS

1. A 30-year-old woman is admitted with new onset of seizures. She had a witnessed generalized tonic-clonic seizure and was evaluated in the ED, where results of physical examination, complete blood count, measurement of serum electrolyte levels, and urine toxicology screen were all normal. She is otherwise healthy,

has no significant personal or family medical history, and takes no medications. Repeat physical examination is also normal. In addition to EEG, which of the following diagnostic tests should be performed next?

A. CT of the head

B. LP

C. MRI of the brain

D. PET

2. A 50-year-old man is admitted to the hospital after having 2 generalized tonic-clonic seizures in a 24-hour period. He has had seizures in the past, which were always attributed to alcohol withdrawal. He has end-stage liver disease secondary to alcoholic cirrhosis and is awaiting a liver transplant. His kidney function is normal. His current medications include propranolol, spironolactone, and furosemide. On physical examination, the patient is awake and alert, and vital signs are normal. Neurologic examination findings are normal. The general physical examination shows jaundice and ascites. The creatinine level is 0.6 mg/dL and blood alcohol level is nondetectable. Electrolyte levels are normal. An MRI of the brain is normal. An EEG is negative.

Which of the following is the best treatment for this patient?

A. Levetiracetam

B. Oxcarbazepine

C. Phenytoin

D. Valproic acid

Answers

1. **C.** For patients with new onset of a seizure and no provocative cause, an EEG and MRI of the brain should be obtained. These tests will help to confirm the diagnosis, predict the risk of recurrence, and rule out any underlying condition (such as a brain tumor). MRI has been shown to be clearly superior to CT in detecting potentially epileptogenic lesions.

2. **A.** Levetiracetam, gabapentin, and pregabalin are preferred in patients with significant liver disease because there is no significant hepatic metabolism and low protein binding.

SUGGESTED READINGS

Fisher RS, Cross JH, French JA, et al. Operational classification of seizure types by the International League Against Epilepsy: Position Paper of the ILAE Commission for Classification and Terminology. *Epilepsia*. 2017;58(4):522–530.

Johnson EL. Seizures and epilepsy. *Med Clin North Am*. 2019;103(2):309–324.

Schachter SC. Seizure disorders. *Med Clin North Am*. 2009;93(2):343–351.

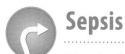

Sepsis

Nathalie Foray, DO, MS and Peter White, MD

A 74-year-old Woman With Cough, Chest Pain, and Shortness of Breath

A 74-year-old female, active cigarette smoker (3/4 to 1 pack of cigarettes per day for 55 years) with hypertension, hyperlipidemia, severe COPD, and type 2 diabetes on insulin therapy and chronic supplemental oxygen presents to the ED with a 1-day history of increased cough, sputum, right-sided pleuritic chest pain, shortness of breath, fevers, and a single shaking chill. Upon arrival to triage, she has a temperature of 102.7°F, her blood pressure is 90/60 mm Hg, heart rate is 120 bpm, respiratory rate is 22 bpm, and S_{PO_2} is 85% on her home oxygen at 2 liters per minute via nasal cannula. She is pale and diaphoretic and has a wet cough. Work of breathing is increased. There is a prominent tracheal tug and pursed lip breathing. Her breath sounds are decreased on the left. There are anterior and lateral crackles with bronchial breath sounds in the right mid chest. No E to A changes are found. Heart PMI is in the epigastrium. Heart tones are distant, regular, and rapid. Neck veins are flat. Abdomen is soft with decreased bowel sounds. Her hands and feet are cool, and there is no pedal edema. Capillary refill time is unable to be measured due to the presence of nail polish.

Chest x-ray reveals an ill-defined large density at the right mid lung. She has a white blood cell count of 22,000 cells/mm³, neutrophil predominant. Lactate is 2.7 mmol/L. She has on her bedside table a sputum cup with purulent yellow phlegm. Additional labs are in process as well as a CT chest PE protocol.

1. What is the clinical syndrome presented?

2. What is the next best step in management?

3. Does she need a CT-PA to exclude pulmonary embolism?

Answers

1. This patient meets criteria for systemic inflammatory response syndrome (SIRS), which consists of leukocytosis, tachycardia, hypoxia, and fever. Sepsis is defined as having SIRS plus a suspected or confirmed infection. She is hypotensive upon initial evaluation, which categorizes her as at least having severe sepsis (sepsis plus underlying organ dysfunction), possibly septic shock (sepsis with hypotension refractory to fluid resuscitation). See Table 26-1 regarding SIRS, sepsis, severe sepsis, and septic shock.

2. The first steps in management are to increase the flow of supplemental O_2 (target S_{PO_2} 90% ± 2%), obtain IV access, and initiate fluid resuscitation. Additionally, obtain labs including lactate and blood cultures, obtain urine analysis with reflex culture, and obtain sputum for Gram stain and bacterial culture. Ideally all cultures are obtained prior to antibiotics, but the priority in septic patients is receiving them. If obtaining cultures delays antibiotic administration by more than 30 minutes, the antibiotic administration trumps drawing blood cultures. Depending on how the patient's clinical condition responds to intervention, the patient may require intensive care monitoring versus admission to the general medical bed. This patient is not a candidate for outpatient treatment.

Table 26-1. SEP-1 Definitions for Sepsis, Severe Sepsis, and Septic Shock

SIRS criteria:	Body temperature <36°C or >38°C
	Heart rate >90 bpm
	WBC >12,000/mm³ or <4000/mm³ or >10% bands
	Respiratory rate >20 bpm or Pa$_{CO_2}$ <32 mm Hg
Sepsis:	≥2 SIRS + proven or suspected infection
Severe sepsis:	Sepsis + organ dysfunction
	SBP <90 mm Hg, MAP <65 mm Hg or fall in SBP >40 mm Hg from baseline
	Cr >2.0 mg/dL or urine output <0.5 mL/kg/h × > 2 h
	Total bilirubin >2 mg/d
Platelet count <100,00/mm³	
INR >1.5 or aPTT >60 s	
	Lactate >2 mmol/L
Septic shock:	Severe sepsis + hypotension requiring vasopressor to maintain MAP >65 mm Hg after completing 30-mL/kg IV fluid bolus

3. The chest x-ray, history, physical examination, and blood test results are consistent with an acute community-acquired bacterial pneumonia (CABP). The chest x-ray explains the patient's hypoxemia without invoking pulmonary embolism. If you subscribe to Occam's razor and look for one unifying diagnosis (CABP) to account for the signs or symptoms, there is no need to obtain a chest CT-PA. If, however, you prefer Hickam's dictum—which says a patient can have "as many diagnoses as they damn well please"—then obtaining a chest CT-PA may be reasonable. Either way, CT-PA to exclude acute PE is low yield in this case.

Sign, Symptoms, Physical Examination, and Diagnostic Studies

The history and physical examination in acutely ill septic patients should focus on identifying the source(s) of infection and looking for signs of shock. Literally go from head to toe. Inspect central venous or peripheral lines or IVs, drains, and incisions for signs of infection. Remember to take down dressing. Mental status evaluation in patients with sepsis/septic shock should not be skipped. The clinical spectrum of toxic metabolic encephalopathy ranges from mild confusion to obtundation. Physiologic stress, in this instance sepsis/septic shock, commonly manifests as dysfunction in the organ(s) with the least resilience. In the elderly this will commonly be the brain.

Bacterial meningitis is a life-threatening illness. Patients experience fevers, headache, photophobia, and nuchal rigidity, and in general these patients appear toxic. They require urgent chest CT scan, LP, and stat antibiotics.

Patients complaining of the acute onset of fever, productive cough, shortness of breath, and lassitude with crackles, bronchial breath sounds, dullness to percussion, egophony, and increased tactile fremitus have pneumonia on examination that should be confirmed on chest x-ray. Pneumonia that causes severe sepsis or septic shock should be obvious on chest imaging.

Bacterial endocarditis will present with a new (or worsening of an existing) murmur and is more likely in patients with a history of IV drug use, indwelling vascular catheters, and/or valvar heart disease. Left sided endocarditis may cause signs of peripheral emboli or embolic stoke. Right sided endocarditis is classically associated with septic pulmonary emboli. Echocardiogram may show valvular vegetations, and the blood cultures should be positive.

Right upper quadrant or epigastric pain, jaundice, rigors, and gram-negative bacteremia is concerning for cholecystitis or ascending cholangitis and warrants abdominal CT or US. Abdominal distension, nausea and vomiting, and diffuse or localized abdominal pain with absent bowel sounds and/or peritoneal signs are suggestive of appendicitis, bowel obstruction and/or perforation, or diverticulitis. The patient needs advanced abdominal imaging. Similarly, patients with a history of alcohol abuse or cholelithiasis complaining of abdominal and abdominal tenderness on physical examination may have pancreatitis and need an abdominal

CT scan. Crampy abdominal pain with watery diarrhea, high fever, elevated WBC count (often >30,000), and recent antibiotic treatment is suggestive of *Clostridium difficile* colitis; PCR for C *difficile* toxin and abdominal x-ray or CT scan should be ordered.

Urinary symptoms with dysuria and flank pain indicate pyelonephritis, nephrolithiasis, and/or hydronephrosis need to be excluded by US or CT imaging.

All of the skin on both sides of the body should be inspected for cellulitis, rash, petechia, purpura, ulcerations, fluctuance, pressure ulcers, or signs of complicated skin or soft tissue infection. Necrotizing fasciitis commonly has bullae and/or areas of skin necrosis, and classically the patient's pain is out of proportion to the infection's appearance. This tip-of-the-iceberg phenomenon becomes apparent with CT imaging. A septic joint should have the four classic signs of infection/inflammation: "calor, dolor, rubor, and tumor" (heat, pain in this case increased by movement, redness, and swelling). Mottling of the skin or livedo reticularis in the extremities is due to increased concentration of deoxygenated hemoglobin caused by inadequate blood flow to the skin. Similarly, cyanosis of the nail beds, ear lobes, lips, or skin is a sign of inadequate oxygen delivery to the peripheral tissues. Feel the hands and feet. Are they warm, cool, or cold? In patients with septic shock mottling, cyanosis and/or cold extremities are ominous signs and imply decreased cardiac output, which is a feature of late-stage septic shock. The capillary refill test is performed by pressing on a fingernail with a glass slide or clear plastic specimen cup for 10 seconds so the nail bed blanches (turns white). Then release the pressure and observe the time it takes for the color to return to the nail bed. Less than 2 seconds is normal. More than 2 seconds is abnormal and, in the setting of a systemic infection, is interpreted as an early sign of shock.

Point-of-care US (POCUS) in Sepsis/Septic Shock

POCUS, performed at the bedside, is an important adjunct to the physical examination. In the chest POCUS can reliably identify pleural effusions (anechoic space between the lung and chest wall or diaphragm), pulmonary edema (B-lines), consolidated lung (gray tissue appearance without significant volume loss, dynamic air bronchograms), atelectatic lung (gray tissue appearance with significant volume loss, static air bronchograms), and pneumothorax (lack of sliding lung, lung point, bar code sign). POCUS can be used to identify ascites and the puncture site for para- and thoracentesis. Other uses for US include guiding central venous and arterial line placement, confirming joint effusion, and locating a puncture site for arthrocentesis. Cardiac POCUS can identify pericardial effusions, evaluate for cardiac tamponade, assess LV and RV size and systolic function, and evaluate the IVC to determine the patient's volume status. In a hypotensive medical patient if the cardiac POCUS is unrevealing (no tamponade, normal RV and LV size and function), the patient almost certainly has a distributive shock—which nearly always is septic shock.

Blood Cultures, Labs, and Imaging Studies

Blood cultures should be obtained in patients with sepsis/septic shock. The culture and sensitivity results guide antibiotic selection and/or de-escalation. However, in a general medical ICU approximately 20% of all blood cultures are positive while approximately 50% of patients with septic shock have positive blood cultures. Obtaining blood cultures should not significantly delay antibiotic administration. The floor or ICU resident when faced with a septic patient will be instructed to "pan-culture" or "round up the usual suspects." This translates into culturing blood, urine, and sputum—and if the patient has an altered mental status, culturing the CSF. If a septic patient has ascites or a pneumonia with a pleural effusion it probably warrants paracentesis or thoracentesis to exclude spontaneous bacterial peritonitis or a complicated parapneumonic pleural effusion, respectively. In sepsis/septic shock, source control is the concept that infected closed-space fluid should be aspirated for cultures and decompressed or drained. A urinary tract infection with hydronephrosis due to an obstructed ureteral nephrolithiasis needs a nephrostomy tube. Ascending cholangitis due to a common bile duct stone needs an ERCP. Intraabdominal abscess requires aspiration for cultures and percutaneous drainage. One exception is pancreatitis with associated peripancreatic fluid collection or a pancreatic pseudocyst; in general it should not be aspirated due to concerns of seeding the fluid with bacteria. Patients with central venous catheters and suspected sepsis should have blood cultures drawn via the line and via a peripheral vein. If either blood culture grows a gram-negative rod, MRSA, or MSSA, or *Candida* or another fungus, the line should be removed and the intradermal portion of the catheter sent for semiquantitative culture. The line can, if needed, be replaced via a new puncture site and preferably after appropriate treatment for at least 24 to 48 hours. It is possible to effectively treat central venous catheters infected with coagulase-negative *Staphylococcus*, but this is generally attempted when access is problematic and it represents salvage therapy.

SSC Guidelines and SEP-1 Bundled Care in Sepsis/Septic Shock

Sepsis is defined in the 2021 International Surviving Sepsis Campaign (SSC) guideline as "a life-threatening organ dysfunction caused by a dysregulated response to infection." This definition of sepsis was proposed in 2016 at the Third International Consensus on Sepsis and Septic Shock. In 2015 the Centers for Medicare and Medicaid Services (CMS) launched SEP-1, which was shorthand for the Severe Sepsis and Septic Shock Management Bundle. CMS was motivated by the high mortality and rising cost associated with severe sepsis and septic shock in their enrollees. SEP-1 is an all-or-none performance measurement bundle with mandatory reporting of SEP-1 performance to CMS by acute care hospitals. It is important to understand these sepsis guidelines and apply them to clinical practice. Internal Medicine residents should understand the details of the

Table 26-2. Surviving Sepsis Campaign: 1-Hour Bundle: Initial Resuscitation for Sepsis/Septic Shock

1. Measure lactate level. Remeasure lactate if initial lactate >2 mmol/L.
2. Obtain blood cultures before administering antibiotics.
3. Administer broad-spectrum antibiotics.
4. Rapid infusion of 30-mL/kg crystalloid for hypotension or lactate ≥4 mmol/L.
5. Apply vasopressors if hypotensive during or after fluid bolus to maintain a mean arterial pressure ≥65 mm Hg.

sepsis monitoring program in their hospital(s), use the hospital's sepsis treatment protocol, and understand their role(s) and responsibilities in the hospital's sepsis response program.

SEP-1 defines sepsis as ≥2 SIRS criteria and suspected or proven infection (Table 26-1). SEP-1 defines severe sepsis as sepsis with ≥1 organ failure (Table 26-1). The 2021 SSC guidelines do not provide an operational definition of sepsis and do not use the term *severe sepsis*. The operational definitions of septic shock for both the SSC guidelines and SEP-1 is sepsis/severe sepsis with persistent hypotension (MAP <65 mm Hg) requiring vasopressor after receiving a 30-mL/kg crystalloid IV fluid bolus or an initial lactate >4 mmol/L. The SSC sepsis/septic shock bundle has the same metrics as the SEP-1 but in a 1-hour bundle. The SSC guidelines acknowledge that completing all the elements in the bundle is aspirational and the goal for antibiotic administration is 1 hour for septic shock and 3 hours for sepsis. SEP-1 requires reassessment of volume status and tissue perfusion 6 hours after completion of the fluid bolus. SSC guidelines recommend that healthcare providers closely monitor patients for response to the interventions in the 1-hour bundle.

SSC Guidelines and SEP-1 Metrics

Initial antibiotics

Antibiotics are life-saving, and every effort should be made to expedite their administration in the treatment of sepsis and septic shock. The goal for administering antibiotics is 1 hour for septic shock and 3 hours for sepsis without hypotension in the SSC guidelines, and 3 hours in SEP-1 for severe sepsis/septic shock. Every hour antibiotic administration is delayed translates into an 8% increase in mortality for patients with sepsis/septic shock. There is considerable pressure to draw blood cultures before antibiotics. If obtaining blood or other cultures delays antibiotic administration by more than 30 minutes, order the antibiotics be given (before drawing blood cultures) and document that obtaining blood cultures would have delayed antibiotic administration, which was "detrimental to the

Table 26-3. SEP-1: Early Management Bundle, Severe Sepsis/Septic Shock (Composite Measure)

3-Hour Resuscitation Bundle

1. Measure serum lactate.

2. Obtain blood cultures prior to antibiotics.

3. Administer broad-spectrum antibiotics.

4. Administer fluid bolus 30 mL/kg crystalloid if MAP <65 mm Hg or initial lactate >4 mmol/L.

6-Hour Septic Shock Bundle

1. Start vasopressors if hypotension persists after initial fluid bolus (septic shock) and maintain MAP >65 mm Hg.

2. Repeat lactate if initial lactate was >2 mmol/L.

3. Reassess tissue perfusion and volume status within 6 hours of completing the fluid bolus.

Time zero: The earliest chart documentation consistent with severe sepsis or septic shock.

Triggers: (1) Provider documentation of severe sepsis of septic shock. (2) ≥2 SIRS criteria plus 1 organ dysfunction when the last metric is positive for severe sepsis or septic shock criteria (all parameters within 6-hour window).

Denominator: Inpatients age ≥18 with an ICD-10-CM Principal or Other Diagnosis Code of sepsis, severe sepsis, or septic shock.

Excluded: Transfers from outside facility, enrollment in a clinical trial, or hospice/palliative care at admission or before 6 hours after time zero.

patient." Similarly document if blood cultures could not be obtained (tried but unable to draw blood specimen and antibiotics given).

Antibiotic selection is initially empiric and should be broad spectrum. SEP-1 has a confusing series of tables outlining what constitutes broad-spectrum antibiotics, and they are not helpful for guiding clinical care. In general, start with a broad-spectrum beta-lactamase antibiotic (piperacillin-tazobactam, meropenem, cefepime) for first-line gram-negative rod coverage and add vancomycin if MRSA coverage is necessary (skin or soft tissue infection, line sepsis, hospital-acquired pneumonia with known MRSA colonization). Review recent culture results and antibiotic treatment to determine if the patient has grown a multidrug-resistant (MDR) organism in the past. If the patient has a history of MDR gram-negative organisms, treatment with 2 antimicrobials with gram-negative coverage may be reasonable. Avoid treatment with double beta-lactamase antibiotics. Once the antibiotic sensitivities are available, de-escalate to one antibiotic. If the patient has CABP start with ceftriaxone unless he or she has structural lung disease and a history of Pseudomonas or another MDR gram-negative rod that will require treatment with an antipseudomonal beta-lactam antibiotic. Add azithromycin or doxycycline for Legionella, Mycoplasma, Chlamydia, etc, coverage if clinically indicated. Patients with nosocomial pneumonias require broad-spectrum gram-negative rod coverage, but if the nasal MRSA PCR is positive they should initially receive MRSA coverage. Intraabdominal infections involving the upper GI tract and biliary system can generally be treated with ceftriaxone or ciprofloxacin and metronidazole and do not require coverage for MRSA or Candida species. Infections involving the colon require broad-spectrum beta-lactam antibiotics, first-line anaerobic coverage, and fluconazole or micafungin. Clostridium difficile can be treated with oral vancomycin or fidaxomicin, but optimal treatment can be nuanced based on initial versus recurrent infection and moderate versus severe versus fulminant disease. If there is a history of penicillin allergy, provided it was not anaphylaxis, it is generally safe to give a carbapenem or a monobactam or opt for a fluoroquinolone. If there is a possibility of tick-borne illness (Rocky Mountain spotted fever, anaplasmosis, ehrlichiosis, babesiosis) add doxycycline. Exposure to rodents or other animals (domestic or wild), their urine/feces, or fleas, flies, or ticks on the animals can be associated with serious, albeit rare, infections including hantavirus pulmonary syndrome (no specific treatment, supportive care); leptospirosis (doxycycline or penicillin); plague (Yersinia pestis; gentamicin and ciprofloxacin); or tularemia (Francisella tularensis; streptomycin, gentamicin, ciprofloxacin).

The status of the patient's immune system may put him or her at risk for opportunistic infections as well as the usual offenders. Immunosuppression can be due to the underlying disease (acute leukemia and neutropenia, common variable immune deficiency and low IgG, HIV/AIDS and low CD4 count) or treatment (cytotoxic medications causing neutropenia or lymphopenia or pancytopenia, chronic steroids [>20 mg per day of prednisone]). Immunosuppression gives an increased susceptibility to Aspergillus and other fungal infections (including Pneumocystis jirovecii, tuberculosis, and nontuberculous mycobacteria), strongyloidiasis and herpes zoster, as well as influenza, Staphylococcus, and Pneumococcus. Anti-TNF drugs increase the risk of TB, bacterial sepsis, histoplasmosis, and other invasive fungi (Legionella, Listeria).

Infectious Disease Consultation

If the patient is in shock or has a life-threatening infection, discuss consulting the Infectious Disease (ID) service with the ICU members. The ID physicians are the experts in treating infections. If your patient is at risk of dying from an infection or has an infection not typically treated by the ICU service (meningitis or other CNS infections, complicated skin and soft tissue infection, endocarditis, osteomyelitis, intra-abdominal sepsis, disseminated fungal infection, etc), consult the ID service.

Antibiotic therapy is evaluated daily for de-escalation based on the culture sensitivity results provided the patient is improving (decreasing or resolution of fevers, normal or improving WBC count, discontinued or decreasing vasopressors). Discontinuation of antibiotics is based on the patient's clinical improvement and the procalcitonin level (<0.05 or decreased by 80% from the peak level). In general, the duration of antibiotics in septic patients is 5 to 7 days but may be longer.

Lactate Clearance and Initial IV Fluid Resuscitation

In patients with sepsis-induced hypoperfusion/shock, the standard recommendation is 30 mL/kg rapid infusion of crystalloid fluid within the first 3 hours for SEP-1 and 1 hour for SSC guidelines. The operational definition of septic shock for both SEP-1 and the SSC guidelines is the need for a vasopressor to keep the MAP >65 mm Hg despite receiving a 30-mL/kg IV fluid bolus. Lactate clearance is used to guide IV fluid resuscitation. If the initial lactate is >2 mmol/L, the lactate should be repeated until it is <2 mmol/L. The goal is normalization of lactate. In SEP-1 repeat lactate is a 6-hour goal for severe sepsis and septic shock.

Sepsis-induced proinflammatory vasodilatory mediators cause peripheral arterial and venous vasodilation coupled with increased endothelial permeability, which results in an intravascular volume deficit. Initially septic patients are predictably volume responsive; hence the need for a rapid IV fluid bolus. The optimal fluid for volume resuscitation in sepsis remains undefined. The current consensus is that colloids and crystalloids are equivalent in sepsis, but due to cost and availability crystalloids are preferred. Hydroxyethyl starches (HES) are never used due to the risk of acute kidney injury and need for hemodialysis. The results from studies comparing normal saline versus balanced physiologic salt solutions (lactated Ringer's, Plasma-Lyte) in severe sepsis and septic shock are mixed. While there is concern that normal saline is associated with increased AKI and mortality, this has not been a consistent finding. The SSC guidelines and SEP-1 do not favor one crystalloid IV fluid solution over another.

The initial crystalloid fluid bolus target is 30 mL/kg based on actual body weight. SEP-1 accepts an IV crystalloid fluid bolus within 10% of goal (27 mL/kg of actual body weight), and prehospital IV crystalloid fluid can be included. If the patient's BMI is >30, SEP-1 does advise using the ideal body weight to calculate the target IV fluid bolus. Similarly, SEP-1 allows the treating clinician to opt out of the 27-mL/kg fluid bolus in patients who are volume overloaded due to chronic kidney disease (stage IV or V or ESRD on dialysis) and heart failure (NYHA Class III and IV). These patient factors (BMI >30, CKD stage IV or V, ESRD on dialysis, NYHA Class III or IV heart failure) must be documented, and typically this is done in the 6-hour sepsis documentation note. In general patients with septic shock should not require >3 L of IV fluids in the first 24 hours. Avoid repeat 500- to 1000-mL fluid bolus after the initial fluid resuscitation unless there is objective evidence the patient remains fluid responsive.

Vasopressors and Target Blood Pressure

Septic shock, despite an initial or early supernormal cardiac output, is characterized by hypotension and vital organ dysfunction due to hypoperfusion and inadequate oxygen delivery. The management of septic shock is focused on early antibiotic administration and, as importantly, on restoring the intravascular volume depletion, as well as maintaining an adequate MAP and organ perfusion. If volume resuscitation with IV fluids fails to restore MAP to >65 mm Hg, vasopressors are needed. The 2021 Surviving Sepsis Campaign recommends norepinephrine as the vasopressor of choice for septic shock, and vasopressin is the preferred choice for a second vasopressor if needed. Alternative vasopressors include epinephrine, phenylephrine, dobutamine, and dopamine. Dopamine has been shown to be inferior to norepinephrine and should be avoided. It is acceptable to start norepinephrine, epinephrine, or phenylephrine via peripheral IV assuming the IV is in a large vein with good blood flow. If the norepinephrine dose is ≥8 ± 2 μg/min and/or it has been infusing for ≥24 hours, most ICU clinicians will opt for central vein delivery. The target MAP for septic shock patients on a vasopressor is ≥65 mm Hg for both SSC guidelines and SEP-1. This is based in part on 2 randomized trials in patients with septic shock. Asfar and colleagues and Ovation showed improved survival when the target MAP was 65–70 mm Hg versus 80–85 mm Hg and 60–65 mm Hg versus usual care, respectively.

Ventilation/Oxygenation Recommendations per the SSC Guidelines

The SSC guidelines recommend high-flow nasal cannula over noninvasive ventilation in those with sepsis-induced hypoxemic respiratory failure. Adhere to the ARDSNET low-tidal-volume protocol for patients with ARDS precipitated by sepsis/septic shock. The principle metrics are tidal volume of 6 mL/kg ideal body weight. Maintain the plateau pressures ≤30 cm water. In addition, in moderate to severe ARDS, use prone ventilation >12 hours per day, and favor intermittent rather than continuous infusion dosing of nondepolarizing neuromuscular blocking medications.

Additional Treatments per SSC Guidelines for Sepsis/Septic Shock

The use of steroids in sepsis/septic shock is not an SEP-1 metric. The 2021 SSC guidelines recommend IV hydrocortisone (200 mg IV per day) in refractory septic shock (increasing vasopressor requirements despite adequate IV fluids and antibiotics). This was based on two metanalyses that showed decreased time on vasopressors but no improvement in mortality or ICU length of stay. SSC guidelines also recommend pharmacologic VTE prophylaxis, RBC transfusion trigger of <7 g/dL, insulin infusion trigger of blood glucose >180 g/dL, and IV $NaHCO_3$ for pH <7.2 and acute kidney injury. SSC does not recommend IV immunoglobins, concurrent pharmacologic and mechanical DVT prophylaxis, IV vitamin C, or NaHCO$_3$ to improve hemodynamics or to decrease vasopressor dose.

TIPS TO REMEMBER

- Use your hospital's sepsis protocol/order set and know who is responsible for completing the 6-hour sepsis documentation note.
- Do not delay antibiotics. Time to administration of antibiotics is the metric most strongly associated with survival in severe sepsis and septic shock.
- Vasopressor of choice in septic shock is norepinephrine, and the target MAP is >65 mm Hg.
- Ensure prompt volume resuscitation with IV crystalloid fluid but do not overdo it. Most patients with sepsis/severe sepsis/septic shock do not need >3 liters of IV fluid in the initial 24 hours of treatment.
- Variance documentation for SEP-1: (1) Unable to draw lactate or blood cultures or patient, power of attorney or healthcare surrogate declined. (2) The 27-mL/kg fluid bolus can include prehospital fluid provided it was crystalloid and rapidly infused. (3) Adjust the fluid bolus for sepsis/septic shock if BMI >30, patient has volume overload/pulmonary edema due to CKD stage IV and V or ESRD on dialysis, or chronic heart failure with NYHA Class III or IV symptoms, but document that not adjusting the fluid administration would be detrimental to the patient.

COMPREHENSION QUESTIONS

1. An elderly woman presents to the ED with a fever, confusion, and a urinalysis with large leukocyte esterase and nitrites. She has been hospitalized 3 times in the past year for the same. Her blood pressure is 100/60, HR is 110, and she is breathing comfortably on room air. All the following should be done except:

   A. Admit to hospital

   B. Draw blood cultures before administering antibiotics, even if this results in a delay of >30 minutes

   C. Double check that the lab has a reflex urine culture

   D. Review previous cultures to tailor antibiotic therapy

2. In patients with septic shock, which of the following vasopressors is considered first line?

   A. Dopamine

   B. Norepinephrine

C. Epinephrine

D. Vasopressin

3. True or False: In patients with septic shock, all patients should receive a 30-cc/kg fluid bolus.

Answers

1. B. Blood cultures should be drawn before administering antibiotics, but if there is a thought that antibiotics would be delayed >30 minutes, it is detrimental to delay antibiotic therapy. At this point, administering antibiotics over obtaining cultures would be appropriate.

2. B. Per the 2021 Surviving Sepsis Campaign, the vasopressor of choice is norepinephrine. Dopamine should be avoided.

3. False. There are exceptions where a 30-cc/kg fluid bolus would not be appropriate (patients with congestive heart failure, ESRD on HD, BMI >30). These patients should have fluid resuscitation tailored to their clinical picture.

SUGGESTED READINGS

Chin-Hong PV, Guglielmo BJ. Common problems in infectious diseases & antimicrobial therapy. In: McPhee S, Papadakis M, Rabow MW, eds. *Current Medical Diagnosis and Treatment 2012*. New York: The McGraw-Hill Companies; 2011.

Dellinger RP, Levy MM, Carlet JM, et al. Surviving Sepsis Campaign: international guidelines for management of severe sepsis and septic shock: 2008. *Intensive Care Med*. 2008;34:17–60.

Evans L, Rhodes A, Alhazzani W, et al. Surviving sepsis campaign: international guidelines for management of sepsis and septic shock 2021. *Intensive Care Med*. 2021;47(11):1181–1247.

Munford RS. Severe sepsis and septic shock. In: Longo D, Fauci A, Kasper D, et al, eds. *Harrison's Principles of Internal Medicine*. 18th ed. New York: The McGraw-Hill Companies; 2012.

Rivers E, Nguyen B, Havstad S, et al. Early goal-directed therapy in the treatment of severe sepsis and septic shock. *N Engl J Med*. 2001;345:1368–1377.

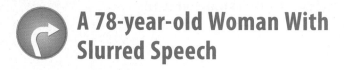

A 78-year-old Woman With Slurred Speech

Wael Dakkak, MD

A 78-year-old female presents to the ED with a 2-hour history of slurred speech, word-finding difficulties, and right-sided weakness and numbness. She denies any vision changes, headache, fever, trauma, chest pain, or abdominal pain. She has a history of hypertension, hyperlipidemia, and atrial fibrillation. Her medications include hydrochlorothiazide, metoprolol, fish oil, and aspirin. She has not taken warfarin for the last 3 years after an incident of diverticular bleeding. She does not smoke or use alcohol. On examination, she is awake yet anxious, with a blood pressure of 194/102 mm Hg, heart rate of 116 bpm, respiratory rate of 20 breaths/min, and oxygen saturation of 96% on room air. Chest auscultation reveals clear lungs and an irregularly irregular rhythm. Abdominal examination reveals a soft, nontender abdomen and normal bowel sounds. Neurologic examination reveals expressive aphasia, left facial droop, right-sided sensory deficits, and right-sided motor strength of 3/5. Left arm and leg sensory and motor examination are normal.

Lab data show hemoglobin 12.6, hematocrit 38, WBCs 10,600, and platelets 186,000. Basic metabolic panel is normal. Point-of-care glucose is 109. CT scan of the head is normal.

1. What is the most likely diagnosis?

2. What is the most likely cause of this new diagnosis?

3. What else should be considered in the differential diagnosis?

Answers

1. This is a 78-year-old with risk factors for stroke (age, hypertension, hyperlipidemia, atrial fibrillation) who presents with sudden onset of focal neurologic findings. A normal head CT scan has ruled out an acute hemorrhage. Thus acute stroke is the most likely diagnosis.

2. Her stroke is most likely embolic, related to not being on anticoagulation for atrial fibrillation.

3. Other potential diagnoses to consider include complex migraine headache, tumor or mass, and toxic-metabolic abnormalities. This case allows for a discussion of acute stroke, including types, presenting signs and symptoms, and management.

STROKE

Acute stroke, commonly called a cerebrovascular accident (CVA), is defined as acute onset of focal neurologic deficit resulting from sudden loss of vascular supply to the affected brain tissue. Stroke is one of the major causes of death and disability in the United States. Strokes can be either ischemic or hemorrhagic. Ninety percent of strokes are ischemic. Transient ischemic attack (TIA) is defined as a focal neurologic deficit lasting less than 24 hours and with the absence of infarction of the brain tissue on imaging (CT/MRI).

Risk factors include hypertension, hyperlipidemia, carotid stenosis, and atrial fibrillation.

Ischemic stroke is further classified as follows: (1) large artery atherosclerosis; (2) cardioembolic; (3) small vessel occlusion (lacunar); (4) stroke of other determined etiology; and (5) stroke of undetermined etiology (cryptogenic).

Large vessel stroke, the major cause of acute stroke, results from atherosclerosis of the cervical or intracranial vessels most commonly affecting the middle cerebral artery (MCA). Cardioembolic stroke results from an arterial embolism arising from the heart, commonly in the setting of atrial fibrillation, left ventricular thrombus, and infective endocarditis. Cardioembolic strokes are often multiple and bilateral, and often affect more than one vascular territory. Lacunar infarcts affect smaller areas of the brain and occur in the setting of hypertension and diabetes. These commonly affect the basal ganglia, internal capsule, corona radiata, and brainstem. Unusual causes of ischemic stroke include vasculopathies, a hypercoagulable state, arterial dissections, and right-to-left vascular shunts. About one-third of ischemic strokes are idiopathic or cryptogenic and can be associated with patent foramen ovale (PFO) and paroxysmal atrial fibrillation.

Hemorrhagic strokes are most commonly caused by hypertension. They commonly affect the basal ganglia, the thalamus, and the pons. Other potential causes include vascular malformations, amyloidosis, bleeding disorders, illicit drug use, and secondary conversion of an ischemic stroke.

Diagnosis

The symptoms of acute stroke are different depending on the intracranial arterial territory involved and the affected area of the brain tissue. Middle cerebral artery stroke results in contralateral hemiparesis and sensory deficits, ipsilateral homonymous hemianopsia, and receptive or expressive aphasia if the dominant hemisphere is affected. Agnosia and neglect may be seen if the nondominant hemisphere is affected. Anterior cerebral artery stroke may present with contralateral weakness (legs > arms) and contralateral sensory deficits, gait apraxia, urinary incontinence, abulia, and altered mentation. Posterior cerebral artery stroke usually presents with contralateral homonymous hemianopsia, visual agnosia, alexia without agraphia, and impaired memory. Vertebrobasilar artery strokes can present with cranial nerve palsies, vertigo, nystagmus, syncope, dysarthria, dysphagia, diplopia, nausea, and even coma. Cardiovascular exam may reveal atrial fibrillation, murmurs, and carotid bruits. The initial assessment involves monitoring hemodynamic stability and establishing the exact time the patient was last seen well.

Because it is impossible to differentiate between ischemic and hemorrhagic stroke based on the physical exam alone, an emergent noncontrast CT scan is the most important diagnostic step to rule out acute hemorrhagic stroke because of its extremely high sensitivity to detect fresh intracranial bleeding. However, CT scan is poorly sensitive for recent ischemia, small strokes, and strokes located in the posterior fossa. Diffusion-weighted MRI has about a 90% sensitivity for acute ischemic strokes and is the most accurate test. However, MRI is time consuming and should not delay treatment if the patient presents within the window of reperfusion therapy. CT angiography (CTA) and magnetic resonance angiography (MRA) are important tools to select patients for mechanical thrombectomy. Complete blood count (CBC), basal metabolic profile (BMP), and coagulation profile are all important initial labs. Further labs include a lipid profile and hemoglobin A1c, which are obtained to assess for risk factors. An ECG should be obtained to assess for cardiac arrhythmia. Cardiac telemonitoring is recommended for all patients with acute stroke. Echocardiography should be obtained especially if a cardioembolic stroke is suspected.

Differential diagnosis
The differential diagnosis list for patients presenting with stroke-like symptoms should include the following:

- Complex migraine headache
- Seizures (Todd's palsy)
- Multiple sclerosis
- Conversion disorder
- Systemic infection/meningitis/encephalitis
- Toxic-metabolic abnormalities (hyper- or hypoglycemia, renal failure, liver failure, illicit drug use)

Treatment

Before starting specific treatment for ischemic stroke it is essential to rule out intracranial hemorrhage by an emergent noncontrast CT scan. Determining the severity of the neurologic deficit by measuring the NIH stroke scale score (NIHSS) is essential to determine the benefit of thrombolysis. IV thrombolysis is not recommended for those with low NIHSS score (0–5).

Treatment for acute ischemic strokes
If the patient presents within 4.5 hours after the onset of stroke, tissue plasminogen activator (TPA) has been shown to reduce disability and should be given if there

is no contraindication to it (Table 27-1). Those who present within >4.5 hours but <6 hours of symptom onset and have intracranial large vessel occlusion on MRA or CTA are eligible for endovascular treatment (mechanical thrombectomy).

Patients presenting within 24 hours after the onset of symptoms and who have a low NIHSS score may benefit from a 21-day course of dual antiplatelet therapy (aspirin, clopidogrel) followed by clopidogrel alone to reduce the risk of recurrent stroke. There is no role for long-term dual antiplatelet therapy in stroke patients.

If symptom onset is greater than 24 hours, aspirin (160–300 mg) daily is indicated to reduce mortality and recurrent stroke.

If TPA therapy was chosen, a blood pressure <180/105 mm Hg should be maintained for the first 24 hours after administration. Such patients are usually admitted to the intensive care unit for blood pressure monitoring and neurologic checks. Similarly, antithrombotic therapy is contraindicated in the first 24 hours after thrombolysis to reduce the risk of hemorrhagic transformation. Permissive hypertension treatment is recommended in the first 48 hours for patients who did not receive thrombolysis or endovascular therapy. BP control is recommended for patients with BP ≥220/120 mm Hg.

According to the 2021 AHA/ASA guidelines, the majority of strokes can be prevented by modulating the vascular risk factors, which include blood pressure control, diet, exercise, and smoking cessation. Anticoagulation is indicated in patients with atrial fibrillation. A goal of BP <130/80 mm Hg is recommended. A high-intensity statin is indicated to reduce stroke recurrence with a goal of low-density lipoprotein (LDL) <70 mg/dL. Adding another lipid-lowering agent is

Table 27-1. Thrombolytic Therapy Contraindications

• Acute or prior intracranial bleeding
• Ischemic stroke in the past 3 months
• Intracranial or intraspinal surgery in the past 3 months
• Head trauma within 3 months
• Gastrointestinal bleeding within 21 days or GI malignancy
• Known intracranial neoplasm
• Suspected aortic dissection
• Infective endocarditis
• BP >185/110 mm Hg
• Coagulopathy: platelet count <100,000/mm³, INR >1.7, aPTT >40 s
• LMWH treatment in the prior 24 hours
• Treatment with DOAC and direct thrombin inhibitors in the last 48 hours

recommended in those who do not achieve this goal. Hemoglobin A1c ≤7% is recommended in patients who have diabetes. Carotid endarterectomy (CEA) is indicated within a couple of weeks for suitable surgical patients with TIA or minor ischemic stroke who have a severe degree of stenosis. PFO closure may be indicated for those with cryptogenic embolic strokes in patients <60 years old.

Treatment for acute hemorrhagic strokes

The goal of the treatment of acute hemorrhagic stroke is to stop the bleeding from propagation and to achieve BP control. Rapid BP control has as a goal systolic BP of less than 140 mm Hg. Any anticoagulation or antiplatelet therapy should be immediately discontinued. Platelet transfusion is indicated if platelets are below 50,000. Heparin should be reversed with protamine; warfarin should be reversed with 4-factor PCC or fresh frozen plasma (FFP) if PCC is unavailable. Intracranial pressure can be treated medically with osmotic therapy or surgically (ventricular drainage) in patients with concomitant hydrocephalus. Surgical decompression and evacuation are reserved for patients with evidence of cerebellar or brainstem compression, and those with life-threatening hemorrhage.

TIPS TO REMEMBER

● An emergent noncontrast CT scan is the best initial test when an acute stroke is suspected to rule out hemorrhagic stroke.

● Therapeutic anticoagulation has no role in the treatment of acute stroke, as it does not decrease the risk of recurrence and is associated with the risk of hemorrhagic transformation.

● Patients who present within a 4.5-hour window and have a high NIHSS score should be treated with TPA if there is no contraindication to thrombolysis.

● If the patient did not receive TPA, a permissive hypertension strategy is preferred in the first 48 hours. However, if the BP is at least 220/120 mm Hg, lowering BP by 15% in the first 24 hours is recommended.

● Avoid antithrombotic agents in the first 24 hours after TPA.

COMPREHENSION QUESTIONS

1. For the case presented at the beginning of the chapter, what is the next best step in management?
   A. TPA
   B. Control her BP
   C. MRI of the brain

2. A 64-year-old male suffered an ischemic stroke 2 weeks ago. The determining cause of his stroke was left internal carotid artery stenosis. He has residual

deficits of minimal right hand weakness. He has stopped smoking. His medications include aspirin, atorvastatin, ramipril, and metoprolol. His vital signs are normal. What is the next step for the secondary prevention of stroke?

A. Add clopidogrel.

B. Add warfarin.

C. Maintain current medication and rehabilitation regimen.

D. Refer for carotid endarterectomy.

3. A 71-year-old female has been diagnosed with a hemorrhagic stroke due to intraparenchymal hemorrhage. Her vital signs include a blood pressure of 166/98 mm Hg. What is the next step in managing this patient's blood pressure?

A. Do nothing. Her blood pressure is at an ideal range to maintain cerebral perfusion.

B. Start IV fluids. Her intravascular volume should be increased to raise the systolic blood pressure to 180 mm Hg.

C. Start IV labetalol. The goal is a systolic blood pressure <140 mm Hg.

Answers

1. **B.** The patient presented with sudden neurologic findings and a negative CT head indicating acute ischemic stroke. She is within the window for TPA, and her NIHSS score is high. However, her BP is 194/102 which doesn't allow the use of TPA. The first step is to reduce BP to <185/110 mm Hg before and during the infusion, and then to control the BP at a goal of 180/105 mm Hg in the immediate 24-hour period. While MRI of the brain confirms the diagnosis of acute ischemic stroke, it should never delay treatment with thrombolysis.

2. **D.** This patient should be referred for carotid endarterectomy. Doing nothing allows the continued stenosis and presumed atherosclerotic disease to place this patient at risk for another stroke. Adding clopidogrel to aspirin increases the risk of bleeding and doesn't offer an additional benefit compared to clopidogrel alone. For secondary prevention of stroke or for those who fail ASA, treatment should be changed to (1) clopidogrel or (2) aspirin plus extended-release dipyridamole. Warfarin is not indicated, as the patient doesn't have atrial fibrillation and the stroke is not cardioembolic.

3. **C.** Blood pressure management differs in the setting of hemorrhagic stroke versus ischemic stroke. For patients with hemorrhagic stroke, the blood pressure should be normalized as soon as possible to potentially avoid worsening the area of hemorrhage. Maintaining the current blood pressure, or adding measures that may increase it, will put the patient at a higher risk for worsening stroke symptoms.

SUGGESTED READINGS

Hankey GJ. Stroke. *Lancet.* 2017;389(10069):641–654.
Kleindorfer DO, Towfighi A, Chaturvedi S, et al. 2021 Guideline for the Prevention of Stroke in Patients With Stroke and Transient Ischemic Attack: A Guideline From the American Heart Association/American Stroke Association. *Stroke.* 2021;52(7):e364–e467.
Knight-Greenfield A, Nario JJQ, Gupta A. Causes of acute stroke: a patterned approach. *Radiol Clin North Am.* 2019;57(6):1093–1108.
Morotti A, Poli L, Costa P. Acute stroke. *Semin Neurol.* 2019;39(1):61–72.
Powers WJ. Acute ischemic stroke. *N Engl J Med.* 2020;383(3):252–260.

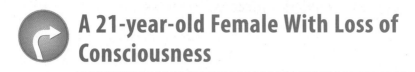

A 21-year-old Female With Loss of Consciousness

Martha L. Hlafka, MD and Susan Thompson Hingle, MD

A 21-year-old college student was brought to the ED by EMS following an episode of loss of consciousness on a hot summer afternoon. She is accompanied by her friends who witnessed the episode. She is awake and alert, and she claims now to be in her usual state of health. She is on the cheer team and lost consciousness just before half time. She felt light-headed and weak prior to the episode with vague abdominal pain and nausea. She has no recollection after that, and the next thing she can remember is that her friends were calling her name when she was lying on the floor. As per the friends, she looked pale initially and had shaky movements of the limbs for a few seconds. She was unconscious for less than a minute. After that, her color returned, and she regained consciousness spontaneously. She was in her usual state of health until a few seconds prior to the episode. She has never lost consciousness in the past. She has a negative review of systems. She takes oral contraceptive pills for birth control. The patient denies tobacco, alcohol, or illicit drug use. She has no significant family history. Vital signs, including orthostatic blood pressure, are normal. Examination, including neurologic examination, is unremarkable. ECG is normal. Urine pregnancy test is negative.

1. What is the diagnosis and next step of action?

Answer

1. Neurocardiogenic (vasovagal) syncope. Discharge from the ED with patient education and precautions to take if she suffers another episode.

CASE REVIEW

The patient in this case description is a young college student cheering for her team on a hot summer day. She had warning signs with presyncopal symptoms, but she remained up on her feet. This led to an episode of brief loss of consciousness, followed by rapid spontaneous recovery. This is a classic description for neurocardiogenic syncope, also known as vasovagal syncope. It is not uncommon to have convulsive activity during syncope, usually lasting less than 15 seconds. It is not a seizure, as the episode was not long enough and she did not have a postictal phase. Neurocardiogenic syncope is the most common type of syncope, and it carries a good prognosis. The description of the episode is diagnostic, and there is no role for further investigation. Reassure and educate the patient on syncope and precautions to take to prevent recurrence. "Always position an unconscious patient in a recovery position, and never make them sit in a chair or hold them in an upright position," as this will not help improve the circulation and regain consciousness.

DEFINITION OF SYNCOPE

Syncope is a clinical diagnosis that can be determined with a thorough history and physical examination. Syncope must have the following characteristics: (1) transient loss of consciousness, (2) loss of postural tone, and (3) complete immediate spontaneous recovery. It is a result of transient global cerebral hypoperfusion. Syncope is only one of many causes of transient loss of consciousness (TLOC), including epilepsy, head trauma, cerebrovascular disease, and psychogenic causes.

Presyncope is the prodromal symptom of near faintness without loss of consciousness. It is more prevalent than syncope, and the symptoms may last for seconds to minutes with light-headedness, warmth, nausea, and blurring of vision. Many patients describe their presyncope symptoms as dizziness, a vague term that may mean different things to different people. It is important to try to differentiate the patient's experience of dizziness as lightheadedness/faintness versus vertigo (spinning sensation). Presyncope and syncope are a spectrum of presentations of the same underlying pathophysiology, so the following discussion applies to both conditions.

PATHOPHYSIOLOGY

Systemic blood pressure is determined by cardiac output and peripheral vascular resistance. To maintain continuous blood supply to the brain regardless of position, a harmonious function of baroreceptors, the autonomic nervous system, cardiac function, blood volume, and patent blood vessels to the brain is needed. Syncope is a result of interruption of any of these tightly coordinated mechanisms, leading to a fall in systemic blood pressure and decrease in global cerebral blood flow.

Based on the underlying pathophysiology, causes of syncope can be organized into three main mechanisms: neurocardiogenic (also known as reflex-mediated or neurally mediated) syncope, orthostatic syncope, and cardiovascular disorders (Figure 28-1). Episodes of loss of consciousness that have no clear cause are considered to be syncope of unknown etiology. It is important to note: a cause is not identified in nearly one-third of the patients presenting with syncope.

APPROACH TO SYNCOPE

Every patient who presents with presumed syncope should be evaluated with a comprehensive history, a physical exam including orthostatic vital signs assessment, and an ECG. Once cause is determined, further investigation and treatment

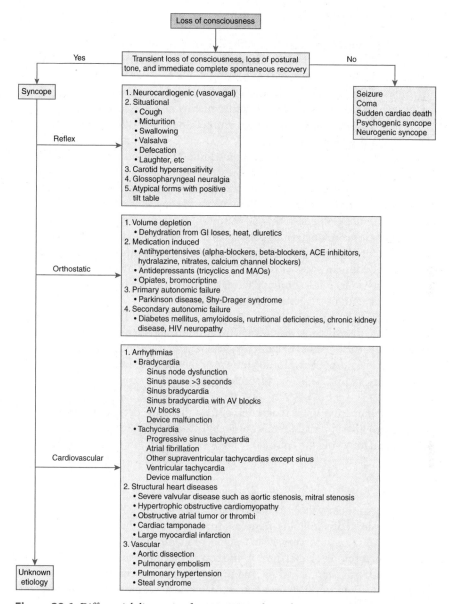

Figure 28-1. Differential diagnosis of nontraumatic loss of consciousness.

is dependent on the patient's individual risk of short-term and long-term morbidity and mortality. History and physical exam alone identify a cause of syncope in 45% of cases. Routine blood testing is not recommended, as it rarely contributes diagnostic information that has not been suggested by the history and physical exam.

History

History is the most important tool in the diagnosis of syncope. The first and foremost challenge in the evaluation of a patient with an episode of loss of consciousness is to differentiate syncope from other possible causes. These include seizures, metabolic causes, intoxication, trauma, and neurovascular disorders. These causes can often be ruled out by a comprehensive history and physical examination.

Syncope is often mistaken for a seizure, as patients with syncope may have convulsive movements that are brief (<15 s) and nonrhythmic, starting after the loss of consciousness. Generalized tonic-clonic movements, tongue biting, and urinary incontinence are rare. In contrast, seizure patients may experience an aura, have a longer duration of unconsciousness, and have generalized tonic-clonic movements that start at the time of loss of consciousness and last approximately 1 minute. Tongue biting is common, as is urinary incontinence. The postictal phase is prolonged and is associated with confusion and sore muscles.

In metabolic causes (hypoglycemia, hypoxia, hyperventilation) and intoxication, loss of consciousness is not due to global cerebral hypoperfusion. Symptoms may last longer unless intervened early; there will be a pre-event history and associated symptoms suggestive of these conditions.

In neurovascular disorders such as vertebrobasilar TIA, stroke, or basilar migraine, loss of consciousness is from brainstem ischemia but not due to global hypoperfusion. Loss of consciousness is associated with neurologic deficits or headaches, and patients do not return to the baseline health status immediately. Because of this, neurovascular loss of consciousness is not considered a true syncope.

In order to rule these diagnoses out and help to determine the cause of syncope, the history should focus on the events prior to the episode, during the episode, and following the episode.

Pre-event

For the pre-episode events, ask about hydration status in the days to weeks prior to the episode: access to fluids, fluid loss from new-onset diabetes, diuretics, diabetes insipidus (neurosurgery, head trauma, or medications), and gastrointestinal losses from vomiting or diarrhea. Acute severe bleeding can cause severe hypovolemia and orthostatic syncope. Inquire about any new medications that may contribute to syncope, such as a new antihypertensive, diuretic, antidepressant, antipsychotic that prolongs QT interval, or CNS depressant. Ask about location, position, situation, and activity engaged in just prior to the event. Inquire about associated symptoms such as nausea, vomiting, pain, palpitations, or shortness of breath. Patients with psychogenic loss of consciousness may provide a positive history for a loss in the family or job or worsening stress leading to exacerbation of their mental health problems.

Event

If there were eyewitnesses, ask about the duration of the event, any movements, color changes, and bladder or bowel incontinence. Pay attention to the point of impact if patients had a fall from loss of postural tone, as this may assist with your assessment and plan. What rescue measures did the eyewitness carry out? Did they have the patient sit in a chair or hold them up in the upright position until the ambulance arrived, or possibly brought them to the ED by bringing them in a seated position in the car? This would prevent reperfusion of the brain, and the patient would then have a longer duration of symptoms and possible complications including watershed infarcts. This could result in needing an extensive battery of tests and a hospital stay.

Post-event

Post-event recovery is fast and complete in syncope. If it is prolonged, think about other conditions that might have led to loss of consciousness. Inquire about bowel and bladder incontinence and tongue biting. Did the patient exhibit any confusion for a prolonged amount of time after regaining consciousness? Does the patient have any persistent neurologic deficits?

Physical Examination

Physical examination is as important as history in the evaluation of syncope. Following are some of the signs that may help to diagnose the cause of syncope.

- Presence/absence of orthostatic hypotension
- Tachypnea and/or hypoxemia: consider pulmonary embolism and congestive heart failure.
- Tachycardia and/or hypotension: consider hypovolemia, pulmonary embolism, aortic dissection, myocardial infarction, arrhythmias, and pulmonary hypertension.
- Signs of Parkinson disease: consider orthostatic syncope.
- Abnormal cardiovascular exam: heart murmurs (consider valvular heart disease, hypertrophic obstructive cardiomyopathy), extra heart sounds (S3, S4, "tumor plop" of atrial myxomas), rhythm abnormalities, signs of systolic heart failure with a high risk of arrhythmias (peripheral edema, elevated jugular venous pulse, diffuse/displaced point of maximal impulse), and arterial bruits.
- Rectal examination is important in hypotensive patients to assess for gastrointestinal bleeding.
- A thorough neurologic examination is indicated in patients presenting with symptoms suggestive of a posterior stroke.

Electrocardiogram

Electrocardiogram is an important tool in the evaluation process to evaluate for a cardiovascular cause of syncope. Every effort should be made to identify a cause from history and physical examination, as they yield the most vital information to assist in reaching a diagnosis. ECG alone has a diagnostic yield of only around 5%, but, when added to the history and physical examination, the diagnostic yield can be up to 50%. It is important to note, however, that a normal ECG does not rule out a cardiac cause unless it happens to be obtained during an episode of syncope or presyncope. Further investigation should be streamlined based on the available information, comorbid conditions, single episode or recurrent syncope, and presence of structural heart disease and high-risk features.

Risk Stratification

Once the diagnosis of syncope is made, it is important to risk stratify the patient to determine further management strategy. Patients with short-term, high-risk features should be admitted to the hospital for evaluation and treatment. High-risk patients (Table 28-1) have an increased short-term mortality, and they should be evaluated in the hospital immediately. Patients with syncope and a history suggesting potentially fatal conditions such as massive pulmonary embolism, subarachnoid hemorrhage, acute severe hemorrhage, acute aortic dissection, acute coronary syndromes, malignant arrhythmias, and severe structural heart diseases fall into the high-risk category.

For those patients who fall into the high-risk category, admission to the hospital for further investigation is warranted. Additional studies for further evaluation are dependent on the features of the patient's presentation.

CAUSES OF SYNCOPE

Orthostatic Hypotension

Syncope or presyncope that occurs upon standing is suggestive of orthostatic hypotension. Orthostatic hypotension is defined as a decrease in systolic blood pressure of at least 20 mm Hg or diastolic blood pressure of at least 10 mm Hg within 3 minutes of standing.

A comprehensive history should be obtained, focusing on potential causes of volume loss. Acute hemorrhage, diarrhea, vomiting, or poor oral intake can contribute to volume depletion. This also may occur in patients with significant third-spacing of fluid in conditions such as liver cirrhosis with portal hypertension, massive inflammation, and malnutrition to name a few. Adrenal insufficiency also should be considered.

Elderly patients are more prone to orthostatic hypotension, possibly due to decreased baroreceptor sensitivity. The elderly are particularly susceptible to orthostasis from drug effects. Medications such as diuretics, anticholinergics,

Table 28-1. High-risk Features Requiring Admission to the Hospital for Further Evaluation and Treatment

History, Physical Examination, and Basic Laboratory Work	ECG Findings
History	Sinus bradycardia <50 beats/min or sinoatrial block, A-V nodal block in the absence of nodal blocking agents
Exertion syncope	
Syncope in supine position	
Palpitation at the time of syncope	QRS duration >120 ms
Acute blood loss	Bifascicular block
Acute shortness of breath	Prolonged or short QT interval
Acute sharp tearing or ripping chest pain with radiation	Nonsustained ventricular tachycardia
Sudden severe worst headache	Preexcitation syndromes such as Wolff-Parkinson-White syndrome
Physical examination	
Severe hypotension	Brugada pattern with RBBB with ST elevation in the anterior leads
Severe hypoxemia	
Pulse deficit	Arrhythmogenic right ventricular dysplasia (ARVD) findings with epsilon wave, inverted T waves, and S-wave upstroke >55 ms in the anterior precordial leads
Past medical history	
Congestive heart failure	
Systolic dysfunction	
Myocardial infarction or coronary artery disease	
Valvular or obstructive cardiac abnormalities or history of arrhythmias	
Family history	
Family history of sudden cardiac death	
Basic laboratory work	
Severe anemia	
Severe electrolyte abnormalities	

alpha blockers, beta blockers, nitrates, and other antihypertensives are common causes of orthostatic symptoms in the elderly.

Patients with underlying autonomic failure are more prone to have orthostatic symptoms due to lack of an effective vasoconstrictor response. In this situation, sympathetic efferent activity is chronically impaired leading to decreased vasoconstrictor response. Primary autonomic failure (Parkinson disease, multiple system atrophy, Shy-Drager syndrome) and secondary autonomic failure from chronic conditions such as diabetes, renal failure, nutritional deficiencies, or amyloidosis are potential causes.

Treatment for orthostatic hypotension is aimed at the underlying cause. Volume expansion is appropriate for those whose symptoms are acute and secondary to dehydration or blood loss. Medications that may be contributing to symptoms should be discontinued or be reduced in dose. For individuals with chronic orthostatic hypotension, increased salt and fluid intake may be helpful. Compression stockings and abdominal binders can help reduce venous pooling. The addition of mineralocorticoids and alpha agonists may be added if nonmedication approaches are not sufficient.

Cardiovascular Syncope

The second most common cause of syncope is cardiovascular in origin. Syncope results from abrupt reduction in cardiac output from either an arrhythmia or mechanical obstruction to the outflow. Arrhythmias cause about 15% of cardiovascular syncope, and it should be suspected if the patient had palpitations or no warning/prodrome. Mechanical obstruction is a relatively less common cause, and patients often complain of presyncope or syncope on exertion associated with some chest discomfort. Ischemic heart disease, acute coronary syndromes, and systolic heart failure are risk factors for arrhythmias. Acute coronary syndrome is unlikely to cause syncope in the absence of an arrhythmia. Mortality rate is high among patients presenting with cardiovascular syncope, and up to nearly one-third of them die in the first year. Patients with suspected cardiovascular syncope are considered high risk and warrant hospital admission for further evaluation.

Atrial tachyarrhythmias, ventricular tachycardia, and bradyarrhythmias all cause decreased cardiac output, resulting in syncope. A careful history of underlying risk factors such as ischemic heart disease or heart failure should be obtained. A family history of syncope or sudden cardiac death is suggestive of Brugada syndrome, long QT syndrome, or hypertrophic obstructive cardiomyopathy (HOCM has a predisposition to ventricular tachycardia). A full list of a patient's medications can also be crucial to determining possible arrhythmogenic drug effects.

Obstructive causes of cardiovascular syncope include structural heart disease such as hypertrophic obstructive cardiomyopathy, severe aortic stenosis, mitral stenosis, or pulmonic stenosis. Syncope that occurs with structural heart disease is often precipitated by exertion. Pulmonary hypertension, particularly in the setting of an acute pulmonary embolus, can also cause significant obstruction to blood flow and decreased cardiac output, resulting in syncope.

Testing and treatment for cardiovascular syncope is based on the probability of a particular cause of syncope. A preliminary ECG in this setting may be diagnostic for an ongoing arrhythmia, prolonged QTc interval, high-grade AV nodal blocks, and pre-excitation syndromes. However, a normal ECG does not rule out a cardiovascular cause of syncope unless it is obtained at the time the patient's symptoms are occurring. An echocardiogram is indicated only if structural heart disease is the suspected cause.

Diagnostic yield of telemetry is low at 16% in hospitalized patients suspected to have arrhythmia as a cause of syncope. If a patient's syncope remains unexplained after admission to the hospital, and no arrhythmias are captured on continuous telemetry, they may require continuous ECG monitoring as an outpatient or additional testing. Table 28-2 lists other possible testing and evaluations that may be utilized in unexplained syncope.

Table 28-2. Testing for Unexplained Syncope

Test	Comments
Targeted blood Testing	Blood testing is of low yield when used routinely. Targeted blood tests are reasonable in select patients when a cause is suggested by the history and physical exam (eg, complete blood count in patients with GI bleeding, BNP and troponin in patients with concern for cardiac syncope).
Echocardiography	Indicated in patients with exertional syncope or clinically suspected structural heart disease.
CT or MRI	May be useful in selected patients with suspected cardiac syncope when there is concern for pulmonary embolus or structural/infiltrative/congenital heart disease.
Ambulatory electrocardiography monitoring	Type of monitoring should be chosen by the frequency and nature of syncopal events. Holter monitors provide continuous recording for 24–72 h, and they are helpful only if symptoms are frequent enough to be recorded in a short time period. For patients with symptoms likely to recur within 2–6 weeks, event monitors, external loop recorders, and external patch recorders can be patient- or auto-triggered for recording. Implantable cardiac monitors are helpful for infrequent symptoms and can be utilized for up to 3 years.
Electrophysiologic studies	Useful in select patients when there is high index of suspicion for arrhythmia.
Tilt table test	Useful for patients if diagnosis is unclear but neurocardiogenic syncope or delayed orthostatic hypotension is suspected. May also be useful to distinguish psychogenic pseudosyncope from true syncope.
Stress testing	May be useful in patients with exertional syncope. Must be done in a closely monitored setting with availability of advanced life support measures.

Treatment for cardiovascular syncope is aimed at the underlying cause. Treatment may include antiarrhythmic medications, a pacemaker, an implantable cardioverter-defibrillator, catheter ablation, or surgical correction for structural heart disease.

TIPS TO REMEMBER

- Syncope is defined as sudden transient loss of consciousness with loss of postural tone and complete spontaneous recovery.
- Syncope is a clinical diagnosis that can be made with a thorough history and physical examination.
- Pre-event, event, and post-event history will help to differentiate syncope from other causes of TLOC, and also help to identify the etiology.
- History, physical examination, and ECG combined has a diagnostic yield up to 50%.
- Neurocardiogenic syncope is the most common cause, and it has a low risk of mortality.
- Syncope from cardiovascular causes has a high mortality rate, reaching up to 30% in 1 year.
- High-risk patients should be admitted to the hospital for further evaluation and management.

COMPREHENSION QUESTION

A 72-year-old gentleman presented with syncope on exertion. He had to walk an extra block this morning to buy milk, as the store next door was closed. At the end of the block he felt light-headed and was trying to lean against the wall; the next thing he remembers he was lying down on the pavement. He was soon picked up by EMS and brought to the ED. There is no eyewitness to describe the episode. He thinks he passed out for a minute and took a few seconds to figure out where he was. He complains of fatigue and increasing dyspnea on exertion. His exercise tolerance is limited to half a block secondary to shortness of breath. He has orthopnea and paroxysmal nocturnal dyspnea. He has no significant past medical history, and the last time he saw a physician was 30 years ago. The rest of the history is not significant. On examination, the patient is afebrile, blood pressure is 102/72 mm Hg, heart rate is 98/min, respiratory rate is 20/min, and oxygen saturation is 94% on room air. He has a laceration on the left temporal area from the fall. JVD is elevated to the angle of the jaw. There is an ejection systolic murmur with late peaking in the second right intercostal space radiating to the carotids. Lungs show bilateral basal rales, and the patient has mild pedal edema. ECG showed left ventricular hypertrophy, biatrial enlargement, and no ischemic ST–T changes. Chest radiograph is significant for cardiomegaly and pulmonary vascular congestion. Basic metabolic profile is normal, and hematocrit is 36.

1. What is the next best step in the evaluation of this patient with syncope and why?
   A. Suture the laceration and discharge, as this is the first episode of syncope.
   B. Work up for syncope as outpatient.
   C. Order a tilt-table test, as he is elderly and probably had a reflex syncope.
   D. Admit to cardiovascular unit for further management of syncope.

Answer

1. **D.** This patient has high-risk features. He has exertional syncope, and the rest of the history, physical examination, and ECG suggests aortic stenosis. He has a high short-term risk of death. He also has decompensated heart failure with fluid overload. His laceration needs to be taken care of, and he should be followed by CT head to rule out intracranial bleed, but he is not a low-risk patient to work up as an outpatient or discharge. Tilt-table test is not an option at this stage with this significant cardiac history.

SUGGESTED READINGS

Albassam OT, Redelmeier RJ, Shadowitz S, et al. Did this patient have cardiac syncope? The Rational Clinical Examination Systematic Review. *JAMA*. 2019;321(24):2448–2457.

Brignole M, Moya A, de Lange FJ, et al. 2018 ESC Guidelines for the diagnosis and management of syncope. *Eur Heart J*. 2018;39(21):1883–1948.

Shen W, Sheldon R, Benditt D, et al. 2017 ACC/AHA/HRS Guideline for the Evaluation and Management of Patients With Syncope. *J Am Coll Cardiol*. 2017;70(5):e39–e110.

Sutton R, Ricci F, Fedorowski A. Risk stratification of syncope: current syncope guidelines and beyond. *Auton Neurosci*. 2021;238:102929.

van Dijk JG, van Rossum IA, Thijs RD. The pathophysiology of vasovagal syncope: novel insights. *Auton Neurosci*. 2021;236:102899.

A 32-year-old Woman With Fever, Chills, and Weakness Status After a Blood Transfusion

Ruchika Goel, MD, MPH, Satyam Arora, MD and Mingmar Sherpa, SBB

A 32-year-old woman is evaluated for fever, chills, and weakness. She had a blood transfusion 10 days prior after she underwent an open reduction and internal fixation of the right femur due to a motor vehicle accident. She has had no significant past medical history except for a C-section 2 years ago, at which time she successfully received a blood transfusion.

On examination, she has a fever of 100.1°F. Blood pressure is 100/64 mm Hg, pulse rate is 110 bpm, and respiration is 20/min. On physical examination, the patient appears uncomfortable and has scleral icterus. The remainder of the examination is unremarkable. There is no evidence of bleeding.

Hemoglobin concentration is 6.2 g/dL compared with a hemoglobin of 8.6 g/dL previously. Platelet and leukocyte count are normal. Direct and indirect Coombs tests are positive. The blood bank identifies a new alloantibody on further testing.

1. What is the most likely diagnosis?
2. What is the next step in management?

Answers

1. Delayed hemolytic transfusion reaction (DHTR).
2. Specific treatment generally is not necessary. Supplemental transfusion of blood lacking the antigen corresponding to the offending antibody may be necessary to compensate for the transfused cells that have been removed from the circulation.

CASE REVIEW

DHTR occurs due to an antibody response primarily to previously sensitized RBC alloantigens, which have a negative alloantibody screen due to low or serologically undetectable antibody levels. This reaction typically occurs 7 to 14 days following a transfusion. The alloantibody is detectable 1 to 2 weeks following the transfusion, and the posttransfusion direct antiglobulin test may become positive due to circulating donor RBCs coated with antibody or complement. These reactions are detected most commonly in the blood bank as a delayed serologic transfusion reaction when a subsequent patient sample reveals a positive alloantibody or a new alloantibody in a recently transfused recipient. The DHTR is the clinical manifestation of the delayed serologic reaction and is associated with jaundice, low-grade fever, and a decrease in hemoglobin levels due to hemolysis. Many delayed hemolytic reactions go undetected because the red cell destruction occurs slowly. Any adverse reaction to the transfusion of blood or blood components should be reported to blood bank personnel as soon as possible. DHTR is more commonly due to alloantibodies against blood group antigens belonging to the Kell, Kidd, Duffy, and Rh blood groups. The specificity of the alloantibody can also be confirmed by elution of these antibodies from the direct Coombs–positive RBCs.

Chills and rigor within 10 minutes of starting a blood transfusion in a 62-year-old man

A 62-year-old man 3 days after total hip arthroplasty with a hemoglobin of 6.5 g/dL was ordered 2 units of RBCs. Transfusion of the first unit was uneventful, but 10 minutes after the start of the second unit the patient complained of chills and rigors. The nursing staff immediately stopped the transfusion and informed the physician on the floor. The pre-transfusion vitals were temperature 36.2°C, pulse 75/min, and blood pressure of 110/70. At the time of symptom development temperature was 38.1°C, pulse 90/min, and blood pressure 115/80.

The clerical check from the blood bank and the file showed that there were no errors. Patient appeared stable. The blood bank workup showed that there was no blood grouping error, and the repeat cross-match and antibody screening from the posttransfusion samples were negative. The direct antiglobulin test (DAT) and urinalysis also were negative.

1. What is the diagnosis

2. What is the next step in management?

3. How can these type of transfusion reactions be prevented?

Answers

1. There are two typical diagnoses for this manner of presentation
   a. Febrile nonhemolytic transfusion reactions (FNHTR)

   b. Bacterial contamination

   The sign and symptoms of both conditions overlap considerably since they can occur within a few minutes of starting a transfusion and have similar clinical features such as chills, rigors, and fever. One of the most important points of differentiation is the presence of hypotension and tachycardia with bacterial contamination, which is unlike the patient's presentation. Hence this is likely a case of a febrile nonhemolytic transfusion reaction (FNHTR), which is a diagnosis of exclusion.

2. The next step in management is to stop the transfusion and send the bag and set along with a sample to the blood bank for workup. In case of

suspected bacterial contamination, send cultures (anaerobic and aerobic) from the patient as well as the bag and start broad-spectrum antibiotics.

3. FNHTRs are typically due to cytokines released by the leukocytes present in the stored blood. Leukoreduction is generally an effective way to reduce the incidence of these type of reactions, although they can still occur. Leukoreduction may be done at various stages of the processing of blood components such as at "pre-storage" (done during the component preparation and before the units is stored). The other is "pre-transfusion" where either at the bedside or in the blood bank the unit is filtered using a leukofilter just before transfusion or issue from the blood bank.

Transfusions

Physiology of anemia

Anemia is defined as a reduction below normal of the number of erythrocytes in the circulation. The World Health Organization defines anemia as a hemoglobin level of less than 13 grams per deciliter in men and less than 12 grams per deciliter in women. Anemia is the most common indication for RBC transfusion among patients. It results from at least 1 of the following 4 factors:

1. Blood loss related to the primary condition or to an operation

2. Diminished erythropoiesis related to the primary illness

3. Hemolysis or red cell breakdown which can be due to a range of clinical etiologies

4. Iatrogenic due to serial blood draws (totaling, on average, approximately 40 mL per day in an ICU setting)

Acute anemia can be due to blood loss or hemolysis. If blood loss is mild, enhanced O_2 delivery is achieved through changes in the O_2–hemoglobin dissociation curve mediated by a decreased pH or increased CO_2 (the Bohr effect). With acute blood loss, hypovolemia dominates the clinical picture and the hematocrit and hemoglobin levels do not reflect the volume of blood lost. Signs of vascular instability appear with acute losses of 10% to 15% of the total blood volume. In such patients, the issue is not just anemia, but hypotension and decreased organ perfusion. When more than 30% of the blood volume is lost suddenly, patients are unable to compensate with the usual mechanisms of vascular contraction and changes in regional blood flow. The patient will prefer to remain supine and will show postural hypotension and tachycardia. If the volume of blood lost is greater than 40% (ie, >2 L in the average-sized adult), signs of hypovolemic shock including confusion, dyspnea, diaphoresis, hypotension, and tachycardia appear. Such patients have significant deficits in vital organ perfusion and require immediate volume replacement. Symptoms associated with more chronic or progressive anemia depend on the age of the patient and the adequacy of blood supply to critical organs.

With chronic anemia, intracellular levels of 2,3-bisphosphoglycerate rise, shifting the dissociation curve to the right and facilitating O_2 unloading. This compensatory mechanism can only maintain normal tissue O_2 delivery in the face of a 2- to 3-g/dL deficit in hemoglobin concentration. Finally, further protection of O_2 delivery to vital organs is achieved by the shunting of blood away from organs that are relatively rich in blood supply, particularly the kidney, gut, and skin.

Indications for Red Blood Cell Transfusion

Despite extensive physiologic data, indications for RBCs are controversial. Before the 1980s, most perioperative transfusion protocols used the "10/30 rule," which held that hemoglobin must exceed 10 grams per deciliter and hematocrit should be higher than 30% before major procedures should occur. RBC transfusion is administered most often to surgical and intensive care patients. This recommendation, which was intended for high-risk anesthesia patients, was incorrectly applied to all transfusion settings, acute or chronic, and became synonymous with the single hemoglobin value 10 grams per deciliter at which transfusion is indicated (Table 29-1).

The Association for Advancement of Blood and Biotherapies (AABB) gives clinical practice guidelines for RBC transfusion. In general, one needs to evaluate the risk-benefit ratio of transfusion. It is good practice to consider the hemoglobin level, the overall clinical context, patient preferences, and alternative therapies when making transfusion decisions regarding an individual patient. Currently, a restrictive RBC transfusion threshold (in which the transfusion is not indicated until the hemoglobin level is 7 g/dL) is recommended for hospitalized adult patients who are hemodynamically stable, including critically ill patients, rather than when the hemoglobin level is 10 grams per deciliter. Per AABB, a restrictive RBC transfusion threshold of 8 grams per deciliter is recommended for patients undergoing orthopedic surgery, cardiac surgery, and those with preexisting cardiovascular disease.

One needs to use clinical judgment with regard to the need for transfusion and consider the following:

- Ability to compensate for anemia
- Rate of ongoing blood loss
- Likelihood of further blood loss
- Evidence of end-organ compromise
- Risk of ischemia: history of coronary artery disease
- Balance of risk versus benefit of transfusion

Blood Group Antigens and Antibodies

At the beginning of the 20th century, Austrian scientist Karl Landsteiner noted that the RBCs of some individuals were agglutinated by the serum from other

Table 29-1. Guidelines for Transfusion and Volume Replacement in Adults

Need based on estimated loss of blood volume

>40% loss (>2000 mL)	30%–40% loss (1500–2000 mL)	15%–30% loss (800–1500 mL)	<15% blood loss (<750 mL)
Rapid volume replacement RBC transfusion is required	Rapid volume replacement with crystalloids or synthetic colloids RBC transfusion may be required	Volume replacement (crystalloids or synthetic colloids) RBC transfusion unlikely, unless preexisting anemia, ongoing blood loss, reduced cardiovascular reserve	May require volume replacement RBC transfusion is not warranted, unless symptomatic with preexisting anemia, severe cardiac and respiratory distress

Need based on hemoglobin concentration

Hgb <7 g/dL	Hgb 7–10 g/dL	Hgb >10 g/dL
RBC transfusion indicated If patient is otherwise stable, should receive 2 U of PRBCs, following which the clinical status and circulating Hgb should be reassessed	Unclear indications Balance of risk versus benefits of transfusion	RBC transfusion not indicated

High-risk patients: >65 and/or those with cardiovascular or respiratory disease may tolerate anemia poorly. Such patients may be transfused when Hgb <8 g/dL.

Data from Murphy MF, Wallington TB, Kelsey P, et al. British Committee for Standards in Hematology, Blood Transfusion Task Force. Guidelines for the clinical use of red cell transfusions. *Br J Haematol*. 2001;113:24.

individuals. Landsteiner explained that the reactions between the RBCs and serum were related to the presence of markers (antigens) on the RBCs and antibodies in the serum. Agglutination occurred when the RBC antigens were bound by the antibodies in the serum. He called the antigens A and B, and depending on which antigen the RBC expressed, blood belonged to either blood group A or

Table 29-2. ABO Blood Groups

Blood Group	Antigen(s) (on the RBC)	Antibodies (in the Serum)	Genotype(s)
A	A antigen	Anti-B	AA or AO
B	B antigen	Anti-A	BB or BO
AB (universal recipient)	A antigen and B antigen	None	AB
O (universal donor)	None	Anti-A and anti-B	OO

blood group B. A third blood group, originally recognized as C by Landsteiner, contained RBCs that reacted as if they lacked the properties of A and B, and this group was later called O. The following year the fourth blood group, AB, was added to the ABO blood group system. These RBCs expressed both A and B antigens (Table 29-2). The naturally occurring ABO antibodies are able to activate complement activity, causing severe immediate hemolytic transfusion reaction, thus making it the most important blood group system.

Rh System

The Rh system is the second most important blood group system in pre-transfusion testing. The Rh antigens are found on a 30- to 32-kDa RBC membrane protein that functions to maintain the integrity of the RBC membrane. This is one of the most polymorphic and immunogenic antigen systems, with more than 40 different antigens. An understanding of the Rh system, particularly the D antigen, is fundamental to understanding pre-transfusion and prenatal testing. The presence of the D antigen confers Rh positivity, while persons who lack the D antigen are Rh negative. Two allelic antigen pairs, E/e and C/c, also are found on the Rh protein. The D antigen is a potent alloantigen. About 15% of individuals lack this antigen. Exposure of these Rh-negative persons to even small amounts of Rh-positive cells, by either transfusion or pregnancy, can result in the production of anti-D alloantibody.

Blood Components

Blood products intended for transfusion are routinely collected as whole blood (450 mL) in various anticoagulants. Most donated blood is processed into components: PRBCs, platelets, and fresh frozen plasma (FFP) or cryoprecipitate. Whole blood is first separated into PRBCs and platelet-rich plasma by slow centrifugation. The platelet-rich plasma is then centrifuged at high speed to yield 1 U of random donor (RD) platelets and 1 U of FFP. Cryoprecipitate is produced by

Table 29-3. Characteristics of Selected Blood Components

Component	Volume (mL)	Content	Clinical Response
PRBC	180–200	RBCs with variable leukocyte content and small amount of plasma	Increase Hb by 1 g/dL and hematocrit by 3%
Platelets	50–70 200–400	5.5×10^{10}/RD unit $>3 \times 10^{11}$/single-donor apheresis product	Increase platelet count by 5000–10,000/μL
FFP	200–250	Plasma protein—coagulation factors, proteins C and S, antithrombin	Increases coagulation factors by 2%
Cryoprecipitate	10–15	Cold insoluble plasma proteins, fibrinogen, factors VIII, vWF	Topical fibrin glue, also 80 IU factor VIII
Whole blood (not readily available as it is routinely processed into components)	350–450	PRBC, platelets, FFP, cryoprecipitate	

Data from Longo DL, Fauci AS, Kasper DL, Hauser SL, Jameson L, Loscalzo J, eds. *Harrison's Principles of Internal Medicine.* 18th ed. New York: McGraw-Hill; 2012

refrigerator-thawing FFP to precipitate the plasma proteins, and then separating it by centrifugation (Table 29-3).

Adverse Reactions to Blood Transfusions

Adverse reactions to transfused blood components occur despite multiple tests, inspections, and checks. Fortunately, the most common reactions are not life-threatening, although serious reactions can present with mild symptoms and signs.

Immune-mediated reactions: Immune-mediated reactions are often due to preformed donor or recipient antibody; however, cellular elements also may cause adverse effects (Tables 29-4 to 29-6).

Table 29-4. Transfusion Reactions

Reaction Type	Symptoms	Cause	Treatment/ Prevention
Hypothermia	Chills, cardiac dysrhythmias	Exposing sinoatrial node to cold fluids	Use of an inline warmer
Electrolyte abnormalities	Renal failure, circumoral numbness, and/or tingling sensation of the fingers/toes	Hyperkalemia—RBC leakage during storage Hypocalcemia—citrate, commonly used to anticoagulate blood components; chelates calcium and inhibits coagulation cascade	Using fresh or washed RBCs
Reaction Type	**Symptoms**	**Cause**	**Treatment/ Prevention**
Iron overload	Symptoms and signs of iron overload affecting endocrine, hepatic, and cardiac functions are common after about 100 U of RBCs has been transfused	Each unit of RBCs contains 200–250 mg of iron	Deferoxamine and deferasirox. Alternative therapies—erythropoietin—and judicious transfusion are preferable
Hypotensive reactions	Drop of at least 10 mm Hg in the absence of other signs/symptoms of other transfusion reactions	Patients on ACE-I. Since blood products contain bradykinin that is normally degraded by ACE, patients on ACE-I may have increased levels of bradykinin that causes hypotension	Usually does not require any intervention—BP returns to normal

Table 29-5. Transfusion-transmitted Infections

Infections	Frequency (United States) (Episodes:Unit)
Hepatitis B	1:220,000
Hepatitis C	1:1,800,000
HIV-1 and -2	1:2,300,000
HTLV-I and -II	1:2,993,000
Malaria	1:4,000,000

Infectious agents rarely associated with transfusion, theoretically possible, or of unknown risk include West Nile virus, hepatitis A virus, parvovirus B19, *Babesia microti, Borrelia burgdorferi, Anaplasma phagocytophilum, Trypanosoma cruzi, Treponema pallidum*, and HHV-8.

Nonimmunologic reactions: Nonimmune causes of reactions are due to the chemical and physical properties of the stored blood component and its additives.

Transfusion-transmitted infections: Transfusion-transmitted viral infections are increasingly rare due to improved screening and testing. Multiple tests performed on donated blood to detect the presence of infectious agents using nucleic acid amplification testing (NAAT), or evidence of prior infections by testing for antibodies to pathogens, further reduce the risk of transfusion-acquired infections.

TIPS TO REMEMBER

- One needs to evaluate the risk-benefit ratio of transfusion on a case by case basis.

- Febrile nonhemolytic transfusion reactions are the most commonly encountered reactions associated with blood transfusion. Non-aspirin antipyretic agents can generally resolve the symptoms.

- Hyperkalemia and hypocalcemia are some of the most common electrolyte abnormalities involved with transfusion.

- Stop the transfusion and notify the blood bank immediately if symptoms are suggestive of an adverse reaction due to transfusion.

Table 29-6. Immune-mediated Reaction Types to Blood Transfusion

Reaction Type	Symptoms	Cause	Frequency	Treatment/ Prevention
Acute hemolytic reaction	Fever, chills, chest/ flank discomfort, tachypnea, tachycardia, hypotension, hemoglobinemia, discomfort at infusion site	ABO incompatibility Clerical errors	1:12,000	Immediately discontinue the transfusion while maintaining venous access for emergency management Treat shock, disseminated intravascular coagulation when appropriate
Delayed hemolytic transfusion reactions	Falling hematocrit and a positive direct Coombs test. Fever, leukocytosis Most commonly occur about 7–14 days following a transfusion, may also develop up to 1 month later	Previous sensitization to RBC alloantigens who have a negative alloantibody screen	1:1000	No specific treatment Supplemental transfusion of RBC lacking the antigen corresponding to the offending antibody
Febrile nonhemolytic transfusion reactions	Fever—rise of 1.0°C from baseline, chills, rigors	Cytokines and antibodies to leukocyte antigens reacting with leukocytes or leukocyte fragments	1–4:100	Non-aspirin antipyretic agents

(Continued)

Table 29-6. Immune-mediated Reaction Types to Blood Transfusion (*Continued*)

Reaction Type	Symptoms	Cause	Frequency	Treatment/ Prevention
Allergic reactions	Rash, laryngeal edema, bronchospasm	Foreign plasma protein in transfused components	1–4:100	Stop the transfusion temporarily. Administer antihistamine. Transfusion can be completed after symptoms resolve
Anaphylactic reactions	Dyspnea, stridor, hypotension, cardiac/respiratory arrest, shock	Anti-IgA	1:150,000	Stop transfusion. Maintain vascular access and administer epinephrine. Glucocorticoids for severe cases
Graft-versus-host reactions	Rash, fever, diarrhea, cytopenia, liver dysfunction 3–4 weeks after transfusion	Donor T lymphocytes recognize host HLA antigens as foreign and mount an immune response in immunodeficient recipients/ immunocompetent recipients who share HLA antigens with the donor	Rare	Can be prevented by irradiation of cellular components before transfusion to patients at risk

(*Continued*)

Table 29-6. Immune-mediated Reaction Types to Blood Transfusion (*Continued*)

Reaction Type	Symptoms	Cause	Frequency	Treatment/ Prevention
Transfusion-related acute lung injury	Respiratory compromise and symptoms of noncardiogenic pulmonary edema within 6 h of transfusion	Antibodies in donor plasma reactive to recipient leukocyte antigens	1:5000	Immediately discontinue the transfusion while preserving venous access
				Patients with mild episodes should respond to oxygen administered by nasal catheter or mask
				If shortness of breath persists after oxygen administration, transfer the patient to an intensive care setting where mechanical ventilation can be administered
				Supportive. Patient usually recovers without sequelae
Posttransfusion purpura	Purpura. Thrombocytopenia 7–10 days after platelet transfusion	Production of antibodies that react to both donor and recipient platelets	Rare	IV immunoglobulins or plasmapheresis to remove antibodies

COMPREHENSION QUESTIONS

1. Which of the following blood levels is considered as an adequate clinical response after 1 U of platelet transfusion?
    A. 1000 to 3000/μL
    B. 5000 to 10,000/μL
    C. 10,000 to 20,000/μL
    D. 20,000 to 25,000/μL

2. An acute hemolytic transfusion reaction occurs due to which of the following?
    A. Presence of an atypical antibody in the recipient that was undetectable in the initial antibody screen
    B. Presence of antibody in the recipient that is directed against HLA antigens on donor leukocytes
    C. ABO mismatch or due to antibodies in the host against the antigens on donor RBCs
    D. Presence of anti-IgA

3. Which of the following electrolyte abnormalities would contribute to circumoral numbness in a patient who has received 4 U of packed red blood cells due to acute blood loss involving a motor vehicle accident?
    A. Hyponatremia
    B. Hypernatremia
    C. Hypomagnesemia
    D. Hypocalcemia

Answers

1. C. Platelets are given as either pool preparations from RD or single-donor apheresis platelets. In an unsensitized patient without increased platelet consumption (from splenomegaly, fever, or DIC), 1 U of transfused pooled RD/single-donor apheresis platelets is anticipated to increase the platelet count by approximately 10,000–20,000/μL.

2. C. Acute hemolytic transfusion reactions may be intravascular (ABO mismatch) or extravascular (due to antibodies in the host against antigens on donor RBCs). Signs and symptoms include hypotension, burning at the infusion site, fever, pain in the lower back or chest, DIC, oliguria, and hemoglobinuria. Infusion of ABO-mismatched blood is most commonly the result of human error, in which the patient blood bank identification number is not matched with the number of the unit of blood to be transfused.

3. D. Citrate is commonly used to anticoagulate blood components. Citrate chelates calcium and thereby inhibits the coagulation cascade. Hypocalcemia may

manifest as circumoral numbness, and tingling sensation of the fingers and toes may result from multiple rapid transfusions. Because citrate is quickly metabolized to bicarbonate, calcium infusion is seldom required in this setting. If calcium is required, it must be given through a separate line.

SUGGESTED READINGS

Carson JL, Guyatt G, Heddle NM, et al. Clinical Practice Guidelines From the AABB: Red Blood Cell Transfusion Thresholds and Storage. *JAMA*. 2016;316(19):2025–2035.

Dean L. *Blood Groups and Red Cell Antigens*. Bethesda: National Center for Biotechnology Information; 2005.

Loscalzo J, Fauci AS, Kasper DL, eds. *Harrison's Principles of Internal Medicine*. 21st ed. New York: McGraw-Hill Professional; 2022.

Owings J, Utter G, Gosselin R. *Basic Surgical and Perioperative Considerations: Bleeding and Transfusions*. New York: WebMD; 2006.

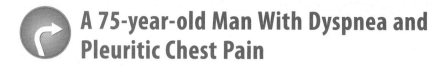

A 75-year-old Man With Dyspnea and Pleuritic Chest Pain

Robert Robinson, MD, MS, FACP

You are called by the ED and told of a 75-year-old male nonsmoker with a history of coronary artery disease and hypertension who presents with pleuritic chest pain with dyspnea. You are asked to admit this patient to the hospital for a lobar infiltrate seen on chest x-ray. The patient is febrile and tachypneic and has a blood pressure of 145/65, a pulse of 115, and an oxygen saturation of 87% on room air. Physical examination shows right lower-extremity edema with tenderness. Laboratory studies show a white blood cell count of 14,000, no evidence of acute renal failure, a negative COVID-19 test, and a positive d-dimer. Blood cultures have been obtained, and ceftriaxone and azithromycin have been started in the ED.

1. What is this patient's risk of a coexisting pulmonary embolism (PE)?

2. How could you diagnose a PE in this patient?

3. When should treatment start for a suspected PE?

4. What are the initial treatment options for PE in hemodynamically stable patients?

5. Is it worthwhile to evaluate this patient for a DVT?

Answers

1. The patient is at moderate risk for a coexisting pulmonary embolism. The patient's Wells score, a clinical risk stratification for venous thromboembolism (VTE) described in Table 30-1, is 4.5 (+3 for signs/symptoms of DVT, +1.5 for tachycardia). Note that pneumonia can cause a positive d-dimer in the absence of VTE.

2. CT pulmonary angiography is the first-line diagnostic test for pulmonary embolism and can evaluate for alternative causes of chest pain and dyspnea as well. Ventilation perfusion (V/Q) scanning is a less accurate alternative diagnostic test for patients with contraindications to CT angiography.

3. Treatment for suspected PE should be initiated while waiting for diagnostic imaging in patients with no contraindications for systemic anticoagulation. If the patient has an absolute contraindication to anticoagulation, an inferior vena cava (IVC) filter can be placed.

4. Initial treatment for VTE in hemodynamically stable patients can be with apixaban, rivaroxaban, low-molecular-weight heparin (LMWH), fondaparinux, or unfractionated heparin (UFH). Warfarin therapy for ongoing treatment for the VTE should be initiated for patients started on LMWH, fondaparinux, or UFH.

Table 30-1. The Simplified Wells Criteria

Risk Factor	Score
Clinical signs/symptoms of DVT	3
No alternative diagnosis other than PE	3
Heart rate >100 beats/min	1.5
Immobilization or surgery within 4 weeks	1.5
History of prior VTE	1.5
Hemoptysis	1
Cancer treated within 6 months	1

5. If there is no PE, identification of a DVT and initiation of treatment to prevent PE is essential. Treatment for DVT is identical to the treatment for PE, so it is reasonable to forgo an ultrasound of the lower extremities in a patient with a confirmed PE. Identifying remaining DVTs is helpful in deciding if an IVC filter should be considered in a hemodynamically unstable patient or patients who would not be able to survive another PE.

CASE REVIEW

This patient is at moderate risk of a pulmonary embolus given a Wells score of 4.5 and is hemodynamically stable. Most of the symptoms can be explained by pneumonia, but the unilateral leg swelling and positive D-dimer is suggestive of a DVT. Ultrasonography, including point of care ultrasonography (POCUS), can be used to quickly determine if a patient has a DVT. CT pulmonary angiography (CTPA) is the most widely available and accurate method to evaluate for PE. If the patient is in renal failure or has a severe allergy to IV contrast, a V/Q scan can be considered. Treatment for a potential VTE should start immediately while waiting for the results of the diagnostic workup.

VENOUS THROMBOEMBOLISM

Risk factors
The primary risk factors for VTE are venous stasis, endothelial injury, and hypercoagulable states. Many patients who develop VTE have more than 1 of these risk factors. See Table 30-2.

Risk stratification
Clinical risk stratification for VTE can be done with the simplified Wells criteria (see Table 30-1).

Table 30-2. Risk Factors for VTE

Venous Stasis	Endothelial Injury	Hypercoagulability
Immobility	Prior DVT	Drugs
Surgery	Leg trauma	Genetic predisposition
CHF	Central vascular catheters	Acquired
Venous obstruction		Malignancy
Morbid obesity		Trauma/burns

Add the points for all risk factors to determine the Wells score. A score greater than 6 puts the patient at high risk, 2 to 6 at moderate risk, and a score of less than 2 represents a low risk for VTE.

VTE prevention

VTE can be prevented with heparin, LMWH, fondaparinux, direct oral anticoagulants (DOACs), and mechanical devices. A VTE prevention strategy should be implemented in all hospitalized patients with 1 or more risk factors for VTE. For patients with intracranial bleeding or major trauma, an IVC filter can be placed for VTE risk reduction. Pharmacologic VTE prevention should be started as soon as feasible after placement of an IVC filter due to the risk of thrombosis of the filter. See Table 30-3.

Diagnosis of pulmonary embolism

CTPA is the fastest, safest, and most accurate method to diagnose PE. In patients with advanced chronic kidney disease or a serious allergy to IV contrast, V/Q scanning is an option. V/Q scanning is not feasible if the patient is unstable or unable to hold their breath for the scan and has reduced accuracy in patients with

Table 30-3 VTE Prevention

Method	Dose
LMWH	Enoxaparin 40 mg SC Daily
	or
	Dalteparin 5000 U SC Daily
UFH	5000 U SC twice daily
Fondaparinux	2.5 mg SC Daily
Rivaroxaban	10 mg PO daily
Apixaban	2.5mg PO twice daily
Pneumatic compression devices	While in bed

Table 30-4. VTE Diagnosis

Test	Sensitivity for PE	Specificity for PE
CT pulmonary angiogram	90%+	96%+
V/Q Scan	77%	73%

COPD, pulmonary fibrosis, or vasculitis. Pulmonary angiography is rarely done due to availability and the risks of this procedure. See Table 30-4.

PE Classification

Patients with PE are risk stratified as high, intermediate, and low risk. Pulmonary emboli are high risk for mortality ("massive") if the systolic blood pressure (SBP) is less than 90 mm Hg or there is a drop in SBP of 40 mm Hg from the patient's usual SBP for 15 minutes or more. In patients with high-risk PEs, ICU care, IV UFH, and catheter-directed thrombolysis are critical components of therapy. Intermediate-risk PEs ("submassive") are characterized by hemodynamic stability with tachycardia, evidence of right ventricular dysfunction, or elevated troponin. These patients should be anticoagulated, closely monitored for deterioration, and considered for thrombolysis. All other patients are characterized as low risk for mortality and are anticoagulated.

In high- and intermediate-risk patients with DVTs, consider an inferior vena cava filter to reduce the risk of additional PEs.

Diagnosis of deep venous thrombosis

History, physical examination, and D-dimer testing lack specificity for the diagnosis of DVT. A rapid diagnosis can be established with POCUS (93% sensitive) or ultrasonography (95% sensitive). Patients with a history of upper extremity surgery, trauma, radiation, or indwelling devices in the upper extremities also should be evaluated for possible upper-extremity DVT.

VTE Treatment

Initial VTE treatment can be UFH, LMWH, fondaparinux, apixaban, or rivaroxaban. IV UFH dosed by protocol is the mainstay of treatment when the patient is unstable or may need discontinuation of therapy for a procedure in the near future. Heparin-based therapy (UFH or LMWH) can be converted to warfarin therapy with a target INR of 2 to 3 for 3 to 6 months for long-term treatment. Long-term treatment with UFH or LMWH may be needed in pregnant patients or patients with malignancy. VTE treatment of a pregnant patient should be done in consultation with the patient's OB provider.

DOACs are a new option with a PO route for initial and long-term therapy. These drugs have been shown to be as effective as warfarin, LMWH, and UFH

Table 30-5. Pharmacologic VTE Treatment Options

Drug	Dose	Notes
LMWH	Enoxaparin 1 mg/kg SC twice daily *or* Enoxaparin 1.5 mg/kg SC daily *or* Dalteparin 200 U SC daily	Transition to PO warfarin for long-term treatment
Intravenous UFH	Weight-based dosing protocol	Preferred agent for patients with a high-risk PE Transition to PO warfarin for long-term treatment
Fondaparinux	7.5–10 mg SC daily based on weight	Transition to PO warfarin for long-term treatment
Rivaroxaban	15 mg PO twice daily for 21 days, then 10 mg PO daily	
Apixaban	10 mg PO twice daily for first 7 days, then 5 mg PO twice daily	

Dose adjustment may be needed if patient has renal impairment.

in the treatment of VTE. Because of this feature, DOAC treatment of VTE can facilitate early hospital discharge and outpatient therapy.

The duration of therapy for an unprovoked VTE is 3 to 6 months. Longer-term therapy may be required for patients with an ongoing risk of a VTE due to pregnancy, malignancy, or clotting disorder. See Table 30-5.

Catheter-directed thrombolysis is an additional treatment option for high- and intermediate-risk PE.

IVC filter placement is a treatment option for patients who have an absolute contraindication for anticoagulation. If this contraindication is temporary, full anticoagulation to prevent thrombosis of the IVC filter should be initiated as soon as possible.

TIPS TO REMEMBER

- History and physical examination are not sensitive for VTE.
- VTE prophylaxis should strongly be considered for all hospitalized patients.

- Treat for VTE while waiting for diagnostic confirmation.
- Risk-stratify patients with known or suspected PE to guide treatment.
- CT pulmonary angiography is the best test for diagnosing PE.

COMPREHENSION QUESTIONS

1. While on duty in the ICU, you receive an unstable patient transferred from the inpatient (non-ICU) internal medicine service. The patient is a 63-year-old female who was admitted for pneumococcal pneumonia 4 days ago. The patient was afebrile and responding well to IV antibiotics. The patient was transferred to the ICU after developing tachycardia, hypotension (BP 94/60), and hypoxia. The inpatient medicine service ordered an ECG, cardiac enzymes, chest x-ray, CBC, blood cultures, and metabolic panel before transferring the patient. The ECG shows sinus tachycardia with a rate of 125. The remainder of the studies are pending.

    Your physical examination of the patient is remarkable for tachypnea, hypotension, tachycardia, and hypoxia. No calf tenderness or edema is present. The patient is afebrile. Review of the chart indicates that the patient was on LMWH for DVT prophylaxis during this hospital stay and no documented contraindications for anticoagulation are present. What is this patient's risk of a PE?

    A. Zero. The patient is on LMWH for DVT prophylaxis
    B. Low
    C. Moderate
    D. High

2. The patient's chest x-ray is unchanged from the admission chest x-ray. Supplemental oxygen and a fluid bolus have been started. What interventions should be ordered while waiting other results? (Choose all that apply.)

    A. Change antibiotics to cover hospital-acquired pneumonia.
    B. D-Dimer assay
    C. Full anticoagulation with IV UFH
    D. POCUS to evaluate for DVT and right ventricular function
    E. CTPA

3. The patient is found to have bilateral pulmonary emboli on CT angiography of the chest, signs of right ventricular overload on POCUS, and multiple large residual clots in the lower extremities. The patient's blood pressure is now 95/60 with a pulse of 90 beats/min. What additional interventions should be considered at this time? (Choose all that apply.)

    A. Catheter-directed thrombolysis
    B. Thrombolytic therapy
    C. Placing an IVC filter
    D. A workup for a hypercoagulable state

Answers

1. C. The patient's Wells score is 3 (tachycardia and immobilization), which is in the moderate risk category. As additional information becomes available, and other alternative diagnoses are excluded, the patient's risk may become higher. VTE prophylaxis reduces, but does not eliminate, the risk of VTE.

2. C, D, and E are all appropriate. The patient is hemodynamically unstable and may have a high-risk PE. Prompt diagnosis with a CTPA, initiation of therapy with IV UFH, and evaluation for RV dysfunction and remaining DVTs are essential in planning the next steps of therapy.

With an unchanged chest x-ray, no fever, and clinical improvement on the initial antibiotic regimen, changing antibiotics does not appear warranted at this time. This could change with additional information such as an elevated WBC, evidence of aspiration by history or examination, or evidence of an infected IV site. A D-dimer assay would not be helpful in this situation.

3. A, B, and C. The patient has a high-risk PE with RV dysfunction and DVTs and should be considered for thrombolytic therapy and placement of an IVC filter. A hypercoagulable workup will be inaccurate in patients with acute thrombosis and should be postponed at this time.

SUGGESTED READINGS

Canakci ME, Acar N, Bilgin M, Kuas C. Diagnostic value of point-of-care ultrasound in deep vein thrombosis in the emergency department. *J Clin Ultrasound.* 2020;48(9):527–531.

Chunilal SD, Eikelboom JW, Attia J, et al. Does this patient have pulmonary embolism? *JAMA.* 2003;290(21):2849–2858.

Dong B, Jirong Y, Liu G, et al. Thrombolytic therapy for pulmonary embolism. *Cochrane Database Syst Rev.* 2006;(2):CD004437.

Habscheid W, Höhmann M, Wilhelm T, Epping J. Real-time ultrasound in the diagnosis of acute deep venous thrombosis of the lower extremity. *Angiology.* 1990;41(8):599–608.

Sostman HD, Stein PD, Gottschalk A, et al. Acute pulmonary embolism: sensitivity and specificity of ventilation-perfusion scintigraphy in PIOPED II study. *Radiology.* 2008;246(3):941–946.

Stein PD, Fowler SE, Goodman LR, et al; PIOPED II Investigators. Multidetector computed tomography for acute pulmonary embolism. *N Engl J Med.* 2006;354(22):2317.

Section II.
Outpatient Medicine

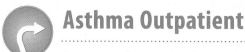

Asthma Outpatient

M. Haitham Bakir, MD, FCCP, DABSM

A 32-Year-old Woman With a Dry Cough and Chest Tightness

A 32-year-old woman presents for the first time to the pulmonary outpatient clinic, complaining of recurrent spells of dry cough and chest tightness, worse with activity (especially fast walking out doors), or exposure to strong odors or perfumes. There has been a gradual increase in cough with wheezing for the past 1 to 2 months. Her medical history is notable only for obesity, GERD, and seasonal allergic rhinitis. The patient notes that previously between attacks of her breathing difficulty (described as shortness of breath with wheezing), she would feel "pretty normal." For the past year, she feels her breathing is worse than usual, especially after gaining 15 pounds when she quit smoking a year ago. Her symptoms now do not seem to fully resolve after attacks. Her current BMI is 31.

The patient had a clear CXR. Pulmonary function testing was ordered. Previously she had been prescribed an albuterol inhaler that helped relieve the symptoms, but the symptoms have become a daily problem, and she ran out of her last prescription due to frequent use. The patient had smoked a half pack of cigarettes per day since the age of 18, up until a year ago when she quit. No pets are in the home, and she denies having any prior or recent exposure to industrial chemicals. There is no family history of emphysema or significant lung or heart diseases.

On examination, she does not appear to be in any distress. She is afebrile, with a heart rate of 76 bpm, blood pressure of 120/76 mm Hg, respiratory rate of 18 per minute, and a resting oxygen saturation of 98%. Lung examination is notable for equal breath sounds bilaterally, no dullness, mild hyperinflation, and mild scattered bilateral wheezing worse with forced expiration. There is no clubbing or edema in her extremities.

1. What is your first impression, and how will you confirm the diagnosis?

2. What are the risk factors for her illness?

Answers

The patient has a prior history of allergic rhinitis. She presents with intermittent chest tightness with a dry cough, which is becoming more frequent. She has a chronic airway disease such as asthma or COPD, rather than parenchymal diseases such as ILD. Her smoking history is less than 10 pack-years, not enough to be at risk for COPD. She demonstrates signs of airflow limitation on examination. In light of her reported intermittent symptoms by history, the patient's most likely primary diagnosis is uncontrolled asthma.

1. She will need blood tests to check her allergy components, such as a CBC with eosinophils and IgE levels. She will need spirometry and full pulmonary function tests. If there is no significant airway obstruction (FEV_1 >65%), she will need evaluation for hyperreactive airway disease, with a methacholine challenge test. An FEV_1 drop by 20% or more with a dose of methacholine under 0.8 mg/dL is considered diagnostic for reactive airway disease. This would suggest an asthma diagnosis (along with the clinical presentation of recurrent cough, wheezing, and chest tightness.) If the FEV_1 is below 65% of predicted, she will need an albuterol treatment with repeat FEV_1 to measure her response to bronchodilators. An improvement of 12% and 200 mL of FEV_1 suggests good bronchodilator responsiveness to the degree seen in asthma.

Case discussion

The patient has intermittent episodes of shortness of breath and wheezing, separated by essentially normal respiratory function. Her history is clinically consistent with a diagnosis of asthma. Her symptom frequency and need for frequent short-acting beta-2 agonists (SABA), along with worsening symptoms with exertion, classify her as having uncontrolled asthma. Obesity with weight gain, GERD, and allergic rhinitis are all common reasons for worsening asthma control. Some features of her presentation of concern include the following: She has not been formally diagnosed with having asthma previously. Her progressive symptoms and smoking history suggest she may be at risk for developing uncontrolled asthma with remodeling effects, which may suggest a poor response to albuterol. She needs a daily controller. There is some concern about developing COPD, although this is less likely due to the amount of smoking she has had.

The patient is not in significant respiratory distress, although her symptoms are not well controlled, so she should continue her use of SABAs as needed. She should control her GERD and should control her allergic rhinitis with an antihistamine or nasal fluticasone. The patient should also consider her need for weight loss. Adding an inhaled corticosteroid (ICS), or short course of oral steroids, would be reasonable if she has acute airway obstruction with an exacerbation.

Asthma is characterized by airflow limitation, which is considered fully reversible in the early stages before developing a remodeling effect from recurrent untreated attacks. Exposed to various risk factors such as allergy, GERD, or smoking exposure, chronically inflamed airways become hyperresponsive, resulting in bronchoconstriction, mucus plugs, and increased inflammation. Asthma is one of the most common chronic diseases globally and affects more than 300 million people, with 3000 deaths a year. Approximately 17% of adults in the United States have bronchial hyperresponsiveness, which is common to all types of asthma. Allergic asthma is characterized by an immediate-phase reaction of mast cells and basophils, as well as a late-phase reaction in which eosinophils become prominent. Biomarkers such as IgE, eosinophil count, exhaled nitric oxide (FeNo), and serum periostin help targeted therapy. Numerous risk factors have been implicated in asthma, and it is believed to result from an interplay between genetic and environmental risk factors (Table 31-1).

Asthma Diagnosis

Asthma is suspected based on a patient's symptoms and medical history. Spirometry and full pulmonary function testing are the preferred methods of measuring airflow limitation and reversibility to establish the diagnosis. An increase in the forced expiratory volume at 1 second (FEV_1) by greater than or equal to 12% with bronchodilator administration is consistent with the reversibility suggestive of asthma. This may not be seen in all asthmatics at each assessment, however. Patients with suspected asthma and otherwise normal spirometry results are

Table 31-1. Risk Factors and Triggers Involved in Asthma

Endogenous Factors	Environmental Factors	Triggers
Genetic predisposition	Indoor allergens	Allergens
Atopy	Outdoor allergens	Upper respiratory tract viral infections
Airway hyperresponsiveness	Passive smoking	Exercise and hyperventilation
Gender	Respiratory infections	Cold air
		Sulfur dioxide
		Drugs (beta blockers, aspirin)
		Stress
		Irritants (household sprays, paint fumes)

Data from Fauci AS, Braunwald E, Kasper DL, et al, eds. *Harrison's Principles of Internal Medicine.* 17th ed. New York: McGraw-Hill; 2008.

candidates for a methacholine bronchial challenge. A 20% decrease in the FEV_1 with gradual administration of 0.8 mg methacholine is considered a positive result.

Some challenges may occur in patients with cough-variant asthma, as they may not have wheezing at all but demonstrate airway responsiveness on methacholine challenge. In exercise-induced bronchoconstriction, physical activity may be the only trigger, usually confirmed with an FEV_1 drop by 20% on spirometry after exercise to 85% of the target heart rate (220 minus the patient's age). Occupational asthma related to workplace exposures should be considered, particularly when symptoms are clearly made worse when at work and improve when away, especially when a temporal association can be made with symptoms being absent before starting employment.

Measurement of asthma control is based on frequency of symptoms, use of albuterol rescue inhalers, and exacerbations. The asthma control test (ACT) is a valid and helpful test, which is easy to apply in clinic. It consists of a set of 5 questions, with rating 1-5 on each question.

The questions include:

1. In the past 4 weeks how often did your asthma keep you from getting as much done at work, school, or home as you would like?

2. During the past 4 weeks, how often have you had shortness of breath?

3. During the past 4 weeks, how often did your asthma symptoms wake you up at night or earlier than usual in the morning?

4. During the past 4 weeks, how often did you use your rescue inhaler or nebulizer?

5. How would you rate your asthma control over the past 4 weeks?

A cut-off score of ≤19 can be used to identify patients with uncontrolled asthma. A cut-off score of >20 can be used to identify patients with well-controlled asthma. A score of 25 identifies patients with completely controlled asthma.

Treatment of Asthma

When the diagnosis of asthma is clearly established, it is important to determine the level of asthma control based on well-defined clinical characteristics. (See Table 31-2.)

Based on the level of control, medication should be adjusted appropriately. The most common reason for uncontrolled asthma is nonadherence to medications, particularly ICSs; this should be assessed. Five treatment steps can guide the revision of the patient's medication regimen, with attention to the various endogenous and environmental triggers (Table 31-3). This should help to better control

Table 31-2. GINA Classification of Levels of Asthma Control

Characteristics	Controlled (All of the Following)	Partly Controlled (Any Measure Present)	Uncontrolled
Assessment of current clinical control over 4 weeks			
Daytime symptoms	None (twice or less per week)	More than twice per week	Three or more features of partly controlled asthma
Limitations of activities	None	Any	
Nocturnal symptoms or awakening	None	Any	
Need for reliever or rescue treatment	None (twice or less per week)	More than twice per week	
Lung function (PEF or FEV_1)	Normal	<80% predicted or personal best (if known)	
Medical management	Maintain lowest dose necessary	Consider stepping up control	Step up control

Data from *Global Strategy for Asthma Management and Prevention,* Global Initiative for Asthma (GINA). www.ginasthma.org. 2021.

asthma and prevent remodeling effects. Signs of poor control of asthma include awakening at night with symptoms, urgent care or ED visits, hospital admissions, increased need for SABAs, and requesting frequent SABA refills.

Before increasing medications, check for proper inhaler technique and adherence to a prescribed regimen. Also consider alternative diagnoses in cases of presumed asthma that do not respond to therapy.

Basic therapy consists of inhaled SABAs (such as albuterol) as a reliever medication at all levels of asthma, resulting in a rapid relief of symptoms. Additionally between steps 2 and 5, as symptoms become uncontrolled, controller medications, starting first with a low-dose ICS, are indicated. If uncontrolled symptoms continue to persist despite inhaled low-dose ICS, adding long-acting beta-2 agonists (LABAs) in combined form (ICS/LABA) may be considered, as well as the use of medium- to high-dose ICS. Although less effective than adding LABAs, leukotriene

Table 31-3. Treatment Steps to Asthma Control

Controller Therapy				
Step 1	**Step 2**	**Step 3**	**Step 4**	**Step 5**
None	Select one:	Select one:	Step 3 + one or more:	Step 4 + one:
	Low-dose ICS	Low-dose ICS + LABA	Medium- or high-dose ICS + LABA	Oral glucocorticoid (lowest dose needed)
	Leukotriene modifier	Medium- or high-dose ICS	Leukotriene modifier, long-acting muscarinic antagonist, tiotropium	Anti-IgE therapy, anti-IL5, anti-TSLP
		Low-dose ICS + leukotriene modifier	Sustained-release theophylline	
		Low-dose ICS + sustained-release theophylline		
Rapid Therapy				
As-needed SABA	As-needed SABA	As-needed SABA	As-needed SABA	As-needed SABA

Data from *Global Strategy for Asthma Management and Prevention*, Global Initiative for Asthma (GINA). www.ginasthma.org. 2022.

modifiers and sustained-release theophylline can also be added in combination with low-dose ICS. If the patient is classified as difficult to treat or refractory, referral to a pulmonary specialist is recommended. Checking biomarkers such IgE or eosinophils and starting biologic agents based on these levels can be helpful. Give monoclonal antibodies to IgE such as omalizumab for allergic asthma, an anti-IL5 such as mepolizumab or benralizumab for eosinophilic asthma, and anti-IL4, anti-IL13, or dupilumab for eosinophilic and allergic asthma. One may use anti-TSLP or tezepelumab as an add-on for severe asthma without phenotypic or biomarker limitations. All biologic agents should be administered in a monthly injection as or biweekly SC injections. Before assuming asthma is refractory make sure nonadherence to the medical regimen has been excluded.

Follow-up

The patient had mild airway obstruction and an FEV_1 of 2.1 L (68%) with a positive methacholine test (FEV_1 dropped by 21%). She was started on an inhaled steroid/budesonide but still showed symptoms such as waking up 3 to 5 times a month and needing an albuterol inhaler 5 to 10 times a week. Her ACT was 16/25. The patient was switched to LABA/ICS in the form of budesonide/formoterol twice daily with some improvement. However, she was still waking up 3 times a month, and her ACT was still 19/25. She was counseled regarding treatment of her obesity and GERD. Her eosinophil count was elevated above 300 cells per microliter on 3 occasions and was above 450 at least once. During this time she had good adherence to her medical management, including the proper use of her inhalers. At this point, the patient qualified for anti-IL5, so she was started on a mepolizumab injection 100 mg SC monthly. After 3 months, the patient did very well, requiring albuterol use 1 to 2 times a week. Spirometry is now normal (FEV_1 89%), and her ACT is 23/25.

Besides thinking about asthma, pay extra attention and look for similar conditions that can imitate severe uncontrolled asthma, such as allergic bronchopulmonary asthma (ABPA) that manifests as uncontrolled asthma with very high IgE, high eosinophils, and bronchiectasis on CXR/HRCT. Cystic fibrosis is consistent with chronic purulent sputum (*Pseudomonas, Staphylococcus aureus*), lifelong symptoms, obstructive lung disease, cystic bronchiectasis on HRCT, elevated sweat chloride, and an abnormal CF gene. Other considerations include Ciliary Dyskinesis, Churg-Strauss Syndrome, or Eosinophilic Granulomatosis with Polyangiitis (EPGA).

TIPS TO REMEMBER

- Asthma is a chronic and multifactorial condition; your approach should be systematic.
- Asthma can present in various manifestations; diagnosis requires good history, examination, and confirmatory tests.
- Control various factors that trigger asthma such as allergy, GERD, obesity, and environmental control to achieve best results and prevent complications.
- Close follow-up is needed to ensure good control; use minimal medications to achieve control with the fewest side effects.

- Counsel the patient, family, and primary care to maintain good control of asthma.

SUGGESTED READINGS

Broaddus VC, Mason RJ, Ernst JD, et al, eds. *Murray & Nadel's Textbook of Respiratory Medicine*. 6th ed. Philadelphia: Elsevier Saunders; 2016.
Crees Z, Fritz C, Huedebert A, et al. *Washington Manual of Medical Therapeutics*. Philadelphia: Wolters Kluwer; 2022.

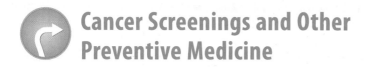

Cancer Screenings and Other Preventive Medicine

Rexanne Lagare Caga-anan, MD

A 68-year-old Man Who Presents to Establish Care

A 68-year-old male presents to the outpatient clinic to establish care. He has not seen a medical provider for the last 10 years because he did not have any medical concerns. He does not have any known medical conditions. His friend just got diagnosed with lung cancer, and his neighbor had some abnormal findings on his prostate screening. The patient is worried about his own risk for cancer because he recently became a father. He is a current cigarette smoker, consuming at least 1 pack a day. He started smoking at the age of 46 when he became a truck driver, as a way to pass the time. He rarely drinks alcohol and reports no drug use. He is adopted, and he does not know the medical history of his biological parents.

He does not have any shortness of breath, cough, or weight changes. There are no changes or problems with his urinary habits. Review of systems and physical exam are unremarkable.

1. Which cancers should he be screened for?

2. Which other preventive measures are appropriate for him?

Answers

1. Because of his 22-pack-year smoking history and age greater than 50, he qualifies for his first annual low-dose lung CT to screen for lung cancer. He will also need to undergo colorectal cancer screening since he is more than 45 years old. Because he is at average risk, he can choose from either stool-based or visualization studies. A discussion regarding the need for prostate cancer screening should be initiated, focusing especially on the harms of false positives, overdiagnosis, and overtreatment.

345

2. Screening for an abdominal aneurysm is warranted because he is more than 65 years old and has smoked more than 100 cigarettes in his lifetime. He will also need to be screened for hypertension, diabetes, and hyperlipidemia, so that his CVD risk can be calculated (to begin discussion about his need for a statin and aspirin for primary prevention of CVD, if indicated). Depression screening should be done as well. Hepatitis C and HIV screening also are recommended.

Screening

Screening is an important aspect of the routine care of the patient. Apart from managing multiple comorbid conditions, addressing key preventive care strategies should be given priority as well. Screening is appropriate if early intervention can decrease morbidity and mortality, and there are screening tests that are safe, acceptable, and adequately sensitive and specific. It is also important to remember that screening applies only to patients without signs or symptoms for a specific disease or condition.

Patients should be informed participants regarding these screening measures, and discussion of not just the benefits but also the potential harm of screening should be included.

The US Preventive Services Task Force (USPSTF) makes evidence-based recommendations to inform clinical practice guidelines for screening and other areas of preventive medicine. These recommendations are frequently changing, so it is important to be aware of these developments as they occur.

Colon Cancer Screening (Updated 2021)

- All average-risk, asymptomatic adults age 45 to 75 years
  - Stool-based tests
    o Highly sensitive fecal immunochemical test (FIT) every year
    o Highly sensitive guaiac-based fecal occult blood test (gFOBT) every year
    o Multitargeted stool DNA test (mt-sDNA, eg, Cologuard) every 3 years
  - Direct visualization tests
    o Colonoscopy every 10 years
    o CT colonography every 5 years
    o Flexible sigmoidoscopy every 5 years
    o Flexible sigmoidoscopy every 10 years + annual FIT
- Adults age 76 to 85 years
    o Selectively screen. Take into consideration the patient's overall health status (life expectancy, comorbid conditions), prior screening history, and preferences.

Special note

- Abnormal results from stool-based tests, CT colonography, and flexible sigmoidoscopy should be followed up with colonoscopy.
- High-risk patients, such as those in the following groups, need earlier or more frequent screening:
  - Prior colorectal cancer, adenomatous polyps, inflammatory bowel disease
  - Personal diagnosis or family history of Lynch syndrome or familial adenomatous polyposis
  - Family history of colorectal cancer (even in the absence of an inherited syndrome)
- The evidence is unclear on whether aspirin reduces the risk of colorectal cancer incidence or mortality.

Lung Cancer Screening (Updated 2021)

- Adults age 50 to 80 years who have a 20-pack-year smoking history and currently smoke or quit within the last 15 years: low-dose lung computed tomography (LDCT) every year.
- Stop screening once the patient has quit smoking for 15 years or has a health problem that limits life expectancy or the ability to have lung surgery.
- One pack-year is the equivalent of smoking an average of 20 cigarettes—1 pack—per day for a year.

Cervical Cancer Screening

As of May 2022, update in progress. Latest guidelines were released in 2018.

- Women age 21 to 29 years: cervical cytology every 3 years
- Women age 30 to 65: cervical cytology every 3 years or high-risk HPV (hrHPV) testing every 5 years or cervical cytology PLUS hrHPV (cotesting) every 5 years

Special note

- Not indicated after a hysterectomy if there is no history of a high-grade precancerous lesion (CIN grade 2 or 3) or cervical cancer

Prostate Cancer Screening (Updated 2018)

- Men age 55 to 69 years
  - Shared decision-making. Discuss potential benefits and harms of screening (false positive results requiring additional testing and possible prostate biopsy; overdiagnosis; overtreatment; treatment complications).

- Men 70 and older
  o Do not screen.
- Prostate-specific antigen (PSA) is the screening test of choice if the patient chooses to undergo screening.

Breast Cancer Screening

As of May 2022, update in progress. Latest guidelines were released in 2016.

- Women age 50 to 74 years
  o Screening mammography every 2 years.
- Women age 40 to 49 years
  o The decision to start screening should be individualized.
  o Women with a parent, sibling, or child with breast cancer are at higher risk and may benefit from beginning screening in their 40s.
- Women age 75 and older
  o No recommendation (insufficient evidence).

Special note

- Offer to prescribe risk-reducing medications (tamoxifen, raloxifene, or aromatase inhibitors) to asymptomatic women age 35 years or older at increased risk for breast cancer.
  o Numerous risk assessment tools, such as the National Cancer Institute (NCI) Breast Cancer Risk Assessment Tool, can be used. Women at greater risk, such as those with at least a 3% risk for breast cancer in the next 5 years, are likely to derive more benefit than harm from risk-reducing medications and should be offered these medications if their risk of harm is low.
  o Increased risk also includes previous atypical ductal or lobular hyperplasia and lobular carcinoma in situ on biopsy.
  o Patients with documented pathogenic mutations in the breast cancer susceptibility 1 and 2 genes (BRCA1/2) and history of chest radiation therapy are at especially high risk for breast cancer.

OTHER PREVENTIVE MEASURES

Abdominal Aortic Aneurysm Screening (Updated 2019)

- Men age 65 to 75 years who have ever smoked (100 or more cigarettes)
  o One-time abdominal duplex ultrasonography

Osteoporosis Screening

As of May 2022, update in progress. Latest guidelines were released in 2018.

- Women 65 years and older
  o Central dual-energy x-ray absorptiometry (DEXA) of the hip and lumbar spine.
- Postmenopausal women younger than 65 who are at increased risk
  o Parental history of hip fracture, smoking, excessive alcohol consumption, low body weight, early menopause, steroid use.
  o Clinical assessment tools (such as FRAX) can be used to determine whom to screen in this population.
- Men
  o No recommendation. Insufficient evidence.

Hypertension Screening (Updated 2021)

- Adults age 18 and older

Prediabetes and Diabetes Screening (Updated 2021)

- Adults age 35 to 70 years who are overweight or obese
  o HgbA1c or fasting plasma glucose

Special note

- Optimal screening interval is not certain, but screening every 3 years may be a reasonable approach in adults with normal blood glucose levels.

Obesity (Updated 2018)

- All adults with a body mass index (BMI) of 30 or higher need to be offered intensive, multicomponent behavioral interventions.

Depression Screening

As of May 2022, update in progress. Latest guidelines were released in 2016.

- All adults, including pregnant and postpartum women

Tobacco Smoking Cessation

- All adults
  o Ask about tobacco use, and advise the patient to stop using tobacco. Provide behavioral interventions and FDA-approved pharmacotherapy (nicotine replacement therapy, sustained-release bupropion, varenicline) for cessation.

Unhealthy Alcohol Use Screening (Updated 2018)

- All adults 18 and older
  - o Screening tools like AUDIT-C

HIV Screening (Updated 2019)

- Adolescents and adults age 15 to 65 years
- Patients older than 65 can be screened if they are at high risk
  - o Sexual risk factors
  - o Injection drug use
- All pregnant persons

Special note

- Recommend pre-exposure prophylaxis (PreP) to persons at high risk of HIV acquisition
  - o Once-daily oral treatment with combined tenofovir disoproxil fumarate and emtricitabine

Hepatitis C Screening (Updated 2020)

- All adults age 18 to 79 years (asymptomatic, without known liver disease)
  - o One-time anti-HCV antibody testing followed by confirmatory PCR

Chlamydia and Gonorrhea Screening (Updated 2021)

- Women who are sexually active age 24 years or younger
- Women 25 years or older who are at increased risk of infection
  - o Previous or coexisting STI
  - o New or more than 1 sex partner
  - o Sex partner with STI
  - o Sex partner who is not monogamous
  - o Inconsistent condom use
- Nucleic acid amplification tests (NAATs) for *Chlamydia trachomatis* and *Neisseria gonorrhoeae* infections are used on urogenital and extragenital sites.
- Urine testing with NAATs is at least as sensitive as testing with endocervical specimens, clinician- or self-collected vaginal specimens, or urethral specimens in clinical settings.

Aspirin for Primary Prevention of Cardiovascular Disease (Updated 2021)

- Adults age 40 to 59 years
  - o In patients whose estimated CVD risk is 10% or greater, use shared decision-making to discuss potential benefits and harms of aspirin use, as well as patients' values and preferences, to inform the decision about initiating aspirin.
- Adults age 60 or older
  - o Do not initiate aspirin for primary prevention of CVD

Statin Use for Primary Prevention of Cardiovascular Disease (Updated 2016)

- Adults age 40 to 75 years with no history of CVD, 1 or more CVD risk factors (dyslipidemia, diabetes, hypertension, smoking), and a calculated 10-year CVD event risk of 10% or greater
  - o Low- to moderate-dose statin when *all* criteria mentioned above are met

Not recommended

- Asymptomatic carotid artery stenosis screening
- Vitamin D supplementation to prevent falls in the community-dwelling adult 65 years or older

COMPREHENSION QUESTIONS

A 64-year-old woman presents to the clinic for her routine annual exam. She has prediabetes (on metformin) and hypertension (on lisinopril). She underwent a total hysterectomy 5 years ago for abnormal uterine bleeding. She has a history of cigarette smoking, but she quit at the age of 52. She had a negative stool DNA test 2 years ago. Her mammogram was negative 2 years ago. She feels well and does not have any acute concerns.

Which of the following statements are true for this patient?

A. She is due for a mammogram and stool DNA test.
B. She is due for a low-dose lung CT and a mammogram.
C. She is due for a stool DNA test and a pap smear.
D. She is due for a mammogram and a pap smear.

Answer: B

The patient is due for her biennial mammogram for breast cancer screening. She will also need to continue her annual low-dose lung CT for lung cancer screening because it has been only 12 years since she quit smoking. Screening can be discontinued after she has quit smoking for 15 years or more.

She will be due for her repeat stool DNA test next year, 3 years from her last test. She no longer needs to get a pap smear for cervical cancer screening even though she is less than 65 years old because she had a hysterectomy for a benign condition.

SUGGESTED READINGS

Qaseem A, Crandall CJ, Mustafa RA, et al; Clinical Guidelines Committee of the American College of Physicians. Screening for Colorectal Cancer in Asymptomatic Average-Risk Adults: A Guidance Statement From the American College of Physicians. *Ann Intern Med.* 2019;171:643–654.

Qaseem A, Lin JS, Mustafa RA, et al; Clinical Guidelines Committee of the American College of Physicians. Screening for Breast Cancer in Average-Risk Women: A Guidance Statement From the American College of Physicians. *Ann Intern Med.* 2019;170:547–560.

U.S. Preventive Services Task Force. Screening for Breast Cancer: U.S. Preventive Services Task Force Recommendation Statement. *Ann Intern Med.* 2009;151:716–726.

U.S. Preventive Services Task Force. www.uspreventiveservicestaskforce.org/uspstf/

A Review of Chronic Kidney Disease

Bemi (Oritsegbubemi) Adekola, MD

1. A 55-year-old Woman With 10-year History of Type 2 Diabetes

This patient was first noted to have proteinuria 4 years earlier; her serum creatinine level then was 1.1 mg/dL. Her urinary protein has progressively increased to 3.1 g/24 h, and her serum creatinine level to 2.1 mg/dL. The estimated glomerular filtration rate (GFR) is 42 mL/min/1.73 m² of body-surface area. Her blood pressure is 150/90 mm Hg, and the glycated hemoglobin level is 8.1 mg/dL. She has 2+ lower extremity edema bilaterally and increasing weight. The medications she is currently taking include glipizide, a calcium channel blocker, a statin, and a thiazide diuretic.

What is the target BP in this patient?

    A. 140/90 mm Hg
    B. 160/80 mm Hg
    C. <130/80 mm Hg
    D. >130/80 mm Hg
    E. 135/85 mm Hg

Is the patient's medication regimen appropriate considering the edema, proteinuria, and eGFR? What additional medications can be added?

    A. Hydralazine, furosemide, insulin for better glycemic control
    B. Olmesartan, furosemide, discontinue thiazide diuretic, low-dose SGLT-2 inhibitor
    C. Spironolactone, discontinue thiazide diuretic, low-dose SGLT-2 inhibitor
    D. Olmesartan, furosemide, discontinue thiazide diuretic, GLP-1 agonist

After 3 months, the patient reports to clinic for follow-up and is noted to have improved home blood pressure to 130/80 mm Hg. Lab work shows eGFR 39 mL/min and potassium 4.6 meq/L. Urine protein creatinine ratio improved to 1.5. Peripheral edema also improved. What additional intervention for proteinuria can be added to her management?

A. Increase GLP1 agonist dose, add nonsteroidal mineralocorticoid receptor antagonist
B. Discontinue SGLT-2 inhibitor
C. Add GLP-1 agonist
D. Add nonsteroidal mineralocorticoid receptor antagonist
E. Reassure patient about slight drop in eGFR
F. Reassure patient that proteinuria is improved and no further intervention is needed

The patient asks why the proteinuria is a bad finding. What is the answer?

A. Proteinuria is bad because it causes edema
B. Proteinuria is bad because it causes frothy urine
C. Proteinuria is bad because it causes progression of CKD
D. Proteinuria is bad because it causes more UTI

Your patient has just been informed that he has chronic kidney disease (CKD). His urine microalbumin creatinine ratio is 29 mg/g. He is worried and wants more information. Please see the definition and use the heat map below to determine the staging and risk category for this patient.

Definition

CKD is defined as abnormalities of kidney structure or function, present for greater than 3 months, with implications for health.

Classification

The heat map below classifies and presents prognoses related to different categories of CKD.

Epidemiology of CKD

CKD by Numbers, per the Centers for Disease Control and Prevention:

- Kidney diseases are a leading cause of death in the United States.
- About 37 million US adults are estimated to have CKD, and most are undiagnosed.

Prognosis of CKD by GFR and albuminuria category

Prognosis of CKD by GFR and Albuminuria Categories: KDIGO 2012			Persistent albuminuria categories Description and range		
			A1	A2	A3
			Normal to mildly increased	Moderately increased	Severely increased
			<30 mg/g <3 mg/mmol	30-300 mg/g 3-30 mg/mmol	>300 mg/g >30 mg/mmol
GFR categories (ml/min/1.73 m²) Description and range	G1	Normal to high ≥90			
	G2	Mildly decreased 60-89			
	G3a	Mildly to moderately decreased 45-59			
	G3b	Moderately to severely decreased 30-44			
	G4	Severely decreased 15-29			
	G5	Kidney failure <15			

Green: low risk (if no other markers of kidney disease, no CKD); Light green: moderately increassed risk; Gray: high risk; Black: very high risk.

Reproduced with permission from KDIGO 2012 Clinical Practice Guideline for the Evaluation and Management of Chronic Kidney Disease. Kidney Int.2013;3(1):3-5.

- Some 40% of persons with severely reduced kidney function (not on dialysis) are not aware of having CKD.
- In the United States, diabetes and high blood pressure are the leading causes of kidney failure, accounting for 3 out of 4 new cases.
- In 2019, Medicare beneficiaries with CKD cost $87.2 billion, and treating patients with ESRD cost an additional $37.3 billion.
- Other causes of kidney disease include glomerulonephritis, chronic interstitial nephritis or obstruction, cystic kidney diseases/hereditary diseases, secondary glomerulonephritis, plasma cell dysplasia/neoplasms, and miscellaneous or unrecorded causes.

Review of Pathophysiology in Chronic Kidney disease

- Loss of greater than 50% renal mass results in the following:
  1. Hemodynamic adaptation, glomerular hypertension, and single nephron hyperfiltration—activating RAAS and worsening systemic hypertension

2. Systemic hypertension, which worsens proteinuria and also triggers RAAS

3. Hyperlipidemia

4. Activation of the renin-angiotensin-aldosterone system and proteinuria

- The above 4 processes result in increased inflammation and oxidative stress with upregulation of inflammatory markers like TGF-beta, VEGF, and IGF-1, and a decrease in NO.

- Increased inflammatory markers and oxidative stress result in changes in the various renal compartments as follows:

  o Glomerular: mesangial cell and podocyte hypertrophy, increased apoptosis, matrix elaboration. Endothelial cells decrease NO production, and activation of adhesion molecules increases.

  o Tubular epithelial cells: matrix elaboration, cytokine and chemokine production, change to mesenchymal cell characteristics, apoptosis.

  o Interstitial cells: proliferation, activation of myofibroblasts leading to increase in matrix elaboration.

  o Vascular cells: decreased NO production, activation of adhesion molecules, matrix elaboration, proliferation of adventitial cells.

- These changes in the 4 renal compartments result in glomerulosclerosis **and interstitial fibrosis**.

It is important to review the above pathophysiology of CKD because the interventions are aimed at slowing each of those initial processes (1–4 above), which in turn will mitigate inflammation and oxidative stress and the other downstream changes in the renal compartments.

Interventions Targeted at Slowing Progression of CKD
Control of Hypertension

1. Control of systemic hypertension slows the rate of progression of CKD. Based on current recommendation, blood pressure should be lowered to less than 130/80 mm Hg in all patients with chronic kidney disease. An early, rapid decline in the GFR may occur if the target blood pressure is achieved abruptly, and in such cases, renal function should be monitored closely until it stabilizes.

2. Angiotensin receptor blockers (ARBs) and angiotensin-converting enzyme (ACE) inhibitors are considered to be the first line of antihypertensive therapy for all patients with CKD, including those with advanced CKD.

3. However, it should be recognized that most randomized trials in which ACE inhibitors or ARBs were used involved relatively young adults who

had well-defined causes of CKD, and the applicability of the findings of those trials to adults older than 70 years of age who have chronic kidney disease is uncertain.

4. A high salt intake blunts the effect of antihypertensive medications and the antiproteinuric effects of ACE inhibitors and ARBs. Thus <2.4 g sodium per day is recommended.

Reduction of Proteinuria

Albuminuria as a marker of kidney damage (increased glomerular permeability), urinary albumin excretion rate (AER) >30 mg/24 h, approximately equivalent to urine ACR >30 mg/g (>3 mg/mmol). However, the urine albumin creatinine ratio (ACR) is more commonly used.

The normal urine ACR in young adults is <10 mg/g (<1 mg/mmol).

Urine ACR 30–300 mg/g (3–30 mg/mmol; category A2) generally corresponds to "microalbuminuria," now referred to as "moderately increased albuminuria."

Urine ACR greater than 300 mg/g (30 mg/mmol; category A3) generally corresponds to "macroalbuminuria," now termed "severely increased." Subsequent proteinuria monitoring should use the urine protein creatinine ratio.

Urine ACR greater than 2200 mg/g (220 mg/mmol) may be accompanied by signs and symptoms of nephrotic syndrome (eg, low serum albumin, edema, and high serum cholesterol).

High urine ACR can be confirmed by urine albumin excretion in a timed urine collection expressed as AER.

Randomized trials in which ARBs were administered in patients with hypertension and type 2 diabetes, proteinuria, and CKD (including those with advanced CKD) showed that there was a significant reduction in the risk of the progression of CKD with decrease in proteinuria (risk reduction of 15% to 37%), cardiovascular events, and death.

A reduction in urinary protein excretion to less than 300 to 500 mg per day is associated with a slowing of the progression of CKD.

Protein intake: Kidney Disease—Improving Global Outcomes (KDIGO) suggests lowering protein intake to 0.8 g/kg/day in adults with diabetes (2C) or without diabetes (2B) and nondiabetics with GFR <30 ml/min/1.73 m2 (GFR categories G4–G5), with appropriate education.

Glycemic Control

Poorly controlled blood glucose levels are associated with an increased risk of nephropathy and cardiovascular complications.

Randomized trials suggest that strict control of blood glucose may prevent the development of diabetic nephropathy and retard the progression from microalbuminuria to proteinuria. No randomized trials have assessed the effect of glycemic control on disease progression in patients with advanced CKD.

Recent studies have shown certain medications (SGLT-2 inhibitors and GLP-1 agonists) designed to treat diabetes also confer renoprotection through a mechanism that differs from those affecting glucose homeostasis.

SGLT-2 Inhibitors

SGLT2 inhibitors in several well-designed clinical trials including CREDENCE were seen to decrease the relative risk of deleterious cardiovascular outcomes by 20% to 30%. The slope in decline in GFR was less than that of placebo. HbA1c, body weight, and blood pressure also decreased. The trial halted earlier after a median time of 2.62 years as the primary outcome was met.

Mechanism: SGLT2 inhibition increases glucose and sodium delivery to the distal renal tubule, which is sensed by the juxtaglomerular apparatus as increased glomerular perfusion. This leads to increased vasoconstriction of the afferent arteriole, which decreases glomerular perfusion and intraglomerular pressure. Although these effects decrease the estimated GFR in the short term, the level of angiotensin II in the circulation decreases, as does the level of atrial natriuretic peptide, with a subsequent decrease in inflammation and an increase in intrarenal oxygenation. Decreased body weight and sympathetic output, decreased uric acid, and perhaps an increase in glucagon also may contribute to the favorable renal profile.

KDIGO recommendation: We recommend treating patients with type 2 diabetes, CKD, and an eGFR ≥ 20 mL/min/1.73 m^2 with an SGLT2 inhibitor (1A class recommendation).

Nonsteroidal Mineralocorticoid Receptor Antagonist

In the FIDELIO-DKD and FIGARO-DKD clinical trials, during a median follow-up of 2.6 years, a primary outcome event occurred in 17.8% of the finerenone group and 21.1% of the placebo group (hazard ratio [HR], 0.82; 95% confidence interval [CI], 0.73–0.93; $P = 0.001$). A key secondary outcome event occurred in 13.0% of the treatment group and 14.8% of the placebo group (HR, 0.86; 95% CI, 0.75–0.99; $P = 0.03$). Overall, the frequency of adverse events was similar in the 2 groups. The incidence of hyperkalemia-related discontinuation of the trial regimen was higher with finerenone than with placebo (2.3% and 0.9%, respectively).

The primary composite outcome was a sustained decrease of at least 40% in eGFR from baseline, or death from renal causes. The key secondary composite outcome was death from cardiovascular causes, nonfatal myocardial infarction, nonfatal stroke, or hospitalization for heart failure.

KDIGO recommendation: We suggest a nonsteroidal mineralocorticoid receptor antagonist with proven kidney or cardiovascular benefit for patients with type 2 diabetes, eGFR 25 mL/min/1.73 m^2, normal serum potassium concentration, and albuminuria ($\geq$30 mg/g [3 mg/mmol]) despite maximum tolerated dose of RAS inhibitor (2A class recommendation).

Further studies of nonsteroidal mineralocorticoid receptor antagonists in nondiabetic CKD patients are underway.

Cardiovascular Disease Management

Given the high risk of cardiovascular disease in patients with CKD, attention should be paid to preventing and treating traditional cardiovascular risk factors in these patients.

Mitigating these risk factors may include the following: smoking cessation, dietary sodium intake <2 g/d, maintaining healthy BMI, exercise if feasible, hypertension control, glycemic control, proteinuria control, and treatment of dyslipidemia especially in the early stages of CKD (stages 1–3A). Fibrates used in treatment of CKD need to be dose adjusted, hyperuricemia. SGLT-2 inhibitors, GLP-1 agonists, and addition of nonsteroidal mineralocorticoid receptor blockers also decrease cardiovascular risk.

2. A Patient With CKD 4 and eGFR 19 mL/min

You are the resident on renal rotation, and this patient is admitted for UTI. There has been a gradual drop in hemoglobin to 7.1 g/dL from ~9g/dL in the last 4 months. The patient has not initiated care with a nephrologist. The corrected calcium is noted to be 8.2 mg/dL and phosphorus is noted to be 5.9 mg/dL.

What are the next steps?
- A. Arrange for urgent blood transfusion, give IV calcium gluconate, advise low-phosphorus diet, 25 vitamin D level pending
- B. Start erythropoietin-stimulating agent, start oral calcium supplement
- C. Order iron panel, order PTH, start active vitamin D, no need for erythropoietin-stimulating agent, advise low-phosphorus diet
- D. Order iron panel, start erythropoietin-stimulating agent, start active vitamin D, advise low-phosphorus diet

Bone and Mineral disorders in CKD

Disorders of mineral and bone metabolism are common in patients with stage IV CKD and may be associated with increased cardiovascular calcification, potentially contributing to an increased risk of complications and death.

CKD is characterized by decreased renal phosphate excretion, with resultant increases in serum phosphate levels. Furthermore, there is decreased conversion of vitamin D to its active form, 1,25-dihydroxyvitamin D (1,25(OH)D3), resulting in decreased levels of circulating 1,25(OH)D3 and serum calcium and decreased intestinal calcium absorption and secretion of parathyroid hormone. High phosphate levels may also increase production by osteocytes of the phosphaturic hormone fibroblast growth factor 23 (FGF-23). FGF-23 inhibits the synthesis of 1,25(OH)D3 and contributes to high levels of parathyroid hormone.

The hyperphosphatemia, hypocalcemia, and decreased levels of active vitamin D are all triggers for synthesis and secretion of PTH.

Hyperparathyroidism is present in more than half of patients who have a GFR of <60 mL/min/1.73 m^2 and is independently associated with increased mortality and an increased prevalence of cardiovascular disease.

Patients with persistently elevated parathyroid hormone levels (secondary hyperparathyroidism) should restrict their intake of dietary phosphate and be treated, in most cases, with a phosphate binder and an active vitamin D analogue if they have normal calcium levels.

Serum levels of 25-hydroxyvitamin D are also decreased in many patients with stage IV CKD and end-stage renal disease, and supplementation is recommended if levels fall below 30 ng/mL.

Electrolyte and Acid–base Abnormality

The kidney is generally able to compensate for a loss of functioning nephrons and maintain euvolemia, electrolyte balance, and acid–base balance until the GFR falls below 30 mL/min/1.73 m^2. When the GFR is below that level, there is impairment in both sodium excretion in response to a sodium load and sodium conservation in response to an acute reduction in sodium intake.

A concomitant impairment in the physiologic processes that allow for maximal concentration or dilution of the urine confers a predisposition to hyponatremia or hypernatremia in these patients.

Most patients with CKD have a nearly normal potassium level, except those with diabetes mellitus or hypoaldosteronism. However, hyperkalemia may result in those treated with ARBs or ACE inhibitors. The current approach, if tolerated, is to continue therapy with the RAAS blocker and potassium-rich diet and initiate potassium-binding medications such as patiromer and sodium zirconium cyclosilicate.

Non–anion gap metabolic acidosis can develop in patients with CKD, owing primarily to reduction in renal ammonia genesis. In addition, in those with advanced kidney disease, there is a decrease in titratable acid (phosphoric acid) excretion.

Anion gap metabolic acidosis occurs in those with advanced CKD approaching end stage due to accumulation of organic acids.

There is evidence that oral sodium bicarbonate supplementation slows the progression of CKD and improves nutritional status. The goal is to keep the bicarbonate level above 22 mEq/L.

Chronic metabolic acidosis also results in demineralization of bone and osteoporosis.

Anemia

Anemia is common in patients with CKD, especially in those with diabetes and those with stage IV disease, more than half of whom have anemia. Deficient erythropoietin synthesis, iron deficiency, blood loss, and a decreased erythrocyte half-life are the major causes of anemia associated with CKD. The use of erythro-poiesis-stimulating agents (ESAs) results in a reduced need for blood transfusions among patients with advanced CKD and is also associated with a reduction in left ventricular hypertrophy. There should be concurrent treatment of iron deficiency and other deficiencies like B_{12} and folate. There is new class of medications for the treatment of anemia in CKD—namely, hypoxia-inducible factor prolyl hydroxy-lase inhibitors. They work by stimulating production of endogenous erythropoi-etin. They are noted to induce lower but more consistent blood erythropoietin levels than ESAs with fewer cardiovascular side effects.

Conclusion

Refer to specialist kidney care services for patients in whom CKD is suspected:

- Abrupt sustained fall in GFR, unexplained acute kidney injury
- A consistent finding of significant albuminuria (ACR >300 mg/g [>30 mg/ mmol] or AER >300 mg/24 h, approximately equivalent to UPCR >500 mg/g [>50 mg/mmol] or PER >500 mg/24 h)
- Progression of CKD from stage 2 to 3A or sharp drop in GFR
- CKD and hypertension refractory to treatment with 4 or more antihyper-tensive agents
- Persistent abnormalities of serum potassium
- Recurrent or extensive nephrolithiasis
- Hereditary kidney disease

At eGFR 20 mL/min or less, discussions are held with patients about prognosis of their CKD diagnosis and choice for renal replacement therapy. (Renal transplan-tation is superior to dialysis.)

If hemodialysis is the identified suitable modality suitable, patients are referred for vascular access placement at eGFR 20 mL/min with a goal to start dialysis with a mature arteriovenous fistula rather than a dialysis catheter.

The home modalities—namely, peritoneal dialysis and home hemodialysis—confer benefits including improved nutrition and improved phosphorus control and improved LVH and volume control.

Table 33-X. Nonpharmacologic Interventions

Distraction	Humor
Massage therapy	Music
Therapeutic touch	Chiropractic manipulation
Pet therapy	Cognitive and behavioral therapies
Local heat or cold	Acupuncture
Education about illness	Transepidermal nerve stimulator unit
Hypnosis	Guided imagery
Biofeedback	Specialized mattress and turning every 2 hours for pressure ulcers

Source: Reproduced with permission from Periyakoil VS, Denney-Koelsch EM, White P, et al. *Primer of Palliative Care.* 7th ed. Chicago: American Association of Hospice and Palliative Medicine; 2019, Table 2.5:53.

Table 33-X. Adjuvant (Opioid-sparing) Pharmacologic Interventions by Pain Type

Drug Class	Notes	Examples
Somatic pain: aching, throbbing, stabbing; examples include bone metastases, wounds, soft tissue tumors, arthritis		
NSAIDs	Limited by GI, renal, and cardiac effects. Increased bleeding risks. Avoid in older adults, advanced renal disease, advanced cirrhosis, heart failure.	Naproxen 500 mg every 12 hours

Ibuprofen 600 mg every 6 hours |
| Acetaminophen | Excessive dosing leads to hepatotoxicity. Maximum daily dose in cirrhosis is 2000 mg per day. | Acetaminophen 650 mg every 6 hours |
| Bisphosphonates | For fracture prevention with osteolytic bone lesions and for patients on long-term steroids. Effective to relieve pain from bone metastases.

Side effects include nausea, fever, renal dysfunction, hypocalcemia, osteonecrosis of the jaw. | Pamidronate, zoledronic acid, etc. |

(Continued)

Drug Class	Notes	Examples
Corticosteroids	Consider time-limited trial. Short-term adverse effects include hyperglycemia, thrush, dyspepsia, insomnia, delirium, anxiety, elevated blood pressure, immunosuppression. Long-term side effects include secondary adrenal insufficiency, proximal myopathy, osteoporosis, osteonecrosis.	Dexamethasone 1–4 mg 2–3 times daily, maximum 16 mg/day. Prednisone 20–30 mg PO 2–3 times daily. Taper rapidly to lowest effective dose. Avoid nighttime dosing if possible.
Neuropathic pain: burning, tingling, shooting, painful numbness; examples include postherpetic neuralgia, diabetic neuropathy, compression radiculopathy		
Anticonvulsants	Side effects include sedation, dizziness, ataxia, peripheral edema. Adjust dosing for renal impairment.	

Source: Reproduced with permission from Periyakoil VS, Denney-Koelsch EM, White P, et al. *Primer of Palliative Care*. 7th ed. Chicago: American Association of Hospice and Palliative Medicine; 2019; Table 2.3:46–48.

Answers to Clinical Vignettes

Vignette 1:

I. C

II. B

III. C

IV. C

Vignette 2: Answer in discussion

Vignette 3: D

SUGGESTED READINGS

Barnett AH, Bain SC, Bouter P, et al. Angiotensin-receptor blockade versus converting–enzyme inhibition in type 2 diabetes and nephropathy. *N Engl J Med.* 2004;351:1952–1961.

Brenner BM, Cooper ME, de Zeeuw D, et al. Effects of losartan on renal and cardiovascular outcomes in patients with type 2 diabetes and nephropathy. *N Engl J Med.* 2001;345:861–869.

Coresh J, Selvin E, Stevens LA. Prevalence of chronic kidney disease in the United States. *JAMA.* 2007;298:2038–2047.

Credence Perkovic V, Jardine MJ, Neal B, et al. Canagliflozin and renal outcomes in type 2 diabetes and nephropathy. *N Engl J Med.* 2019;380:2295–2306.

de Brito-Ashurst I, Varagunam M, Raftery MJ, Yaqoob MM. Bicarbonate supplementation slows progression of CKD and improves nutritional status. *J Am Soc Nephrol.* 2009;20:2075–2084.

El-Achkar TM, Ohmit SE, McCullough PA, et al. Higher prevalence of anemia with diabetes mellitus in moderate kidney insufficiency: the Kidney Early Evaluation Program. *Kidney Int.* 2005;67:1483–1488.

Esnault VLM, Ekhlas AMR, Delcroix C, et al. Diuretic and enhanced sodium restriction results in improved antiproteinuric response to RAS blocking agents. *J Am Soc Nephrol.* 2005;16:474–481.

Go AS, Chertow GM, Fan D, et al. Chronic kidney disease and the risks of death, cardiovascular events, and hospitalization. *N Engl J Med.* 2004;351:1296–1305.

Hou FF, Zhang X, Zhang GH, et al. Efficacy and safety of benazepril for advanced chronic renal insufficiency. *N Engl J Med.* 2006;354(2):131–140.

Jafar TH, Stark PC, Schmid CH, et al. Progression of chronic kidney disease: the role of blood pressure control, proteinuria, and angiotensin-converting enzyme inhibition: a patient-level meta-analysis. *Ann Intern Med.* 2003;139:244–252.

KDOQI. KDOQI clinical practice guideline and clinical practice recommendations for anemia in chronic kidney disease: 2007 update of hemoglobin target. *Am J Kidney Dis.* 2007;50:471–530.

KDOQI. KDOQI clinical practice guideline and clinical practice recommendations for diabetes and chronic kidney disease. *Am J Kidney Dis.* 2007;49(Suppl 2):S12–S154.

Keith DS, Nichols GA, Gullion CM, et al. Longitudinal follow-up and outcomes among a population with chronic kidney disease in a large managed care organization. *Arch Intern Med.* 2004;164:659–663.

Kestenbaum B, Sampson JN, Rudser KD, et al. Serum phosphate levels and mortality risk among people with chronic kidney disease. *J Am Soc Nephrol.* 2005;16:520–588.

Kidney Disease: Improving Global Outcomes (KDIGO) CKD-MBD Work Group. KDIGO clinical practice guideline for diagnosis, evaluation, prevention, and treatment of chronic kidney disease-mineral and bone disorder (CKD-MBD). *Kidney Int Suppl.* 2009;113:S1–130.

Kidney Disease: Improving Global Outcomes (KDIGO) Diabetes Work Group. KDIGO 2022 clinical practice guideline for diabetes management in chronic kidney disease. *Kidney Int.* 2022;102(5S):S1–S127.

Kosiborod M, Cavender MA, Fu AZ, et al. Lower risk of heart failure and death in patients initiated on sodium-glucose cotransporter-2 inhibitors versus other glucose-lowering drugs: the CVD-REAL study (comparative effectiveness of cardiovascular outcomes in new users of sodium-glucose cotransporter-2 inhibitors). *Circulation.* 2017;136:249–259.

Lewis EJ, Hunsicker LG, Bain RP, Rohde RD. The effect of angiotensin-converting-enzyme inhibition on diabetic nephropathy. *N Engl J Med.* 1993;329:1456–1462.

Lewis EJ, Hunsicker LG, Clarke WR, et al. Renoprotective effect of the angiotensin-receptor antagonist irbesartan in patients with nephropathy due to type 2 diabetes. *N Engl J Med.* 2001;345:851–860.

Locatelli F, Fishbane S, Block GA, Macdougall IC. Targeting hypoxia-inducible factors for the treatment of anemia in chronic kidney disease patients. *Am J Nephrol.* 2017;45(3):187–199.

National Kidney Foundation. End stage renal disease in the United States, 2019.

O'Hare AM, Kaufman JS, Covinsky KE, et al. Current guidelines for using angiotensin-converting enzyme inhibitors and angiotensin II-receptor antagonists in chronic kidney disease: is the evidence base relevant to older adults? *Ann Intern Med.* 2009;150:717–724.

Ruggenenti P, Cravedi P, Remuzzi G. Proteinuria: increased angiotensin-receptor blocking is not the first option. *Nat Rev Nephrol.* 2009;5:367–368.

UK Prospective Diabetes Study (UKPDS) Group. Intensive blood-glucose control with sulphonylureas or insulin compared with conventional treatment and risk of complications in patients with type 2 diabetes (UKPDS 33). *Lancet.* 1998;352:837–853.

Umanath K, Lewis JB. Update on diabetic nephropathy: core curriculum 2018. *Am J Kidney Dis.* 2018;71:884–895.

Whelton PK, Carey RM, Aronow WS. 2017 ACC/AHA/AAPA/ABC/ACPM/AGS/APhA/ASH/ASPC/ NMA/PCNA Guideline for the Prevention, Detection, Evaluation, and Management of High Blood Pressure in Adults: Executive Summary: A Report of the American College of Cardiology/American Heart Association Task Force on Clinical Practice Guidelines. *Hypertension.* 2017;71:1269–1324.

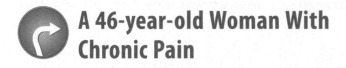

A 46-year-old Woman With Chronic Pain

Jacob Varney, MD and Stacy Sattovia, MD, MBA

Ms. Q is a 46-year-old female with a past medical history significant for depression, gastroesophageal reflux, and a motor vehicle accident 7 years ago. Over the last 3 years she has developed worsening low back pain that she feels is limiting her ability to carry out her activities of daily living. She works as a heavy equipment operator at a local factory. She denies fevers, chills, weight loss, and bladder or bowel habit changes. She denies radicular pain, numbness, and weakness in her legs. Her vital signs include a blood pressure of 128/65, heart rate of 72 bpm, respiratory rate of 16/min, and temperature of 37.2°C. She is seeing you for the first time for pain control and is requesting opioid medication.

1. What is your differential diagnosis?

2. What are the key elements of the history and physical examination?

3. What diagnostic evaluation should be done for this patient?

4. What are the best treatment strategies for her pain?

Answers

Summary: This is a 46-year-old female with a history of depression, motor vehicle accident, and an occupation that involves heavy machine operation presenting with nonspecific low back pain that appears to be chronic in nature.

1. Subacute on chronic mechanical axial low back pain is the most likely diagnosis. Within this category, specific causative pathologies could include lumbar facet arthropathy, discogenic pain / annular fissure, sacroiliitis, and myofascial pain. Separate from this category and less likely considerations include neoplasm, infection, and fracture.

2. Obtaining information to rule out neoplasm, infection, and fracture is key. A history of bacteremia or other disseminated infection as well as immunosuppression may heighten your suspicion for infection. Inquiring about fevers and chills is thus important. A history of IV drug use raises concern for diskitis. A history of incarceration or prior tuberculosis may suggest tuberculosis of the spine (Pott's disease). In addition, a history of unexplained weight loss or known malignancy may increase your concern for a neoplasm or complication of a malignancy. Pain at rest, especially at night, suggests possible infection or malignancy as well. A recent history of trauma as well as risk factors for osteoporosis would increase your concern for fracture.

   Physical examination should focus on location of tenderness on examination—percuss over each spinous process. True tenderness over the spine itself raises concern for neoplasm, infection, or fracture. Muscle tenderness is most likely seen in nonspecific back pain as well as fibromyalgia, myositis, and chronic muscle strain. A straight leg raise, performed with the patient supine, with the knee in full extension is considered positive for nerve root compression if contralateral radiation of pain is elicited.

3. Numerous guidelines provide recommendations about diagnostic evaluation. The focus is primarily on identification of patients who are at high risk for pathology such as tumor, infection, and fracture. None of the guidelines advocate routine use of imaging, especially at the initial evaluation. Imaging is recommended primarily for those patients who exhibit red flags, such as fever, weight loss, pain waking a patient from sleep, or bowel or bladder incontinence. If red flags do exist, a plain film can be diagnostic of fracture, but for evaluation of infection and malignancy, MRI is typically recommended.

4. Because there are no red flags present on this patient's history or physical examination, she is most likely experiencing chronic, nonspecific back pain. Back pain is a common reason for seeking primary care services and a leading chronic pain condition in the United States. The approach to chronic pain will thus be discussed in detail.

CHRONIC PAIN IN AN AMBULATORY SETTING

The World Health Organization estimates that 20% of the world's population has some type of chronic pain. Chronic pain is defined as "pain lasting longer than 3 months or beyond the expected period of healing of tissue pathology." Characteristically, the nature and severity of the pain is not necessarily correlated with the degree of tissue injury. Specifically low back pain accounts for a majority of musculoskeletal and chronic pain visits to primary care.

Chronic pain typically affects all areas of a patient's life and can lead to significant loss of function, both physically and emotionally. In addition, there is a large burden to society due to this loss of function and productivity with studies indicating that the "total cost of chronic pain exceeds $210 billion annually in the United States."

Pathophysiology

Research done in osteoarthritis suggests that osteoarthritis is similar to other chronic pain states associated with "peripheral tissue injury and repair." As injury and remodeling occurs, "physiologic mechanisms of pain operate at the local joint level, the dorsal root ganglion level and higher brain processing centers." The release of inflammatory mediators leads to sensitization of the nociceptive system creating "heightened sensitivity to noxious stimuli [hyperalgesia] and to pain in response to non-noxious stimuli [allodynia]." This sensitization can occur at any of these 3 levels. The nervous system demonstrates plasticity, and in response to tissue injury and repair, it can (among other mechanisms) (1) upregulate or downregulate receptor expression, (2) alter neuronal firing thresholds, and (3) lead to "subsequent abnormal sensation of pain, unrelated to inflammation."

In addition, it is accepted that chronic pain is a complex interplay of "individuals' unique previous histories, any physiologic abnormalities, cognitive perceptions of nociception, emotional factors, coping styles, and social and financial resources." Concurrent anxiety or depression can impair a patient's ability to cope with their pain.

Approach to Chronic Pain Management

Chronic pain management requires a multimodal approach focusing on both pain and function. This may include physical, cognitive, pharmacologic, or interventional therapies. When indicated and available, physical and occupational therapy, cognitive behavioral therapy, exercise, weight loss, massage, yoga, pilates, mindfulness-based stress reduction, low-level laser therapy, acupuncture, and/or biofeedback should be implemented. All patients should receive education related to their disease process, treatment planning, and expected outcomes. The Pain, Enjoyment, and General Activity (PEG) scale (Figure 33-1) can be used to assess the effect of pain on a patient's function and also improvement after interventions are implemented. Realistic goals for improvement in pain and function should be discussed, such as a 30% improvement in PEG score from baseline. None of the most commonly prescribed treatments are, by themselves, sufficient to eliminate chronic pain. Physicians should evaluate patients for comorbidities such as uncontrolled anxiety or depression and provide appropriate management.

Pharmacologic Management

Pharmacologic therapy is tailored to the individual patient based on diagnosis and comorbidities. Whenever possible, treatments specific for the etiology and nature of pain should be implemented, such as tryptans for migraines and gabapentin for neuropathic pain. Prescribers must weigh the expected benefit versus risk for each treatment, keeping in mind patient-specific details such as past history, renal and hepatic function, age, and current medications.

Excluding cancer-related pain and palliative care settings such as end-of-life, opioid medications are not first-line treatment for chronic pain. In a systematic review, opioids did not differ from nonopioid medication in pain reduction, and nonopioid medications were better tolerated, with greater improvements in physical function.

The PEG (Pain, Enjoyment, General Activity) Scale, created by Dr. Charles Cleeland, is used to assess the impact of a person's pain on their quality of life. They respond to the following questions using a 10 point Likert scale (with 0 being no pain and 10 being pain as bad as one can imagine):

1) What number best describes your pain on average for the past week?
2) What number best describes how, during the past week, pain has interfered with your enjoyment of life?
3) What number best describes how, during the past week, pain has interfered with your general activity?

The PEG score is used to track a person's pain over time. If the treatment regimen is successful, then pain scores should decrease over time.

Figure 34-1. PEG scale assessing pain intensity and interference (Pain, Enjoyment, General Activity. (Reproduced with permission from Krebs EE, Lorenz KA, Bair MJ, et al. Development and initial validation of the PEG, a three-item scale assessing pain intensity and interference. J Gen Intern Med. 2009;24(6):733-8.)

Acetaminophen is an appropriate first-line analgesic for mild to moderate pain due to conditions such as osteoarthritis and low back pain, with attention to maximum daily dose limits to avoid hepatotoxicity. Nonsteroidal anti-inflammatory drugs (NSAIDs) also are considered first-line agents in osteoarthritis and low back pain and are thus highly recommended, with likely higher magnitude of benefit compared with acetaminophen. NSAIDs have several limiting side effects including NSAID gastropathy, major coronary events, and exacerbation of renal failure and congestive heart failure.

Antidepressant drugs including tricyclic antidepressants (TCAs) and selective serotonin norepinephrine reuptake inhibitors (SNRIs) such as duloxetine and milnacipran have been shown to be more effective than placebo, particularly in neuropathic pain but also in fibromyalgia, back pain, and headaches. Antidepressant agents, specifically TCAs, carry the risk of arrhythmias, hypertension, and postural hypotension—with concern for falls in elderly patients. SNRIs have a more preferable side-effect profile, but attention must be paid to doses and interactions with other medications that can increase serotonin levels and lead to increased risk for serotonin syndrome.

Anticonvulsant agents, specifically gabapentin, pregabalin, and oxcarbazepine, have good evidence for use in chronic neuropathic pain and fibromyalgia. Gabapentin and pregabalin inhibit peripheral nerve calcium channels, helping to abate excess peripheral nerve calcium influx in the setting of neuropathy. Anticonvulsant drugs can cause somnolence, confusion, weight gain, fatigue, blurred vision, dizziness, and peripheral edema, with higher risk of side effects with pregabalin compared to gabapentin and at higher doses. Skeletal muscle relaxants are frequently prescribed but with little evidence of effectiveness beyond adjuvant therapy with NSAIDs for acute pain relief. Somnolence is the prominent side effect of muscle relaxants. Topical agents include topical NSAIDs such as diclofenac for localized osteoarthritis, topical lidocaine for neuropathic pain, and topical capsaicin for musculoskeletal and neuropathic pain.

History of the Opioid Epidemic

Multiple factors led to increased opioid use for the treatment of acute and chronic pain in the 1990s and 2000s. With intent to improve pain evaluation and treatment, pain was labelled the "fifth vital sign" in 1995. National organizations published standards for pain management and reduced regulatory scrutiny. Consumption of opioids in the United States increased from ~47,000 kg in 2000 to ~165,000 in 2012. Patients taking opioids as prescribed experienced adverse effects, and opioid dependence became more common. Ultimately, opioid-related deaths increased sharply in 2016, with overdoses due to illegally manufactured fentanyl representing the greatest contribution to the increase, followed by heroin and then prescription medications. In 2017, the US government declared the opioid epidemic a public health emergency.

Review of Opioid Use Disorder

While patients and providers are often appropriately concerned about opioid addiction, it is important to distinguish opioid use disorder from expected changes related to opioid use as prescribed or other phenomenon. **Tolerance** is a physiologic adaptation in the context of continued exposure to a drug, resulting in reduced effectiveness of the medication. Physiologic **dependence** is a state of adaptation to a drug class, characterized by a withdrawal syndrome that can be provoked by abrupt cessation, rapid dose reduction, decreasing blood level of the drug, or administration of an antagonist. **Pseudoaddiction** is a controversial term, defined as an iatrogenic syndrome of behaviors due to inadequate pain management, with phases including (1) insufficient prescription of analgesics to manage the primary pain stimulus, (2) increasing demands by the patient for improved pain control, associated with behavioral changes to convince others of pain severity, and (3) mistrust between the treating team and the patient. **Substance use disorder** (formerly, "addiction") is a "treatable, chronic medical disease involving complex interactions among brain circuits, genetics, the environment, and an individual's life experiences" that is characterized by craving for the substance, loss of control of the amount or frequency of use, compulsion of use, and use despite consequences.

Opioid use disorder (OUD) diagnostic criteria are described below:

DSM-5-TR Diagnostic Criteria for OUD

A. A problematic pattern of opioid use leading to clinically significant impairment or distress, as manifested by at least two of the following, occurring within a 12-month period:

1. Opioids are often taken in larger amounts or over a longer period than was intended.

2. There is a persistent desire or unsuccessful efforts to cut down or control opioid use.

3. A great deal of time is spent in activities necessary to obtain the opioid, use the opioid, or recover from its effects.

4. Craving, or a strong desire or urge to use opioids.

5. Recurrent opioid use resulting in a failure to fulfill major role obligations at work, school, or home.

6. Continued opioid use despite having persistent or recurrent social or interpersonal problems caused or exacerbated by the effects of opioids.

7. Important social, occupational, or recreational activities are given up or reduced because of opioid use.

8. Recurrent opioid use in situations in which it is physically hazardous.

9. Continued opioid use despite knowledge of having a persistent or recurrent physical or psychological problem that is likely to have been caused or exacerbated by the substance.

10. Tolerance, as defined by either of the following:

    a. A need for markedly increased amounts of opioids to achieve intoxication or desired effect.

    b. A markedly diminished effect with continued use of the same amount of an opioid.

    Note: This criterion is not considered to be met for those taking opioids solely under appropriate medical supervision.

11. Withdrawal, as manifested by either of the following:

    a. The characteristic opioid withdrawal syndrome (refer to Criteria A and B of the criteria set for opioid withdrawal).

    b. Opioids (or a closely related substance) are taken to relieve or avoid withdrawal symptoms.

    Note: This criterion is not considered to be met for those taking opioids solely under appropriate medical supervision.

Specify if:

In early remission: After full criteria for opioid use disorder were previously met, none of the criteria for opioid use disorder have been met for at least 3 months but for less than 12 months (with the exception that Criterion A4, "Craving, or a strong desire or urge to use opioids," may be met).

In sustained remission: After full criteria for opioid use disorder were previously met, none of the criteria for opioid use disorder have been met at any time during a period of 12 months or longer (with the exception that Criterion A4, "Craving, or a strong desire or urge to use opioids," may be met).

Specify if:

On maintenance therapy: This additional specifier is used if the individual is taking a prescribed agonist medication such as methadone or buprenorphine and none of the criteria for opioid use disorder have been met for that class of medication (except tolerance to, or withdrawal from, the agonist). This category also applies to those individuals being maintained on a partial agonist, an agonist/antagonist, or a full antagonist such as oral naltrexone or depot naltrexone.

In a controlled environment: This additional specifier is used if the individual is in an environment where access to opioids is restricted.

Coding based on current severity/remission: If an opioid intoxication, opioid withdrawal, or another opioid-induced mental disorder is also present, do not use the codes below for opioid use disorder. Instead, the comorbid opioid use disorder is indicated in the 4th character of the opioid-induced disorder code (see the coding note for opioid intoxication, opioid withdrawal, or a specific opioid-induced mental disorder). For example, if there is comorbid opioid-induced depressive disorder and opioid use disorder, only the opioid-induced depressive disorder code is given, with the 4th character indicating whether the comorbid opioid use disorder is mild, moderate, or severe: F11.14 for mild opioid use disorder with opioid-induced depressive disorder or F11.24 for a moderate or severe opioid use disorder with opioid-induced depressive disorder.

Specify current severity/remission:

(F11.10) Mild: Presence of 2-3 symptoms.
(F11.11) Mild, In early remission
(F11.11) Mild, In sustained remission
(F11.20) Moderate: Presence of 4-5 symptoms.
(F11.21) Moderate, In early remission.
(F11.21) Moderate: In sustained remission
(F11.20) Severe: Presence of 6 or more symptoms.
(F11.21) Severe, In early remission.
(F11.21) Severe, In sustained remission.

Safer Opioid Prescribing

Regarding chronic noncancer pain, opioids are associated with small improvements in pain and function compared with placebo. There is increased risk of harms at short-term follow up. Evidence for long-term benefit is very limited. There is evidence for dose-dependent long-term risk of serious harms. Co-prescription of opioids with benzodiazepines and gabapentinoids might increase risk of overdose.

When considering the initiation or continuation of opioids for chronic pain, there are several steps to keep in mind.

- Check that non-opioid therapies have been attempted or optimized
- Assess baseline pain and function
- Discuss expected benefits and risks
- Evaluate for risk of harm or misuse

  o Assess for risk factors including sleep apnea, pregnancy, renal or hepatic insufficiency, age >65, mental health conditions, history of alcohol or substance use disorder, history of nonfatal overdose.

  o Check urine drug screen

  o Review prescription drug monitoring program (PDMP) data.

- Set criteria for stopping or continuing opioids.
- Schedule initial reassessment within 1-4 weeks
- For initiation, prescribe short-acting opioids at the lowest dose provide supply to match the scheduled reassessment.

At the return visit, continue opioids only after confirming clinically meaningful improvements in pain and function without significant risks of harm.

- Determine whether to continue, adjust, taper, or stop opioids, tapering, 10% of total daily morphine milligram equivalent per month is reasonable for chronic opioid use and mild adverse effects, sudden or abrupt tapering should be avoided.
- Assess pain and function, comparing results with baseline
- Evaluate for signs of over-sedation or overdose risk, if positive, taper opioids.
- Check PDMP
- Screen for opioid use disorder if indicated; start or refer for treatment if positive.
- Optimize non-opioid therapies
- Calculate opioid dosing morphine milligram equivalent (MME)

  o If >50 MME per day in total, consider offering naloxone and increase frequency of follow-up

- o Avoid >90 MME per day or carefully justify; consider specialist referral.

Side effects of opioids include nausea, constipation, dizziness, and somnolence. Among opioid side effects, only constipation persists at consistent doses. Notably, respiratory depression is always preceded by sedation. Constipation can be managed with medications to counteract slowed peristalsis, such as stimulant laxatives (senna). Rarely, patients maintained on very high-dose opioid therapy chronically can begin to experience opioid-induced hyperalgesia. This "occurs when patients taking opioids become hypersensitive to nociceptive stimuli … postulated to result from changes in the peripheral and central nervous system that lead to facilitation of nociceptive pathways." If providers are unaware of this phenomenon, they can continue to escalate doses in the setting of little relief and actually increase pain symptomatology. Management of opioid-induced hyperalgesia typically involves opioid taper, opioid rotation, and/or addition of a NMDA antagonist.

In addition to traditional opioids (morphine, hydrocodone, hydromorphone, etc), prescribers should be aware of unique properties of certain opioids. Tramadol's initial form inhibits the reuptake of serotonin and norepinephrine, similar to other SNRI's. It is hepatically metabolized by cytochrome P450 enzyme 2D6 to a metabolite with opioid agonism. Notably, each patient's CYP2D6 activity is genetically based and the range across a population varies considerably. Possible side effects of tramadol include seizures, serotonin syndrome, drug-drug interactions, and hypoglycemia. In a similar way, codeine is a prodrug, metabolized by the same CYP2D6 enzyme, into morphine.

Buprenorphine is a partial mu opioid agonist that has commonly been used to treat opioid use disorder. It has been shown to provide similar analgesic effect when compared with traditional full agonist opioids such as morphine, with a reduced risk for respiratory depression. Side effects such as nausea, vomiting, and constipation are much less common with buprenorphine compared with traditional full opioid agonists. It has been FDA approved for use in acute pain, chronic pain, opioid use disorder, and opioid dependence, although the approval varies based on the formulation of buprenorphine product. Clinicians should consider buprenorphine in lieu of traditional full opioids, especially for patients at high risk of adverse effects.

TIPS TO REMEMBER

- Chronic pain is difficult to manage, and therapy must be tailored to each individual patient and the underlying diagnosis.
- Currently available treatments provide modest improvements in pain and minimum improvements in physical and emotional functioning, so expectation setting is an important component of each treatment plan.
- Optimization of nonpharmacologic therapy and non-opioid therapy is essential. Nonpharmacologic and local, interventional therapies should be

Table 34-1.

Generic Name	Route of Administration Dosing	Brand Names	For the Treatment of	Formulation Considerations
Buprenorphine (monoprodact)	Sublingual Tablets Daily	Generic versions available similar to Subutex ±	Opioid withdrawal and opioid use disorder	Some risk for diversion or misuse; Requires daily compliance
Buprenorphine and Balosone	Sublingual tablets and film Daily	Generic versions available in addition to Suboxone, Cassipa, Zabsolv, Bunavail	Opioid withdrawal and opioid use disorder	Lower potential for misuse and diversion (compared to monoproduct); Requires daily compliance
Buprenorphine extended-release	Extended-release Iojection (Monthly)	Sublocade	Moderate to severe opioid use disorder in patients who have initiated treatment with transmacosal buprenorphine followed by dose adjustment for a minimum of 7 days	No risk for patient diversion or misuse, Requires patients to be on a stable dose of transmucosal buprenorphine for at least 7 days; Monthly instead of daily medication compliance; Less fluctuation in buprenorphine levels (compared to daily doses)

(Continued)

| Buprenorphine extended-release | Extended-release Injection (Weekly or Monthly) | Brixadi | Moderate to severe opioid use disorder in patients who have initiated treatment with a single dose of transmucosal buprenorphine or who are already being treated with buprenorphine | Tentative approval from FDA (not currently eligible for marketing in the U.S. became of exclusivity considerations). No risk for patient diversion or misuse; only a single prior dose of transmecosal buprenorphine required prior to initiation; Weekly or Monthly instead of daily medication compliance, Less fluctuation in buprenorphine levels (compared to daily doses) |
| Buprenorphine hydrochloride | Subcutaneous Implant (Every 6 months) | Probuphine Implant | Treatment of opioid use disorder in patients who have achieved and sustained prolonged clinical stability on low-to-moderate doses of a transmucosal buprenorphine (i.e., no more than 8 mg per day) | Requires prolonged stability on 8 mg per day or less transmucosal buprenorphine; No risk for patient diversion or misuse; Physician training required for implant insertion and removal; Insertion site should be examined one week after insertion; Implant must be removed after 6 months; Risks associated with improper insertion and removal; Currently only FDA approved (or a total treatment duration of one year fone insertion per arm); Less fluctuation in buprenorphine levels (compared to daily dones) |

*Some patients may experience withdrawal/cravings when switched to a differne firmulation.

± Subutes was discontinued.

Table content was derived from FDA labels. Labels and label updates can be accessed at https://www.accessdata.fda.gov/scripts/cder/def/index.cfm.

Reproduced with permission from Crotty K, Freedman KI, Kampman KM. Executive Summary of the Focused Update of the ASAM National Practice Guideline for the Treatment of Opioid Use Disorder J Addict Med 2020;14(2):99-112.

considered, as many systemic pharmacological treatments have unwanted side effects and complications.

● Opioid risks and benefits should be discussed, and if they are continued or initiated, short-term follow-up to identify improvements in function or side effects is prudent.

COMPREHENSION QUESTIONS

1. A 52-year-old man with a history of hypertension presents to your acute care clinic with a 3-day history of severe low back pain. He has been unable to perform his occupation as a mail carrier during these 3 days and is seeking relief of his symptoms. He is interested in opioid therapy as this "happens a few times every year" and he believes "pain pills" will help prevent his symptoms from recurring. He has no fever, chills, weakness, numbness, or change in bladder or bowel habits. On examination, he is an obese gentleman with no spinal tenderness, but significant bilateral muscle tenderness. In addition to nonpharmacologic therapies such as physical therapy, what is your first line of therapy?

    A. Oral opioid
    B. NSAID
    C. Muscle relaxant
    D. Intravenous opioid

2. A 35-year-old woman with a history of chronic abdominal pain is referred to your clinic from a local emergency department for continued opioid therapy and monitoring. She has not had a single primary care provider in adulthood. She is status postcholecystectomy and 2 exploratory laparotomies for severe abdominal pain with little change in her symptoms. On examination, she has vital signs within the normal range and diffuse tenderness to abdominal palpation. There is no rebound or guarding. What is the next best step?

    A. Refill opioid medications
    B. Obtain a thorough social history
    C. Abdominal CT scan
    D. Abdominal ultrasound

Answers

1. **B.** This 52-year-old gentleman most likely has acute, nonspecific low back pain, with intermittently recurrent symptoms. He has no elements on history or physical examination that would suggest infection, malignancy, or trauma. The best first line of therapy is NSAIDs. Patient education regarding the most effective treatment for low back pain and counseling about weight loss and exercise may benefit this patient as well.

2. **B.** This 35-year-old female illustrates the complexity of chronic pain. Obtaining further information about contributing social and personal factors may be helpful to determine the next best therapeutic plan for her. She may benefit from social services to help address social stressors or counseling and therapy for a contributing (and possibly undiagnosed) psychiatric condition. Her care will most likely require repeat, frequent visits to establish rapport and explore contributors to her chronic pain.

SUGGESTED READINGS

Ahrq.gov systematic reviews (Opioid treatments for chronic pain 2020; Systematic Review on Nonopioid Pharmacologic Treatments for Chronic Pain: Surveillance Report 3 Literature Update Period: January 2022 through April 1, 2022; Nonopioid Pharmacologic Treatments for Chronic Pain.

Cdc.gov/opioids

Crotty K, Freedman KI, Kampman KM. Executive Summary of the Focused Update of the ASAM National Practice Guideline for the Treatment of Opioid Use Disorder J Addict Med 2020;14(2):99-112.

Dalal S, Chitneni A, Berger AA, et al. Buprenorphine for Chronic Pain: A Safer Alternative to Traditional Opioids. Health Psychol Res. 2021;9(1):27241.

Dowell D, Haegerich TM, Chou R. CDC Guideline for Prescribing Opioids for Chronic Pain--United States, 2016. JAMA. 2016 Apr 19;315(15):1624-45.

Greene MS, Chambers RA. Pseudoaddiction: Fact or Fiction? An Investigation of the Medical Literature. Curr Addict Rep. 2015;2(4):310-317.

Hale M, Garofoli M, Raffa RB. Benefit-Risk Analysis of Buprenorphine for Pain Management. J Pain Res. 2021;14:1359-1369.

Jones MR, Viswanath O, Peck J, Kaye AD, Gill JS, Simopoulos TT. A Brief History of the Opioid Epidemic and Strategies for Pain Medicine. Pain Ther. 2018;7(1):13-21.

Krebs EE, Lorenz KA, Bair MJ, et al. Development and initial validation of the PEG, a three-item scale assessing pain intensity and interference. J Gen Intern Med. 2009;24(6):733-738.

LeBlond RF, Brown DD, DeGowin RL. *DeGowin's Diagnostic Evaluation*. 9th ed. New York: McGraw-Hill; 2009.

Lee M, Silverman S, Hansen H, Patel V, Manchikanti L. A comprehensive review of opioid-induced hyperalgesia. *Pain Physician*. 2011;14:145–161.

McPherson ML. *Demystifying Opioid Conversion Calculations*. 2nd ed. 2018.

Noble M, Treadwell JR, Tregear SJ, et al. Long-term opioid management for chronic non-cancer pain [review]. *Cochrane Database Syst Rev*. 2010;(1):CD006605.

Office of National Drug Control Policy. Epidemic: responding to America's prescription drug abuse crisis. 2011 prescription drug abuse prescription plan. www.whitehouse.gov/ondcp/prescription-drug-abuse.

Smith TJ, Hillner BE. The Cost of Pain. *JAMA Netw Open*. 2019;2(4):e191532.

Sofat N, Ejindu V, Kiely P. What makes osteoarthritis painful? The evidence for local and central pain processing. *Rheumatology*. 2011;50:2157–2165.

Turk DC, Wilson HD, Cahana A. Treatment of chronic non-cancer pain. *Lancet*. 2011;377:2226–2235.

Webster L, Gudin J, Raffa RB, et al, Understanding Buprenorphine for Use in Chronic Pain: Expert Opinion. *Pain Medicine*. 2020;21(4): 714–723.

Weissman DE, Haddox DJ. Opioid pseudoaddiction--an iatrogenic syndrome. Pain. 1989;36(3):363-366.

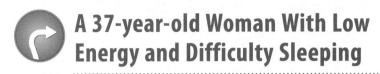

A 37-year-old Woman With Low Energy and Difficulty Sleeping

Dorcas Adaramola, MD, MPH and Tiffany I. Leung, MD, MPH

A 37-year-old woman presents to establish care with you in the office today. She complains of low energy levels and difficulty sleeping, especially in the last 4 weeks. She admits that she has had episodes of similar situations on and off in the past. She has gained 10 lb over the past 2 weeks. She reports a family history of alcoholism in her mother and her older brother, and completed suicide in her father. She thinks her mother was hospitalized for a suicide attempt many years ago, but she does not know any more details. When you ask about her social history, she hesitates in giving her answer, and then becomes tearful as she tells you with great difficulty that she was in a physically and sexually abusive marriage for 10 years. The marriage finally ended over 1 year ago, but the patient still expresses guilt about its end and says she feels worthless every day. She recalls that she always enjoyed watching her favorite TV shows but recently has been unable to focus on them and they simply do not seem enjoyable anymore. She admits that she has had suicidal thoughts on and off in the recent past but has none currently. She has never had a suicide attempt. She drinks 3 beers nightly. Her vital signs and complete physical examination are normal except for a low mood and tearful affect.

1. What is the most likely diagnosis?

2. What is the next appropriate step in evaluation?

3. What therapeutic options can you offer to this patient?

Answers

1. This patient presents with classic symptoms of major depressive disorder (MDD) and meets diagnostic criteria for MDD, according to the fifth edition of the *Diagnostic and Statistical Manual of Mental Disorders, Revised* (DSM-5). She has depressed mood, insomnia, loss of energy, feelings of worthlessness, weight gain, and recurrent suicidal ideation without a specific plan. These symptoms have been present for 4 weeks, which is longer than the 2-week period required to meet DSM-5 criteria for MDD. She has multiple risk factors for MDD, most notably a family history of mood disorders and stressful life events, including a difficult marriage and history as a victim of intimate partner violence. She also has unhealthy alcohol use that needs further evaluation and directed management.

2. The next appropriate step is to evaluate her depressive symptoms in an objective manner to guide diagnosis, evaluate severity, and establish a baseline of severity that can later be compared to assess the treatment response to pharmacologic and behavioral therapies. Multiple rating scales and scores exist to assist with quantifying the severity of depression symptoms and their level of functional impairment. Most residents are now able to access these through the use of applications on their phones.

3. Therapeutic options for an episode of major depression include a wide variety of pharmacologic and behavioral therapies. Among pharmacologic therapies, selective serotonin reuptake inhibitors (SSRIs) are considered first-line agents in the treatment of an episode of major depression. The choice of SSRI depends in part on the side effect profiles for each medication in this class, as common side effects for each medication can be targeted to some of the specific symptoms that the patient is experiencing. It is important to recognize that all SSRIs are not immediately effective and must be titrated to a dose that will have maximum therapeutic effect over several weeks. Close follow-up is important to ensure that patients are deriving maximum benefit possible from adequate doses of medication, and if ineffective, the medication may be switched to an alternative agent. Eight weeks on a prescribed pharmacologic therapy is considered an adequate trial of a SSRI medication. SSRIs as a class carry a black box warning of initially increasing suicidal ideations, particularly in ages 16 to 34, and also have the potential to interact with other medicines due to their effects on the cytochrome P450 systems of liver metabolism. Additional pharmacologic agents exist and are alternatives for treatment of MDD as well.

The most common and well known of behavioral therapies is cognitive behavioral therapy (CBT), which is a form of therapy where awareness of dysfunctional thoughts as sources of depressed mood and appropriate coping techniques for these thoughts are fostered. Typically, a combination of pharmacologic therapy and CBT is the most effective treatment for MDD. Practically, affordable mental health services for the most vulnerable patients can often be challenging to access, and maintaining a supportive role as patient advocate can be vital to maintaining a therapeutic physician–patient relationship.

CASE REVIEW

This case clearly describes a patient with symptoms of untreated depression and with multiple risk factors for depression, including a family history of mood disorders and a personal history of excessive alcohol use and intimate partner violence. She clearly meets diagnostic criteria for a major depressive episode as defined in DSM-5 (Table 35-1). Additionally, a family history of completed and attempted suicide increases the patient's risk of suicide, even if she has never had a suicide attempt prior to her visit. Of her risk factors, the most modifiable is to abstain or at least limit alcohol consumption. It is important to recognize that substance abuse is a common comorbid condition in patients with mental health disorders, and intoxication or withdrawal from recreational or illicit substances can exacerbate the symptoms of a mood disorder, especially depression. According to the DSM-5, depressive disorders are categorized into different types including disruptive mood dysregulation disorder, major depressive disorder, persistent depressive disorder (dysthymia), substance/medication-induced depressive disorder, depressive disorder due to another medical condition, and other specified depressive disorder. Exploring all these would be beyond the scope of this text, which will focus primarily on the management of major depressive disorder in a primary care setting.

Table 35-1. Criteria for Major Depressive Episode (*Diagnostic and Statistical Manual of Mental Disorders, Revised*)

Five or more of the following symptoms (1 of which is depressed mood or loss of interest or pleasure) have occurred together for a 2-week period and represent a change in previous functioning:

1. Depressed mood most of the day, nearly every day as self-reported or observed by others
2. Diminished self-interest or pleasure in all or almost all activities most of the day, nearly every day
3. Significant weight loss when not dieting, or weight gain; or decrease or increase in appetite nearly every day
4. Insomnia or hypersomnia nearly every day
5. Psychomotor agitation or retardation nearly every day
6. Fatigue or loss of energy nearly every day
7. Feelings of worthlessness or excessive or inappropriate guilt nearly every day
8. Diminished ability to concentrate or think every day
9. Recurrent thoughts of death, recurrent suicidal ideation without a specific plan

The symptoms cause clinically significant distress or impairment in social, occupational, or other areas of functioning

The symptoms are not due to the direct physiologic effects of a substance (drug or medication) or a general medical condition

The symptoms are not better accounted for by bereavement, or the symptoms persist for more than 2 months or are characterized by marked functional impairment, morbid preoccupation with worthlessness, suicidal ideation, psychotic symptoms, or psychomotor retardation

MAJOR DEPRESSIVE DISORDER

Diagnosis

Major depressive disorder is defined by the DSM-5 as consisting of the presence of 5 or more of the following symptoms present over a 2-week period and representing a change from previous functioning with at least 1 of the symptoms being either (1) depressed mood or (2) loss of interest or pleasure.

1. Depressed mood most of the day, nearly every day, as indicated by either subjective report (eg, feels sad, empty, hopeless) or observation made by others (eg, appears tearful).
2. Markedly diminished interest or pleasure in all, or almost all, activities most of the day, nearly every day.
3. Significant weight loss when not dieting or weight gain such as >5% of body weight in one month or decrease or increase in appetite nearly every day.
4. Insomnia or hypersomnia nearly every day.
5. Psychomotor agitation or retardation nearly every day.
6. Fatigue or loss of energy nearly every day.
7. Feelings of worthlessness or excessive or inappropriate guilt (which may be delusional) nearly every day, but not merely self-reproach or guilt about being sick.
8. Diminished ability to think or concentrate, or indecisiveness, nearly every day.
9. Recurrent thoughts of death (not just fear of dying), recurrent suicidal ideation with or without a specific plan.

The symptoms cause significant distress or impairment in important areas of function and are not attributable to a substance or medical condition.

Pathophysiology and Epidemiology

The neurobiologic pathways affected in depression are complex and incompletely elucidated. Neuroendocrine abnormalities resulting from alterations in these pathways can explain some symptoms of depression. Genetic predisposition for developing depression can account for 40% to 50% of the risk for developing depression, but no specific gene for depression has been identified. Physical and emotional stress, as well as drugs and other ingested substances, also influence the pathways involved in depression. First-line therapeutic agents target pathways involved in serotonin and norepinephrine reuptake, and, with time, neurobiologic pathways of the brain adapt to the changes produced by antidepressant medications and ideally result clinically in mood elevation. More detailed neurobiologic pathways are beyond the scope of this text.

The prevalence of major depression is approximately 5%, with about 15% of the population experiencing depression at least once during their lifetime. Milder forms of depression can have up to a 15% to 20% prevalence, and this excludes other mixed mood disorders that include symptoms that overlap with depression, such as bipolar disorder. Depression affects up to 10% of patients at any given time. Women are twice as likely as men to have depression. Depression is commonly underdiagnosed and undertreated. In the United States, an estimated $55.1 billion in lost productivity per year is attributed to all mood disorders, including depressive disorders, bipolar disorders, and depression associated with medical illness or substance abuse. About 10% to 15% of cases of depression can be explained by general medical illness or substance use. Depressive disorders manifest in about 20% to 30% of patients with cardiac disease; 25% to 50% of patients with cancer, with certain cancers being associated with a much higher prevalence; 8% to 27% of patients with diabetes mellitus; 22% to 45% of patients with HIV infection; and roughly 20% of patients with left-hemispheric stroke.

Rarely, a patient will present to their primary care physician with a chief complaint of depressed mood. More commonly, an associated complaint is the first symptom identified, and more detailed history including a thorough review of symptoms is necessary to reveal symptoms of depression. Common symptoms include low energy levels and low motivation, poor sleep, lack of interest in previously enjoyable activities, and poor concentration. However, it is important to recognize that symptoms of depression are rarely the same between individual patients. Depression screening and diagnostic tools, which will be discussed further in this chapter, can be helpful to assess for symptoms of depression in a systematic, objective manner. A detailed medical history is important to identify potentially treatable etiologies of secondary depression or comorbid illness that, if better controlled, can improve symptoms of depression.

A careful review of medications and use of other substances is important to identify iatrogenic etiologies for depressive symptoms (Table 35-2). It is also important to ask the patient in a nonjudgmental manner about important components of the social and family history that may increase risk for and contribute to depression (Table 35-3). The family history should include mental health disorders, suicide attempts or completions, and substance abuse including alcoholism. The social history should address the patient's personal history of substance dependence or abuse, significant life events, as well as screening for intimate partner violence, which can include physical, verbal, or sexual abuse. Substance abuse history is essential, as intoxication or withdrawal from a substance also can cause depressive symptoms.

Multiple depression screening tools exist for use at the point of care. The shortest is the Primary Care Evaluation of Mental Disorders (PRIME-MD), which is a 2-item screening tool that asks the following 2 questions:

1. Over the past 2 weeks have you felt down, depressed, or hopeless?
2. Over the past 2 weeks have you felt little interest or pleasure in doing things?

Table 35-2. Secondary Causes of Depression

Medications	Other substances
Antihypertensive drugs (eg, beta blockers)	Psychostimulants, such as cocaine and amphetamines
Anticholesterolemic agents	
Antiarrhythmic agents (eg, digoxin)	Heroin and other opiates
Glucocorticoids	Ethanol
Antimicrobials (eg, mefloquine)	Marijuana and related synthetic cannabinoids
Systemic analgesics (eg, opioid analgesics)	
Antiparkinsonian medications (eg, levodopa)	Phencyclidine
Anticonvulsants	Hypothyroidism
Contraceptive medications	Hypogonadism

Table 35-3. Risk Factors for Depression

Older age (including associated neurologic conditions, such as Alzheimer disease and parkinsonism)

Recent childbirth

Neurologic conditions (multiple sclerosis, traumatic brain injury)

Stressful life events

Personal or family history of depression

Comorbid medical conditions (diabetes, coronary artery disease, stroke, obesity, HIV infection, cancer, hepatitis C)

Comorbid mental health conditions (eating disorders, anxiety disorders, somatoform disorders, psychotic disorders, personality disorders)

Chronic fatigue syndrome or fibromyalgia

Alarm symptoms[a]

- Past history of suicide attempts
- Profound hopelessness
- Substance abuse
- Social isolation

[a]Immediate mental health evaluation may be indicated if these significant risk factors are identified.

A positive response, which is an answer of yes to any of the items, has a sensitivity of 96% and a specificity of 57%. More lengthy screening tools and depression scales exist that can be used in specific clinical situations. For example, the Geriatric Depression Scale (GDS) is intended for patients over 65 years of age, and the Edinburgh Postnatal Depression Scale is intended for use in postpartum women. The benefit of using a depression scale that assesses a more detailed inventory of symptoms is that the same scale may then be used to follow treatment responses. Common tools used to screen for depression and follow treatment response include the Patient Health Questionnaire (PHQ-9) and the Beck Depression Inventory (BDI). The PHQ-9 and its score interpretation are included here (Tables 35-4 and 35-5). The 2-item screening tool is more efficient and can perform as well as the longer instruments, but it does not provide the level of detail needed to follow treatment response.

It is important to screen for risk of self-harm or harm to others through direct, nonjudgmental inquiry. Some depression scales, such as PHQ-9 and BDI, include questions about suicidal or homicidal ideation or intent, which, if marked affirmatively, should prompt more detailed questioning of the patient's imminent risk for harmful behaviors in order to guide triage and emergent psychiatric management.

Examine the patient for signs of a medical condition, substance use, or withdrawal that may be the cause of depressive symptoms. A social history indicating substance use can guide the physical examination, with attention to signs of withdrawal from or intoxication with the suspected substance(s). Attention to signs of intimate partner violence also is essential, including, for example, a detailed examination of injuries at varying stages of healing for which the patient is unable to adequately account.

Laboratory studies should be ordered judiciously based on the clinical suspicion for secondary causes of depression (Tables 35-2 and 35-3). Because a patient frequently presents with varied symptoms of depression, symptoms should guide indicated laboratory analyses. Common tests that are performed in a primary care setting include thyroid-stimulating hormone, comprehensive metabolic panel, complete blood count, and free and total testosterone levels, although this list is by no means exhaustive.

Treatment

Of primary importance is to be able to recognize when a patient may need referral to a psychiatrist, or urgent psychiatric evaluation including possible hospitalization. These situations include suicidal or homicidal ideation, with or without intent and a plan. If initial depression screening indicates the presence of a depressive episode, pharmacologic and behavioral therapies may be recommended. Initial treatment choices should be selected based on the clinical context of the patient's depressive disorder (Table 35-6). First-line therapy is often an adequate trial of a SSRI. However, SNRIs, atypical antidepressants, and serotonin modulators can be

Table 35-4. Patient Health Questionnaire

Over the *last 2 weeks*, how often have you been bothered by any of the following problems?

	Not at All	Several Days	More Than Half the Days	Nearly Every Day
1. Little interest or pleasure in doing things	0	1	2	3
2. Feeling down, depressed, or hopeless	0	1	2	3
3. Trouble falling or staying asleep, or sleeping too much	0	1	2	3
4. Feeling tired or having little energy	0	1	2	3
5. Poor appetite or overeating	0	1	2	3
6. Feeling bad about yourself— or that you are a failure or have let yourself or your family down	0	1	2	3
7. Trouble concentrating on things, such as reading the newspaper or watching television	0	1	2	3
8. Moving or speaking so slowly that other people could have noticed? Or the opposite—being so fidgety or restless that you have been moving around a lot more than usual	0	1	2	3
9. Thoughts that you would be better off dead or of hurting yourself in some way	0	1	2	3
If you checked off *any* problems, how *difficult* have these problems made it for you to do your work, take care of things at home, or get along with other people?	Not difficult at all	Somewhat difficult	Very difficult	Extremely difficult

Table 35-5. PHQ-9 and Proposed Treatment Actions

PHQ-9 Score	Depression Severity	Proposed Treatment Actions
1–4	None	None
5–9	Mild	Watchful waiting; repeat PHQ-9 at follow-up
10–14	Moderate	Treatment plan, considering counseling, follow-up, and/or pharmacotherapy
15–19	Moderately severe	Immediate initiation of pharmacotherapy and/or psychotherapy
20–27	Severe	Immediate initiation of pharmacotherapy and, if severe impairment or poor response to therapy, expedited referral to a mental health specialist for psychotherapy and/or collaborative management

reasonable alternatives depending on the comorbid illness and side effect profiles desired. TCAs and MAOIs are not recommended as first-line agents due to concerns about safety and side-effect profiles. They are preferably managed in consultation with a psychiatrist. Combination therapy with pharmacologic therapy and psychotherapy, specifically CBT, can be a more effective method of treating depression. In CBT, patients learn and practice techniques, including role playing, imagery, problem-solving skills, and guided discovery, with the goal of identifying and modifying dysfunctional beliefs.

Close follow-up after initiation of medical therapy is essential. Initial follow-up within 2 weeks can be helpful to evaluate acceptance of the medication, to reinforce educational messages, to reassess suicidality, and to address adverse events. Evidence of response to antidepressant medication is a 50% reduction in PHQ-9 score by 6 weeks. Continued follow-up for a minimum of 6 to 9 months on drug therapy should be considered. Patient counseling regarding expectations of treatment response must be clear in order to optimize treatment adherence.

Treatment-resistant depression can occur in up to 40% of patients, but treatment resistance or nonresponse should be differentiated from inadequate treatment or pseudoresistance. First, adherence to the recommended treatment regimen should be assessed, as patients with depression are at risk for nonadherence to all treatment modalities, including antidepressants. Nonadherence to antidepressant medication occurs in approximately 28% of patients after 1 month

Table 35-6. Medications for Treatment of Depression

Drug Class	Benefits	Side Effects	Notes
Selective serotonin reuptake inhibitor (SSRI) (citalopram, escitalopram, fluoxetine, fluvoxamine, paroxetine, sertraline)	Effective, well tolerated	Nausea, diarrhea, decreased appetite, anxiety, nervousness, insomnia, somnolence, sweating, impaired sexual function	Contraindicated with MAOIs Use with caution when also taking hepatically metabolized drugs If mental status changes occur while on SSRI, check electrolytes to rule out syndrome of inappropriate antidiuretic hormone (SIADH)
Serotonin and selective norepinephrine reuptake inhibitor (SNRI) (venlafaxine, duloxetine, mirtazapine)	Venlafaxine: effective, well tolerated Mirtazapine may be effective when other agents have not been	Venlafaxine: nausea, dry mouth, anorexia, constipation, dizziness, somnolence, insomnia, nervousness, sweating, abnormalities of sexual function, cardiovascular effects Mirtazapine: weight gain, somnolence, dizziness, increased cholesterol, elevated liver transaminases, orthostatic hypotension, agranulocytosis	Venlafaxine: contraindicated with MAOIs Monitor blood pressure Taper slowly due to potential for withdrawal syndrome Duloxetine: may be hepatotoxic with alcohol Mirtazapine: use caution with renal impairment; contraindicated with MAOIs; avoid benzodiazepines. Check fasting glucose and lipids

(Continued)

Table 35-6. Medications for Treatment of Depression (*Continued*)

Drug Class	Benefits	Side Effects	Notes
Dopamine reuptake inhibitor (bupropion)	Less weight gain, fewer adverse effects on sexual functioning, approved for smoking cessation	Lowers seizure threshold, may exacerbate eating disorders, anorexia, rash, sweating, tinnitus, tremor, abdominal pain, agitation, anxiety, dizziness, insomnia, myalgia, nausea, palpitations, pharyngitis, urinary frequency	Contraindicated when there is a personal or family history of seizures, or with MAOIs, or with a history of bulimia or anorexia Use with caution with other drugs that may lower seizure threshold and in patients with impaired hepatic function
5-HT$_2$ receptor antagonist (trazodone)	May be used for insomnia Fewer adverse effect on sexual functioning; lower incidence of postural hypotension than TCAs, but higher than SSRIs	Somnolence, dry mouth, nausea, dizziness, constipation, asthenia, light-headedness, blurred vision, confusion, abnormal vision, priapism	Contraindicated with certain medications (carbamazepine, triazolam, alprazolam) Use with caution in cardiovascular, cerebrovascular, and seizure disorders Related medication nefazodone was removed from the market due to severe hepatotoxicity

(Continued)

Table 35-6. Medications for Treatment of Depression (*Continued*)

Drug Class	Benefits	Side Effects	Notes
Tricyclic antidepressant (TCA) (nortriptyline, amitriptyline, doxepin, desipramine, imipramine, clomipramine)	Desipramine least sedating Amitriptyline and doxepin may be taken at bedtime to aid with sleep Desipramine may be stimulating	Dry mouth, dizziness, nervousness, constipation, nausea, sedation, anticholinergic and orthostatic hypotension, may cause tardive dyskinesia and the neuroleptic malignant syndrome	Contraindicated with MAOIs, or in patients with prolonged QT interval or on drugs that may prolong QT interval Use with caution in patients with cardiovascular disease and arrhythmia, patients prone to urinary retention and on thyroid medications May precipitate attacks in narrow-angle glaucoma Monitor EKG and orthostatic blood pressure changes
Monoamine oxidase inhibitor (MAOI) (phenelzine, isocarboxazid, tranylcypromine)	May be effective when other agents have not been May be more effective in patients with atypical depression (hypersomnolence, hyperphagia, and rejection sensitivity)	Dizziness, headache, drowsiness, insomnia, hypersomnia, fatigue, weakness, tremors, twitching, myoclonic movements, hyperreflexia, constipation, dry mouth, gastrointestinal disturbances, elevated liver transaminases, weight gain, postural hypotension, edema, sexual disturbances	Infrequently used in primary care Contraindicated when there is a history of cerebrovascular and cardiovascular disease, pheochromocytoma, liver disease; many drug interactions Increases risk for hypertensive crisis and serotonin syndrome (hypertension, hyperthermia, tachycardia, death) Extensive patient education is required

(*Continued*)

Table 35-6. Medications for Treatment of Depression (*Continued*)

Drug Class	Benefits	Side Effects	Notes
5HT$_{A1}$ receptor partial antagonist (buspirone)	May be used in second- and third-line treatment to augment antidepressant therapy in treatment-resistant depression	Insomnia, dizziness, headache, light-headedness, nausea, gastrointestinal side effects	Use with caution when also taking hepatically metabolized drugs
Atypical antipsychotics (olanzapine, aripiprazole, quetiapine)	May be used in third-line treatment to augment antidepressant therapy in treatment-resistant depression. Specialty referral is likely needed	Olanzapine is most likely to have side effects of weight gain, insulin resistance, elevated cholesterol, sedation	Check fasting glucose and lipids at baseline and annually. Check EKG in patients >40 years old or with cardiac risk factors

and 44% after 3 months. Specific patient educational messages that promote adherence include the following 5 messages:

1. Take the medication daily.
2. Antidepressants must be taken for 2 to 4 weeks for a noticeable effect.
3. Continue taking the medicine even if feeling better.
4. Do not stop taking the antidepressant without checking with the physician.
5. Provide specific instructions regarding what to do to resolve questions regarding antidepressants.

Second, an adequate trial is considered 8 weeks of treatment with an optimal dose of an antidepressant medication. Subsequent management may include switching to an alternative medication of the same class (eg, switch to a different SSRI) or to a different class of medication (eg, selective norepinephrine reuptake inhibitor [SNRI] or bupropion), combining with another medication (eg, bupropion), or augmenting with another class of medication (eg, buspirone or atypical antipsychotics) or with psychotherapy.

Complementary and alternative medicines also have been considered in the treatment of mild depression. Dietary supplements including omega-3 fatty acids, St. John's wort, and valerian are alternative treatments for depression. Complementary health practices that can be used in the treatment of depression include regular exercise, massage, yoga, and relaxation techniques. When compared head to head with antidepressants, physical exercise has been shown to reduce depressive symptoms by as much as 40% compared with antidepressants in the same study that reduced standardized tool scores by 50%. When seasonal worsening of depressive symptoms are recognized, light therapy is an important intervention that is effective in the treatment of depressive symptoms. Recognizing insomnia as a separate disorder, if present, and targeting this with multimodality interventions can determine successful treatment of depression. It is important to recognize that complementary medicines and practices are not regulated or well studied, and supplements can potentially interact with numerous prescription medicines. Careful discussion of the benefits and risks of each of these therapies is essential to guide an informed decision regarding their use.

TIPS TO REMEMBER

- Depression is common in the general population and incurs significant direct and indirect health care costs in the United States.
- Depression is frequently underdiagnosed and undertreated. Screening for depressive symptoms using evidence-based tools should be incorporated into routine clinical practice. Close follow-up and monitoring are necessary to ensure adherence to therapy and adequate treatment response.
- In patients with severe major depression and a score >20 on PHQ-9, refer to a psychiatrist.

COMPREHENSION QUESTIONS

1. A 55-year-old woman with diabetes, a history of depression, and a history of sexual abuse in childhood presents after being lost to follow-up when her primary care provider moved. She states that she has not taken any medications for more than 1 year. What is the next best step in evaluation in the office?

    A. Check hemoglobin A1c to evaluate diabetes control.

    B. Start an antidiabetic medication.

    C. Start an antidepressant medication.

    D. Both B and C.

    E. Screen for depression to guide further management.

2. A 32-year-old man with a history of alcoholism and depression sees you for a 4-week follow-up after starting low-dose sertraline for symptoms meeting criteria for an episode of MDD, without suicidal thoughts or ideation. His PHQ-9 score was 21 at his initial office visit. His current PHQ-9 score is 13, and he reports that he is taking his antidepressant daily and that his energy levels have improved slightly. What is the next best step in management?

    A. No change in medication dose, and recommend follow-up in 4 weeks.

    B. Increase medication dose, and recommend follow-up in 4 weeks.

    C. Change medication because sertraline was ineffective, and recommend follow-up in 4 weeks.

    D. Refer to a psychiatrist because he has treatment-resistant depression.

3. A 25-year-old female presents to the emergency department via ambulance after she was found unconscious on her bedroom floor by her roommate. Paramedics report that when she was found, there were empty, unlabeled prescription bottles scattered on the bedroom floor. She was intubated for airway protection and treated in the ambulance with the usual medications in a suspected case of poisoning with an unknown substance, and IV fluids were started. She is hypotensive and tachycardic, and an ECG shows a QRS duration of 134 milliseconds. What is one of the likely substances that was overdosed based on the limited information available so far?

    A. Benzodiazepine

    B. Beta blocker

    C. Acetaminophen

    D. Tricyclic antidepressant

    E. SSRI

Answers

1. **E.** The next best step in evaluation is to use a depression screening questionnaire, such as PHQ-9 or BDI, to establish a baseline of severity of depressive symptoms and their impact on overall function. Adequate treatment of depression will be essential to satisfactory management of diabetes, a common comorbid condition and risk factor for depression.

2. **B.** The next best step in management is to optimize the dose of sertraline for treatment response. He is demonstrating some improvement in symptoms based on self-reported symptoms and reassessment with the PHQ-9 scale; however, his response can be improved. Increasing sertraline and reevaluating with the PHQ-9 in 4 weeks is the most reasonable option. Not changing the dose is not appropriate because his treatment response is not optimal. Changing medication or referring for specialist evaluation and management of his depression suggests that he has treatment-resistant depression, which he does not have because he has not tried an adequate trial of first-line treatment as of this office visit.

3. **D.** In this case, it is unclear how many substances this patient may have over-dosed, and a broad workup and management for suspected substances to guide therapeutic management and monitoring is necessary. Additionally, it is important to contact the local Poison Control Center (800-222-1222) for assistance in managing suspected poisonings. In this case, at a minimum, one of the suspected substances should include tricyclic antidepressants, and monitoring for cardiac arrhythmias should be instituted, because they may be preceded by a prolonged QRS complex over 100 ms.

SUGGESTED READINGS

American College of Physicians. ACP depression care guide: team-based practices for screening, diagnosis, and management in primary care settings. American College of Physicians. Accessed March 2012. depression.acponline.org

Fancher TL, Kravitz RL. In the clinic. Depression. *Ann Intern Med.* 2010;152:ITC51–ITC15.

Longo D, Fauci A, Kasper D, et al. *Harrison's Principles of Internal Medicine.* 18th ed. New York: The McGraw-Hill Companies; 2012.

WEBSITES

Search for mental health centers supported by county public health departments and other local mental health resources:

National Association of State Mental Health Directors: www.nasmhpd.org/mental_health_resources. cfm#State

National Suicide Hotlines USA: www.suicidepreventionlifeline.org (toll-free, available 24 hours a day, 7 days a week); 1-800-SUICIDE (784-2433); 1-800-273-TALK (8255); TTY: 1-800-799-4TTY (4889).

National Domestic Violence Hotline: www.thehotline.org; 1-800-799-SAFE (7233); TTY: 1–800–787–3224.

National Institutes of Mental Health: www.nimh.nih.gov/health/topics/depression/

A 36-year-old Man With a Request for a Diabetes Screening

Vanessa Williams, MD and Michael Jakoby, MD, MA

A 36-year-old man presents to clinic as a new patient. He has not seen a physician since he turned 18 years old and would like a general health checkup. The patient denies any known chronic health problems. However, his father and older brother have been diagnosed with type 2 diabetes, and the patient would like to be screened for diabetes mellitus. Physical examination is unremarkable except for weight of 108 kg and height of 175 cm (BMI 35.2 kg/m²). Blood pressure on multiple measurements during the visit averages 142/96 mm Hg. Hemoglobin A1c (HbA1c) is measured and found to be 6.7%, and morning fasting plasma glucose is 138 mg/dL.

The patient returns to the office 3 months later to discuss further management of his type 2 diabetes mellitus. He modified his diet and participated in an exercise program for 3 months, but his HbA1c remains 6.7%. He is started on metformin and adjusted to 1000 mg twice daily without side effects. Three months later, capillary blood glucose (CBG) measurements are consistently below 130 mg/dL, and HbA1c improves to 6.0%.

Two years later, HbA1c has steadily increased to 7.5% despite compliance with diet, exercise, and metformin. Dilated fundoscopy and foot examination are unremarkable, and urine albumin/creatinine ratio remains below 30 mg/g. Initially, HbA1c improves with the addition of glipizide to metformin. Semaglutide is then started 1 year later due to worsening glycemic control. Two years later, the patient returns to discuss additional treatment options. Despite taking maximal effective doses of metformin (1000 mg BID), glipizide (20 mg BID), and semaglutide (1 mg weekly), HbA1c is now 8.5% and fasting CBG measurements fall mostly in the range of 160 to 210 mg/dL.

1. Who should be screened for type 2 diabetes mellitus?

2. How should type 2 diabetes mellitus initially be managed?

3. What regular screening is necessary for patients with type 2 diabetes mellitus?

4. What additional therapies can be added if metformin monotherapy is ineffective?

5. What is the next step in management for patients with progressively worsening glycemic control despite multiple oral medications or glucagon-like peptide-1 (GLP-1) analog therapy?

Table 36-1. Risk Factors for Type 2 Diabetes Mellitus

Physical inactivity
First-degree relative with diabetes
High-risk ethnicity (African American, Latino, Native American, Asian American, Pacific Islander)
Women with history of gestational diabetes or baby weighing >9 lb
Hypertension (treated or screening blood pressure ≥140/90 mm Hg)
HDL <35 mg/dL or triglycerides >250 mg/dL
Polycystic ovary syndrome (PCOS)
Cardiovascular disease
Pre–diabetes mellitus
Conditions associated with insulin resistance (obesity, acanthosis nigricans)

Answers

1. All adults with BMI ≥25 kg/m^2 and 1 or more risk factors as presented in Table 36-1 should be screened annually. Individuals age 45 years or older without risk factors should be screened every 3 years.
2. Therapeutic lifestyle change (TLC), which consists of diet and aerobic exercise, and metformin are the initial interventions for type 2 diabetes mellitus.
3. Complete physical examination including dilated fundoscopy and foot examination with monofilament evaluation should be performed at least annually. Hemoglobin A1c (HbA1c) should be checked at 3-month intervals if diabetes mellitus is uncontrolled and at 6-month intervals if glycemic control is at target. Fasting lipid panel and urine albumin/creatinine ratio should also be checked at least annually.
4. Sulfonylureas, thiazolidinediones (TZDs), dipeptidyl peptidase-IV (DPP-4) inhibitors, glucagon-like peptide-1 (GLP-1) analogs, sodium-glucose cotransporter-2 (SGLT-2) inhibitors, and insulin are all potential add-on therapies to metformin (see Appendix 1). The decision on next best therapeutic option should be individualized for each patient based on a variety of factors.
5. Insulin therapy is required when combinations of alternative therapies fail to keep HbA1c ≤7%. Basal insulin alone or the combination of basal and prandial insulin may be required.

CASE REVIEW AND DIAGNOSIS

Overview

Type 2 diabetes mellitus is caused by impaired insulin signaling in key organ systems such as skeletal muscle, liver, and adipose tissue and relative insulinopenia.

More than 37 million Americans have been diagnosed with diabetes mellitus, with approximately 95% of patients qualifying for a diagnosis of type 2 diabetes mellitus. It is estimated that 8.5 million Americans have diabetes mellitus but are currently undiagnosed.

All adult patients with BMI ≥25 kg/m² and 1 or more risk factors (see Table 36-1) should be screened at least annually for type 2 diabetes mellitus. Patients older than 45 years should be screened every 3 years regardless of risk.

The American Diabetes Association (ADA) recommends that the diagnosis of diabetes mellitus be made based on the results of 2 concordant screening tests, which include hemoglobin A1c (HbA1c) ≥6.5%, fasting plasma glucose ≥126 mg/dL (after minimum 8-h fast), and/or 2-hour plasma glucose ≥200 mg/dL during a 75-g oral glucose tolerance test. However, patients can be diagnosed with diabetes mellitus if they present with symptoms of hyperglycemia, such as polyuria and polydipsia, and a random plasma glucose ≥200 mg/dL.

Monitoring for Complications

Before starting treatment, patients with newly diagnosed type 2 diabetes mellitus should undergo screening for complications of hyperglycemia, including microvascular complications (retinopathy, neuropathy, and nephropathy) and macrovascular complications (coronary artery disease, cerebrovascular disease, and peripheral artery disease), as this population of patients is at increased risk for vascular complications even before being diagnosed. For example, in the Diabetes Prevention Program, more than 10% of patients with newly diagnosed type 2 diabetes mellitus already had some degree of retinopathy at the time of diagnosis.

A complete physical examination and dilated fundoscopic evaluation should be performed at least once a year. A foot examination that includes monofilament testing and evaluation of vibratory sensation and proprioception should be performed at routine office visits, at least annually. Blood pressure should be measured at each visit and treated to goal of <130/80 mm Hg. Patients who have diabetes mellitus with proteinuria and hypertension should be managed with a regimen that includes either an angiotensin-converting enzyme (ACE) inhibitor or an angiotensin receptor blocker (ARB).

HbA1c is a marker of glycemic control over the previous 2 to 3 months and strongly correlates with the risk of microvascular complications. It should be checked every 3 months in patients starting or changing glucose-lowering therapy or who have not achieved HbA1c <7%. HbA1c may be checked every 6 months when glycemic control is at goal and stable. Target HbA1c for most patients is ≤7.0%, although some patients may be able to achieve HbA1c ≤6.5% without significant risk of hypoglycemia. For patients with frequent hypoglycemia, hypoglycemia unawareness, or limited life expectancy, a higher HbA1c (eg, ≤8.0%) is acceptable.

Fasting lipid profile (total cholesterol, HDL cholesterol, LDL cholesterol, and triglycerides) should be checked at least once yearly. Target LDL is <100 mg/dL for patients with diabetes mellitus and no other risk factors for cardiovascular disease. However, patients with diabetes mellitus who have other risk factors for cardiovascular disease should be managed to a target LDL <70 mg/dL, while those patients who have had multiple cardiovascular events have a target of <55 mg/dL. Other lipid targets are HDL >40 mg/dL in men and >50 mg/dL in women, and triglycerides <150 mg/dL. HMG CoA reductase inhibitor ("statin") therapy is indicated in all patients with diabetes mellitus who have a history of cardiovascular disease or who are ≥40 years with baseline LDL cholesterol >70 mg/dL. Therapy should be considered in diabetic patients under age 40 with baseline LDL cholesterol >100 mg/dL.

Patients should be screened annually for proteinuria by measurement of urine albumin to creatinine ratio on a spot urine sample. A ratio of 30 to 300 mg/g is considered moderately increased albuminuria, and a ratio >300 mg/g indicates severely increased albuminuria. Several factors can lead to spurious elevation of the ratio, such as vigorous exercise, menstruation, or urinary tract infection. An abnormal result should be confirmed on at least two additional urine samples obtained within 3 to 6 months of the initial abnormal test.

Treatment

Diabetes management requires a team including physicians, certified diabetes educators, and dietitians. Lifestyle modification (healthy diet and regular aerobic exercise) and metformin are recommended as initial therapy for most patients in guidelines published by the ADA, the American Association of Clinical Endocrinology (AACE), the American College of Endocrinology, and the European Association for the Study of Diabetes. However, patients with an initial HbA1c >7.5% may require initial treatment with metformin and a second therapeutic agent, depending on the degree of hyperglycemia. The determination of this second therapeutic agent should be personalized to each patient's case. Dietitians can help patients choose appropriate foods, particularly when they face multiple restrictions such as low-sodium diet for hypertension and low-fat diet for dyslipidemia. The Centers for Disease Control recommends 150 minutes of exercise per week, with a target heart rate of 70% of maximum predicted for age.

Type 2 diabetes mellitus is a slowly progressive disease, primarily due to a steady decline in beta-cell function on a background of increased insulin resistance. In the United Kingdom Prospective Diabetes Study (UKPDS), fewer than half of patients maintained HbA1c <7% in their original treatment arms 3 years after randomization. Patients should be educated regarding the natural history of type 2 diabetes and advised that changes in treatment are likely to be required to maintain appropriate glycemic control. Depending on the decrement in glycemic control, combinations of oral medications, oral medications and GLP-1 analogs, oral medications and insulin, or insulin monotherapy may be required to improve blood glucose control.

Metformin is a drug from the biguanide class that lowers glucose primarily by decreasing hepatic glucose output. Metformin is highly potent at reducing plasma glucose but does not cause hypoglycemia or weight gain. The most common side effect is gastrointestinal upset that may manifest as abdominal discomfort, nausea, bloating, cramping, or diarrhea. In updated US Food and Drug Administration (FDA) labeling, metformin is contraindicated in patients with eGFR <30 mL/min/1.73 m^2 and not recommended to be initiated if eGFR is between 30 and 45 mL/min/1.73 m^2. Risks and benefits of metformin should be considered carefully in patients whose GFR falls below 45 mL/min/1.73 m^2. It is typically started at 500 mg twice daily and then advanced in 500-mg weekly increments to the maximally effective dose of 1000 mg twice daily. Metformin dose should be reduced to no more than a 1000-mg cumulative daily dose if GFR falls below 45 mL/min/1.73 m^2. Clinical conditions that are considered potential contraindications to metformin include severe liver disease, unstable heart failure, alcohol abuse, and past history of lactic acidosis while taking metformin. However, a recent meta-analysis found use of metformin in patients with type 2 diabetes and moderate renal failure, liver failure, or heart failure was associated with reduced all-cause mortality. As monotherapy, metformin lowers HbA1c by 1% to 2%.

Sulfonylureas are the oldest class of oral diabetes medications. They act by binding to the sulfonylurea receptor (SUR-1), inhibiting potassium efflux, and increasing transmembrane potential. Voltage-gated calcium channels are then activated, and insulin release is increased for any given plasma glucose level. The second-generation sulfonylureas glipizide, glimepiride, and glyburide are the most commonly prescribed sulfonylureas. Anticipated improvement in HbA1c is 1% to 2%, particularly when sulfonylureas are used as initial therapy. Weight gain and hypoglycemia are the two most common side effects of treatment with sulfonylureas. Metabolites of sulfonylureas are renally excreted, and metabolites of glyburide have glucose-lowering activity, making it appropriate to use glipizide or glimepiride in patients with chronic renal insufficiency. There is evidence from the University Group Diabetes Program that first-generation sulfonylureas (eg, tolbutamide) increase risk of cardiovascular disease, although second-generation agents do not appear to increase cardiovascular event rates, CVD mortality, or all-cause mortality in patients with type 2 diabetes.

Nateglinide and repaglinide are a part of the meglitinide class and bind to the sulfonylurea receptor at sites distinct from sulfonylurea class drugs. They are also insulin secretagogues but have a shorter duration of activity than sulfonylureas and are dosed before each meal. Blood glucose-lowering potency is similar to somewhat lower than the sulfonylureas and metformin, although meglitinides have a better safety profile compared with sulfonylureas in patients with renal impairment, particularly repaglinide. Meglitinides have similar potential as sulfonylureas to cause weight gain but a lower risk than sulfonylureas of causing hypoglycemia.

Thiazolidinediones (TZDs) are agonists of peroxisome proliferator–activated receptor gamma (PPAR-γ) that improve hyperglycemia primarily by improving the insulin sensitivity of skeletal muscle. Troglitazone has been withdrawn from the market due to hepatotoxicity, and rosiglitazone was withdrawn from retail pharmacies and restricted to a special access program for a period of time due to concern for increased risk of cardiovascular events such as myocardial infarction. Pioglitazone is the most common TZD in clinical use. Anticipated improvement in HbA1c is 0.5% to 1.5%, including when pioglitazone is used as a second-line agent. Weight gain and edema are the most common untoward effects of therapy, and TZDs are contraindicated when patients are predisposed to fluid retention (eg, heart failure, hepatic insufficiency). There is an extensive body of evidence that TZDs decrease bone density and predispose to low-trauma fractures, especially in women, and controversy that TZDs may increase risk of bladder carcinoma and diabetic macular edema.

Dipeptidyl peptidase 4 (DPP-4) inhibitors are a relatively new class of insulin secretagogue. Glucagon-like peptide-1 (GLP-1) is an incretin-class hormone that augments prandial insulin release, and these drugs increase GLP-1 levels by inhibiting DPP-4, the enzyme that inactivates GLP-1. Sitagliptin, saxagliptin, and linagliptin are the currently available DPP-4 inhibitors in the United States. HbA1c improves by 0.5% to 0.8% when DPP-4 inhibitors are used as monotherapy. DPP-4 inhibitors are generally well tolerated, and they do not cause weight gain or hypoglycemia. DPP-4 inhibitors appear to have no measurable effects on CVD event rates, CVD mortality, all-cause mortality, or progression of renal disease, although the FDA has added a warning about an increased risk of hospitalization for heart failure to labeling for saxagliptin. Linagliptin is the only DPP-4 inhibitor that does not require dose adjustment in patients with reduced eGFR.

GLP-1 analogs, which include exenatide, liraglutide, semaglutide, and dulaglutide, are the other class of incretin mimetics for management of type 2 diabetes. GLP-1 is a hormone secreted by L-cells in the ileum in response to carbohydrate intake. Prandial insulin is consequently increased in a glucose-dependent manner. GLP-1 also delays gastric emptying, inhibits glucagon release, and acts on satiety centers in the hypothalamus to reduce food intake. It is quickly degraded by the enzyme DPP-4, making it difficult to utilize as a diabetes therapy. However, GLP-1 analogs have been developed that are resistant to degradation by DPP-IV and have significantly longer half-lives. Almost all these agents are administered subcutaneously, with frequency of administration ranging from twice daily to once weekly. Semaglutide is now available as a once-daily oral preparation. These medications are approved as add-on therapies for patients failing to control hyperglycemia adequately with oral medications and lifestyle changes. Anticipated improvement in HbA1c is 1% to 2%. Weight loss is also common with these agents, particularly when added to treatment with metformin. Liraglutide, semaglutide, and dulaglutide have been shown to reduce the risk of major adverse cardiovascular events and progression of diabetic nephropathy (see Table 36-2).

Table 36-2. Effect on Major Adverse Cardiovascular Events (MACE), Diabetic Nephropathy, and Hospitalizations for Heart Failure (HF) With Reduced Ejection Factor (HFrEF) From GLP-1 Agonists and SGLT-2 Inhibitors

Medication	Trial(s)	MACE*	New/ Worsening Nephropathy	Hospitalizations for HF
GLP-1 Agonists				
Liraglutide	LEADER (2016)	Significant reduction (HR 0.87)	Significant reduction (HR 0.78)	No difference
SC Semaglutide	SUSTAIN-6 (2016)	Significant reduction (HR 0.74)	Significant reduction (HR 0.64)	No difference
Dulaglutide	REWIND (2019)	Significant reduction (HR 0.88)	Significant reduction (HR 0.85)	No difference
SGLT-2 Inhibitors				
Canagliflozin	CANVAS (2013) CANVAS-R (2017)	Significant reduction (HR 0.86)	Significant reduction (HR 0.73)	Significant reduction (HR 0.67)
Dapagliflozin	DECLARE-TIMI 58 (2019)	No difference (later subgroup analysis showed benefit in patients without previous MI)	Significant reduction (HR 0.53)	Significant reduction (HR 0.73)
Empagliflozin	EMPA-REG (2015)	Significant reduction (HR 0.86)	Significant reduction (HR 0.87)	Significant reduction (HR 0.65)
Ertugliflozin	VERTIS CV (2020)	No difference	No difference	Significant reduction (HR 0.7)

Note: Other GLP-1 agonists not listed (eg, lixisenatide, exenatide, oral semaglutide) have not been shown to have benefit in these outcomes.

*MACE is a composite endpoint that included the first occurrence of death from cardiovascular causes, nonfatal myocardial infarction (MI), and nonfatal stroke.

Most patients experience mild nausea and abdominal discomfort at start of treatment with GLP-1 receptor analogs, which resolves spontaneously, although up to 5% to 10% of patients may not be able to tolerate this therapeutic class due to persistent gastrointestinal side effects. There is also concern for increased risk of acute pancreatitis in GLP-1 analog–treated patients, although rates from postmarketing surveillance are similar to the background rate for all patients with diabetes. Liraglutide was associated with benign and malignant C-cell tumors in rodents, so it is contraindicated in patients with a personal or family history of medullary thyroid cancer or multiple endocrine neoplasia type 2A or 2B.

The SGLT-2 inhibitor class of glucose-lowering medications includes canagliflozin, empagliflozin, dapagliflozin, and ertugliflozin. These agents decrease the renal threshold for glucose excretion by inhibiting glucose reabsorption in the proximal tubule, resulting in increased glucosuria that in turn reduces plasma glucose levels. Due to their mechanism of action, SGLT-2 inhibitors do not cause hypoglycemia. Reduction in HbA1c from baseline is 0.5% to 1.0%, depending on baseline level of hyperglycemia and whether these drugs are used as initial or add-on therapy. Multiple randomized controlled trials have demonstrated that SGLT-2 inhibitors reduce rates of major adverse cardiovascular events, particularly for patients with established atherosclerotic cardiovascular disease, and hospitalizations for heart failure with reduced ejection fraction (see Table 36-2). Recent meta-analyses also indicate that SGLT-2 inhibitors reduce progression of diabetic kidney disease and all-cause mortality.

Glucosuria caused by SGLT-2 inhibitors increases rates of cystitis and vulvovaginal candidiasis. Osmotic diuresis may result in volume contraction and predispose to hypotension, particularly in patients taking other blood pressure–lowering medications. Diabetic ketoacidosis (DKA) occurs more often in patients taking SGLT-2 inhibitors than other noninsulin therapeutics for type 2 diabetes, and the absence of typical hyperglycemia (plasma glucose >250 mg/dL) may delay diagnosis of DKA. Some studies also show increased risks of fractures and lower limb amputations in patients treated with SGLT-2 inhibitors compared with other classes of diabetes medications.

Acarbose and miglitol are alpha-glucosidase inhibitors. Alpha-glucosidases are enzymes in the small intestines that break down complex polysaccharides into monosaccharides. These drugs delay glucose absorption to the distal small bowel and better match glucose absorption with prandial insulin release. Improvement in HbA1c is modest (approximately 0.5%), and the drugs are often poorly tolerated due to frequent occurrence of gastrointestinal side effects including abdominal pain, flatulence, and diarrhea.

Insulin is the most effective therapy for controlling hyperglycemia and is always an option for patients who are unable to achieve adequate glycemic control with lifestyle changes and oral medications. The odds of requiring insulin for successful management increase substantially with increasing duration of type 2 diabetes mellitus. Declining insulin secretory reserve is an important part of the natural history of type 2 diabetes, and most patients will require therapy with insulin, often both prandial and basal preparations, to achieve and maintain desirable glycemic control. Unfortunately, insulin may be delayed for several years due to patient or health care provider reluctance to start treatment despite suboptimal glycemic control. In a retrospective study conducted in the United Kingdom, 25% of patients delayed initiating insulin for 18 months and 50% of patients delayed starting insulin for almost 5 years despite HbA1c ≥8% and treatment with multiple oral medications.

American Association of Clinical Endocrinologists (AACE) guidelines recommend starting insulin for patients with HbA1c ≥7.5% 3 months after adding a third oral agent or GLP-1 analog if glucose control fails to improve and immediately for patients with HbA1c >9.0% or symptoms of hyperglycemia. Appendix 2 contains a complete list of currently available insulins and their pharmacokinetics. Many patients may achieve good glycemic control by adding a basal insulin (NPH, insulin detemir, insulin glargine, insulin degludec) to oral medications and adjusting the dose in a stepwise manner to achieve morning fasting glucose 80 to 110 mg/dL. Hypoglycemia and weight gain are the most common adverse effects of insulin therapy.

Patients should be prepared for the possibility that insulin will be required for optimal glycemic control early in the course of treatment. The patient in this vignette requires both prandial and basal insulin to restore good blood glucose control. The most common approaches are to use premixed insulin with fixed ratios of NPH insulin and prandial insulin (eg, NovoLog® 70/30 mix, Humalog® 75/25 mix, Humalog® 50/50 mix) or basal/bolus insulin combining a rapid-acting insulin analog (lispro, aspart, or glulisine) dosed before meals with a basal insulin analog (glargine, detemir, or degludec) dosed once daily.

Insulin doses are adjusted to achieve premeal and bedtime blood glucose measurements in the range of 80 to 130 mg/dL for most nonpregnant adults. When prandial insulin is prescribed, insulin secretagogues such as sulfonylureas and meglitinides are typically stopped. Insulin may be combined with agents that reduce total daily insulin requirements including metformin, SGLT-2 inhibitors, GLP-1 receptor analogs, and thiazolidinediones. Because patients with type 2 diabetes mellitus are insulin resistant, total daily insulin doses of ≥1 unit/kg body weight are not uncommon.

TIPS TO REMEMBER

- Type 2 diabetes mellitus is caused by relative insulinopenia in the setting of significant insulin resistance.

- Diagnostic criteria for type 2 diabetes mellitus include fasting plasma glucose ≥126 mg/dL after an 8-hour fast, 2-hour glucose ≥200 mg/dL on a 75-g oral glucose tolerance test, random glucose ≥200 mg/dL with symptoms of hyperglycemia (eg, polyuria, polydipsia), and hemoglobin A1c (HbA1c) ≥6.5%.

- Initial therapy for most patients includes lifestyle modification (diet and exercise) and metformin; multiple therapies may be required if HbA1c is >7.5% at initial presentation, and insulin is recommended if HbA1c is >10.0% or with presenting symptoms of hyperglycemia.

- Type 2 diabetes mellitus is a progressive disease with loss of beta-cell function over time resulting in the need for multiple oral medications, GLP-1 analog therapy, and/or insulin to maintain satisfactory glycemic control.

- The general goal of glycemic therapy is to maintain HbA1c ≤7%. However, some patients can be managed more aggressively if risk of hypoglycemia is low, while other patients may need to be managed with higher HbA1c targets for safety in the setting of hypoglycemia unawareness or limited life expectancy.

SUGGESTED READINGS

American Diabetes Association Professional Practice Committee. 11. Chronic kidney disease and risk management: standards of medical care in diabetes – 2022. *Diabetes Care.* 2022;45(suppl 1): S175–S184.

American Diabetes Association Professional Practice Committee. 12. Retinopathy, neuropathy, and foot care: standards of medical care in diabetes – 2022. *Diabetes Care.* 2022;45(suppl 1):S185–S194.

American Diabetes Association Professional Practice Committee. 2. Classification and diagnosis of diabetes: standards of medical care in diabetes – 2022. *Diabetes Care.* 2022;45(suppl 1):S17–S38.

American Diabetes Association Professional Practice Committee. 4. Comprehensive medical evaluation and assessment of comorbidities: standards of medical care in diabetes – 2022. *Diabetes Care.* 2022;45(suppl 1):S46–S59.

American Diabetes Association Professional Practice Committee. 6. Glycemic targets: standards of medical care in diabetes – 2022. *Diabetes Care.* 2022;45(suppl 1):S83–S96.

American Diabetes Association Professional Practice Committee. 9. Pharmacologic approaches to glycemic treatment: standards of medical care in diabetes – 2022. *Diabetes Care.* 2022;45(suppl 1):S125–S143.

Amori RE, Lau J, Pittas AG. Efficacy and safety of incretin therapy in type 2 diabetes: systematic review and meta-analysis. *JAMA.* 2007;298:194–206.

Bailey CJ, Turner RC. Metformin. *N Engl J Med* 1996;334:574–583.

Brown E, Rajeev SP, Cuthbertson DJ, Wilding JPH. A review of the mechanism of action, metabolic profile, and haemodynamic effects of sodium-glucose co-transporter-2 inhibitors. *Diabetes Obes Metab.* 2019;21(suppl 2):9–18.

Centers for Disease Control and Prevention. National Diabetes Statistics Report website. www.cdc.gov/diabetes/data/statistics-report. Accessed February 10, 2022.

Crowley MJ, Diamantidis CJ, McDuffie JR, et al. Clinical outcomes of metformin use in populations with chronic kidney disease, congestive heart failure, or chronic liver disease: a systematic review. *Ann Intern Med.* 2017;166(3):191–200.

Dormandy J, Blattacharya M, van Troostenburg de Bruyn AR, et al. Safety and tolerability of pioglitazone in high-risk patients with type 2 diabetes: an overview of data from PROactive. *Drug Saf.* 2009;32(3):187–202.

Fong DS, Contreras R. Glitazone use associated with diabetic macular edema. *Am J Ophthalmol.* 2009;147(4):583–586.

Garber AJ, Handelsman Y, Grunberger G, et al. Consensus statement by an American Association of Clinical Endocrinologists/American College of Endocrinology on the comprehensive type 2 diabetes management algorithm – 2020 executive summary. *Endocr Pract.* 2020;26(1):107–139.

Groop L. Sulfonylureas in NIDDM. *Diabetes Care.* 1992;15:737–747.

Grundy SM, Stone NJ, Baily AL, et al. 2018 AHA/ACC/AACVPR/AAPA/ABC/ACPM/ ADA/AGS/ APhA/ASPC/NLA/PCNA guideline on the management of blood cholesterol: a report of the American College of Cardiology/American Heart Association task force on clinical practice guidelines. *Circulation.* 2019;139(25):e1082–e1143.

Haahr H, Heise T. A review of the pharmacological properties of insulin degludec and their clinical relevance. *Clin Pharmacokinet.* 2014;53:787–800.

Habib ZA, Havstad SL, Wells K, et al. Thiazolidinedione use and the longitudinal risk of fractures in patients with type 2 diabetes mellitus. *J Clin Endocrinol Metab.* 2010;95(2):592–600.

Hirsch IB, Bergenstal RM, Parkin CG, et al. A real-world approach to insulin therapy in primary care practice. *Clin Diabetes.* 2005;23:78–86.

International Expert Committee. International Expert Committee report on the role of the A1C assay in the diagnosis of diabetes. *Diabetes Care.* 2009;32:1327–1334.

Inzucchi SE, Berganstal RM, Buse JB, et al. Management of hyperglycemia in type 2 diabetes – a patient-centered approach: position statement of the American Diabetes Association (ADA) and the European Association for the Study of Diabetes (EASD). *Diabetes Care.* 2012;35:1364–1379.

Kanie T, Mizuno A, Takaoka Y, et al. Dipeptidyl peptidase-4 inhibitors, glucagon-like peptide 1 receptor agonists and sodium-glucose co-transporter-2 inhibitors for people with cardiovascular disease: a network meta-analysis. *Cochrane Database Syst Rev.* 2021;10(10):CD013650.

Knowler WC, Barrett-Connor E, Fowler SE, et al. Diabetes Prevention Program Research Group. Reduction in the incidence of type 2 diabetes with lifestyle intervention or metformin. *N Engl J Med.* 2002;346:393–403.

Malaisse WJ. Pharmacology of the meglitinide analogs: new treatment options for type 2 diabetes mellitus. *Treat Endocrinol.* 2003;2:401–414.

Meinert CL, Knatterud GL, Prout TE, Klimt CR. A study of the effects of hypoglycemic agents on vascular complications in patients with adult-onset diabetes. *Diabetes.* 1970;19(Suppl):789–830.

Nathan DM, Buse JB, Davidson MB, et al. Medical management of hyperglycemia in type 2 diabetes: a consensus algorithm for the initiation and adjustment of therapy: a consensus algorithm for the initiation and adjustment of therapy. *Diabetes Care.* 2008;31:1–11.

Richter B, Bandeira-Echtler E, Bergerhoff K, et al. Dipeptidyl peptidase-4 (DPP-4) inhibitors for type 2 diabetes mellitus. *Cochrane Database Syst Rev.* 2008;2008(2):CD006739.

Rubino A, McQuay LJ, Gough SC, et al. Delayed initiation of subcutaneous insulin therapy after failure of oral glucose-lowering agents in patients with type 2 diabetes: a population-based analysis in the UK. *Diabet Med.* 2007;24:1412–1418.

Scirica BM, Bhatt DL, Braunwald E, et al. Saxagliptin and cardiovascular outcomes in patients with type 2 diabetes mellitus. *N Engl J Med.* 2013;369(14):1317–1326.

Shyangdan DS, Royle P, Clar C, et al. Glucagon-like peptide analogues for type 2 diabetes mellitus. *Cochrane Database Syst Rev.* 2011;2011(10):CD006423.

Turner RC, Cull CA, Frighi V, Holman RR. Glycemic control with diet, sulfonylurea, metformin, or insulin in patients with type 2 diabetes mellitus: progressive requirement for multiple therapies (UKPDS 49). *JAMA.* 1999;281:2005–2012.

UKPDS Study Group (UKPDS 16). Overview of six years' therapy of type 2 diabetes – a progressive disease. *Diabetes.* 1995;44:1249–1258.

US Department of Health and Human Services. *2008 Physical Activity Guidelines for Americans.* www. health.gov/PAGuidelines/guidelines/default.aspx. Accessed December 26, 2023.

Van de Laar FA, Lucassen PLB, Akkermans RP, et al. Alpha-glucosidase inhibitors for type 2 diabetes mellitus. *Cochrane Database Syst Rev.* 2005;2005(2):CD003639.

Varvaki Rados D, Catani Pinto L, Reck Remonti L, et al. The association between sulfonylurea use and all-cause and cardiovascular mortality: a meta-analysis with trial sequential analysis of randomized clinical trials. *PLoS Med.* 2016;13(4):e1001992.

Weyer C, Bogardus C, Mott DM, Pratley RE. The natural history of insulin secretory dysfunction and insulin resistance in the pathogenesis of type 2 diabetes mellitus. *J Clin Invest.* 1999;104:787–794.

Yki-Jarvinen H. Drug therapy: thiazolidinediones. *N Engl J Med.* 2004;351:1106.

Zelniker TA, Wiviott SD, Raz I, et al. SGLT2 inhibitors for primary and secondary prevention of cardiovascular and renal outcomes in type 2 diabetes: a systematic review and meta-analysis of cardiovascular outcome trials. *Lancet.* 2019;393(10166):31–39.

A 75-year-old Man Diagnosed With Metastatic Non-small Cell Lung Cancer

Jacob Varney, MD and Vajeeha Tabassum, MD, FACP

John is a 75-year-old man married to Mary, 74-years-old, for 43 years. They have just moved to live close to their daughter and have always had active lifestyles. They invested their retirement funds in a condominium near a golf course. Despite John's history of hypertension, coronary artery disease, diabetes, 25-pack-year smoking history, and chronic kidney disease stage G3b, John was doing well at home until about 2 months ago when he noticed shortness of breath on exertion. Mary had suffered a fall around the same time with a fracture of her hip requiring hospitalization. Initially, John and his family attributed his shortness of breath to high humidity, increased physical demands in caring for Mary, and ongoing anxiety.

A few days ago, John's pain and shortness of breath increased and became persistent at rest. He went to the emergency department and was diagnosed with subsegmental pulmonary emboli with a left hilar mass, bilateral hilar and mediastinal lymphadenopathy, and multiple hypodense liver lesions. The physician in the ED calls you to admit the patient. She tells you she shared with John and Mary that there were findings concerning for cancer.

1. **In addition to performing a routine admission history and physical exam, what additional assessments are warranted at this time?**

    A. Decision-making capacity

    B. Advance directives

    C. Information preferences

    D. Code status

    E. All of the above

    F. None of the above

Answer: E. All of the above

All patients making medical decisions should be assessed for whether or not they have capacity to make the specific medical decision in question. The Aid for Capacity Evaluation (ACE) is a validated instrument for decision making capacity assessment. While completing advance directives is always voluntary, it is often

409

prudent and encouraged to appoint a healthcare power of attorney. It is important to know if prior documents exist and whether they are congruent with a patient's current wishes. Regarding information preferences, it is best practice to assess a) what a patient already knows, b) what they would like to know, and c) who else should know prior to disclosing medical information. Code status discussions are often best after a full shared understanding of the patient's condition, prognosis, treatment options, and expected outcome, but a brief assessment and default determination is frequently performed on admission. For additional suggestions on code status conversations, refer to "Fast Fact" #365 and #366. The "GO-FAR" calculator helps predict neurologic outcomes following cardiac arrest and can assist in informed decision-making.

Following admission, John's liver biopsy confirms metastatic squamous cell carcinoma. You arrange for John, Mary, and their daughter to meet you at the bedside in the afternoon.

2. What techniques or tools should be used to disclose new medical information?

Answer:

The "Ask – Tell – Ask" technique is a simple way to engage with patients and help optimize the effectiveness of the conversation. The first "ask" can represent asking for permission, asking what someone already knows, or asking what they want to know. "Tell" refers to disclosing new information or clarifying understanding. The second "ask" can check for understanding or inquire about what the patient thinks about information you disclosed.

When breaking bad news, SPIKES is a commonly employed framework [insert chart / summary of SPIKES; **S**et up the interview. Assess the patient's **P**erception. Obtain the patient's **I**nvitation (ask for permission). Give **K**nowledge and information to the patient. Address the patient's **E**motion with empathetic responses. **S**ummarize and discuss next steps.]

While John, Mary, and their daughter were saddened to learn his diagnosis, they express interest in meeting with an oncologist to explore his treatment options and prognosis.

PALLIATIVE CARE

Palliative care is "the active holistic care of individuals across all ages with serious health-related suffering due to severe illness and especially of those near the end of life. It aims to improve quality of life of patients, their families, and their caregivers." The palliative model of care recognizes the importance of symptom control, relief of suffering, and support for the best quality of life for patients and their families, regardless of the stage of illness or continuation of life sustaining treatment. While palliative care has been associated with oncology, patients with a serious illness due to any disease process may benefit from palliative care assessment and interventions. Table 37-1 compares the characteristics of curative and palliative care.

CASE REVIEW

John and Mary completed staging workup confirming stage IV disease with multiple metastatic sites and met with their oncologist, who openly shares that while John's cancer is incurable, he has treatment options that would prolong his life. The oncologist introduces a multidisciplinary and multimodal approach, with discussion at tumor board conference, consideration for radiation therapy and surgery if indicated, and palliative care referral. Based on John's values and goals, disease state, and good performance status, they decided to start on first line immunotherapy. John tolerates immunotherapy with only mild side effects; he returns to golfing and enjoying time with his family. While John begins to feel as if he is "winning" in his "battle" against his

Table 37-1. Characteristics of Curative Versus Palliative Care Models

Curative Model	Palliative Model
The primary goal is cure	The primary goal is relief of suffering
The objective of analysis is the disease process	The objective of analysis is the patient and the family
Symptoms are treated primarily as clues to the diagnosis	Distressing symptoms are treated as entities in themselves
Primary value is placed on measurable date, for example, lab tests	Both measurable and subjective dates are valued
This model tends to devalue information that is subjective, immeasurable, or unverifiable	This model values the patient's experience of an illness
Therapy is medically indicated if it eradicates or slows progression of disease	Therapy is medically indicated if it controls symptoms and relieves suffering
The patient's body is differentiated from the patient's mind	The patient is viewed as a complex being comprising physical, emotional, social, and spiritual dimensions
Death is the ultimate failure	Enabling a patient to live fully and comfortably until he or she dies is a success

cancer, Mary wonders if they are doing enough to prepare for John's future and the inevitable end of his life.

John and Mary meet with the palliative care team, including the palliative medicine physician, nurse, and social worker. At the first meeting, the patient's understanding of the diagnosis and purpose of treatment is reviewed and clarified, a comprehensive symptom assessment is performed, and an expanded social history sheds light on John's work and military history, hobbies, faith tradition, and family structure. When John references his cancer "battle," the team explores this analogy and advises caution in the setting of incurable illness. The team uses questions from the "Serious Illness Conversation Guide" to elicit John and Mary's hopes and worries, sources of strength, and acceptable burdens of treatment. Finally, the team assesses for prior advance directives, assists in the completion of a power of attorney for healthcare, and provides contacts for resources in the community.

Several months later, John notices increasing fatigue, cough, and dyspnea. Despite initial response to treatment, restaging imaging shows disease progression, and he is started on second-line immunotherapy.

Palliative interventions are primarily designed to provide comfort, not cure disease or extend life. Because palliative interventions control distressing symptoms and provide psychological and spiritual support, they may prolong a patient's life and improve its quality.

The essential components of hospice and palliative care include:

- A collaborative, interdisciplinary approach to caring for the patient and family. Core members of a palliative care team include a physician, nurse, social worker, and a chaplain or bereavement specialist.
- Helping the patient and family understand the patient's illness and prognosis.
- Alleviating the suffering of patients and families by focusing on all aspects of total pain: physical, emotional, spiritual, and social.
- Assessing symptoms and providing pharmacologic and nonpharmacologic management.
- Assessing patient values and goals, and aligning treatment to match these goals.
- Helping patients cope with the psychosocial and spiritual questions or distress associated with serious illness.
- Helping patients and families make the transition from health to illness to death to bereavement.

Table 37-2 lists a set of core principles for end-of-life care that were published by the Milbank Report in December 1999, which are embraced by a substantial number of medical societies and the Joint Commission on the Accreditation of Healthcare Organizations.

Table 37-2. Core Principles of End-of-life Care

Respect the dignity of both the patient and caregivers
Be sensitive to and respectful of the patient's and family's wishes
Use the most appropriate measures that are consistent with patient choices
Encompass alleviation of pain and other physical symptoms
Assess and manage psychological, social, and spiritual or religious problems
Offer continuity (eg, the patient should be able to receive continued care by primary care provider or specialist providers, if so desired)
Provide access to any therapy that may realistically be expected to improve the patient's quality of life, including alternative or nontraditional treatments
Provide access to palliative and hospice care
Respect the right to refuse treatment
Respect the physician's professional responsibility to discontinue some treatments when appropriate, with consideration for both patient and family preferences
Promote clinical and evidence-based research on providing care at the end of life

Several months later, John begins to have back pain. He is found to have vertebral metastases with associated compression fracture. He receives radiation and is started on opioid-sparing ("adjuvant") analgesics such as NSAIDs and bisphosphonates, which help with his pain. Due to progression of disease, his treatment plan is again modified, but he has used all possible biologic treatments available per National Comprehensive Cancer Network (NCCN) guidelines; he starts cytotoxic chemotherapy. He is no longer able to golf.

John and Mary meet with the palliative care team again. John is noticing increased side effects from chemotherapy, with fatigue, nausea, and neuropathy. The team provides evidence-based treatments in line with the National Comprehensive Cancer Network (NCCN) Palliative Care guidelines. Due to ongoing dyspnea, cough, and worsening back pain, John is started on short acting opioids. See [New Table] for a summary of symptom management interventions to consider.

The team explores how John and Mary are coping with John's illness and provides counseling. While supporting John's desire to live as long as possible while his quality of life is acceptable, they help John and Mary anticipate and plan for the future, considering end of life care settings, preferred place of death, and introducing hospice services. They share that hospice is a care program for patients who are expected to die in 6 months or less. Hospice includes visits from nurses, nurse aids, social worker, chaplain, bereavement services under the guidance of a physician. John begins to acknowledge his situation gradually and begins completing a number of tasks, including financial planning, making adjustments to his will and estate planning, and visiting with cherished family and friends.

A few months later, John is admitted to the hospital with confusion, progressive generalized weakness, and headaches. He is found to have brain metastases with leptomeningeal carcinomatosis. His oncologist shares that due to his poor performance status, he is no longer a candidate for chemotherapy.

He suggests that John meet with the hospice team to discuss services that could help him remain at home and provide assistance for Mary. The oncologist promises that he will be available to discuss any concerns. Mary then asks about the charges for hospice care. The physician reassures Mary that, in his case, hospice services are covered in full by Medicare and discusses the core principles of end-of-life care with John and his family. Mary agrees to talk with the hospice representative. The physician arranges for the referral. Mary cries quietly and thanks the physician for supporting them.

The hospice representative arrives, asks about John and Mary's situation, describes the hospice services that are offered, and tailors it to their needs. She emphasizes how the program focuses on keeping patients at home and avoiding readmission to the hospital, controlling pain and other symptoms with a focus on quality of life and relieving suffering. She shares that medications such as opioids are only started or increased when indicated for symptom management. She also discusses how health aids can intermittently assist with bathing and caregiving needs. Mary indicates a preference for John's primary care doctor to act as the hospice attending of record, who is supported by the hospice medical director.

John is discharged from the hospital to hospice home care. John remains comfortable as his condition declines over 3 weeks before he dies peacefully at home amidst family and friends. Mary is very grateful to the physicians involved and the hospice program.

Table 37-3 describes some of the roles that physicians who practice hospice and palliative care play.

Everyone involved in this process—patient, family members, and health care professionals—struggles with the challenging task of envisioning meaningful roles for a person who is dying but who may continue to live for several months. Researchers have identified some activities described as developmental tasks of dying patients. These tasks may help support a sense of meaning for persons during the final stages of their lives. However, caution should be taken as to not place burdens by insisting that dying patients engage in these activities. Listed in Table 37-4 are some of the activities described as developmental tasks.

The case of the 75-year-old man—follow-up: Over the next several months, the hospice bereavement counselor and trained hospice volunteers contact Mary at regular intervals and invite her to bereavement support groups.

Mary also has regular follow-up visits scheduled with her primary care doctor. She misses John deeply, however is more involved with life after 3 months and is extremely thankful for the team effort.

Table 37-3. Role of Physicians Practicing Hospice and Palliative Medicine

Care for patients

Provide guidance and support as patients make the transition from curative to palliative care

Provide competent assessments and diagnosis

Provide information about diagnosis, prognosis, and treatment options

Provide guidance during the process of making treatment decisions

Respect the patient's beliefs, values, and goals

Provide skilled, effective interventions that meet the patient's needs

Collaborate with the patient's attending physician and with members of the interdisciplinary team to achieve outcomes that meet the patient's needs

Offer caring presence

Support the patient's search for a renewed sense of meaning, purpose, and hope

Serve as an advocate to help patients receive needed services

Participate in teaching and research activities to improve the standards of patient care

Care for family members

Provide guidance and support as families make transition from curative to palliative goals for continued care

Provide information about diagnosis, prognosis, and treatment options

Provide guidance during the process of making treatment decisions so that the patient's wishes are honored

Adjust therapies to meet the capabilities of family members, and teach patient care techniques

Provide ongoing emotional support and reassurance

Care for self

Attain professional competence

Seek peer support

Learn stress management techniques and practice self-care activities, including taking time for exercise, interactions with family members, and vacations

Table 37-4. Development Tasks of People Who Are Dying

Develop a renewed sense of personhood and meaning
Find meaning of life through life review and personal narrative
Develop a sense of worthiness, both in the past and in the current situation
Learn to accept love and caring from other people
Bring closure to personal and community relationships
Say goodbye to family members and friends with expressions of regret, gratitude, appreciation, and affection
Ask for and grant forgiveness to estranged friends and family members so that reconciliation can occur
Say goodbye to community relationships
Bring closure to worldly affairs
Arrange for the transfer of fiscal, legal, and social responsibilities

TIPS TO REMEMBER

- Anyone with a serious illness, regardless of life expectancy or receipt of treatments with curative intent, can receive palliative care.
- Anyone with a terminal illness—with an expected prognosis of 6 months or less—qualifies for hospice care.
- In almost all states, Medicare pays all charges related to hospice care.
- Explore the patient's beliefs, values, and goals and make recommendations regarding treatment decisions in light of these.

COMPREHENSION QUESTIONS

1. Which factor best differentiates palliative care from hospice?
    A. Patient / surrogate declines life sustaining treatment
    B. Patient lacks decision making capacity
    C. Patient's prognosis is expected to be 6 months or less
    D. Patient requests increased symptom management (ie, increase in opioids)

2. Which of the following are true regarding transitioning to hospice?
    A. Patient must agree with hospice philosophy of care
    B. Patient may not remain full code
    C. Patient must stop all prior routine medications (antihypertensives, antidepressants, etc)
    D. Patient may not receive antibiotics

3. When a terminally ill patient is losing weight because of difficulties in swallowing, which of the following is the most appropriate first step?
   A. Surgical resection of the obstructing lesion
   B. Assess for the presence of oral candidiasis
   C. Placement of an esophageal stent
   D. Radiation therapy

Answers

1. **C.** While patients on hospice may lack decision making capacity, decline life sustaining treatment, and/or request improved symptom management, they are only eligible for hospice enrollment if they have a terminal diagnosis, for which life expectancy is expected to be 6 months or less.

2. **A.** Patients and families entering hospice should agree with the hospice philosophy of care, which is to promote patient and family quality of life while accepting that the terminal illness will continue to progress. While a full code status may be incongruent with the hospice philosophy of care, it is not required for a patient to transition to DNR status prior to hospice enrollment. Under Medicare guidelines, patients must discontinue treatments for the terminal illness that are intended to prolong life. However, patients who are not actively dying often continue medications such as antidepressants or antihypertensives, as withholding them could contribute to new or worsening symptoms. Patients on hospice who have symptoms from minor, non-life limiting infections such as a urinary tract infection may receive appropriate antibiotics.

3. **B.** Impaired oral intake could be a consequence of dry mouth, altered taste or small, stomatitis, odynophagia, dysphagia, severe constipation, bowel obstruction, nausea, vomiting or uncontrolled pain, or dyspnea. Clinicians should focus on the identifiable treatable causes of difficulty swallowing. After triaging for common and more easily reversible problems, further evaluation for other problems could be considered if medically appropriate and in line with the patient's goals of care.

SUGGESTED READINGS

Baile WF, Buckman R, Lenzi R, et al. SPIKES—a six-step protocol for delivering bad news: application to the patient with cancer. *Oncologist.* 2000;5(4):302–311.

Bernacki R, Hutchings M, Vick J, et al. Development of the Serious Illness Care Program: a randomised controlled trial of a palliative care communication intervention. *BMJ Open.* 2015;5(10):e009032.

Center to Advance Palliative Care. www.capc.org. Accessed December 26, 2023.

Ebell MH, Jang W, Shen Y, Geocadin RG; Get With the Guidelines–Resuscitation Investigators. Development and validation of the Good Outcome Following Attempted Resuscitation (GO-FAR) score to predict neurologically intact survival after in-hospital cardiopulmonary resuscitation. *JAMA Intern Med.* 2013;173(20):1872–1878.

Education in Palliative and End of Life Care (EPEC). www.epec.net. Accessed December 26, 2023.

End of Life—Palliative Education Resource Center. www.eperc.mcw.edu. Accessed December 26, 2023.

Goldish A, Rosielle DA. Language for routine code status discussions #365. *J Palliat Med.* 2019;22(1):98–99.

Goldish A, Rosielle DA. Recommending a do not resuscitate order for patients with advanced illness #366. *J Palliat Med.* 2019;22(1):100–101.

Hui D, Zhukovsky DS, Bruera E. Serious illness conversations: paving the road with metaphors. *Oncologist.* 2018;23(6):730–733.

Maxwell TL, Martinez JM, Knight CF. The hospice and palliative medicine approach to life-limiting illness. In: Storey P, Levine, J, Shega J. *Unipac Series.* Glenview: Mary Ann Liebert; 2008:1–71.

National Hospice and Palliative Care Organization (includes state-specific advance directives). www.nhpco.org. Accessed December 26, 2023.

NCCN. *The National Comprehensive Cancer Network Palliative Care Guidelines.* www.nccn.org. Accessed December 26, 2023.

Paladino J, Koritsanszky L, Nisotel L, et al. Patient and clinician experience of a serious illness conversation guide in oncology: a descriptive analysis. *Cancer Med.* 2020;9(13):4550–4560.

Palliative Care Network of Wisconsin. /www.mypcnow.org. Accessed December 26, 2023.

Quill TE, Periyakoil V, Denney-Koelsch E, et al. AAHPM *Primer of Palliative Care.* 7th ed. Chicago: American Academy of Hospice and Palliative Medicine; 2019.

Radbruch L, De Lima L, Knaul F. Redefining palliative care—a new consensus-based definition. *J Pain Symptom Manage.* 2020;60(4):754–764.

Sessums LL, Zembrzuska H, Jackson JL. Does this patient have medical decision-making capacity? *JAMA.* 2011;306(4):420–427.

Vital Talk. www.vitaltalk.org. Accessed December 26, 2023.

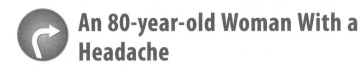

An 80-year-old Woman With a Headache

Noupama N. Mirihagalle, MD and Siegfried W. B. Yu, MD, FACP

An 80-year-old female presents to the outpatient clinic complaining of headache in the bilateral frontal and temporal regions. She says the headache has been present for at least a couple of years but has recently become worse over the past few months. It is described as squeezing in character with muscle tightness, graded around 8/10 in severity. She notes occasional nausea without vomiting. No sensitivity to light or sound is noted. She denies having any problems with vision, eye tearing, swallowing, speech, or neck pain. No bladder or bowel movement problems are noted. No complaints of new numbness or weakness are noted. The headache occurs throughout most of the day, every day, and it can happen any time. She has a background of hip arthritis, with prior hip replacement, and has been on chronic oral narcotic therapy. Due to the increase in headache severity, she has been taking more of her pain medication, without much benefit.

On examination, she is anxious and in mild distress due to the headache. She is afebrile, with a heart rate of 78 bpm and a blood pressure of 130/85 mm Hg. She is alert and oriented, and speech and expression are intact. Palpation of her temporal regions bilaterally does not elicit tenderness. Her face appears symmetric. Fundoscopy does not reveal papilledema. Cardiac examination and lung examination are normal. Normal sensory function is noted with light touch. Muscle strength is graded as 5/5 throughout with deep tendon reflexes 1+ throughout. There is pain with internal and external rotation of her right hip. Gait and stance including tiptoe and heel walking are normal but unsteady on tandem walk. Romberg sign is negative. Finger-to-nose testing does not reveal ataxia.

1. In light of her reported symptoms by history, what is the patient's most likely primary diagnosis?

2. What may be the precipitating factor in this case?

3. What management decision would you need to make at this time?

Answers

1. The patient's baseline chronic headache seems to have worsened with her increased narcotic pain medication use, which she originally started for her arthritic pain. In light of her reported symptoms by history, and lack of other striking features on her history and examination, the patient's most likely primary diagnosis is a medication-overuse headache, with a likely underlying preceding tension-type headache (TTH).

2. Narcotic pain medications are the likely precipitating factor.

3. It would be reasonable to attempt a taper off of her narcotic pain medications and reassess her symptoms. Due to her age, it would be also appropriate to exclude secondary causes of her headache.

CASE REVIEW

Although the character of the patient's headache does not appear to suggest a very specific cause, her presentation forces one to think about the various potential causes of headache. Because of her advanced age, it is important that we start by excluding specific secondary causes of headache, such as temporal arteritis, and vascular dissection. Migraine-type symptoms, such as aura, laterality, nausea, and vomiting, are not present, but likewise, because of her age at onset, these symptoms would still prompt a search for a secondary cause of the headache. Likewise, a thorough physical examination, with careful attention to neurologic function, is important for assessing the cause of the headache. Ultimately, the most prominent feature of her history was the increased use of narcotic pain medication, which is the most likely cause. In order to fully exclude other causes of headache, however, it would be appropriate to assess inflammatory markers, such as the erythrocyte sedimentation rate (ESR), and an advanced imaging study, such as CT or MRI, because of her advanced age.

HEADACHES

Pathophysiology

Headache may originate from one of the following mechanisms of pain perception: (1) pain that is the result of a normal physiologic response from a healthy nervous system or (2) pain that results when pain-producing pathways are damaged or activated inappropriately. Pain, in general, usually occurs when peripheral nociceptors are stimulated in response to tissue injury, visceral distention, or other factors. In regard to headache, the scalp, middle meningeal artery, dural sinuses, falx cerebri, and proximal segments of the large pial arteries are the pain-producing structures. The primary structures involved in primary headache include the large intracranial vessels and dura mater, the peripheral terminals of the trigeminal nerve that innervate these structures, the caudal portion of the trigeminal nucleus (the trigeminocervical complex), and the pain modulatory systems in the brain that receive input from the trigeminal nociceptors. The trigeminovascular system is composed of the trigeminal innervation of the large intracranial vessels and respective dura mater (see Figure 38-1). It is not surprising that lacrimation and nasal congestion are prominent in the trigeminal

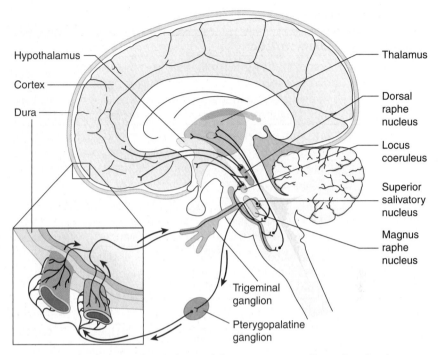

Hypothalamus

Cortex

Dura

Thalamus

Dorsal raphe nucleus

Locus coeruleus

Superior salivatory nucleus

Magnus raphe nucleus

Trigeminal ganglion

Pterygopalatine ganglion

Figure 38-1. Brainstem pathways that modulate sensory input. (Reproduced with permission from Fauci AS, Braunwald E, Kasper DL, et al, eds. *Harrison's Principles of Internal Medicine.* 17th ed. New York: McGraw-Hill; 2008.)

autonomic cephalgias (TACs), such as cluster headache and paroxysmal hemicranias, as well as some migraine headaches.

Diagnosis

A thorough history is the most important way to differentiate among the different causes of headache, which are many (Table 38-1). A classification dividing the headache types into primary headache (those in which headache and its associated features are the primary disorder) and secondary headache (those in which the headaches are secondary to another distinct disorder) has been developed by the International Headache Society (IHS). See Table 38-2 for common causes of headache.

PRIMARY HEADACHES

Primary headache disorders often result in significant disability and decreased quality of life. Among them, the most common are TTH, migraine headache, and idiopathic stabbing headache.

Table 38-1. Differential Diagnosis of Headache

Disease	Characteristics
Tension-type headache	Common; duration 30 min–7 days; typically bilateral, nonpulsating pressing quality; mild to moderate in intensity without prohibiting activity; no nausea, vomiting, no more than one of photophobia or phonophobia (anorexia may occur)
Cluster headache	Uncommon; sudden onset; duration, minutes to hours; severe and sharp or stabbing quality, repeats over a course of weeks, and then disappears for months or years; often unilateral tearing and nasal congestion; pain is severe, unilateral, and periorbital; more common in men
Frontal sinusitis	Usually worse when lying down; associated with nasal congestion; tenderness over affected sinus
Cervical spondylosis	Worse with neck movement; posterior distribution; pain is neuralgic and sometimes referred to vertex or forehead; more common in elderly patients
Greater occipital neuralgia	Occipital location; tenderness at base of skull; pain is neuralgic in character and sometimes referred to vertex or forehead; more common in elderly patients
Postconcussion syndrome	History of antecedent head trauma; vertigo (often positional), light-headedness, or giddiness; poor concentration and memory; lack of energy; irritability and anxiety
Trigeminal neuralgia	Brief episodes of sharp, stabbing pain with trigeminal nerve distribution
TMJ dysfunction	Pain generally involves the TMJ and temporal areas and is associated with symptoms when chewing
Medication-induced headache	Chronic headache with a few features of migraine; tends to occur daily; HRT and hormonal contraceptives are frequent culprits
Subarachnoid hemorrhage	Explosive onset of severe headache; 10% preceded by "sentinel" headaches
Acute or chronic subdural	History of antecedent trauma; may have subacute onset; altered level of consciousness or neurologic deficit, hematoma may be present
Meningitis	Fever; meningeal signs
Encephalitis	Associated with neurologic abnormalities, confusion, altered mental state, or change in level of consciousness
Intracranial neoplasms	Worse on awakening; generally progressive; aggravated by coughing, straining, or changing position

(Continued)

Table 38-1. Differential Diagnosis of Headache (*Continued*)

Disease	Characteristics
Benign intracranial hypertension (pseudotumor cerebri)	Often abrupt onset; associated with nausea, vomiting, dizziness, blurred vision, and papilledema; may have CN VI palsy; headache aggravated by coughing, straining, or changing position
Temporal arteritis	Occurs almost exclusively in patients aged over 50; associated with tenderness of scalp or temporal artery, and jaw claudication; visual changes
Acute severe hypertension	Marked BP elevation (systolic ≥210 mm Hg; diastolic ≥120 mm Hg); may have symptoms of encephalopathy (eg, confusion, irritability)
CO poisoning	May be insidious or associated with dyspnea; occurs more commonly in the colder months
Acute glaucoma	Associated with blurred vision, nausea, vomiting, and seeing halos around lights; ophthalmologic emergency
Carotid dissection	Cause of stroke; can be spontaneous or following minor trauma or sudden neck movement; unilateral headache or face pain; ipsilateral Horner syndrome; ophthalmologic emergency

BP, blood pressure; CN VI, cranial nerve VI; CO, carbon monoxide; HRT, hormone replacement therapy; TMJ, temporomandibular joint.

Data from Wilson JF. In the clinic. Migraine. *Ann Intern Med.* 2007;147(9):ITC11-1–ITC11-6.

Table 38-2. Common Causes of Headache

Primary Headache Type	%	Secondary Headache Type	%
Migraine	16	Systemic infection	63
Tension-type	69	Head injury	4
Cluster	0.1	Vascular disorders	1
Idiopathic stabbing	2	Subarachnoid hemorrhage	<1
Exertional	1	Brain tumor	0.1

Data from Olesen J, Goadsby PJ, Ramadan N, et al. *The Headaches.* Philadelphia: Lippincott Williams & Wilkins; 2005.

Tension Headache

TTH describes a chronic headache syndrome characterized by bilateral, tight, band-like discomfort, with pain that builds slowly, fluctuates in severity, and may persist continuously for many days. It can be episodic or chronic (>15 days in a month). An approach to TTH may clearly delineate them based on the absence of nausea, vomiting, photophobia, phonophobia, osmophobia, throbbing, and aggravation with movement. This simplifies TTH in contrast to migraine headache; however, other definitions allow for degrees of nausea, photophobia, and phonophobia. TTH may represent a primary disorder of central nervous system pain modulation.

Migraine Headache

Migraine headache is the second most common cause of headache and is usually associated with triggers. It is episodic and has features such as light, sound, and movement sensitivity, as well as nausea and vomiting. It affects 15% of women and 6% of men. It is a syndrome of recurring headache, which is generally benign, and associated with other symptoms of neurologic dysfunction. A useful mnemonic for the symptoms of migraine headache is POUND. P indicates a pulsatile quality of headache. O indicates 1-day duration (<4 hours suggests TTH). U indicates unilateral location. N indicates the presence of nausea or vomiting. D indicates a disabling intensity. The presence or absence of these features can be used to formulate the probability that the headache is a migraine headache versus a TTH (see Table 38-3).

Idiopathic Stabbing Headache

Idiopathic stabbing headache is also known as primary stabbing headache. Ophthalmodynia periodica is a relatively uncommon headache syndrome. Most patients have another coexisting primary headache disorders such as migraine or cluster headache. This headache is characterized by transient, sharp head pains typically lasting for a few seconds, occurring anywhere in the head though typically outside trigeminal regions. Patients may also report nausea, vomiting, and photophobia but no cranial autonomic symptoms. Symptoms of primary stabbing headache may also be due to secondary causes; these need to be excluded with neuroimaging and other diagnostic testing prior to the diagnosis. Common differential diagnosis of idiopathic stabbing headache includes subtypes of trigeminal autonomic cephalgias (TACs), such as cluster headache, paroxysmal hemicranias, and short-lasting unilateral neuralgiform headache attacks with conjunctival injection and tearing (SUNCT). These are characterized by relatively short-lasting attacks of head pain with associated lacrimation, conjunctival injection, or nasal congestion (see Table 38-4).

Table 38-3. Elements of Patient History for Clinical Diagnosis of Migraine Versus Tension-type Headache

Clinical Feature	Sensitivity (%)	Specificity (%)	Positive Likelihood Ratio	Negative Likelihood Ratio
Nausea or vomiting	42–60	81–93	6	0.62
Duration 4–72 h	74	53	1.6	0.49
Pounding or throbbing character	64–87	22–83	3.8	0.43
Unilateral head pain	65–75	60–85	4.3	0.41
Disabling for usual activities	59–87	52–76	2.5	0.54
Presence of ≥4 of the above symptoms	29	100	23	0.71
Presence of ≥3 of the above symptoms	80	94	13	0.21
Presence of ≥2 of the following 3 symptoms: nausea, photophobia, and headache-related disability (any day in the previous 3 months)	81	75	3.25	0.25

Other Headaches

Other variants of headache include medication-overuse headache, which typically occurs in the context of overuse of narcotic or barbiturate-containing analgesics, which results in a daily or near-daily headache that is refractory. This headache should be strongly considered in patients using these types of medications. This is not likely a separate headache entity, but a consequence of overuse of this type of medication. Likewise, another broad diagnosis is chronic daily headache (CDH) that is present when a patient experiences headache more than 15 days per month, and while it may include medication-overuse headaches, it may also be caused by secondary causes of headache, such as trauma, infection, inflammation, low cerebrospinal fluid (CSF) volume headache, and raised CSF pressure headache.

Table 38-4. Clinical Features of the Trigeminal Autonomic Cephalgias

	Cluster Headache	Paroxysmal Hemicranias	SUNCT
Gender	M > F	F = M	F ~ M
Pain type	Stabbing, boring	Throbbing, boring, stabbing	Burning, stabbing, sharp
Severity	Excruciating	Excruciating	Severe to excruciating
Site	Orbit, temple	Orbit, temple	Periorbital
Attack frequency	1/alternate day to 8/day	1–40/day (>5/day for more than half the time)	3–200/day
Duration of attack	15–180 min	2–30 min	5–240 s
Autonomic features	Yes	Yes	Yes (prominent conjunctival injection and lacrimation)[a]
Migrainous features[b]	Yes	Yes	Yes
Alcohol trigger	Yes	No	No
Cutaneous triggers	No	No	Yes
Indomethacin effect	—	Yes[c]	—
Abortive treatment	Sumatriptan injection or nasal spray, oxygen	No effective treatment	Lidocaine (IV)
Prophylactic treatment	Verapamil, methysergide, lithium	Indomethacin	Lamotrigine, topiramate, gabapentin

SUNCT, short-lasting unilateral neuralgiform headache attacks with conjunctival injection and tearing.

[a]If conjunctival injection and tearing not present, consider SUNA.

[b]Nausea, photophobia, or phonophobia; photophobia and phonophobia are typically unilateral on the side of the pain.

[c]Indicates complete response to indomethacin.

Secondary causes of headache are many, and it is paramount that these are appropriately excluded before assuming a headache is due to a primary cause. Much of this can be determined by a thorough history and physical examination. Some major causes to take note of include meningitis, intracranial hemorrhage, brain tumor, temporal arteritis, and glaucoma. It is important to assess for alarm features that suggest headache due to secondary, non-benign causes (see Table 38-5).

The physical examination should be directed to evaluate features suggestive of a secondary headache. This includes evaluation of blood pressure, the presence of fever, meningeal signs or other signs of infection, neurologic deficits, visual acuity changes, increased intraocular pressure, and mental status changes. As noted above, combined with thorough history-taking, a thorough physical examination plays an essential role in the diagnosis of headache syndromes.

Depending on the clinical impression, and what causes of headache are necessary to confirm and exclude, laboratory testing should proceed in an evidence-based manner. For example, for a patient with a new-onset headache after 50 years of age, it would be important to obtain an ESR to exclude

Table 38-5. "Red Flag" or Alarm Features That Suggest Headache Is Due to Non-benign, Secondary Causes

Daily headache
Dizziness, syncope, discoordination, blurred vision or focal neurologic abnormality
Sudden, explosive onset
Headaches associated with maneuvers that increase or decrease intracranial pressure (pain worse with coughing or movement)
Change in personality or mental status
Headache awakens person from sleep
Onset after 50 years of age
Signs or symptoms of systemic illness (fever, chills, weight loss)
Meningeal signs
Diastolic blood pressure >120 mm Hg
Diminished pulse or tenderness of temporal artery
Papilledema
Necrotic or tender scalp lesions
Increased intraocular pressure

secondary causes of headache such as temporal arteritis and other vasculitides. If elevated, this would lead to a temporal artery biopsy to confirm the diagnosis. On the other hand, if fever and neck rigidity were the prominent features, performing a lumbar puncture would be more important to establish the diagnosis. Laboratory testing may also need to be done if the patients' symptoms are severe enough to cause significant metabolic derangements that may require correction.

Advanced neuroimaging, such as MRI, should be performed particularly in patients with atypical headache features, substantial changes in headache pattern, or symptoms or signs of neurologic abnormalities. It is also important to note, however, that certain instances may occur in which serious causes of headache exist and neuroimaging may be normal (see Table 38-6).

Treatment

Once the diagnosis is clearly established, treatment may be pursued. TTH can generally be managed with simple analgesics such as acetaminophen, NSAIDs, or aspirin. For chronic TTH, amitriptyline is the only proven treatment. Other pharmacologic treatments such as other tricyclics, selective serotonin reuptake inhibitors, and benzodiazepines have not been shown to be effective. Relaxation can be effective.

For mild to moderate migraine headaches not associated with vomiting, over-the-counter analgesics such as acetaminophen, aspirin, or NSAIDs (alone or in combination) may be sufficient. Standard treatment for severe acute migraine headache, however, typically includes the use of triptan medications (see Table 38-7), although other classes of medications can be used with good

Table 38-6. Serious Causes of Headache in Which Neuroimaging Findings May Be Normal

Giant cell or temporal arteritis
Glaucoma
Trigeminal or glossopharyngeal neuralgia
Lesions around sella turcica
Warning leak of aneurysm (sentinel bleed)
Inflammation, infection, or neoplastic invasion of leptomeninges
Cervical spondylosis
Pseudotumor cerebri
Low intracranial pressure syndromes (cerebrospinal fluid leaks)

Table 38-7. Short-term Drug Treatment for Migraine and Migraine-specific Medications

Agent (Route)	Mechanism of Action	Dosage	Notes
Sumatriptan (subcutaneous)	Selective serotonin (5-HT1B/1D) agonist	6 mg at onset (may repeat after 1 h; maximum 12 mg/day)	Rapid onset of action; little sedation; treatment of choice for moderate-severe attacks; not effective if given during aura; contraindicated in patients with CAD, uncontrolled hypertension, or strictly basilar or hemiplegic migraine; pregnancy category C
Sumatriptan (oral)	Selective serotonin (5-HT1B/1D) agonist	25–100 mg at onset (may repeat after 2 h; maximum 200 mg/day)	Well tolerated; little sedation; less rapid onset; may be used again for recurrent headache; no evidence of teratogenicity
Sumatriptan (nasal)	Selective serotonin (5-HT1B/1D) agonist	20 mg at onset (may repeat after 2 h; maximum 40 mg/day)	Well tolerated; little sedation; speed of action and effectiveness similar to oral sumatriptan; useful when nonoral route of administration needed; no evidence of teratogenicity
Almotriptan (oral)	Selective serotonin (5-HT1B/1D) agonist	6.25–12.5 mg at onset (maximum 25 mg/day)	Similar efficacy to oral sumatriptan

(Continued)

Table 38-7. Short-term Drug Treatment for Migraine and Migraine-specific Medications (*Continued*)

Agent (Route)	Mechanism of Action	Dosage	Notes
Eletriptan (oral)	Selective serotonin (5-HT1B/1D) agonist	20–40 mg at onset (may repeat after 2 h; maximum 80 mg/day)	Highly effective oral triptan; rapid onset of action; slightly higher efficacy compared with oral sumatriptan
Frovatriptan (oral)	Selective serotonin (5-HT1B/1D) agonist	2.5 mg at onset (may repeat after 2 h; maximum 7.5 mg/day)	Well tolerated; little sedation; effective for prevention of menstrual migraine
Naratriptan (oral)	Selective serotonin (5-HT1B/1D) agonist	1.0–2.5 mg at onset (may repeat after 4 h; maximum 5 mg/day)	Possibly lower risk for headache recurrence than other oral triptans; relatively lower efficacy and incidence of side effects than other triptans
Rizatriptan (oral)	Selective serotonin (5-HT1B/1D) agonist	5–10 mg at onset (may repeat after 2 h; maximum 30 mg/day)	Available in a fast-melt preparation, which may be no faster in providing pain relief than the regular tablet; slightly higher efficacy compared with oral sumatriptan
Zolmitriptan (oral)	Selective serotonin (5-HT1B/1D) agonist	1.25–2.5 mg at onset (may repeat after 2 h; maximum 10 mg/day)	Similar efficacy to oral sumatriptan; also available in a rapidly dispersing tablet formulation
Dihydroergotamine (nasal)	Nonselective serotonin agonist	1 spray (0.5 mg) into each nostril (may repeat after 15 min; maximum 4 sprays/day, 8/week)	No sedation; should not be used with a 5-HT1B/1D; pregnancy category X

(*Continued*)

Table 38-7. Short-term Drug Treatment for Migraine and Migraine-specific Medications (*Continued*)

Agent (Route)	Mechanism of Action	Dosage	Notes
Dihydroergotamine (all other routes)		1 mg SC/IM/IV (may repeat after 1 h; maximum 2 mg/dose, 3 mg/attack, 6 mg/week)	Useful in status migrainosus; contraindicated in patients with CAD; pregnancy category X
Lasmiditan (oral)	Selective serotonin 1F receptor agonist	50–100 mg (no benefits of repeating for the same migraine attack, may increase 100–200 mg in subsequent attacks)	Approved by FDA in 2019; most common adverse effect is dizziness, which is dose dependent

effectiveness (see Table 38-8). For those with contraindications to, or who do not tolerate triptans, a calcitonin gene-related peptide (CGRP) antagonist or lasmiditan may be effective. Less effective nonspecific short-term drug treatments for migraine include acetaminophen, chlorpromazine, prochlorperazine, topical lidocaine, isometheptene-containing preparations, and codeine combinations. Codeine and other narcotics have a high potential for "rebound" headaches and opiate dependence and should generally be avoided. Conflicting evidence for migraine treatment exists for ergotamine/caffeine oral preparations, and dexamethasone or other corticosteroids.

It is important to note that triptans do not have a class effect; therefore, lack of efficacy or intolerance of side effects to one triptan does not predict a patient's response to other triptans. The dose may need to be repeated in order to be effective. Triptans are contraindicated in patients with coronary artery disease (CAD) or uncontrolled hypertension. Antiemetic agents can be used in conjunction with analgesics and migraine-specific medications to address migraine-associated nausea and vomiting. In particular, metoclopramide may address both pain and nausea symptoms.

Preventive migraine treatments are indicated in several situations. Patients with frequent disabling migraine headaches (>4 per month) or headaches that

Table 38-8. Short-term Drug Treatment for Migraine and Non-migraine-specific Medications

Agent (Route)	Mechanism of Action	Dosage	Notes
Naproxen and other NSAIDs (oral)	Inhibits cyclooxygenase, decreases prostaglandin synthesis	500 mg at onset (may repeat after 6–8 h)	Well tolerated; treatment of choice for mild to moderate attacks; may be given with antiemetic; avoid in pregnancy after 32-week gestation; pregnancy category B
Aspirin/ metoclopramide (oral)	Blocks dopamine receptors in CTZ; increases response to acetylcholine in upper GI tract	650/10 mg at onset (may repeat after 3–4 h)	Antinausea effect; elderly are more likely to develop dystonic reactions than younger adults; use lowest recommended doses initially; pregnancy category C (D in third trimester)
Butorphanol (nasal)	Opiate agonist–antagonist	1 spray in 1 nostril (may repeat after 1 h)	Well-tolerated rescue medication; risk for opiate dependence; pregnancy category C
Metoclopramide/ diphenhydramine (intravenous)	Blocks dopamine receptors in CTZ	20–25 mg over 20 min (may repeat after 1 h)	Antinausea effect; recent RCT showed equal effectiveness to sumatriptan; pregnancy category C

last longer than 12 hours are generally candidates for preventive treatments. Migraine attacks that cause significant disability, contraindications to acute therapies or serious adverse effects of acute therapies, menstrual migraines, neurologic impairments such as hemiplegic migraine, migraine with brainstem aura, and migrainous infarctions qualify for preventive treatments (Table 38-9). Other available options, which have lower efficacy and/or limited strength of evidence for prophylactic migraine therapy, include fluoxetine, verapamil, naproxen, feverfew, riboflavin, magnesium, and ACE inhibitors/angiotensin II receptor blockers.

Table 38-9. Preventive Drug Treatment for Migraine With Medium-to-high Efficacy

Agent	Mechanism of Action	Dosage	Notes
Amitriptyline	Inhibits norepinephrine	Amitriptyline, 30–150 mg PO qd	Anticholinergic effects, dry mouth, drowsiness; weight gain
Divalproex sodium, other anticonvulsants (eg, sodium valproate, gabapentin, topiramate)	Unknown	Divalproex sodium, 250–500 mg PO bid	Bone marrow suppression, liver inflammation, alopecia, tremors, weight loss with topiramate
Propranolol, other non-ISA beta-adrenergic antagonists (eg, timolol, atenolol, metoprolol, nadolol)	Beta-adrenergic antagonists	Propranolol, 120–240 mg PO qd in divided doses	Fatigue, bradycardia, hypotension (check blood pressure and heart rate before prescribing)
Methysergide	Selective serotonin agonist (5-HT2); constricts cranial and peripheral blood vessels	4–8 mg PO qd	Limited by side effect concerns— retroperitoneal fibrosis, pulmonary fibrosis, nausea, vomiting—no longer available in the United States

Treatment of the TAC primary headache category is reviewed in Table 38-4. Treatment of secondary headaches from a variety of causes should be targeted to the particular etiology at hand.

Chronic daily headache (CDH) that has evolved from medication-overuse headache is usually due to the overuse (>10 days per month for >3 months) of ergotamine tartrate, triptans, analgesics (especially those combined with barbiturates), narcotics, and possibly benzodiazepines. Some physicians think that even simple analgesics taken more than 15 days a month for more than 3 months can cause a daily headache syndrome. The overuse of triptan drugs is now becoming a common cause of this syndrome. In order to obtain control of these headaches, the medications have to be discontinued. Not only does the overuse of these medications cause the daily headache, but the daily use of these medications also prevents

other medications from working effectively. Treatment may require hospitalization with supervised withdrawal, and treatment with IV dihydroergotamine
combined with an antiemetic, such as metoclopramide. NSAIDs, beta blockers,
calcium channel blockers, and tricyclics do not cause a withdrawal syndrome.

TIPS TO REMEMBER

- A thorough history is the most important way to differentiate among the different causes of headache, which are many.
- A useful mnemonic for the symptoms of migraine headache is POUND. P
  indicates a pulsatile quality of headache. O indicates 1-day duration (<4 hours
  suggests TTH). U indicates unilateral location. N indicates the presence of
  nausea or vomiting. D indicates a disabling intensity.
- Overuse of narcotic or barbiturate-containing analgesics resulting in refractory
  daily or near-daily headaches should be strongly considered in patients using
  these drugs.
- The overuse of triptan drugs (more than 3 days a week, for 2 or more weeks) is
  now becoming a common cause of medication-overuse headache.
- It is important to assess for alarm features that suggest headache due to a
  secondary, nonbenign cause.
- There are serious causes of headache that exist and for which neuroimaging
  may be normal.
- For migraine treatment, codeine and other narcotics have a high potential for
  "rebound" headaches and opiate dependence and should generally be avoided.
- It is important to note that triptans do not have a class effect; therefore, lack of
  efficacy or intolerance of side effects to one triptan does not predict a patient's
  response to other triptans.
- Triptans are contraindicated in patients with CAD or uncontrolled
  hypertension.
- Preventive migraine treatment should be considered in patients with frequent
  disabling migraine headaches (>4 per month) and may reduce frequency by
  one-third to one-half.

COMPREHENSION QUESTIONS

1. A 25-year-old man presents to the clinic complaining of severe headaches near
his frontal sinus region that have been more frequent over the past week. They occur
multiple times a day, and he notes some associated tearing and nasal stuffiness.

Between the short attacks he feels okay. The headaches are described as sharp in character. No fever noted. He has not responded to nasal spray given at his last visit. On examination you don't find any sign of sinus tenderness or nasal congestion.

What is the diagnosis?

A. Migraine headache

B. Acute sinusitis

C. Brain tumor

D. Cluster headache

2. A 60-year-old woman presents to the clinic with 10 days of headaches that are severe. They are pounding in character, primarily on the right side, and are associated with some difficulty chewing her food. She is trying to read you a list of medications she has brought with her; however, she is having difficulty seeing out of her right eye.

What test would best confirm your diagnosis?

A. ESR

B. Temporal artery biopsy

C. MRI

D. Antineutrophilic cytoplasmic antibody (ANCA)

3. A 50-year-old man complains of sudden headache associated with tearing neck pain, dizziness, and vomiting. On your neurologic examination, you find leftward rapid eye movements, with drooping of his eyelid. He has lost sensation to his left face, and his right arm and leg. What is going on?

A. Paroxysmal hemicrania

B. Complicated migraine

C. Vertebral artery dissection

D. Normal pressure hydrocephalus

Answers

1. **D**. Based on the clinical features in this patient's history, the headache is not compatible with the typical migraine character of symptoms. Remember the mnemonic POUND. P indicates a pulsatile quality of headache. O indicates 1-day duration (<4 hours suggests TTH). U indicates unilateral location. N indicates the presence of nausea or vomiting. D indicates a disabling intensity. Although there is some suggestion of nasal congestion, the patient's history of short, frequent headaches without fever and examination findings absent for sinus tenderness do not suggest the problem is acute sinusitis. Brain tumor, though not fully excluded, would be expected to produce identifiable neurologic deficits and/or signs and symptoms of increased intracranial pressure.

2. B. The patient has a number of "red flags" in her history including her age, associated vision impairment, and a constellation of findings suggestive of temporal arteritis. ESR would be useful supportive testing; however, it would not necessarily be the best test to confirm the diagnosis. The association between giant cell arteritis and ANCA remains obscure despite several published studies.

3. C. This patient also has a number of "red flags" in his history, including his age, explosive onset, and neurologic deficits. The tearing neck pain, suggesting dissection, may be the etiology in light of the associated symptoms. Paroxysmal hemicrania is one of the TACs and is characterized by multiple short headaches affecting the orbit or temple, which are throbbing, boring, or stabbing in character. Complicated migraine would have a pain presentation of migraine character, which does not fit with this patient, and would have associated neurologic deficits. The patient's symptoms and findings do not fit with normal pressure hydrocephalus either, which is not in the differential diagnosis for headache. Furthermore, the headache is slow in onset and associated with symptoms of walking difficulty, slowing of mental function, and urinary incontinence.

SUGGESTED READINGS

Brian A, Crum M, Benarroch EE, Brown RD Jr. Neurology. Part II: general principles from the level of the cerebral cortex through the neuraxis to muscle. In: Ghosh AK, ed. *Mayo Clinic Internal Medicine Board Review*. 9th ed. New York: Oxford University Press; 2010.

Goadsby PJ, Ruskin NH. Headache. In: Fauci AS, Braunwald E, Kasper DL, et al, eds. *Harrison's Principles of Internal Medicine*. 17th ed. New York: McGraw Hill; 2008:95–106.

Wilson JF. In the clinic. Migraine. *Ann Intern Med*. 2007;147(9):ITC11-1–ITC11-16.

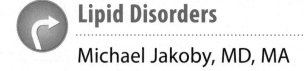

Lipid Disorders

Michael Jakoby, MD, MA

A 26-year-old Woman With Abdominal Pain

A 26-year-old female presents to the ED for evaluation of abdominal pain. Her history is notable for 2 episodes of acute pancreatitis occurring at ages 12 and 15 years. The patient was recently started on an oral contraceptive. Examination is notable for clusters of flesh-colored papules on extensor surfaces of the extremities and torso. Blood drawn in the ED is reported as "lipemic" by the laboratory.

1. What is the cause of lipemia?

2. What is the most likely etiology of abdominal pain?

3. What are appropriate treatment options for this patient?

Answers

1. The report of lipemic serum indicates significant hypertriglyceridemia, with a triglyceride level greater than 1000 mg/dL. The flesh-colored papules are eruptive xanthomas, a cutaneous indicator of hypertriglyceridemia. Severe hypertriglyceridemia that predisposes to acute pancreatitis is sometimes referred to as *chylomicronemia syndrome.*

2. Given knowledge of lipemic serum and 2 episodes of acute pancreatitis during adolescence, the patient most likely has hypertriglyceridemia-induced acute pancreatitis on this presentation. Oral estrogens such as the ethinyl estradiol in oral contraceptives may substantially increase triglyceride levels in susceptible women such as this patient. The patient's history of pancreatitis in adolescence implies lifelong hypertriglyceridemia and a diagnosis of Fredrickson's type I hyperlipoproteinemia due to deficiency of lipoprotein lipase (LPL), apo-lipoprotein CII, or compound heterozygosity for LPL and apo-CII deficiencies. The Fredrickson classification of dyslipidemias is presented in Table 39-1.

3. If the patient has mild pancreatitis with absence of worrisome features such as fever or hypothermia, tachycardia, tachypnea, leukocytosis or leukopenia, and

Table 39-1. Fredrickson Classification of Hyperlipidemias

Phenotype	Lipoprotein Abnormality	Lipid Abnormality
I	Chylomicrons	Hypertriglyceridemia
IIa	LDL	Hypercholesterolemia
IIb	VLDL and LDL	Combined hyperlipidemia
III	Chylomicron remnants and IDL	Combined hyperlipidemia
IV	VLDL	Hypertriglyceridemia
V	Chylomicrons and VLDL	Hypertriglyceridemia

multiorgan dysfunction on the Modified Marshall scoring system, then bowel rest (fasting), hydration, and treatment with pain medications and antiemetics is sufficient. In a recent study comparing conservative management and IV insulin for patients with triglyceride-induced acute pancreatitis, triglyceride levels improved by 45% in the first 24 h after admission and by nearly 80% on hospital day 4. If the patient has severe acute pancreatitis, an IV insulin, glucose, and potassium infusion or plasmapheresis may be utilized to expedite the improvement in triglyceride levels. Once the patient is able to eat, a low-fat (<10%–15% of daily calories from fat) diet and pharmacotherapy for triglycerides are indicated. The fibric acid derivatives fenofibrate and gemfibrozil are mainstays of pharmacotherapy.

CASE REVIEW

Lipids are sparingly soluble molecules that include cholesterol, fatty acids, and their derivatives. They are transported in the circulation by lipoprotein particles composed of proteins called apolipoproteins and phospholipids. Human plasma lipoproteins are classified into 5 major classes based on density: chylomicrons (least dense), very low-density lipoprotein (VLDL), intermediate-density lipoprotein (IDL), LDL, and HDL. A sixth class called lipoprotein(a) [Lp(a)] resembles LDL in lipid composition and has density that overlaps that of both LDL and HDL. Physical properties of lipoprotein particles are presented in Table 39-2.

There are three major lipid metabolic pathways. In the exogenous pathway, dietary long-chain fatty acids and cholesterol are esterified and assembled into chylomicrons as triglycerides and cholesterol esters, respectively. The primary structural protein on chylomicrons is apolipoprotein B48 (apo-B48). Chylomicrons are secreted into the lymphatic circulation by small bowel enterocytes and enter the venous circulation from the thoracic duct. Triglycerides are hydrolyzed to non-esterified fatty acids by the activity of the enzyme lipoprotein lipase (LPL), with apo-CII on chylomicrons serving as an essential cofactor.

Table 39-2. Physical Properties of Lipoproteins

Lipoprotein	Lipid Composition*	Apolipoproteins	Origin
Chylomicrons	TG 90%; chol 3%	B48; CI, CII, CIII; E	Intestine
VLDL	TG 55%; chol 20%	B100; CI, CII, CIII; E	Liver
IDL	TG 30%; chol 35%	B100; CI, CII, CIII; E	VLDL metabolism
LDL	TG 10%; chol 50%	B100	IDL metabolism
HDL	TG 5%; chol 20%	AI, AII, AIV; CI, CII, CIII; E	Liver, intestine
Lp(a)	TG 10%; chol 50%	B100; apo(a)	Liver

*Balance of composition is protein and phospholipid.
chol, cholesterol; HDL, high-density lipoprotein; IDL, intermediate-density lipoprotein; LDL, low-density lipoprotein; Lp(a), lipoprotein (a); TG, triglycerides; VLDL, very low-density lipoprotein.

Triglyceride-depleted chylomicrons are called chylomicron remnants and are cleared by the LDL receptor–like protein (LRP) in an interaction with apo-E.

Hepatic triglycerides and cholesterol esters are assembled into VLDL particles and secreted into the portal venous circulation in the endogenous lipid pathway. The main structural protein on VLDL particles is apo-B100, a high-affinity ligand for the LDL receptor. Triglycerides are hydrolyzed by LPL (with apo-CII as cofactor) to create triglyceride-depleted IDL. IDL can be cleared by binding to either LRP or LDL receptor or can undergo further removal of triglyceride by LPL or hepatic lipase to create cholesterol ester–enriched LDL particles. Apo-B100 is the only structural protein on LDL particles, and LDL is cleared by interaction of apo-B100 with LDL receptors expressed by liver and extrahepatic tissues.

HDL is the key lipoprotein in the reverse cholesterol pathway. Nascent HDL is secreted from the liver and small intestines as small apo-AI-containing discs. The discs acquire free cholesterol from peripheral tissues through activity of the cholesterol efflux regulatory protein ABC1. Cholesterol is then esterified by the enzyme lecithin:cholesterol acyltransferase (LCAT), with apo-AI serving as cofactor. At this time, the particles are termed HDL3. Larger HDL2 particles are formed by the acquisition of apolipoproteins and lipids released from delipidated chylomicrons and VLDL particles. HDL2 is converted back to HDL3 after removal of triglycerides by hepatic lipase or transfer of cholesterol esters to apo-B100-bearing lipoproteins (VLDL, IDL, or LDL particles) catalyzed by cholesterol ester transport protein (CETP), resulting in reverse cholesterol transport.

Lipid disorders are usually multifactorial in etiology and reflect the effects of uncharacterized genetic influences coupled with diet, inactivity, tobacco, alcohol, and comorbid conditions such as obesity and diabetes mellitus. However, some lipid abnormalities can be linked to specific causes, such as severe elevations of

Table 39-3. Differential Diagnosis of Major Lipid Disorders

Lipid Abnormality	Primary Disorders	Secondary Disorders
Cholesterol	Polygenic, familial hypercholesterolemia (FH), familial defective apo-B100	Hypothyroidism, nephrotic syndrome
Triglycerides	LPL deficiency, apo-CII deficiency, familial hypertriglyceridemia	Diabetes mellitus, obesity, metabolic syndrome, alcohol, medications (eg, oral estrogen)
Combined	Familial combined hyperlipidemia, type III hyperlipoproteinemia	Diabetes mellitus, obesity, metabolic syndrome, hypothyroidism, nephrotic syndrome
Low HDL	Familial a-lipoproteinemia, Tangier disease, LCAT deficiency	Diabetes mellitus, metabolic syndrome, hypertriglyceridemia, smoking

LDL cholesterol caused by inactivating LDL receptor mutations in familial hypercholesterolemia (FH) or severe triglyceride elevations in LPL deficiency states. The differential diagnosis of major lipid disorders is presented in Table 39-3.

Diagnosis

Hypertriglyceridemia is defined as a triglyceride level >150 mg/dL after a fast of 8 h or longer. In an analysis of adults ages ≥20 years who participated in National Health and Nutrition Examination Surveys (NHANES) conducted 2007 to 2014, the overall prevalence of hypertriglyceridemia was nearly 26%. Prevalence was higher in selected subgroups, with a high of 39.5% in patients with diabetes who were prescribed an HMG-CoA reductase inhibitor ("statin"). Most patients with moderate hypertriglyceridemia (150–499 mg/dL) have acquired factors that predispose to triglyceride elevations (Table 39-4). Moderate to severe (500–999 mg/dL) hypertriglyceridemia may be due to either acquired factors or reflect a primary disorder of triglyceride metabolism, and severe hypertriglyceridemia (≥1000 mg/dL) is usually caused by primary triglyceride disorders with monogenetic or polygenetic causes. Primary triglyceride disorders are presented in Table 39-5.

Patients with moderate hypertriglyceridemia rarely have signs or symptoms of their lipid abnormality. Patients with moderate to severe hypertriglyceridemia or more commonly severe hypertriglyceridemia may have overt clinical manifestations. Cutaneous xanthomas may be present at triglyceride levels ≥500 mg/dL and can indicate the type of triglyceride disorder, particularly in cases of Fredrickson

Table 39-4. Acquired Etiologies of Hypertriglyceridemia

Disease states

- Obesity
- Metabolic syndrome
- Type 2 diabetes mellitus
- Chronic renal disease (chronic renal failure, nephrotic syndrome)
- Hypothyroidism
- Pregnancy (typically third trimester)
- Multiple myeloma
- Systemic lupus erythematosus

Medications

- Thiazide diuretics
- Oral estrogens
- SERMS (tamoxifen, raloxifene)
- Beta blockers
- Glucocorticoids
- Immunosuppressants (cyclosporine, sirolimus, everolimus)
- Retinoids (isotretinoin, bexarotene, acitretin)
- Antiretrovirals (stavudine, ritonavir)
- Antipsychotic agents (olanzapine, clozapine)

Table 39-5. Primary Disorders of Triglyceride Metabolism

Phenotype*	Genetics	TG level (mg/dL)	Xanthomas
Type I	Monogenic	≥1000	Eruptive
Type V	Polygenic	≥1000	Eruptive
Type IV	Polygenic	≥500	Eruptive
Type III	Homozygous for apoE2 allele	≥500	Tuberoeruptive and palmar
Type IIb	Polygenic	≥500	Tuberous

*Fredrickson classification.

type III hyperlipoproteinemia, which is characterized by tuberoeruptive and palmar xanthomas. Severe hypertriglyceridemia may be complicated by the chylomicronemia syndrome, with manifestations including xanthomas, lipemia retinalis, hepatosplenomegaly, abdominal pain, dyspnea, and impaired cognition. The appearance of a plasma sample refrigerated overnight may help distinguish a patient's lipid disorder; in type I hyperlipoproteinemia the supernatant is creamy due to accumulation of chylomicrons and the infranatant is clear, but in type V hyperlipoproteinemia the supernatant is creamy along with a cloudy infranatant due to accumulation of both chylomicrons and VLDL particles. If the laboratory reports lipemic serum, triglyceride level is almost certainly >1000 mg/dL.

Indications to check triglyceride levels are as part of standard health screening, as part of management of patients with cardiovascular disease (CVD) or risk factors for CVD (diabetes mellitus, hypertension, tobacco use), in evaluation of patients with xanthomas, in evaluation of acute pancreatitis, as part of screening for potential familial etiologies of hypertriglyceridemia, and for monitoring the response to triglyceride lowering medications. Although fasting is often not required for measurements of cholesterol, initial lipid panels or those ordered to diagnose hypertriglyceridemia should be obtained after an 8- to 12-hour fast. A nonfasting triglyceride level greater than or equal to 400 mg/dL should prompt subsequent measurement of fasting lipids. Multiple lines of evidence indicate an association between hypertriglyceridemia and increased risk of cardiovascular disease, including Mendelian randomization studies that avoid potential confounding factors such as components of the metabolic syndrome and trials of HMG-CoA reductase inhibitors in high-risk patients. A recent retrospective longitudinal study of individuals at low to moderate risk for CVD found significantly increased risks of both all-cause mortality and CVD events in patients with high (150–500 mg/dL) and very high (>500 mg/dL) triglyceride levels compared to individuals with normal (<150 mg/dL) triglycerides.

Treatment

The goal of management in patients with hypertriglyceridemia is to reduce risks of acute pancreatitis and CVD. The risk of acute pancreatitis begins to increase at triglyceride levels above 500 mg/dL and is increased substantially when levels are greater than 1000 mg/dL, particularly in patients with a history of acute pancreatitis. Professional society treatment guidelines for lipid management to reduce CVD risk uniformly recognize a fasting triglyceride level above 150 mg/dL as elevated, and the 2016 European Society of Cardiology and European Atherosclerosis Society guidelines specifically recognize a triglyceride level below 150 mg/dL as desirable.

An overview of treatment options for hypertriglyceridemia is presented in Table 39-6. Fortunately, there are several nonpharmacologic interventions that improve triglyceride levels significantly. For example, exercise has been

Table 39-6. Treatment Options for Hypertriglyceridemia

Lipid-lowering medications

- Fibrates (fenofibrate and gemfibrozil)
- Marine omega-3 fatty acids
- Niacin
- HMG CoA reductase inhibitors

Nonpharmacologic interventions

- Aerobic exercise
- Weight loss
- Reduce consumption of total and saturated fat
- Reduce consumption of carbohydrates
- Increase consumption of fiber
- Reduce or eliminate alcohol
- Good glycemic control in cases of diabetes mellitus
- Change oral estradiol to topical
- Stop exacerbating medications when possible

demonstrated to reduce triglyceride levels by 15% to 25% independent of weight loss, and the American College of Cardiology recommends 150 minutes of moderate-intensity exercise weekly or 75 minutes of weekly high-intensity exercise for patients with hypertriglyceridemia. Weight reduction has significant effects on fasting triglyceride level; in a study of obese men, a slightly more than 10% weight loss from baseline reduced fasting triglycerides by approximately 40%. In the LIPGENE study, isocaloric diets that were either low fat or enriched in polyunsaturated fatty acids (PUFA) resulted in significant reductions in triglyceride levels compared to the high-saturated-fat control diet as well as a shift from small, dense LDL to larger, more buoyant particles. A study evaluating alcohol cessation and LDL particle distribution documented an approximately 45% improvement in triglyceride level and more favorable LDL particle size profile after 4 weeks of abstinence from alcohol in patients with hypertriglyceridemia. For patients with type 2 diabetes, there is a significant association between rising HbA1c and triglyceride levels, and triglycerides are approximately 40% higher in patients with HbA1c above 8% compared to patients with HbA1c below this threshold. Dietary changes, lifestyle modifications, and improved glycemic control in patients with diabetes are important interventions that improve triglyceride levels in patients with hypertriglyceridemia.

Fibric acid derivatives ("fibrates") are the mainstays of triglyceride-lowering pharmacotherapy and reduce triglyceride levels through effects on the transcription factor peroxisome proliferator activated receptor α (PPAR-α) that result in increased lipoprotein lipase activity, increased β-oxidation of long chain fatty acids, reduced VLDL production, and reduced expression of apo-CIII. Fibrates reduce triglycerides as much as 50% to 70% from baseline. The 2 fibrates available in the United States are fenofibrate and gemfibrozil, with fenofibrate generally preferred due to once-daily dosing and lower risk of adverse interactions with statins or other medications compared to gemfibrozil. Omega-3 fatty acids and niacin are somewhat less potent than fibrates but still achieve significant (25%–45%) reductions in triglyceride levels from baseline. Omega-3 fatty acids primarily reduce triglyceride levels by increasing fatty acid β-oxidation and reducing VLDL production, while niacin reduces VLDL production by inhibiting the activity of hormone sensitive lipase in adipose tissue and the enzyme diacylglycerol transferase-2 I hepatocytes. All the HMG-CoA reductase inhibitors reduce triglyceride levels, although only in hypertriglyceridemic patients and in proportion to reduction in LDL levels. Dosing information for fibrates, omega-3 fatty acid preparations, and niacin is presented in Table 39-7, and dosing information for statins is presented separately in Table 39-12.

Evidence that lowering triglyceride levels significantly reduces CVD risk is mixed. The results of key trials for fibrates, omega-3 fatty acids, and niacin are

Table 39-7. Medications for Management of Hypertriglyceridemia

Class and Drugs	Dosing
Fibrates	
Nanocrystal fenofibrate	48–145 mg daily with or without food
Micronized fenofibrate (generic)	67–200 mg daily with food
Nonmicronized fenofibrate (generic)	54–160 mg daily with food
Choline fenofibrate	45–135 mg daily with or without food
Gemfibrozil	600 mg twice daily 30 min before food
Omega-3 fatty acids (EPA and DHA)	
OTC fish oil concentrate capsules	Varies depending on triglyceride level
Lovaza	2 g twice daily or 4 g daily
EPA only	
Icosapent ethyl	2 g twice daily with food
Niacin	
Regular release	Up to 6 g daily in 3 divided doses
Niaspan (extended release)	1–2 g at bedtime

EPA, eicosapentaenoic acid; DHA, docosahexaenoic acid; OTC, over the counter.

Table 39-8. Selected Cardiovascular Outcomes Trials for Triglyceride-lowering Medications

Study	Drug	Statin	CVD Risk Reduction
Helsinki Heart Study	Gemfibrozil	No	Yes
VA-HIT	Gemfibrozil	No	Yes
FIELD	Fenofibrate	No	No
ACCORD	Fenofibrate	Yes	No
Coronary Drug Project	IR-niacin	No	No
AIM-HIGH	ER-niacin	Yes	No
HPS2-THRIVE	ER-niacin	Yes	No
JELIS	Icosapent ethyl	Yes	Yes
REDUCE-IT	Icosapent ethyl	Yes	Yes

ER, extended release; IR, immediate release.

presented in Table 39-8. In general, trials evaluating fibrates as monotherapy have demonstrated CVD risk reduction, but no benefit of fibrates has been observed when they are used in combination with statins. A recent meta-analysis of fibrate trials found no effects on all-cause mortality, CVD mortality, or stroke but a small reduction in coronary events rate. Low-dose (1 g/d) omega-3 fatty acids have not been shown to reduce CVD risk, but studies of icosapent ethyl 1.8 grams per day (JELIS) and 4 grams per day (REDUCE-IT) added to statins have shown significant reductions in CVD events. Neither studies of niacin alone or in combination with statins have shown significant reductions in CVD events (see Table 39-8).

A young male with low HDL cholesterol
A 25-year-old male is referred due to persistently low HDL cholesterol level. For the past 3 years, annual lipid panels have been notable for HDL levels of 20 to 25 mg/dL. A lipid panel was initially checked due to a family history of premature CVD. Total cholesterol is less than 200 mg/dL, triglycerides are less than 150 mg/dL, and LDL is in the range of 110 to 125 mg/dL. The patient does not smoke or take any prescription medications. He has no CVD symptoms or history, but his father has been treated for CVD and also has low HDL cholesterol.

1. What is the patient's most likely lipid disorder?

2. What is the next appropriate step in management?

Answers

1. This patient's persistently low HDL cholesterol level is due to primary familial hypoalphalipoproteinemia 1, an autosomal dominant disorder characterized by

HDL cholesterol levels below the 10th percentile for age and gender in the proband and at least 1 first-degree relative. The condition is caused by mutations in the apo-A1 gene, and gene mutation frequency is approximately 1:400. Familial hypoalphalipoproteinemia has been identified as a risk factor for CVD.

2. There are no HDL treatment targets in published lipid management guidelines due in large part to limited therapeutic options and an absence of trial data for patients with isolated low HDL cholesterol. Nonpharmacologic interventions including regular moderate-intensity exercise, weight loss in overweight or obese individuals, smoking cessation, and diets reduced in processed carbohydrates and saturated fats and high in polyunsaturated fats are advisable since they reduce CVD risk (though typical HDL increases are 5%–10% from baseline). Regular and moderate alcohol consumption also raises HDL cholesterol levels, but there are no recommendations to encourage alcohol intake in nondrinkers. Niacin is the best available pharmacologic intervention for low HDL and increases HDL levels by 15% to 25%. Given the patient's family history of early CVD, it would be reasonable to consider reducing LDL cholesterol with an HMG-CoA reductase inhibitor.

CASE REVIEW

Diagnosis

There is controversy regarding lipid screening in adults, mostly due to a lack of demonstrated benefit for younger adults. However, it is appropriate to obtain a screening lipid panel when young adults age 20 years or older establish care with a primary care provider, and all individuals with a family history of dyslipidemia or CVD should be screened. A fasting (8–12 h without food) lipid panel is preferred to avoid the need to reevaluate patients with hypertriglyceridemia on a nonfasting lipid profile, although the prognostic value of fasting and nonfasting LDL cholesterol measurements is similar. AHA/ACC recommendations for measuring LDL and non-HDL cholesterol from the latest guidelines are presented in Table 39-9.

Table 39-9. AHA/ACC Recommendations for Measuring LDL and non-HDL Cholesterol in Adults Age 20 Years or Older

- Measurement of either fasting or nonfasting lipid panels is effective to determine baseline LDL cholesterol and CVD risk
- A fasting lipid panel should be obtained if triglyceride level is >400 mg/dL on a nonfasting lipid panel
- If LDL cholesterol calculated from the Friedewald equation at <70 mg/dL, a directly measured LDL cholesterol level should be obtained
- An initial fasting lipid panel should be obtained for patients with a family history of genetic lipid disorder of premature CVD

For patients at low risk for CVD and who do not require lipid lowering treatment, repeat lipid profiles should be obtained at 3- to 5-year intervals. There are no definitive studies that provide guidance on what age to stop lipid screening in patients without CVD and who are not on lipid lowering medications.

Obesity, metabolic syndrome, physical inactivity, tobacco use, diabetes mellitus, hypertriglyceridemia, and certain medications (eg, androgens, progestins, beta blockers, and benzodiazepines) are the most common causes of low HDL cholesterol. There are several monogenic disorders in addition to familial hypoalphalipoproteinemia that cause low HDL cholesterol, and selected characteristics of these conditions are presented in Table 39-10. Patients with familial apo-AI deficiency have undetectable levels of apo-AI and severely reduced levels of HDL cholesterol. LCAT deficiency patients exhibit the combination of corneal opacities, target cell hemolytic anemia, and proteinuria with eventual renal failure, while the "fish eye" variant of LCAT deficiency manifests only with dense corneal opacification. Tangier disease patients are distinguished by enlarged and orange tonsils. Patients with apo-AI Milano have low HDL levels but no increased risk of cardiovascular disease.

The reciprocal relationship between HDL cholesterol level and CVD risk has been well established since it was first published out of Framingham Heart Study data in the late 1970s and confirmed in multiple other cohorts. HDL cholesterol level is a component of the Framingham Risk Score and ACC/AHA Heart Risk Calculator. The antiatherogenic properties of HDL appear to arise primarily from its central role in reverse cholesterol transport, moving excess cholesterol out of peripheral tissues and returning it to the liver for biliary excretion. However, preclinical research indicates that HDL and apo-AI have effects on inflammation, oxidation of LDL, nitric oxide production, and expression of endothelial adhesion molecules that might also reduce occurrence of atherosclerosis and risk of CVD.

Treatment

There are limited options for raising HDL cholesterol. Nonpharmacologic interventions such as aerobic exercise, weight loss, smoking cessation, reduced overall

Table 39-10. Genetic Disorders Causing Low HDL Cholesterol Level

Disorder	Mutation	Inheritance	HDL (mg/dL)
Familial hypoalphalipoproteinemia	Apo-AI	Dominant	20–30
Familial apo-AI deficiency	Apo-AI	Recessive	<5
Apo-AI Milano	Apo-AI	Dominant	~10
LCAT deficiency	LCAT	Recessive	<10
Fish-eye disease	LCAT	Recessive	<10
Tangier disease	ABCA1	Recessive	<5

fat intake (but increased consumption of polyunsaturated fats), and moderate alcohol consumption tend to produce only modest (5%–10%) improvements in HDL level from baseline. Fibrates (see Table 39-7) raise HDL 10% to 20% from baseline but only during treatment of hypertriglyceridemia. HMG-CoA reductase inhibitors, especially high-potency statins such as rosuvastatin and atorvastatin, may raise HDL cholesterol levels by 5% to 10% from baseline, particularly at high doses. Niacin is presently the most effective pharmacologic intervention for raising HDL, with increases of 15% to 25% from baseline at doses of at least 1000 to 2000 mg daily. There are no specific HDL cholesterol treatment targets for patients with low HDL levels. Low HDL frequently occurs with other atherogenic risks such as hypertriglyceridemia, elevated remnant lipoprotein levels, increased small, dense LDL, obesity, insulin resistance, and diabetes mellitus, and treatment of these problems may lead to secondary improvements in HDL level and reduced CVD risk.

Recent clinical trials of HDL-raising therapies call into question whether increasing HDL cholesterol improves cardiovascular outcomes. Two secondary prevention trials of niacin added to statins, AIM-HIGH (Atherothrombosis Intervention in Metabolic Syndrome with Low HDL/High Triglycerides: Impact on Global Health Outcomes) and HPS2-THRIVE (Heart Protection Study 2: Treatment of HDL to Reduce Incidence of Vascular Events), failed to show significant reductions in the combined endpoint of nonfatal myocardial infarction, stroke, coronary artery disease death, and coronary revascularizations (referenced in Table 39-6). Inhibitors of the enzyme CETP (cholesterol ester transferase protein) are potent agents for raising HDL levels, but cardiovascular event and all-cause mortality rates were higher during treatment with the CETP inhibitor torcetrapib and atorvastatin compared with atorvastatin alone in the ILLUMINATE (Study Examining Torcetrapib/Atorvastatin and Atorvastatin Effects on Clinical CV Events in Patients with Heart Disease) trial, and adding the CETP inhibitor dalcetrapib to best evidence-based lipid lowering therapy in the dal-OUTCOMES (Dalcetrapib Outcomes Study) had no effect on CVD event rates or mortality.

A young male with severe hypercholesterolemia and coronary artery disease

A 31-year-old male is referred for lipid management after recently undergoing three-vessel coronary artery bypass surgery. The patient's father experienced an acute myocardial infarction at age 39 years and required bypass surgery for management. The patient has no history of hypertension, diabetes, or tobacco use. Examination revealed a generally fit-appearing young man with bilateral tendon xanthomas. Preoperative fasting lipid panel was notable for total cholesterol

331 mg/dL, HDL cholesterol 44 mg/dL, LDL cholesterol 266 mg/dL, and triglycerides 104 mg/dL.

1. What is the patient's primary lipid disorder?
2. What are the most appropriate therapeutic options?

Answers

1. The severity of hypercholesterolemia, personal history of premature CVD, family history of CVD, and presence of tendon xanthomas indicates heterozygous familial hypercholesterolemia (FH). FH is an autosomal dominant disorder caused by inactivating mutations of the LDL-receptor that has a gene frequency of approximately 1:500. Plasma total and LDL- cholesterol typically exceed 300 mg/dL and 250 mg/dL, respectively. Premature CVD is common with onset before age 45 years in men and 55 years in women. Most affected patients have tendon xanthomas, and other findings on examination include xanthelasmas and premature corneal arcus. Homozygous FH is rare (approximately 1 per 1,000,000 population) and leads to much more severe hypercholesterolemia (total cholesterol >600 mg/dL, LDL cholesterol >500 mg/dL) and very early CVD. Homozygous FH patients develop planar xanthomas at areas of skin trauma, such as elbows and knees, in addition to the other manifestations of heterozygous FH.

2. HMG-CoA reductase inhibitors ("statins") remain the cornerstone of cholesterol-lowering pharmacotherapy, with proprotein convertase subtilisin/kexin type 9 (PCSK9) inhibitors, ezetimibe, bempedoic acid, and bile acid sequestrants ("resins") as potential alternatives or adjunctive therapies. Dosing information for statins by LDL-reducing potency is presented in Table 39-12, and information for other drugs is presented in Table 39-11. A highly potent statin is the initial treatment of choice for this patient. Since he has very high-risk CVD, the goal of lipid management is an LDL cholesterol less than 70 mg/dL. The patient's very high baseline LDL cholesterol level makes it almost certain the he will require a second cholesterol-lowering medication to achieve his LDL cholesterol goal, and PCSK9 inhibitors are the most potent adjunctive therapeutic class, with the strongest evidence of clinical benefit when added to treatment with a statin. Ezetimibe is more convenient and cost effective than PCSK9 inhibitors, however, and there is also evidence of clinical benefit when ezetimibe is added to a statin.

CASE REVIEW

Diagnosis

The differential diagnosis of hypercholesterolemia is presented in Table 39-3. In addition to FH, familial defective apo-B100 (FDB) is a well characterized

Table 39-11. Alternatives to Statins for Treatment of Hypercholesterolemia

Medication	Dosing
PCSK9 inhibitor antibodies	
Alirocumab	75–150 mg every 2 weeks or 300 mg monthly
Evolocumab	
	140 mg every 2 weeks or 420 mg monthly
PCSK9 inhibitor small interfering RNA	
Inclisiran	284 mg initially, repeat in 3 months, then every 6 months
Ezetimibe	10 mg daily
Bile acid sequestrants	
Colesevelam	1.875 g twice daily
Cholestyramine	8–16 g daily in two divided doses
Colestipol granules	5–30 g daily in two divided doses
Colestipol tablets	2–16 g daily in two divided doses
Bempedoic acid	180 mg daily

PCSK9, proprotein convertase subtilisin/kexin type 9.

monogenic cause of severe hypercholesterolemia. FDB is caused by mutations in the apo-B100 gene that reduce the affinity of apo-B100 for the LDL receptor. Prevalence is slightly less than FH at 1:700 to 1:1000. LDL levels range from 160 to 300 mg/dL, and premature CVD is common. Unlike FDB, patients with FDB do not develop tendon xanthomas. Most cases of severe hypercholesterolemia do not have a clear genetic cause and are considered polygenic. Hypothyroidism and nephrotic syndrome are 2 important secondary causes of severe hypercholesterolemia.

There is abundant evidence from animal models, epidemiologic cohort studies, the natural history of monogenic disorders of LDL cholesterol, Mendelian randomization trials, and randomized controlled trials of LDL reducing medications that LDL cholesterol plays a central role in the development of atherosclerosis and CVD. Naturally occurring and experimentally induced elevations of LDL and other apo-B containing lipoproteins cause atherosclerosis in all mammalian species. Exposure to elevated LDL cholesterol levels precedes the onset of CVD. There is a consistent relationship between the magnitude of LDL exposure and risk of CVD, and the results of over 30 randomized controlled trials with more than 200,000 participants and approximately 30,000 CVD events demonstrate that reducing LDL cholesterol levels significantly reduces the risk of CVD, with

Table 39-12. HMG CoA Reductase Inhibitors and Magnitude of LDL Cholesterol Reduction from Baseline

High Intensity (≥50%)	Moderate Intensity (30%–45%)	Low Intensity (<30%)
Atorvastatin (40–80 mg)	Atorvastatin (10–20 mg)	Simvastatin (10 mg)
Rosuvastatin (20–40 mg)	Rosuvastatin (5–10 mg)	Pravastatin (10–20 mg)
	Simvastatin (20–40 mg)	Lovastatin (20 mg)
	Pravastatin (40–80 mg)	Fluvastatin (20–40 mg)
	Lovastatin (40–80 mg)	
	Fluvastatin XL (80 mg)	
	Fluvastatin 40 mg (BID)	
	Pitavastatin (1–4 mg)	

the most recent trials also demonstrating that reduction in CVD risk is proportionate to reduction in LDL cholesterol level.

The latest AHA/ACC recommendations on screening lipid levels in adults is presented in Table 39-9. Patients who are being treated for primary or secondary prevention of CVD should have fasting lipids measured. A fasting lipid panel should be obtained approximately 6 to 8 weeks after medication is started or adjusted. Once a patient is at therapeutic target and medications are no longer being adjusted, fasting lipids can be monitored annually or more frequently as needed for individuals at high risk of medication nonadherence.

Treatment

Therapeutic lifestyle changes (TLC), including saturated fat-restricted diet, regular aerobic exercise, and weight loss typically reduce LDL cholesterol by 10% to 15% from baseline. However, most patients need TLC combined with cholesterol-lowering medications to achieve their LDL cholesterol treatment targets. Initial choice of pharmacotherapy depends on factors including primary or secondary CVD prevention, LDL cholesterol treatment goal, history of intolerance to statins, renal impairment, and impaired liver function.

HMG-CoA reductase inhibitors sorted by anticipated reduction in LDL cholesterol from baseline are presented in Table 39-12, and alternatives to statins for treating hypercholesterolemia are presented in Table 39-11. Statins remain the foundational class of lipid-lowering drugs for management of hypercholesterolemia. In patients with clinical CVD who require secondary prevention, as in this case, current AHA/ACC multispecialty guidelines advise starting treatment with a high-intensity statin or maximally tolerated statin therapy with a goal of reducing LDL cholesterol by 50% or more from baseline. Patients with a history of multiple CVD events or 1 CVD event and multiple high-risk comorbidities (eg, hypertension, diabetes mellitus, tobacco use) are considered to have very high risk for CVD and should be treated with statins, or the combination of a CoA reductase inhibitor and a nonstatin medication to a goal of LDL cholesterol less than 70 mg/dL. Recent trials demonstrating better clinical outcomes or improvement in degree of atherosclerosis for patients randomized to aggressive LDL cholesterol lowering treatment are presented in Table 39-13.

Treatment to reduce LDL cholesterol for primary prevention of CVD has been demonstrated to be beneficial, particularly for patients with significant CVD risk factors such as diabetes mellitus, hypertension, tobacco use, or family history of premature CVD. However, apparently healthy individuals with untreated LDL cholesterol below 130 mg/dL but C-reactive protein above 2 mg/L have also been shown to benefit from statin treatment in the JUPITER trial. In a meta-analysis of 27 trials of statin therapy for patients at low-risk for CVD, there was a significant reduction in CVD event rate that far exceeded complications of treatment with statins. The AHA/ACC multispecialty guidelines recommend treating patients age 40 to 75 years who have diabetes mellitus and baseline LDL cholesterol greater than or equal to 70 mg/dL with a moderate-intensity statin; patients with additional CVD risk factors (eg, hypertension) should be treated with a high-intensity statin. For adults with a 10-year CVD risk of at least 7.5%, current guidelines advise treatment with a moderate-intensity statin unless a coronary artery calcium (CAC) score has been obtained as part of risk assessment and is zero (except for cigarette smokers or patients with a family history of early CVD). All adults with baseline LDL cholesterol greater than or equal to 190 mg/dL should be treated with a high-intensity statin.

Management of LDL cholesterol to reduce CVD risk is an important consideration in patients with chronic kidney disease (CKD). Patients with nondialysis CKD and CVD should be treated with maximally tolerated statin therapy; patients with nondialysis CKD have reductions in all-cause mortality, CVD mortality, and CVD event rate on statins that is comparable to patients without CKD. Since patients with nondialysis CKD but no known CVD commonly have other CVD risk factors (eg, diabetes mellitus, hypertension), treatment with moderate-intensity statins for primary CVD prevention is often indicated according to current AHA/ACC multispecialty guidelines. Atorvastatin is preferred because it does not require dose adjustments for renal impairment. However, patients with end-stage renal disease (ESRD) have not been shown to significantly benefit from lipid-lowering therapy, and both the Kidney Disease: Improving Global Outcomes guidelines and National Kidney Foundation Kidney Disease Outcomes Quality Initiative (KDOQI) recommend that statin therapy not be routinely started for ESRD patients.

Statin-associated muscle symptoms (SAMS) are a poorly understood problem that may cause patients to stop taking their statin. Affected patients typically

Table 39-13. Randomized Controlled Trials Demonstrating Benefit of Aggressive LDL Cholesterol-reducing Treatment

Trial	Intervention	Outcome
High-intensity statin		
PROVE IT	Atorvastatin 80 mg vs pravastatin 40 mg	Significant reduction in composite endpoint[a]
TNT	Atorvastatin 10 mg vs 80 mg	Significant reduction in composite endpoint[b]
SATURN	Atorvastatin 80 mg vs rosuvastatin 40 mg	No difference in reduction of percent atheroma volume
JUPITER	Rosuvastatin 20 mg vs placebo	Significant reduction in composite endpoint[c]
IMPROVE-IT	Simvastatin + ezetimibe vs simvastatin monotherapy	Significant reduction in composite endpoint[d]
FOURIER	Evelocumab + statin vs statin monotherapy	Significant reduction in the composite endpoint[d]

[a]Composite endpoint of all-cause mortality, myocardial infarction, unstable angina requiring hospitalization, revascularization within 30 d of randomization, and stroke.

[b]Composite endpoint of CV death, nonfatal MI, resuscitation after cardiac arrest, and stroke.

[c]Composite endpoint of MI, stroke, arterial revascularization, hospitalization for unstable angina, or CV death.

[d]Composite endpoint of CV death, nonfatal MI, nonfatal stroke, unstable angina requiring rehospitalization, and coronary revascularization.

complain of symmetric proximal muscle soreness that may be accompanied by weakness and functional impairment. Although a meta-analysis of randomized controlled trials failed to find a significant difference in muscle related complications between treatment and placebo arms, some studies used run-in periods to eliminate patients with apparent statin intolerance, and only 1 study specifically asked patients about muscle problems. However, an internet-based survey of current and former statin users found that 25% and 60%, respectively, reported muscle symptoms that they attributed to their statin, and the most common reason patients stopped statin treatment was side effects. Cholestatic liver disease, hypothyroidism, vitamin D deficiency, and exercise are risk factors for SAMS, although in some studies graduated exercise protects skeletal muscle from potential adverse effects of statins. Fluvastatin, pravastatin, and pitavastatin are the CoA reductase inhibitors least likely to cause SAMS, and alternate day dosing of longer-acting statins (rosuvastatin and atorvastatin) improves tolerability in patients with muscle symptoms while preserving LDL-lowering effectiveness. Fortunately, rhabdomyolysis is rare and almost always occurs only when patients taking statins are co-treated with gemfibrozil, cyclosporine, or a protease inhibitor.

Persistent elevations of transaminase levels, defined as greater than or equal to 3-fold above the upper limit of the laboratory reference range, occur in only about 1% of statin-treated patients and are generally not attributable to the medications. Severe elevations of transaminases to greater than or equal to 10-fold above the upper limit of the reference range occur in only 0.1% of patients, and almost all cases are due to adverse drug interactions. Consequently, the US Food and Drug Administration no longer recommends routine screening of liver function during treatment with statins; testing should be performed only prior to initiation of treatment if there is a clear clinical indication.

TIPS TO REMEMBER

- A lipid panel should be obtained in all adults age 20 years or more when they are seen for primary care, have a family history of hyperlipidemia, or have a family history of CVD.

- Hypertriglyceridemia is found in approximately 25% of patients, and a non-fasting triglyceride level above 400 mg/dL should prompt follow-up with a fasting lipid panel.

- Triglyceride levels are responsive to nonpharmacologic interventions including weight loss, exercise, and reductions in intake of saturated fat and carbohydrates. Fibrates, marine-derived omega-3 fatty acids, niacin, and high-potency statins are primary pharmacotherapy options.

- There is a strong inverse relationship between HDL cholesterol level and CVD risk. While low HDL cholesterol most commonly occurs due to obesity, metabolic syndrome, and diabetes mellitus, hypoalphalipoproteinemia has a gene frequency greater than familial hypercholesterolemia (FH).

- Although most cases of severe hypercholesterolemia are polygenic, FH is distinguished by autosomal dominant inheritance, early CVD, and tendon xanthomas. HMG-CoA reductase inhibitors remain first-line therapy for hypercholesterolemia, although adjunctive treatment with PCSK9 inhibitors and ezetimibe has been demonstrated to reduce the risk of events in patients with CVD and LDL-cholesterol greater than 70 mg/dL.

COMPREHENSION QUESTIONS

1. Which of these interventions reduces the risk of CVD?
   A. Adding niacin to a statin
   B. Adding a fibrate to a statin
   C. Adding a PCSK9 inhibitor to a statin

D. All of the above

E. None of the above

2. Which patients do *not* benefit from treatment with statins?

A. Patients with chronic renal insufficiency

B. Patients with end-stage renal disease

C. Patients with hypertension

D. Patients with type 2 diabetes mellitus

E. All of the above

3. Which interventions significantly lower triglyceride levels?

A. Regular exercise

B. Fibric acid derivatives

C. Improving glycemic control in patients with diabetes mellitus

D. High-dose fish oil

E. All of the above

Answers:

1. **C.** The addition of the PCSK9 inhibitor evolocumab to statin therapy reduced the composite primary outcome in the FOURIER trial. There is no evidence that adding niacin or fibrates to treatment with statins reduces CVD risk compared with statin monotherapy.

2. **B.** Patients with chronic kidney disease who do not require dialysis clearly benefit from lipid-lowering therapy, but guidelines for management of patients with end-stage renal disease specifically recommend against treatment with statins. Statins reduce risk of CVD for patients with both type 2 diabetes mellitus and hypertension.

3. **E.** All of the interventions reduce triglyceride levels by 15% or more from baseline.

SUGGESTED READINGS

ACCORD Study Group. Effects of combination lipid therapy in type 2 diabetes mellitus. *N Engl J Med.* 2010;362:1563–1574.

AIM-HIGH Investigators. Niacin in patients with low HDL cholesterol receiving intensive statin therapy. *N Engl J Med.* 2011;365:2255–2267.

Arca M, Veronesi C, D'Erasmo L, et al. Association of hypertriglyceridemia with all-cause mortality and atherosclerotic cardiovascular events in a low-risk Italian population: the TG-REAL retrospective cohort analysis. *J Am Heart Assoc.* 2020;9(19):e015801.

Ayaori M, Ishikawa T, Yoshida H, et al. Beneficial effects of alcohol withdrawal on LDL particle size distribution and oxidative susceptibility in subjects with alcohol-induced hypertriglyceridemia. *Arterioscler Thromb Vasc Biol.* 1997;17(11):2540–2547.

Barter PJ, Caulfield M, Eriksson M et al. Effects of torcetrapib in patients at high risk of coronary events. *N Engl J Med.* 2007;357:2109–2122.

Bhatt DL, Steg PG, Miller M, et al. Cardiovascular risk reduction with icosapent ethyl for hypertriglyceridemia. *N Engl J Med.* 2019;380:11–22.

Birjmohun, RS, Hutten BA, Kastelein JJP, Stroes ESG. Efficacy and safety of high-density lipoprotein-cholesterol increasing compounds: a meta-analysis of randomized controlled trials. *J Am Coll Cardiol.* 2005;45:185–197.

Bornfeldt KE. Triglyceride lowering by omega-3 fatty acids: a mechanism mediated by N-acyl taurines. *J Clin Invest.* 2021;131(6):e147558.

Bouitbir J, Daussin F, Charles AL, et al. Mitochondria of trained skeletal muscle are protected from deleterious effects of statins. *Muscle Nerve.* 2012;46(3):367–373.

Cannon CP, Blazing MA, Giugliano RP, et al. Ezetimibe added to statin therapy after acute coronary syndromes. *N Engl J Med.* 2015;372:2387–2397.

Cannon CP, Braunwald E, McCabe CH, et al. Intensive versus moderate lipid lowering with statins after acute coronary syndromes. *N Engl J Med.* 2004;350:1495–1504.

Catapano AL, Graham I, De Backer G, et al. 2016 ESC/EAS guidelines for the management of dyslipidaemias. *Eur Heart.* 2016;37:2999–3058.

Charles EC, Olson KL, Sandhoff BG, et al. Evaluation of cases of severe statin-related transaminitis within a large health maintenance organization. *Am J Med.* 2005;118(6):618–624.

Cholesterol Treatment Trialist Collaborators, Mihaylova B, Emberon J, et al. The effects of lowering LDL cholesterol with statin therapy in people at low risk of vascular disease: meta-analysis of individual data from 27 randomized trials. *Lancet.* 2012;380(9841):581–590.

Cohen JD, Brinton EA, Ito MK, Jacobsen TA. Understanding Statin Use in America and Gaps in Patient Education (USAGE): an internet-based survey of 10,138 current and former statin users. *J Clin Lipidol.* 2012; 6(3):208–215.

Coronary Drug Project Research Group. Clofibrate and niacin in coronary heart disease. *JAMA.* 1975;231(4):360–381.

D'Agostino RV, Vasan RS, Pencina MJ, et al. General cardiovascular risk profile for use in primary care: the Framingham Heart Study. *Circulation.* 2008;117:743–753.

Dhindsa S, Sharma A, Al-Khazaali A, et al. Intravenous insulin versus conservative management in hypertriglyceridemia-associated acute pancreatitis. *J Endocr Soc.* 2019;4(1):bvz019.

Doran B, Guo Y, Xu J, et al. Prognostic value of fasting versus nonfasting low-density lipoprotein cholesterol levels on long-term mortality: insight from the National Health and Nutrition Examination Survey III (NHANES-III). *Circulation.* 2014;130(7):546–553.

Fan W, Philip S, Granowitz C, et al. Prevalence of US adults with triglycerides ≥ 150 mg/dL: NHANES 2007-2014. *Cardiol Ther.* 2020;9(1):207–213.

Ference BA, Ginsberg HN, Graham I, et al. Low-density lipoproteins cause atherosclerotic disease. 1. Evidence from genetic, epidemiologic, and clinical studies. A consensus statement from the European Atherosclerosis Society Consensus Panel. *Eur Heart J.* 2017;38(32):2459–2472.

FIELD study investigators. Effects of long-term fenofibrate therapy on cardiovascular events in 9795 people with type 2 diabetes mellitus (the FIELD study): randomized controlled trial. *Lancet.* 2005;366(9500):1849–1861.

Frick MH, Elo O, Haapa K, et al. Helsinki Heart Study; primary-prevention trial with gemfibrozil in middle-aged men with dyslipidemia. *N Engl J Med.* 1987;317:1237–1245.

Ganga HV, Slim HB, Thompson PD. A systematic review of statin-induced muscle problems in clinical trials. *Am Heart J.* 2014;168(1):6–15.

Genest JJ Jr, Martin-Munley SS, McNamara JR, et al. Familial lipoprotein disorders in patients with premature coronary artery disease. *Circulation.* 1992;85:2025–2033.

Goff DC Jr, Lloyd-Jones DM, Bennett G, et al. 2013 ACC/AHA guideline on the assessment of cardiovascular risk. *Circulation.* 2014;129:S49–S73.

Gordon DJ, Probsfield JL, Garrison RJ, et al. High-density lipoprotein cholesterol and cardiovascular disease. Four prospective American studies. *Circulation.* 1989;79:8–15.

Gordon T, Castelli WP, Hjortland MC, et al. High density lipoprotein as a protective factor against coronary heart disease. The Framingham Study. *Am J Med.* 1977;62:707–714.

Grundy SM, Stone NJ, Bailey AL, et al. 2018 AHA/AACVPR/AAPA/ABC/ACPM/ADA/AGS/ASPC/ NLA/PCNA Guideline on the management of blood cholesterol: a report of the American College of Cardiology/American Heart Association Task Force on Clinical Practice Guidelines. *Circulation.* 2019;139:e1082–e1143.

Hartwich J, Malec MM, Partyka L, et al. The effect of the plasma n-3/n-6 polyunsaturated fatty acid ratio on the dietary LDL phenotype transformation – insights from the LIPGENE study. *Clin Nutr.* 2009;28:510–515.

HPS2-THRIVE Collaborative Group. Effects of extended-release niacin with laropiprant in high-risk patients. *N Engl J Med.* 2014;371:203–212.

Jellinger PS, Handelsman Y, Rosenblit PD, et al. American Association of Clinical Endocrinologists and American College of Endocrinology guidelines for management of dyslipidemia and prevention of cardiovascular disease: executive summary. *Endocr Pract.* 2017;23(4):479–497.

Jørgensen AB, Frikke-Schmidt R, West AS, et al. Genetically elevated non-fasting triglycerides and calculated remnant cholesterol as causal risk factors for myocardial infarction. *Eur Heart J.* 2013;34:1826–1833.

Jun M, Foote C, Lv J, et al. Effects of fibrates on cardiovascular outcomes: a systematic review and meta-analysis. *Lancet.* 2010;375(9729):1875–1884.

Kamanna VS, Kashyap ML. Mechanism of action of niacin. *Am J Cardiol.* 2008;101(8A):20B–26B.

KDIGO Clinical Practice Guideline for lipid management in chronic kidney disease. *Kidney Int.* 2013;3(Suppl):263–305.

Khera AV, Plutzky J. Management of low levels of high-density lipoprotein-cholesterol. *Circulation.* 2013;128:82–88.

LaRosa JC, Grundy SM, Waters DD, et al. Intensive lipid lowering with atorvastatin in patients with stable coronary disease. *N Engl J Med.* 2005;352(14):1425–1435.

LaRosa JC, Grundy SM, Waters DD, et al. Intensive lipid lowering with atorvastatin in patients with stable coronary disease. *N Engl J Med* 2005;352:1425–1435.

Laufs U, Parhofer KG, Ginsberg HN, Hegele RA. Clinical review on triglycerides. *Eur Heart J.* 2020;41(1):99–109c.

Mullugeta Y, Chawla R, Kebede T, Worku Y. Dyslipidemia associated with poor glycemic control in type 2 diabetes mellitus and the protective effect of metformin supplementation. *Indian J Clin Biochem.* 2012;27(4):363–369.

Nicholls SJ, Ballantyne CM, Barter PJ, et al. Effect of two intensive statin regimens on progression of coronary disease. *N Engl J Med.* 2011;365:2078–2087.

Nordestagaard BG. Triglyceride-rich lipoproteins and atherosclerotic cardiovascular disease: new insights from epidemiology, genetics, and biology. *Circ Res.* 2016;118(4):547–563.

Olefsky J, Reaven GM, Farquar JW. Effects of weight reduction on obesity. *J Clin Invest.* 1974;53(1):64–76.

Palmer SC, Craig JC, Navaneethan SD, et al. Benefits and harms of statin therapy for persons with chronic kidney disease: a systematic review and meta-analysis. *Ann Intern Med.* 2012;157(4):263–275.

Ridker PM, Danielson E, Fonseca FAH, et al. Rosuvastatin to prevent vascular events in men and women with elevated C-reactive protein. *N Engl J Med.* 2008;359:2195–2207.

Rubins HB, Robins SJ, Collins D, et al. Gemfibrozil for the secondary prevention of coronary heart disease in men with low levels of high-density lipoprotein cholesterol. *N Engl J Med.* 1999;341:410–418.

Sabatine MS, Giugliano RP, Keech AC, et al. Evolocumab and clinical outcomes in patients with cardiovascular disease. *N Engl J Med.* 2017;376:1713–1722.

Sanchez RJ, Ge W, Wei W, et al. The association of triglyceride levels with incidence of initial and recurrent acute pancreatitis. *Lipids Health Dis.* 2021;20(1):72.

Sarnak MJ, Bloom R, Munter P, et al. KDOQI US commentary on the 2013 KDIGO Clinical Practice Guidelines for lipid management in CKD. *Am J Kidney Dis.* 2015;65(3):354–366.

Schwartz GG, Olsson AG, Abt M et al. Effects of dalcetrapib in patients with recent acute coronary syndrome. *N Engl J Med.* 2012;367:2089–2099.

Smith CC, Bernstein LI, Davis RB, et al. Screening for statin-related toxicity: the yield of trans-aminase and creatinine kinase measurements in a primary care setting. *Arch Intern Med.* 2003;163(6):688–692.

Staels B, Dallongeville J, Auwerx J, et al. Mechanisms of action of fibrates on lipid and lipoprotein metabolism. *Circulation.* 1998;98:2088–2093.

Stein EA, Lane M, Laskarzewski P. Comparison of statins in hypertriglyceridemia. *Am J Cardiol.* 1998;81(4A):66B–69B.

Third Report of the National Cholesterol Education Program (NCEP) Expert Panel on Detection Evaluation, and Treatment of High Blood Cholesterol in Adults (Adult Treatment Panel III) Final Report. *Circulation.* 2002;106(25):3143–3421.

Virani SS, Morris PB, Agarwala A, et al. 2021 ACC Expert Decision Pathway on the management of ASCVD risk reduction in patients with persistent hypertriglyceridemia: a report of the American College of Cardiology Solution Set Oversight Committee. *J Am Coll Cardiol.* 2021;78(9):960–993.

Weintraub MS, Rosen Y, Otto R, et al. Physical exercise conditioning in the absence of weight loss reducing fasting and postprandial triglyceride-rich lipoprotein levels. *Circulation.* 1989;79:1007–1014.

Yokoyama M, Origasa H, Matsuzaki M, et al. Effects of eicosapentaenoic acid on major coronary events in hypercholesterolemic patients (JELIS): a randomized open-label, blinded endpoint analysis. *Lancet.* 2007;369(9567):1090–1098.

Zotou E, Magkos F, Koutsari C, et al. Acute resistance exercise attenuates fasting and postprandial triglyceridemia in women by reducing triglyceride concentrations in triglyceride-rich lipoproteins. *Eur J App Physiol.* 2010;110(4):869–874.

A 56-year-old Woman With Chronically Elevated Blood Pressure

John M. Flack, MD, MPH, Ashley Hill, DNP, Asad Cheema, MD and Priyanka Bhandari, MD

A 56-year old woman has a 15-year history of hypertension that has been drug-treated for the entire time. Her antihypertensive drug regimen has been unchanged over the last 2 years and consists of hydrochlorothiazide 12.5 milligrams per day and lisinopril 20 milligrams per day. She takes glipizide for glucose control. She underwent training on self-measurement of BP at home, and her home BP device was also successfully calibrated. Home BP readings (12 averaged BP readings per week, 6 distinct measurements) have averaged 144/86 mm Hg over the past 1 month. BP in the office today averages 141/84 mm Hg (seated) and 138/86 mm Hg (after 1 min standing). Over the past 1 year, all BP readings have been greater than 140/84 mm Hg. There have been no changes to her antihypertensive drug regimen. Her most recent laboratory testing showed normal thyroid function, electrolytes, and blood count; hemoglobin A1C was 8.4% and estimated glomerular filtration rate was 42 mL/min/1.73 m2. Urine albumin:creatinine ratio was 340 milligrams per gram (macroalbuminuria).

Questions

1. What is this patient's on-treatment BP target?
2. What diet and lifestyle modifications are appropriate for this patient?
3. Is the patient on comorbidity-indicated hypertension drugs?
4. How can we optimize this patient's antihypertensive drug regimen?
5. What diabetes drugs should be favored given this patient's hypertension and chronic kidney disease (CKD)?

Hypertension is the most common clinical condition for which patients seek care in ambulatory clinics. More than 100 antihypertensive drugs have been approved for treatment of this condition by the US Food and Drug Administration (FDA). One of the more vexing problems has been obtaining accurate office BP measurements, as most clinics have not adopted standard measurement protocols. Among drug-treated hypertensives, inadequate therapeutic intensity is problematic and relates to initiating therapy with only a single drug, and when BP elevations are encountered, the clinician does not intensify the drug regimen (therapeutic inertia). Importantly, most patients with hypertension have other comorbidities that influence drug selection and patient monitoring. This chapter will provide an overview of diagnosis, evaluation, and treatment of hypertension in ambulatory clinic settings.

Blood Pressure Measurement

Accurate BP measurement is essential to diagnosing and managing hypertension. This, however, cannot be accomplished in any setting unless there is adherence to a standard measurement protocol. Overwhelmingly, the errors made during BP measurement bias BP readings upward, leading to overdiagnosis as well as over-treatment of hypertension. Table 40-1 displays an easily implemented standard BP measurement protocol.

Nicotine, exercise, and food consumption should be avoided within 30 minutes of BP measurement. The use of validated (and calibrated) BP measurement devices is recommended; a list of these devices can be accessed at www.validatebp.org. Each BP measurement session should consist of at least 2 BP measurements separated by ~1 minute and averaged. Also, BP at the initial visit should be measured in both arms as well as both in the seated and standing position (after 1 min of standing); subsequent BP measurements should occur in the arm with the highest BP reading. We change our practice approach when SBP falls 10 or more mm Hg upon standing. Accordingly, in this situation, we use standing not seated BP to determine treatment adequacy.

Measuring BP at home is a great strategy for engaging patients. Patients must be trained on the steps to accurately measure BP, ideally using validated and calibrated devices. At each BP measurement, 2 readings should be obtained and averaged. A minimum of 12 BP measurements representing 6 different measurement sessions should be collated and averaged prior to making diagnostic and therapeutic decisions. Thus, a measurement schedule might be once in the morning and once in the evening for 3 consecutive or nonconsecutive days of the week. The average of these 6 averaged BP measurements can be used for monitoring

Table 40-1. Seven Steps to Obtain Accurate Blood Pressure Measurements

1. No conversation (talking or active listening adds 10 mm Hg)
2. Empty bladder (full bladder adds 10 mm Hg)
3. Use correct cuff size (too small of a cuff adds 2–10 mm Hg)
4. Place cuff on bare arm (cuff over clothing adds 5–50 mm Hg)
5. Support arm at heart level (unsupported arm adds 10 mm Hg)
6. Keep legs uncrossed (crossed legs add 2–8 mm Hg)
7. Support back and feet (unsupported back and feet add 6 mm Hg)

Adapted from www.heart.org/en/news/2018/05/01/aha-ama-launch-high-blood-pressure-initiation.

and therapeutic decisions. A patient training video on BP measurement can be accessed by patients at targetbp.org/tools_downloads/self-measured-blood-pressure-video/. We also instruct patients to measure their BP in both seated and standing positions when orthostatic hypotension has been detected in the clinic.

Ambulatory BP monitoring (ABPM) can be used to supplement BP readings obtained in the clinic as well as to confirm home BP monitoring readings. Ambulatory BP monitors are typically programmed to obtain BP readings every 15 to 30 minutes during the day and every 15 minutes to 1 hour at night while the individuals carry out their daily activities. Overall 24-hour average BP levels as well as daytime and nighttime BP levels plus the day/night difference in BP are readily calculated from technically satisfactory recordings.

Blood Pressure Classification

Table 40-2 displays the most recent American College of Cardiology/American Heart Association (ACC/AHA) BP classification scheme. A patient is always classified according to the highest SBP or DBP category if they are not concordant.

These BP classifications have both diagnostic and therapeutic implications. When BP is elevated, lifestyle modifications should be implemented to the degree possible. And although hypertension is diagnosed when BP is consistently at least130/80 mm Hg, the vast majority (~70%) of hypertensives do not qualify for pharmacologic therapy until BP consistently breaches 140/90 mm Hg. Table 40-3 displays the hypertensive thresholds for clinic, home, and ambulatory BP readings.

Diagnosing Hypertension

The accurate diagnosis of hypertension and optimal therapeutic decision-making depend on careful BP measurement. The American College of Cardiology (ACC)/

Table 40-2. Blood Pressure (mmHg) Categories in Adults

BP Category	SBP		DBP
Normal	<120	and	<80
Elevated	120–129	and	<80
Hypertension			
Stage 1	130–139	or	80–89
Stage 2	≥140	or	≥90

Based on average of ≥2 BP readings on ≥2 occasions.
Adapted from Whelton PK, Carey RM, Aronow WS, et al. 2017 ACC/AHA/APA/ABC/ACPM/AGS/APhA/ASH/ASPC/NMA/PCNA guideline for the prevention, detection, evaluation and management of high blood pressure in adults. *Hypertension.* 2018;71:e13–e115.

Table 40-3. Equivalent Blood Pressure Levels Across Different Measurement Modalities

		ABPM		
Clinic	Home BP	Daytime	Nighttime	24 Hours
130/80	130/80	130/80	110/65	125/75
140/90	135/85	135/85	120/70	130/80

ABPM, ambulatory blood pressure monitoring.
Reproduced with permission from Whelton PK, Carey RM, Aronow WS, et al. 2017 ACC/AHA/APA/ABC/ACPM/AGS/APhA/ASH/ASPC/NMA/PCNA guideline for the prevention, detection, evaluation and management of high blood pressure in adults. Hypertension. 2018;71(6): e13-e115.

American Heart Association 2018 guidelines consider either a systolic blood pressure (SBP) reading greater than or equal to 130 mmHg and/or diastolic blood pressure (DBP) reading greater than or equal to 80 mmHg or more as thresholds for diagnosing hypertension in noninstitutionalized, ambulatory, community-living adults. In most situations, the diagnosis of hypertension should not be made based on a single set of BP readings. The average of 2 readings (separated by 1–2 min) on more than 2 occasions should be obtained prior to making the diagnosis of hypertension. In most situations, office BP elevations ideally should be confirmed by self-measured home BP readings or 24-hour ambulatory BP monitoring. However, when BP exceeds 160/110 mm Hg on a single visit, immediate pharmacologic treatment is indicated.

Drug Therapy Initiation BP Thresholds and on-Treatment BP Targets

Risk stratification is essential to initiating drug therapy at the appropriate BP threshold as well as assigning the correct on-treatment BP target. Table 40-4 displays the appropriate BP targets for drug-treated hypertensive patients. Most patients, irrespective of whether drug therapy is initiated at the 130/80 or 140/90 mm Hg threshold, have an on-treatment target of BP below 130/80 mm Hg.

A general approach is to determine if there are high-risk conditions present that would qualify the patient for drug therapy at the 130/80 mm Hg threshold. When no high-risk conditions are identified, then the 10-year ASCVD risk should be calculated (www.cvriskcalculator.com) and if greater than or equal to 10% then high-risk is confirmed. Post–kidney transplant patients require a more nuanced approach. The BP initiation threshold for the first month post-transplant is 160/90 mm Hg with the BP target below 160/90 mm Hg; after the first month the BP target is the same as others with CKD (<130/80 mm Hg). This approach is recommended to ensure adequate graft blood flow to prevent clotting.

Table 40-4. Drug Treatment Initiation Thresholds and on-Treatment Target BP

	BP Initiation Threshold	BP Target
Known CVD Diabetes CKD* ASCVD 10-year risk ≥10%	≥130/80	<30/80
≥65 years	≥SBP 130	<130
All other hypertensives	≥140/90	<130/80

ASCVD, atherosclerotic cardiovascular disease; CKD, chronic kidney disease; CVD, cardiovascular disease.

*Estimated glomerular filtration rate <60 mL/min/1.73m^2 and/or urine albumin:creatinine ratio ≥300 mm Hg/g *or* post–kidney transplant.

Adapted from Whelton PK, Carey RM, Aronow WS, et al. 2017 ACC/AHA/APA/ABC/ACPM/AGS/APhA/ASH/ASPC/NMA/PCNA guideline for the prevention, detection, evaluation and management of high blood pressure in adults. *Hypertension*. 2018;71:e13–e115.

Hypertension Control Data

Although the 2018 ACC/AHA guideline adopted a lower BP threshold for the diagnosis of hypertension (≥130/80 mm Hg), it remains commonplace to report hypertension control rates using the threshold of less than 140/90 mm Hg. There is sound justification for doing so. First, this allows the identification of time trends when compared with older data. Second, only a minority of hypertensives actually qualify for antihypertensive drug therapy at the 130/80 mm Hg threshold.

Hypertension control rates in the United States have been falling since 2015. Among drug-treated hypertensives, fewer than 25% report taking more than 2 antihypertensive drugs with ~40% only taking a single agent. The most commonly used single drug class, by far, is a renin angiotensin system (RAS) blocker—an ACE (angiotensin-converting enzyme) inhibitor or angiotensin receptor blocker (ARB). Approximately one-third of drug-treated hypertensives are not controlled to below 140/90 mm Hg, and roughly 40% of these uncontrolled drug-treated hypertensives report taking only a single antihypertensive drug.

Initial Evaluation of Hypertension

Table 40-5 displays our recommendations for initial diagnostic and laboratory testing in patients with established hypertension. Our recommendations are similar though not identical to those in the ACC/AHA hypertension guideline. Accordingly, we added hemoglobin A1C to the basic tests because it is superior to

Table 40-5. Recommended Diagnostic and Laboratory Testing

Basic	Hemoglobin AC
	Lipid panel
	Serum creatinine/eGFR
	Serum sodium, potassium, calcium, glucose
	Thyroid-stimulating hormone
	Complete blood count
	Uric acid
	Urine albumin:creatinine ratio
	Electrocardiogram
Optional	Echocardiogram
	Chest x-Ray

eGFR, estimated glomerular filtration rate.

Adapted and modified from Whelton PK, Carey RM, Aronow WS, et al. 2017 ACC/AHA/APA/ABC/ACPM/AGS/APhA/ASH/ASPC/NMA/PCNA guideline for the prevention, detection, evaluation and management of high blood pressure in adults. *Hypertension.* 2018;71:e13–e115.

fasting glucose for the early detection of prediabetes and diabetes. We also measure uric acid in our patients and offer allopurinol to those with levels higher than 5.5, as this drug lowers BP, appears to reduce stroke and heart attack risk, and also forestalls the decline in eGFR. Finally, we measure albuminuria in all patients so that we can detect CKD in those with preserved GFR when the urine albumin:creatinine ratio is greater than 300 milligrams per gram.

Therapeutic Principles

Once the diagnosis of hypertension has been confirmed, diet and lifestyle modifications should be implemented to the degree possible. Antihypertensive drug therapy should be initiated with either 1 or 2 medications. There is no compelling rationale for initiating more than 2 antihypertensive drugs in a drug-naïve patient irrespective of their BP elevation.

Most patients with stage 1 hypertension (140/90 mm Hg or higher) should receive two antihypertensive medications with complementary mechanisms of action. The ACC/AHA hypertension guideline recommends 1 of 4 antihypertensive drugs for initial therapy: *A* (ACE or ARB), *C* (calcium antagonist), or *D* (thiazide-like > thiazide). Two-drug therapy can be initiated with any combination of these 3 antihypertensive drug types. Drugs should be uptitrated roughly monthly until BP control is achieved. Aim for doses that minimally are in the middle of the FDA daily approved dose range unless only lower doses are tolerated. Minimize encountering consistent BP elevations but not intensifying drug therapy.

Hypertension Treatment

Diet and lifestyle modifications are indicated for all persons with elevated BP or higher. Thus, all qualifying for drug therapy should, to the degree possible, have received dietary and lifestyle interventions by the time that drug therapy has been initiated. Table 40-6 lists diet and lifestyle modifications that effectively lower BP.

Place most emphasis on dietary sodium reduction and the least emphasis on weight loss—mostly because the former is rapidly effective in lowering BP and the latter is hard for many patients to accomplish, and the BP-lowering effect is variable. Most dietary sodium comes form the consumption of processed foods. Counsel patients to minimize or eliminate added salt (~30% of total intake) as well as to reduce the frequency of high-sodium foods by 25% to 50%. When high-sodium foods are consumed, reduce the total amount consumed by the same percentage.

A logical 3-step approach to constructing a hypertensive drug regimen (or deconstructing an existing suboptimal regimen) is displayed in Figure 40-1.

First, ensure that comorbidity-indicated drugs are included in the regimen. For our patient with diabetes, there is no specific drug class, per se, that is favored. However, given that she has chronic kidney disease (CKD) as evidenced by depressed

Table 40-6. Diet and Lifestyle Interventions With Proven BP-lowering Efficacy

- Dietary sodium reduction
  - Average US adult consumes ~3.4 g (150 mmol) per day
  - Strategies to reduce dietary sodium intake
    - Consume high-sodium foods 25%–50% less frequently
    - Consume 25%–50% smaller portion sizes of high-sodium foods
- Moderation of alcohol intake
  - No more than 2 drinks per day (men) or 1 drink per day (women)
- Weight loss
  - Hard to accomplish
- Increased physical activity
  - Aerobic exercise
  - Isometric exercise
  - Resistance training (avoid heavy weightlifting)

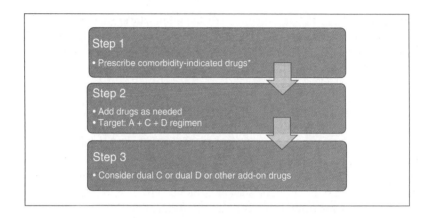

*Atrial fibrillation	ARB or ACE
Aortic disease	Beta blocker
Chronic kidney disease	ACE or ARB
-Post–kidney transplant	Calcium antagonist
Heart failure	
-Reduced EF	GDMT beta blockers
	Aldosterone antagonists
	ARNI (ACE or ARB if ARNI not available)
-Preserved EF	ARNI
Secondary stroke prevention	Thiazide or thiazide-like diuretic
	ACE
	ARB
Stable ischemic heart disease	GDMT beta blockers
	ACE or ARB
-Angina	GDMT beta blockers
-Post-MI or ACS	GDMT beta blockers
Aortic insufficiency	Avoid drugs that drugs that slow the HR (beta blockers, non-DHP calcium antagonists)

A, ACE inhibitor or ARB; ACE, angiotensin-converting enzyme inhibitor; ACS, acute coronary syndrome; ARB, angiotensin receptor blocker; ARNI, angiotensin receptor neprilysin inhibitor; C, calcium antagonist; D, thiazide-like or thiazide diuretic; DHP, dihydropyridine; EF, ejection fraction; GDMT, guideline-directed medical therapy (carvedilol, metoprolol succinate, bisoprolol); HR, heart rate; MI, myocardial infarction.

Adapted from Whelton PK, Carey RM, Aronow WS, et al, 2018.

ACC/AHA/APA/ABC/ACPM/AGS/APhA/ASH/ASPC/NMA/PCNA guideline for the prevention, detection, evaluation and management of high blood pressure in adults. *Hypertension.* 2018;71:e13–e115.

Figure 40-1. Three-step approach to constructing effective hypertension drug regimens.

kidney function (EGFR <60 mL/min/1.73 m² and urine albumin:creatinine ratio >300 mg/g), either an ACE inhibitor or an ARB is indicated. She is on an ACE inhibitor that has been prescribed at the middle of the FDA-approved daily dose range. Second, add additional drugs as needed to achieve the target BP (<130/80 mm Hg). Above and beyond comorbidity-indicated drugs, the target regimen is A (ACE or ARB) + C (calcium antagonist) + D (thiazide-like > thiazide); given that she is already on a submaximal ACE inhibitor dose, a logical question is whether to uptitrate this medication. Most antihypertensive drugs, save the calcium antagonists, have flat dose-response curves and many (though not ARBs) have dose-related side effects. Doubling her dose of lisinopril will result in only modest incremental BP lowering. A highly effective strategy for optimization of her drug regimen would be to discontinue the underdosed HCTZ—the normal daily dose range for this drug is 25 to 50 milligrams. HCTZ loses its effectiveness when the EGFR drops below 45 mL/min/1.73 m², so even HCTZ doses within the recommended daily dose range may not effectively lower her BP. Accordingly, substituting 1 of the more potent thiazide-like diuretics (chlorthalidone 12.5–25 mg/d or indapamide 1.25–2.5 mg/d) would be a good strategy. Chlorthalidone effectively lowers BP down to EGFR ~20 mL/min/1.73 m² while indapamide is effective down to ~30 mL/min/1.73 m². When the GFR is less than 30 mL/min/1.73 m², consider the use of a loop diuretic (eg, furosemide twice daily or metolazone). If a third drug is ultimately needed, the addition of a calcium antagonist is logical; dihydropyridine calcium antagonists should be used almost exclusively in patients already prescribed beta blockers; nondihydropyridine calcium antagonists are contraindicated in beta blocker–treated patients.

Dual diuretic therapy means the addition of a second agent with diuretic properties, typically after the prescription of a thiazide or thiazide-like diuretic. Aldosterone antagonists and epithelial sodium channel (ENAC) inhibitors (eg, amiloride) are the usual add-on diuretics. In hypertensive patients without heart failure, these drugs can be used in patients with EGFR greater than 45 mL/min/1.73 m²; in patients with reduced ejection fraction heart failure where the clinical benefits of using aldosterone antagonists is greater, they can be used down to an eGFR of 30 mL/min/1.73 m². All patients, especially those with CKD (eGFR <60 mL/min/1.73 m²), and particularly those on other RAS antagonists—beta blockers, ACE inhibitors, ARBs—should be periodically monitored for hyperkalemia when potassium-sparing diuretics are prescribed.

Dual calcium antagonist therapy means adding a second calcium antagonist to the drug regimen of a patient already prescribed a calcium antagonist. Accordingly, a dihydropyridine and a nondihydropyridine calcium antagonist calcium blocker may be combined. However, this combination is not recommended for patients treated with beta blockers and/or with reduced ejection fraction heart failure (or even asymptomatic left ventricular dysfunction). The most common dual calcium antagonist combination is verapamil plus amlodipine.

Other add-on antihypertensive agents beyond comorbidity-indicated drugs and the $A + C + D$ regimen include nitrates, beta blockers, alpha blockers, and minoxidil. Central adrenergic inhibitors such as poorly tolerated clonidine are rarely used. Eschew the use of hydralazine in most patients.

The influence of race on antihypertensive drug selections should be de-emphasized. Differences in antihypertensive drug response—both between races and within a racial group—are confined to single-drug therapy; combination drug therapy is recommended for most patients with stage 2 hypertension. There are no racial differences in BP response to well-selected combination drug therapy (eg, ACE or ARB + thiazide diuretic or ACE or ARB + calcium antagonist). Third, the established racial drug selection paradigm (use diuretics and calcium block-ers preferentially to other drug classes in African Americans) is not only a poor strategy for attaining BP control in this high-risk population but also overly com-plicates, for no good reason, the treatment of hypertension in an increasingly diverse and multiracial world. The most exemplary rates of hypertension control to below 140/90 mm Hg in the published literature are from the Kaiser Perma-nente system. Control rates exceed 80% for African Americans and Whites and, although the control rates are slightly higher in Whites, the disparity by race is impressively in the low to mid single digits. Kaiser Permanente's locally tailored approach uses a therapeutic algorithm that focuses on combination drug therapy and avoidance of therapeutic inertia and is agnostic to race—at least in regard to selection of drug therapy. The Kaiser Permanente approach epitomizes character-istics of successful hypertension control programs—multidisciplinary team-based care and patient engagement beyond office visits.

TIPS TO REMEMBER

- The effective treatment of hypertension in ambulatory settings requires patience mixed with persistence in uptitrating medications approximately monthly when BP remains above goal.
- Most patients with established hypertension at or above 140/90 mm Hg should be initiated on 2 drugs.
- Accurately measuring BP through the implementation of a standard measure-ment protocol is essential to obtaining accurate office BP readings.
- Optimal CVD risk reduction depends not only on effective BP lowering but also on simultaneous identification and management of all treatable cardiovas-cular risk factors.

SUGGESTED READINGS

Agarwal R, Sinha AD, Cramer AE, et al. Chlorthalidone for hypertension in advanced chronic kidney disease. *N Engl J Med.* 2021;385(27):2507–2519.

American Heart Association. *Blood Pressure and the New ACC/AHA Hypertension Guidelines* https://www.sciencedirect.com/science/article/pii/S1050173819300684. Accessed December 26, 2023.

Bartolome RE, Chen A, Handler J, et al. Population care management and team-based approach to reduce racial disparities among African Americans/Blacks with hypertension. *Perm J.* 2016;20:53–59.

Derington CG, King JB, Herrick JS, et al. Trends in antihypertensive medication monotherapy and combination use among U.S. adults, National health and Nutrition Examination Survey 2005 – 2016. *Hypertension.* 2020;75(4):973–981.

Egan BM, Li J, Sutherland SE, et al. Hypertension control in the United States 2009 to 2018: factors underlying falling control rates during 2015 to 2018 across age and race-ethnicity groups. *Hypertension.* 2021;78:578–587.

Flack JM, Buhnerkempe MG. Race and antihypertensive drug therapy: edging closer to a new paradigm. *Hypertension.* 2022;79(2):349–351.

Flack JM. Better implementation of what is known will reverse falling hypertension control rates. *Hypertension.* 2021;78:588–590.

Muntner P, Carey RM, Gidding S, et al. Potential U.S. population impact of the 2017 ACC/AHA high blood pressure guideline. *J Am Coll Cardiol.* 2018;71:109–118.

Whelton PK, Carey RM, Aronow WS, et al. 2017 ACC/AHA/APA/ABC/ACPM/AGS/APhA/ASH/ASPC/NMA/PCNA guideline for the prevention, detection, evaluation and management of high blood pressure in adults. *Hypertension.* 2018;71:e13–e115.

A 59-year-old Man Requesting a Checkup for a Scalp Laceration

A 59-year-old male presents to the clinic in the summer after an ED follow-up for a scalp laceration after a bar fight. He has not received any medical care in the last 6 years. His medical history includes hypertension and anxiety, both untreated. He smokes a pack of cigarettes a day and drinks at least 6 beers on a daily basis. He has a remote history of IV drug use and incarceration. He does not recall getting routine vaccinations since moving to the area 8 years ago. He has a new female sexual partner, and he does not use condoms. There is no history of sexually transmitted disease.

Which vaccines can be offered to this patient?

Answer

The ED records should be reviewed to ensure that he received Td or Tdap because of the non-clean wound that he sustained, since it has been at least 5 years since his last vaccination. After that, he will require a booster dose with either Td or Tdap every 10 years. He will need pneumonia vaccination even though he is younger than 65 because of his smoking status and chronic alcoholism. He can either get a single dose of PCV20 (therefore completing his pneumonia vaccination), or 1 dose of PCV15, followed by 1 dose of PPSV23 at least a year later, followed by 1 final dose of PPSV23 at age 65. Because he is more than 50 years old, vaccination for herpes zoster is recommended. He can get the 2-dose Shingrix 2 to 6 months apart. In addition, universal vaccination for hepatitis B is recommended for adults age 19 to 59, so he should get the 3-dose series at 0, 1, and 6 months. If he is found to have liver disease due to his alcoholism, he will also qualify to get the hepatitis A vaccine. The influenza vaccine is not recommended in the summer.

ADULT IMMUNIZATIONS

Immunizations are a vital part of the routine care that is provided to all adult patients. They are one of the cornerstones of preventive medicine and should be addressed regularly.

In November 2021, the Advisory Committee on Immunization Practices (ACIP) approved the 2022 Recommended Adult Immunization Schedule for Ages 19 Years or Older in the United States.

If a vaccination series is interrupted, there is no need to restart or add doses. Doses should not be given earlier than the recommended intervals to allow for a complete immunologic response.

Influenza Vaccination

- Quadrivalent inactivated influenza vaccine (IIV4): IM
- Quadrivalent recombinant influenza vaccine (RIV4): IM (*not* egg based)
- Quadrivalent live attenuated influenza vaccine (LAIV4): intranasal
- High-dose quadrivalent inactivated or recombinant influenza vaccines (HD-IIV4 or HD-RIV4)

  o Adults ≥65 years

  o Immunodeficiency states (congenital and acquired)

Indications

- All adults: 1 dose annually (ideally by the end of October)

Special Notes

- Avoid LAIV4 in adults 50 and older, immunocompromised patients and their close contacts, and pregnancy.
- Egg allergy is not a contraindication. Administer in a medical setting under supervision of a healthcare provider who can recognize and manage severe allergic reactions.
- Severe allergic reaction (ie, anaphylaxis) after a previous dose to any influenza vaccine or to a vaccine component (excluding egg): contraindicated.
- History of Guillain-Barré syndrome within 6 weeks of previous dose: contraindicated.

Pneumococcal vaccination

- 23-valent pneumococcal polysaccharide vaccine (PPSV23): Pneumovax
- 20-valent pneumococcal conjugate vaccine (PCV20): Prevnar 20

- 15-valent pneumococcal conjugate vaccine (PCV15): Vaxneuvance
- 13-valent pneumococcal conjugate vaccine (PCV13): Prevnar 13
  o No longer recommended in the 2022 ACIP guidelines

Indications

- Age 65 years or older (no previous pneumococcal vaccination)
  o One dose PCV15, then 1 dose PPSV23 at least a year later
  or
  o One dose PCV20
- Age 65 years or older who received PPSV23 first
  o PCV 15 or PCV 20 at least a year later.
- Age 19 to 64 with risk factors (alcoholism, cigarette smoking, chronic heart/liver/lung disease, diabetes)
  o One dose PCV15, then 1 dose PPSV23 at least a year later, followed by 1 dose PPSV23 at age 65 (at least 5 years from the last dose)
  or
  o One dose PCV20
- Age 19 to 64 with CSF leak/cochlear implant or immunocompromising condition (chronic renal failure, congenital or acquired asplenia, immunodeficiency or immunosuppression, malignancy, nephrotic syndrome)
  o One dose PCV 15, then 2 doses PPSV23 (5 years apart) at least 8 weeks later, followed by 1 dose PPSV23 at age 65 (at least 5 years from the last dose)
  or
  o One dose PCV 20

Special Notes

- PCV is recommended before PPSV23 because of a better response to serotypes common to both vaccines if given in this order.
- PCV stimulates mucosal immunity, preventing nasal colonization of *Streptococcus pneumoniae*, leading to indirect herd immunity and emergence of replacement strains.
- Because of widespread PCV use in children, the serotypes present in PCV13 have nearly disappeared, which is why this is no longer recommended in adults.

Tetanus, diphtheria, and pertussis (Tdap) vaccination

- All adults
  o One dose Tdap, then Tdap or Td every 10 years

- Pregnancy
  - o One dose Tdap during *each* pregnancy at 27 to 36 weeks
- Wound management
  - o Clean and minor wounds
    - ⊙ One dose Tdap or Td if more than 10 years from last dose
  - o All other wounds
    - ⊙ One dose Tdap or Td if more than 5 years from last dose

Varicella vaccination

- Two-dose VAR vaccine 4 to 8 weeks apart

Indications

- All adults with no evidence of immunity
- Health care personnel

Special Note

- VAR is a live, attenuated virus
- Contraindicated in pregnancy and immunocompromising conditions

Zoster vaccination

- Two-dose recombinant zoster vaccine (RZV) (Shingrix) 2 to 6 months apart

Indications

- All adults 50 years or older, regardless of previous herpes zoster or receipt of live zoster vaccine (Zostavax)
- Age 19 years or older who are or will be immunodeficient or immunosuppressed because of disease or therapy

Special Note

- More than 99% of Americans born before 1980 have had varicella
- Patients who have neither experienced varicella nor received varicella vaccine are not at risk for herpes zoster
- Evidence of immunity confirms the need for RZV

Hepatitis B Vaccination

- Three-dose series (Engerix-B or Recombivax HB) at 0, 1, and 6 months
  or
- Three-dose series hepatitis A and B (Twinrix) at 0, 1, and 6 months

Indications

- All adults age 19 to 59 years
- Adults age 60 years and older at risk for HBV infection
  - Chronic liver disease (including fatty liver disease and AST/ALT more than twice the upper limit of normal)
  - HIV infection
  - Sexual exposure risk
  - Current or recent injection drug use
  - Percutaneous or mucosal risk for exposure to blood (eg, household contacts of HBsAg-positive persons; health care and public safety personnel; patients on dialysis; patients with diabetes)
  - Incarceration
  - Travel in countries with high or intermediate endemic hepatitis B
- Adults age 60 years and older requesting vaccination (regardless of risk)

Hepatitis A vaccination

- Two-dose series (Havrix or VAQTA) at least 6 months apart
  or
- Three-dose series hepatitis A and B (Twinrix) at 0, 1, and 6 months

Indications

- At risk for hepatitis A infection
  - Chronic liver disease
  - HIV infection
  - Men who have sex with men
  - Injection or noninjection drug use
  - Persons experiencing homelessness
  - Travel in countries with high or intermediate endemic hepatitis A

- o Close, personal contact with international adoptee
- o Pregnancy (if at risk)
- o Settings exposure
- Any adult requesting protection from HAV

Measles, Mumps, Rubella

- One-dose MMR: if no evidence of immunity
- Adults born after 1957
- Nonpregnant women of childbearing age
- Two-dose MMR 28 days apart: if no evidence of immunity
- Health care personnel
- Students in post–secondary education institutions
- International travel

Special Notes

- MMR is a live, attenuated virus
- Contraindicated in pregnancy and immunocompromising conditions
- Evidence of immunity includes vaccination records or positive IgG titers
- Individuals born before 1957 are considered immune to measles and mumps, except health care workers

Human papillomavirus vaccination

- Initial vaccination: 3-dose series at 0, 1–2 months, 6 months

Indications

- All adults (not just females) through age 26 years
- Some adults age 27–45 years: based on shared clinical decision-making

Meningococcal vaccination

- One-dose MenACWY-D
  o First-year college students who live in residential housing or military recruits
- Two-dose MenACWY-D 8 weeks apart; revaccinate every 5 years
  o Anatomic or functional asplenia, HIV infection, persistent complement component deficiency, use of complement inhibitor (eculizumab)

Haemophilus influenzae type b vaccination

- One-dose Hib
  - o Anatomic or functional asplenia (including sickle cell disease)
- Three-dose Hib 4 weeks apart starting 6–12 months after successful transplant, regardless of Hib vaccination history
  - o Hematopoietic stem cell transplant

COMPREHENSION QUESTION

A 29-year-old female presents to the clinic to establish care. She has bronchial asthma (on formoterol-budesonide inhaler) and depression (on fluoxetine). She does not smoke, drink alcohol, or use recreational drugs. She just graduated from nursing school and plans to start working next month. She has not seen a medical provider since she last saw her OB at the age of 25. She has a 4-year-old daughter. She feels well and does not have any acute concerns.

Which one of the following statements is true?
A. She may need vaccination for tetanus, pneumonia, and HPV.
B. She may need vaccination for pneumonia, MMR, and varicella.
C. She may need vaccination for HPV, herpes zoster, and hepatitis B.
D. She does not need any vaccines at this point.

Answer: B

She will need pneumonia vaccination because she has asthma, which is a chronic lung disease. Because she is going to be a health care worker, she will need to get her antibodies checked for hepatitis B, measles, mumps, rubella, and varicella. If she has no evidence of immunity, she will need to get vaccinated for HBV, MMR, and varicella. The vaccine for herpes zoster is not indicated for patients before the age of 50. Tdap is given to all pregnant patients with each pregnancy, so she received her Tdap 4 years ago and will not need to have a booster until 6 years later.

SUGGESTED READINGS

Anderson TC, Masters NB, Guo A, et al. Use of recombinant zoster vaccine in immunocompromised adults aged ≥19 years: recommendations of the Advisory Committee on Immunization Practices — United States, 2022. *MMWR Morb Mortal Wkly Rep.* 2022;71:80–84.

Grohskopf LA, Alyanak E, Ferdinands JM, et al. Prevention and control of seasonal influenza with vaccines: recommendations of the Advisory Committee on Immunization Practices, United States, 2021–22 Influenza Season. *MMWR Recomm Rep.* 2021;70(No. RR-5):1–28.

Kobayashi M, Farrar JL, Gierke R, et al. Use of 15-valent pneumococcal conjugate vaccine and 20-valent pneumococcal conjugate vaccine among U.S. adults: updated recommendations of the

Advisory Committee on Immunization Practices — United States, 2022. *MMWR Morb Mortal Wkly Rep.* 2022;71:109–117.

Murthy N, Wodi AP, Bernstein H, et al. Advisory Committee on Immunization Practices Recommended Immunization Schedule for Adults Aged 19 Years or Older — United States, 2022. *MMWR Morb Mortal Wkly Rep.* 2022;71:229–233.

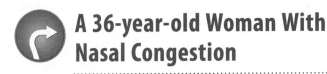

A 36-year-old Woman With Nasal Congestion

Alyssa Ray, MD, Morton Machir, MD, Ahmed Khan, MD and Sheryll Mae C. Soriano, MD

A 36-year-old female presents with a 5-day history of clear nasal discharge, nasal congestion, and frontal headaches associated with nonproductive cough. There is no reported fever. Previously when the patient experienced the same symptoms, she noted improvement with antibiotics. She has seasonal allergies and uses loratadine as needed. Vital signs are within normal limits. There is mild maxillary tenderness present on examination. The nares are patent with a clear mucoid discharge. There is no pharyngeal or tonsillar erythema or exudates, and the lungs are clear to auscultation. What is the most appropriate next step?

CASE REVIEW

The patient most likely has acute rhinosinusitis; therefore, symptomatic treatment is recommended. Symptomatic treatments with systemic or local nasal decongestants, saline nasal washes, and NSAIDs have been shown to have some benefit in alleviating symptoms. Antibiotics are unlikely to be effective in most patients who have acute rhinosinusitis, as studies have shown no difference in the duration of symptoms between those who were treated with antibiotics and those who were not. Imaging studies such as CT scans and plain films of sinuses with or without aspiration of sinus/nasal discharge for gram stain and culture are indicated only in cases where a patient is predisposed to atypical infections such as fungal or pseudomonal infections, seen mainly in the immunocompromised. Therefore, it is recommended not to give antibiotics or perform imaging studies in patients with acute rhinosinusitis.

NONSPECIFIC INFECTIONS OF THE UPPER RESPIRATORY TRACT

The "common cold," which is also known as infective rhinitis or nasopharyngitis, encompasses the nonspecific and usually benign uncomplicated upper respiratory tract infections (URIs).

Etiology

Viruses are the major pathogens causing URIs. The most common etiologic agents are the rhinoviruses, coronaviruses, influenza A and B viruses, parainfluenza, and adenoviruses. In addition, respiratory syncytial virus (RSV) is a well-recognized cause of URIs in the pediatric population, and also in the elderly and immunocompromised. Bacterial pathogens are uncommon causes of URI. However, the most common bacterial causes are *Streptococcus pneumoniae*, *Chlamydia pneumoniae*, *Haemophilus influenzae*, *Moraxella catarrhalis*, and *Mycoplasma pneumoniae*. Secondary bacterial infections may complicate viral URIs in 0.05% to 2% of cases and may present as rhinosinusitis, otitis media, or pharyngitis. These often present with a worsening of symptoms after an initial improvement, particularly in patients at the extremes of age and those who are chronically ill.

Viruses (including SARS-CoV-2) and bacterial infections may be transmitted via contact with droplets, aerosols, and fomites. Therefore, hand washing, respiratory hygiene, and vaccinations are essential measures that can be employed to decrease transmission.

Clinical Manifestations and Diagnosis

The principal signs and symptoms of nonspecific URIs include rhinorrhea, nasal congestion, cough, and sore throat. Less commonly, fever, malaise, sneezing, myalgia, conjunctivitis, fatigue, lymphadenopathy, and hoarseness may occur. Physical examination findings are frequently benign and nonspecific. Although diagnostic modalities such as PCR of nasopharyngeal swabs are available to identify viral pathogens, the lack of specific effective treatment for most etiologic agents makes them less useful. Molecular testing for influenza viruses and SARS-CoV-2, the etiological agent of COVID-19, are significant exceptions. In addition, molecular testing strategies are used for epidemiologic purposes.

Treatment

Prescribing antibiotics has been a common practice in the outpatient setting for URIs. However, antibiotics have no role in uncomplicated URIs. Their misuse leads to antimicrobial resistance and the manifestation of adverse effects. Symptomatic treatment with over-the-counter decongestants with or without antihistamines consistently alleviates symptoms. Other symptomatic treatments such as lozenges with topical anesthetics, dextromethorphan, NSAIDs, saline sinus irrigation, and topical intranasal steroids may be used.

ACUTE SINUSITIS

Acute sinusitis or rhinosinusitis is inflammation, with or without infection, of the 4-paired sinuses surrounding the nose (maxillary, ethmoid, sphenoid, and frontal sinuses). Acute sinusitis overlaps with signs and symptoms of URIs.

URIs, most often viral, are frequently the precursor of sinusitis. Sinusitis also follows the seasonal pattern seen in common colds—the peak is seen in winter. Maxillary and anterior ethmoid sinuses are most commonly affected in adults. Cigarette smoke is a major risk factor for developing bacterial rhinosinusitis due to its effect of reducing the efficiency of the mucociliary clearance of the upper airways. Other risks for sinusitis are allergic rhinitis, cystic fibrosis, asthma, and immunosuppression.

Etiology

Allergies, viral, bacterial, and fungal infections can cause rhinosinusitis. Viral sinusitis resolves without treatment. Superinfection with bacteria occurs in 0.5% to 1% of URIs, resulting in acute bacterial rhinosinusitis (ABRS). The most common bacterial pathogens implicated are *S. pneumoniae* and nontypeable *H. influenzae* (especially in smokers). *Staphylococcus aureus* is the cause of ABRS about 10% of the time. Anaerobes rarely cause sinusitis but may gain entry through the premolar teeth adjacent to the maxillary sinuses. Fungal sinusitis is very rare, but it can be invasive as seen in rhinocerebral mucormycosis and *Aspergillus* when it occurs. Fungal sinusitis may affect immunocompromised patients and patients with poorly controlled diabetes mellitus.

Diagnosis

Acute sinusitis by definition has a duration of less than 4 weeks. A URI usually precedes acute sinusitis—hence the overlapping constellation of signs and symptoms of rhinorrhea, nasal congestion, postnasal drip, cough, facial pressure, and headache. Less common symptoms include tooth pain and fever. Distinguishing viral from bacterial sinusitis is difficult in the ambulatory setting. However, persistence of symptoms, high fever on presentation, and worsening of symptoms after initial improvement should raise suspicion for a bacterial etiology. Acute nosocomial sinusitis manifests atypically, such as with persistent fever, and should be suspected in intubated, hospitalized patients, especially those with nasogastric tubes in place for long periods. The purulence of nasal secretion is not sensitive in distinguishing between bacterial and viral sinusitis.

Complications of acute sinusitis are rare and include preseptal cellulitis, orbital cellulitis, subperiosteal abscess, osteomyelitis, meningitis, intracranial abscess, and cavernous sinus thrombosis. Cellulitis may present with painful and diminished eye movements, high fever, and periorbital edema/ erythema. Tenderness over the frontal sinus with soft tissue swelling (Pott puffy tumor) may suggest the presence of a subperiosteal abscess of the frontal bone.

Chronic rhinosinusitis lasts more than 12 weeks and manifests as constant nasal and sinus congestion with intermittent episodes of increased severity. Chronic rhinosinusitis can be caused by structural abnormalities of the sinuses, presence of uncontrolled allergies, and nasal polyposis. Rhinosinusitis may persist for years, with individuals getting flares secondary to acute viral or bacterial infection.

Treatment

Discussion in this section mainly focuses on the treatment of acute, uncomplicated sinusitis in the ambulatory setting.

Symptom relief and facilitation of sinus drainage with the use of nasal saline irrigation and topical or oral nasal decongestants are recommended as the initial treatment for mild to moderate symptoms of short duration (<10 days). Bacterial sinusitis is less common, and especially if symptoms last less than 7 days, the sinusitis is likely to be viral. Persistent acute sinusitis (symptoms lasting >10 days), along with the presence of purulence, facial pain, and nasal obstruction, is more likely to be bacterial. Additionally, patients with initial improvement but who then develop a second worsening or double worsening have a higher likelihood of a superimposed bacterial sinusitis. However, it is important to note that even in patients who fulfilled these criteria, still, only 40% to 50% had true bacterial sinusitis. Most patients with uncomplicated ABRS will resolve by day 15 regardless of antibiotics. The number needed to treat with antibiotics is around 14 for a mild improvement in symptoms severity and length. The number needed to harm for mild adverse events such as nausea, vomiting, diarrhea, and allergic reaction is 8. The American Academy of Otolaryngology–Head and Neck Surgery 2015 guidelines recommend watchful waiting for 7 days at the same level of recommendation as treatment with antibiotics. Antibiotics in patients who are watchful waiting should be considered if there is failure to improve within 7 days of symptomatic therapy or clinical worsening during this period.

Amoxicillin has shown to be effective in the treatment of bacterial sinusitis. Beta-lactamase–producing organisms including *S pneumoniae*, *Moraxella*, and non-typeable *H influenzae* have all increased in prevalence. Local antibiograms and risk factors of the individual patient should be considered when prescribing antibiotics. Current guidelines recommend amoxicillin or amoxicillin-clavulanic acid at the same level. The use of antibiotics in persistent and severe community-acquired acute bacterial rhinosinusitis is recommended. (Please refer to Table 42-1 for recommended antibiotic treatment.)

A CT scan of the sinuses or sinus radiography is not helpful in acute disease due to the high prevalence of similar abnormalities among patients with acute viral sinusitis. In evaluating persistent and chronic sinusitis, CT of the sinuses is the radiographic study of choice. Sinus aspiration or lavage may be considered in chronic and complicated cases. In chronic rhinosinusitis, treatment with sinus hygiene with daily saline irrigation and treatment of underlying allergies with daily topical steroids is helpful to prevent exacerbations. In patients that fail conservative treatment, an ENT consultation should be acquired in consideration of surgical management.

Table 42-1. Treatment and Diagnostic Guidelines for Acute Sinusitis

Diagnostic Criteria	Treatment Recommendation
Moderate symptoms (eg, nasal purulence/ congestion or cough) for >7 days *or* Severe symptoms of any duration, including unilateral/ focal facial swelling or tooth pain	**First line**
	Amoxicillin, 1.5–3.5 g per day divided in 2 or 3 times daily PO for 10 days
	Penicillin allergy: trimethoprim–sulfamethoxazole 800/160 mg 1 DS tablet PO BID for 10–14 days
	Second line
	Amoxicillin–clavulanate 500/125 mg BID PO for 10 days
	Second- or third-generation cephalosporins (eg, cefuroxime 250 or 500 mg BID or cefaclor, 250 or 500 mg TID PO) for 10 days
	Doxycycline (200 mg day 1, and then 100 mg BID PO for 2–10 days)
	Macrolides (eg, clarithromycin 500 mg BID or azithromycin 500 mg daily PO for 5 days)
	Fluoroquinolones (eg, ciprofloxacin 500 mg BID, levofloxacin 500 mg daily PO) for 10 days

PHARYNGITIS

Sore throat is among the top 10 common chief concerns encountered in the ambulatory setting. The sore throat could be a symptom of a URI caused by a drip that irritates the posterior pharynx. Sore throat from pharyngitis can be due to viral or bacterial infection. Sore throat may also be due to gastroesophageal reflux disease (GERD).

Epidemiology

Viral and group A beta-hemolytic streptococcal (GABHS) pharyngitis peaks in the winter and early spring. It has peak occurrences at 5 and 15 years of age, with diminishing risk above 20 years.

Diagnosis

Respiratory viruses are the most common cause of pharyngitis. Adenovirus and rhinoviruses account for 80% of cases. Coronaviruses, most notably SARS-CoV-2, influenza, parainfluenza, respiratory syncytial virus, herpes viruses, coxsackievirus, Epstein-Barr virus, and HIV are less common causes. Exudative tonsillitis can

be seen in adenovirus (more commonly than in GABHS pharyngitis), coxsackievirus, and Epstein-Barr virus pharyngitis.

GABHS, group G or C *Streptococcus, Chlamydia, Mycoplasma, Neisseria gonorrhea,* and *Corynebacterium diphtheriae* are bacterial causes of acute
pharyngitis.

Associated symptoms are not reliable predictors of the etiologic agent. The
presence of conjunctivitis, coryza, stomatitis, viral exanthem, diarrhea, and
ulcerative lesions or sores may point to a viral cause. Exudative pharyngitis with
fever, fatigue, posterior cervical lymphadenopathy, and splenomegaly is seen in
infectious mononucleosis. In GABHS and non-GABHS pharyngitis, there is an
absence of coryzal symptoms such as cough.

Fusobacterium necrophorum is an important cause of pharyngitis, as it can
rarely cause a septic thrombophlebitis (Lemierre syndrome) in adolescents and
young adults. Lemierre syndrome presents with worsening pharyngitis and neck
swelling from suppurative thrombophlebitis of the internal jugular vein. In addition, bacteremia with metastatic infection such as lung abscesses may occur. This
disease requires intensive care, including antibiotics with anaerobic coverage and
surgical drainage.

Treatment

The primary task of the physician is to distinguish GABHS pharyngitis from other
causes. Identifying GABHS pharyngitis and starting treatment will improve symptoms, reduce spread, and reduce complications such as peritonsillar abscess, post-
streptococcal glomerulonephritis, and rheumatic fever. The necessity of this task
led to the development of the 4-point Centor criteria. One point is given for each
of the following: subjective or documented fever (temperature >38.1°C/100.5°F),
absence of cough, tonsillar exudates, and tender anterior cervical lymphadenopathy. Each score corresponds to recommended testing and treatment (Table 42-2).
Fulfillment of 3 or 4 criteria has a positive predictive value of 28% to 35%, whereas
the absence of 3 or 4 criteria has a negative predictive value of about 80% for
GABHS infection.

The rapid streptococcal antigen detection test has a high degree of specificity
(90%–95%) but a sensitivity range of 77% to 92% when compared with standard
blood agar throat culture. (However, the latter will also identify colonized patients
who may not be infected.) The rapid antigen test is more cost-effective and is
therefore recommended. Tests for other pathogens such as the heterophile agglutination assay in suspected infectious mononucleosis and gonorrhea cultures also
are available. HIV can present as a sore throat as part of an acute retroviral syndrome, making assessment of risk factors for sexually transmitted infections of
importance to determine the necessity of testing for HIV.

Treatment failure occurs in 11% to 45% of penicillin V–treated patients.
Alternative antibiotics such as amoxicillin appear to be effective with lower rates

Table 42-2. Clinical Predictors for GABHS Infection by Centor Criteria

Centor Score	Recommended Testing	Treatment
0	No test	Symptomatic
1	No test	Symptomatic
2	Rapid streptococcal antigen detection test	If positive, penicillin V[a] or amoxicillin[b]
3	Rapid streptococcal antigen detection test	If positive, penicillin V[a] or amoxicillin[b]
	No test	Empiric penicillin V[a] or amoxicillin[b]
4	No test	Empiric penicillin V[a] or amoxicillin[b]

[a]Penicillin V 500 mg BID for 10 days.
[b]Amoxicillin 40 mg/kg per day for 10 days.

of treatment failure (5%–10%). Other second-line agents are first-generation cephalosporins (eg, cephalexin 250–500 mg 4 times daily for 10 days). The carrier state does not require treatment. Testing for cure in GABHS pharyngitis is unnecessary.

TIPS TO REMEMBER

● The common cold and acute sinusitis are commonly of viral etiology; particular attention to hand washing is important in decreasing transmission.

● Antibiotic use in uncomplicated URIs and acute sinusitis of less than 7 days' duration has no proven benefit, and instead may facilitate emergence of antibiotic resistance. Therefore, its routine use is not recommended.

● Amoxicillin or amoxicillin–clavulanic acid are used in acute sinusitis with moderate to severe symptoms of more than 10 days' duration.

● CT of the sinuses is the preferred imaging modality in persistent, chronic, or complicated sinusitis.

● Antibiotics are not recommended for patients presenting with acute pharyngitis with none or only 1 of the following features (Centor criteria): fever, tender cervical lymphadenopathy, tonsillar exudate, and absence of cough.

● Rapid streptococcal antigen testing is a cost-effective diagnostic test when used with Centor criteria, but throat culture remains the gold standard diagnostic test for GABHS pharyngitis.

- The first-line antibiotic of choice in patients with GABHS is penicillin V 500 mg BID or amoxicillin 250 to 500 mg 4 times daily for 10 days.

COMPREHENSION QUESTIONS

1. A 46-year-old man with well-controlled hypertension is seen in the clinic due to a 5-day history of nasal congestion, rhinorrhea, sore throat, and nonproductive cough. He denies fever, history of allergic rhinitis, or sick contacts. His current medications include hydrochlorothiazide and ibuprofen for occasional body aches. He says antibiotics have helped in his past episodes. On physical examination, his temperature is 37.4°C (99.4°F). There is clear nasal discharge, mildly congested turbinates, and no pharyngeal exudate or cervical lymphadenopathy, and he has clear lungs.

What treatment has shown symptomatic benefit in patients with the above concerns?

2. A 28-year-old woman presents with a 2-week history of sinus congestion. It started initially with sneezing, rhinorrhea, and nasal congestion. She self-treated with over-the-counter oral pseudoephedrine and diphenhydramine, and initially felt better. However, her nasal congestion returned with yellowish nasal secretions, which have increased, and she started to have low-grade fevers, headache, and facial fullness. On physical examination, her temperature is 37.3°C (99.2°F). Her turbinates are swollen and erythematous with a thick yellow nasal discharge and she has left maxillary tenderness. What is the most appropriate next step in managing this patient?

3. A 23-year-old female day care teacher presents with a 2-day history of a sore throat associated with pain on swallowing, rhinorrhea, nonproductive cough, and generalized body aches. There is no associated rash or fever. She has no past medical history or allergies. She has no new sexual contacts and does not use IV drugs. Her vital signs are normal. There is no cervical lymphadenopathy. There are bilateral white tonsillar exudates present. What is the best next step?

4. A 34-year-old woman is evaluated for a 4-day history of sore throat, malaise, and low-grade fever. She denies nasal discharge or cough. She has not had any contact with persons who are ill. She has no drug allergies. On physical examination, temperature is 38.5°C (101.3°F). She has clear lungs. The oropharynx is erythematous with minimal whitish exudates, but tonsils are not enlarged. She has tender anterior cervical lymphadenopathy. What is the most appropriate management?

5. A 19-year-old male has a 3-day history of a sore throat, malaise, increasing fatigue, low-grade fever, and nonproductive cough. He has no known drug

allergies and takes no medications. His girlfriend had these same symptoms 2 weeks ago but has now recovered. On physical examination, temperature is 38.5°C (101.3°F). The patient has clear lungs, and there is a faint macular rash on his torso. He has no tonsillopharyngeal exudates but has bilateral posterior nontender cervical lymphadenopathy. Rapid streptococcal antigen test is negative. What should be done next?

Answers

1. The patient has a URI, most likely viral in etiology. Treatment for URIs is mainly supportive with nasal decongestants such as pseudoephedrine, topical intranasal steroids, and saline irrigation of sinuses—which has been shown to lessen the severity of symptoms, although it does not shorten the duration of the illness. Antihistamines, ascorbic acid, zinc, and echinacea have all shown mixed results, and therefore there is insufficient evidence to support their use. Pseudoephedrine is safe in patients with adequately controlled hypertension.

2. This patient meets the criteria for acute rhinosinusitis. She has had symptoms of more than 1 week. Her illness started as a common cold and improved with nasal decongestants. However, her symptoms subsequently worsened ("double sickening phenomenon"). Since her symptoms are more severe (fever and facial pain) and have exceeded 10 days, she will likely benefit from antibiotics (amoxicillin, or doxycycline for 5–7 days) that cover *S pneumoniae* and *H influenzae* to reduce the duration of symptoms. Of note, the character of the nasal discharge or presence of facial pain is not a reliable sign of acute bacterial rhinosinusitis.

3. This patient is at very low risk for GABHS because her Centor score is 1 (based on the presence of tonsillar exudates). Conservative management to reduce her symptoms is sufficient. The 4-point Centor criteria were developed to guide the management of acute pharyngitis in distinguishing GABHS infection from other causes. It assigns 1 point for each of the following: fever, absence of cough, presence of tender cervical lymphadenopathy, and tonsillar exudates (see Table 42-2).

4. Her Centor score is 4; therefore, empiric treatment without testing is warranted. Amoxicillin for 10 days should be started.

5. The patient meets 2 of the Centor criteria (fever, cervical lymphadenopathy); therefore, doing a rapid streptococcal antigen test is warranted. The test was, however, negative. The diagnosis of infectious mononucleosis should be considered in patients presenting with pharyngitis associated with fever and lymphadenopathy, most often involving the posterior cervical lymph nodes. A heterophile antibody (monospot) test to diagnose infectious mononucleosis is indicated in this patient.

He also has a rash, and his girlfriend was recently sick. He has had possible exposure to Epstein-Barr virus, which is the etiologic agent for infectious mononucleosis (also known as the "kissing disease"). Further questioning to determine risk of HIV based on sexual practices—and if high risk, consideration of testing for HIV in addition to testing for infectious mononucleosis—is warranted.

SUGGESTED READINGS

Alguire P, Kroenke K, Ende J, et al. *MKSAP 15 General Internal Medicine.* Philadelphia: American College of Physicians; 2010.

Centor R, Allison J, Cohen S. Pharyngitis management: defining the controversy. *J Gen Intern Med.* 2007;22:127–130.

Chow AW et al. Evaluation of acute pharyngitis in adults. In: Calderwood S, Baron E, eds. UpToDate. 2012.

Longo D, Fauci A, Kasper D, et al. *Harrison's Principle of Internal Medicine.* 18th ed. New York, NY: McGraw-Hill; 2011.

Patel ZM, Hwang PH. Acute sinusitis and rhinosinusitis in adults: clinical manifestations and diagnosis. In: Calderwood S, Baron E, eds. UpToDate. 2012.

Patel ZM, Hwang PH. Uncomplicated acute sinusitis and rhinosinusitis in adults: Treatment. In: Calderwood S, Baron E, eds. UpToDate. 2012.

Pichichero, Michael E. Treatment and prevention of streptococcal pharyngitis in adults and children. In: Calderwood S, Baron E, eds. UpToDate. 2012.

Rosenfeld RM, Piccirillo JF, Chandrasekhar SS, et al. Clinical Practice Guideline (Update): Adult Sinusitis. *Otolaryngol Head Neck Surg.* 2015;152(2_suppl):S1–S39.

Shulman ST, Bisno AL, Clegg HW, et al. Clinical Practice Guideline for the Diagnosis and Management of Group A Streptococcal Pharyngitis: 2012 Update by the Infectious Diseases Society of America. *Clin Infect Dis.* 2012;55(10):e86–e102.

Turner B, Williams S, Taichman D. In the clinic. Acute sinusitis. *Ann Intern Med.* 2010;153: ITC3-3–ITC3-16.

A 22-year-old Woman With Urinary Frequency and Suprapubic Pain

Noupama N. Mirihagalle, MD, Muralidhar Papireddy, MD and Susan Thompson Hingle, MD

A 22-year-old female presents to the ED with 3 days of increased urinary frequency and suprapubic pain after micturition. She has no fevers, chills, flank pain, nausea, vomiting, or urethral discharge. There have been no similar complaints in the past. She is sexually active and uses a barrier mode of contraception. She has no history of sexually transmitted diseases. She has no allergies to medications or food. Physical examination is unremarkable. Spot urinary pregnancy test is negative. Urinalysis is significant for 12 white blood cells (WBCs) and 3 red blood cells (RBCs), and the urine is nitrite positive. She has no primary care physician.

1. What is the diagnosis and the next step of action?

Answer

1. Simple or uncomplicated urinary tract infection. Prescribing a short course (3 days) of trimethoprim–sulfamethoxazole or nitrofurantoin (5 days) is the next step, as she has an uncomplicated lower urinary tract infection that can be managed as an outpatient. She does not need admission to the hospital or need imaging, as she has a simple UTI.

CASE REVIEW

Urinary tract infection is one of the most common infections encountered by physicians. Clinical presentation could range from annoying urinary symptoms to severe sepsis and death. Further management depends on the severity of the infection and risk factors for multidrug-resistant (MDR) organisms. In the above case, the patient is a sexually active young female with no systemic symptoms, comorbid conditions, or risk factors for MDR organisms. Lower urinary tract infections are common among sexually active women due to the anatomy of the female urinary tract. Short antibiotic therapy without further imaging is the best course of management for this patient.

URINARY TRACT INFECTIONS

Urinary tract infections are classified on an anatomic basis into lower and upper UTIs. Lower urinary tract infections include urethritis, cystitis, prostatitis, and epididymitis. Upper urinary tract infections include pyelonephritis. We will discuss topics related to cystitis and pyelonephritis in this section.

Simple or uncomplicated UTIs are urinary tract infections occurring in men and women without evidence of infection extension beyond bladder. Patients with evidence of infection beyond the bladder (such as fever, rigors, chills, flank pain, or pelvic or perineal pain specifically in males, which can suggest prostatitis) are considered complicated UTI. Patients with underlying urologic abnormalities (nephrolithiasis, strictures, and stents), immunocompromised patients, and male patients are not automatically considered as complicated UTIs. Those patients do need close follow-up and a low threshold to be treated as complicated UTIs.

Common Organisms Causing UTIs

Common organisms include *Escherichia coli, Proteus, Klebsiella, Pseudomonas,* enterococci, *Staphylococcus, Chlamydia* (suspect in patients with history of STDs), and *Candida* (in patients with indwelling Foley catheter or immunosuppression).

Cystitis

Cystitis is the infection/inflammation of the urinary bladder. Patients present with urinary frequency, urgency, dysuria, suprapubic discomfort/pain, and hematuria. Physical examination may be positive for suprapubic tenderness.

Cystitis is a clinical diagnosis, and routine urinalysis or reflex cultures are not required unless there is a recurrence. Urinalysis is considered positive if any of the following are present: nitrite positive, leukocyte esterase (LE) positive, or greater than 10 WBC/hpf. Men are treated for longer duration due to the concern of prostatitis. Empiric treatment is per Tables 43-1 and 43-2.

Pyelonephritis

Pyelonephritis is an infection of the kidney/upper tracts. Patients present with fevers, chills, rigors, nausea/vomiting, and flank pain along with symptoms of cystitis. Elderly patients may present with confusion and vague abdominal pain with or without symptoms of cystitis. Costovertebral angle tenderness is a common physical finding in pyelonephritis. Urinalysis, urine cultures, and blood cultures should be done prior to starting antibiotics.

Pyelonephritis is a clinical diagnosis. There is no need for imaging on presentation. CT of the abdomen and pelvis is the image of choice. Get imaging if the patient remains febrile for more than 48 hours after being on appropriate antibiotic therapy. Consider early imaging in patients with diabetes or immunosuppression to look for complications of pyelonephritis including perinephric abscess, gangrenous pyelonephritis, emphysematous pyelonephritis, or papillary necrosis. Consider cyst abscess in patients with underlying cystic kidney disease. Patients with urinary tract obstructions or other abnormalities, recent urinary tract instrumentation, or diabetes mellitus are at increased risk of those complications.

Table 43-1. Empiric Treatment of Simple Cystitis

Empiric antibiotics for women
First-line therapy
Trimethoprim–sulfamethoxazole (TMP-SMX) double-strength PO bid × 3 days *or* nitrofurantoin 100 mg PO bid × 5 days
Trimethoprim 100 mg PO bid × 3 days *or* fosfomycin 3 g × 1 dose (less efficacy compared with TMP-SMX or quinolones)
Second-line therapy
Amoxicillin–clavulanate 500 mg PO bid × 5–7 days
Cefpodoxime 100 mg PO BID × 5–7 days
Cephalexin 250–500 mg PO QID × 5–7 days
Cefdinir 300 mg PO BID × 5–7 days
Third-line therapy
Ciprofloxacin 250 mg PO bid × 3 days
Levofloxacin 250 mg daily for 3 days
Beta-lactams 3–7 days

UA shows pyuria (WBC >10/hpf) or is positive for LE or nitrites with or without positive urine cultures. Complete occlusion of the ureter may give a normal UA or negative cultures, as the infected part is compartmentalized. Blood cultures are positive in up to 20% of patients, but it has no prognostic significance.

Criteria for admission to the hospital depend on clinical condition. If the patient is in sepsis or dehydrated from poor oral intake due to severe nausea/vomiting and not able to take oral medication, then he or she should be admitted for IV antibiotics, hydration, and close monitoring. Otherwise, he or she can be managed in the outpatient setting with close monitoring. Start empiric antibiotics as in Table 43-2. De-escalate to appropriate antibiotics on availability of sensitivities. The patient may need urgent urologic intervention if there are signs of ureteral obstruction or perinephric fluid collections. Young women often present with severe flank pain and systemic symptoms that last longer than the other groups of patients due to degree of inflammation. Patients may be discharged if they are afebrile for more than 24 hours and are able to tolerate PO antibiotics.

Asymptomatic Bacteriuria (ASB)

Urine cultures growing more than 100,000 colony-forming units (cfu) without symptoms of UTI are labeled as ASB. ASB increases with age and is more

Table 43-2. Empiric Treatment of Pyelonephritis and Complicated Cystitis

Empiric antibiotics for outpatient treatment
Ciprofloxacin 500 mg PO bid or levofloxacin 750 mg PO daily × 7 days
Trimethoprim–sulfamethoxazole (TMP-SMX) double-strength PO bid for 14 days
If presenting to the ED, may use 1 dose of ceftriaxone 1 g IV and discharge on quinolones or TMP-SMX
Empiric antibiotics for inpatient treatment
Intravenous ciprofloxacin 400 mg q12h
Intravenous levofloxacin 750 mg daily
Intravenous ceftriaxone 1 g daily
Intravenous piperacillin–tazobactam 3.375 g q6h
For patients presenting with severe sepsis, or if there is suspicion for urinary tract obstruction, patient should receive carbapenems to cover for extended-spectrum beta-lactamases (ESBL) *plus* vancomycin, daptomycin, or linezolid to cover for methicillin-resistant staphylococcus aureus (MRSA), until the culture sensitivities are available

Treat complicated pyelonephritis for 5–14 days depending on the antibiotic chosen and patient's response to treatments.

common in women. Screening for ASB is performed only in pregnant women and patients going for urologic procedures that may cause mucosal bleeding. Some experts screen and treat asymptomatic bacteriuria within the first 3 months after a transplant, while others do not. If someone else did the culture and you have the results, stick to the same principles. Do not treat culture results alone, except for those special populations listed above.

Patients With Indwelling Bladder Catheter

There is no need for routine screening for UTI. Patients may not have typical symptoms. Screen for UTI if the patient has fevers, flank pain, suprapubic pain, hematuria, or sepsis. In these cases, remove the indwelling catheter and repeat the cultures via a new catheter or midstream urine sample for UA and urine cultures. Treat for 7 to 14 days if criteria for catheter-associated UTI are met. Candiduria is common with indwelling catheters, especially if patients are on antibiotics or are diabetic. Replace the Foley catheter and repeat the cultures. If still positive, treat with fluconazole 200 mg PO for two weeks for both cystitis and pyelonephritis.

Table 43-3. Prophylactic Measures for Recurrent Urinary Tract Infections

Antibiotics for prophylaxis postcoital or continuous
Nitrofurantoin 50–100 mg
Trimethoprim–sulfamethoxazole, 40–200 mg (3 times weekly is also effective) (category C medication, may cause adverse events to the fetus)
Cephalexin 250 mg (125 mg is also effective if taken daily)
Fosfomycin 3 g every 7–10 days
Nonantimicrobial prophylaxis
Reduction in frequency or abstinence of intercourse (not a feasible strategy)
Avoid spermicide or spermicide-coated barrier method of contraception
Urinate after intercourse
Cranberry juice or tablets (recent RCT showed no benefit)
Topical estrogens in postmenopausal women (not systemic)

Avoid the use of a long-term catheter if not indicated. Intermittent catheterization is better than an indwelling catheter, if feasible.

Recurrent Cystitis and Prophylaxis

Recurrent UTI refers to 2 or more infections in 6 months or 3 or more than three infections in 1 year. Most recurrences are due to reinfection. They are considered a relapse of the same infection if symptoms develop within 2 weeks from the completion of treatment. Obtain urine cultures and treat a relapse with broad-spectrum antibiotic such as the quinolones. If the symptoms recur after a month, use a short course of first-line agents (but a different antibiotic).

Prophylactic antibiotics (Table 43-3) may be considered if the patient is in agreement.

Other behavioral and biologic agents for prophylaxis are mentioned in Table 43-3.

TIPS TO REMEMBER

- Significant bacteriuria as defined for various collection methods:
  - For clean catheter sample in men and women: 100 cfu/mL
  - For clean catheter sample or midstream urine for catheter-associated UTI: 1000 cfu/mL; catheter removed within last 48 hours
  - For midstream urine in men for UTI: 10,000 cfu/mL

- For midstream urine in women for UTI: 100,000 cfu/mL
- For midstream urine in both men and women for ASB: 100,000 cfu/mL

- Pyuria: WBC >10 in unspun midstream urine. LE positivity suggests WBCs are present in the urine. May repeat UA if WBCs are not seen but LE is positive, but it is a good enough indicator for pyuria if the patient has symptoms of UTI.

- Nitrites: Enterobacteriaceae reduce nitrate to nitrite. Suggest bacteriuria >100,000 cfu/mL. There can be false positives with beet consumption or with use of phenazopyridine.

- Treat simple UTI with a short course of trimethoprim–sulfamethoxazole or nitrofurantoin or fosfomycin as first-line agents. Quinolones and beta-lactams are second-line agents.

- If there is a complicated UTI, treat for 10 to 14 days. Outpatient treatment of complicated UTIs are 10 to 14 days of trimethoprim-sulfamethoxazole or quinolones. Treat with a longer duration of antibiotics in men, due to the concern of prostatitis.

- Severe pyelonephritis needs admission to the hospital and treatment with IV antibiotics such as ceftriaxone or quinolones. If the patient has severe sepsis from UTI or you suspect obstruction, use carbapenems for extended-spectrum beta-lactamase (ESBL)–producing *E. coli* plus cover for methicillin-resistant staphylococcus aureus (MRSA) until the sensitivities are available

- Use ampicillin, cephalosporins, or trimethoprim–sulfamethoxazole in pregnant women. Do not use trimethoprim–sulfamethoxazole in late pregnancy and early nursing mothers to prevent neonatal jaundice. Do not use quinolones or tetracyclines.

- Imaging of the GU tract is not necessary unless the patient is critically ill on presentation or if there is no improvement of symptoms in 48 hours despite appropriate antibiotic therapy.

- Men do not need imaging with their first UTI, but they will need further evaluation to rule out structural abnormalities if the treatment fails or the patient has a repeat infection.

- Think about chronic prostatitis in a man with ASB or in one who has had recurrent UTIs with no other structural abnormalities.

- Do not treat candiduria in a patient with an indwelling Foley catheter. First, remove the catheter and repeat the midstream urine cultures before or after insertion of a new Foley catheter.

- Routine UA and cultures should be ordered only if the patient is a pregnant woman or for any patient about to undergo urologic procedures. Only these patients should be treated for bacteriuria without symptoms.

- Do not order routine UA. Most diagnoses are clinical, and the labs should be ordered only to confirm or refute your diagnosis.

COMPREHENSION QUESTION

1. A 57-year-old man presents with nausea, vomiting, and fevers for 1 day. He also complains of dark urine. He had burning micturition for one day a few days ago, along with colicky abdominal pain radiating to the groin. He had a similar episode 2 weeks ago that improved with levofloxacin 500 mg PO daily for 7 days. Urine culture was done at that time, but the results are not available. Physical examination is significant for a temperature of 102.6°F, heart rate of 116 bpm, BP 112/70 mm Hg, saturating 98% on room air, and respiratory rate of 20/min. There is costovertebral angle tenderness on the right. CBC is significant for elevated WBCs at 15,000 cells/mm³ with a left shift. Urine is dark with increased specific gravity, otherwise unremarkable. Urine and blood cultures are sent. What is the best next step of action?

    A. Admit to medicine floor, start fluids and IV meropenem, and obtain a CT of the abdomen and pelvis with renal protocol.

    B. Switch to PO ciprofloxacin and discharge home.

    C. Do a rectal examination, and if the prostate examination is unremarkable, discharge with PO Bactrim.

    D. Admit; call Urology and Infectious Disease consults for the management of pyelonephritis.

Answer

1. A. The patient probably has a renal calculus that is acting as a nidus for recurrent infection. If the calculus is completely occluding the ureter, the UA can be normal. The patient in this case has sepsis and needs to be admitted to the hospital for IV antibiotics, hydration, and closer monitoring. He needs imaging to look for complications of pyelonephritis and hydronephrosis that may need surgical intervention, as there is a concern of stone impaction. Patients in sepsis should be covered for ESBLs until the sensitivities are available. Carbapenems are the preferred agents. Antibiotics should be switched as per the sensitivities available from urine or blood cultures.

SUGGESTED READINGS

Barbosa-Cesnik C, Brown MB, Buxton M, et al. Cranberry juice fails to prevent recurrent urinary tract infection: results from a randomized placebo-controlled trial. *Clin Infect Dis.* 2011 1;52(1):23–30.

Gupta K, Hooton TM, Naber KG, et al. International clinical practice guidelines for the treatment of acute uncomplicated cystitis and pyelonephritis in women: a 2010 update by the Infectious Diseases Society of America and the European Society for Microbiology and Infectious Diseases. *Clin Infect Dis.* 2011;52:e103–e120.

Hooton TM. Clinical practice. Uncomplicated urinary tract infection. *N Engl J Med.* 2012;366(11):1028–1037.

Hooton TM, Bradley SF, Cardenas DD, et al. Diagnosis, prevention, and treatment of catheter-associated urinary tract infection in adults: 2009 international clinical practice guidelines from the Infectious Diseases Society of America. *Clin Infect Dis*; 2010;50:625–663.

McMurray BR, Wrenn KD, Wright SW. Usefulness of blood cultures in pyelonephritis. *Am J Emerg Med*. 1997;15(2):137–140.

Nicolle LE, Bradley S, Colgan R, et al. Infectious Diseases Society of America guidelines for the diagnosis and treatment of asymptomatic bacteriuria in adults. *Clin Infect Dis*. 2005;40:643–654.

Section III.
Transitions of Care

A 76-year-old Man Discharged After an Upper GI Bleed

Christine Y. Todd, MD, FACP, FHM and Harini Rathinamanickam, MD, FACP

A 76-year-old man with an eighth-grade education, who is chronically antico-agulated on warfarin for a history of paroxysmal atrial fibrillation, is admitted to the hospital with an upper GI bleed. His warfarin is reversed with vitamin K, and upper endoscopy reveals an actively bleeding duodenal ulcer. A *Campylobacter*-like organism (CLO) test confirms the ulcer was caused by *Helicobacter pylori*, and the patient is then placed on a proton pump inhibitor and appropriate antibiotics. After discussion with the GI consultants, the hospitalists advise the patient as he is being discharged to follow up with his primary care physician (PCP) and that he can restart his warfarin in 6 weeks.

When the patient arrives for his outpatient follow-up visit, his PCP is surprised to hear that her patient was in the hospital. No discharge summary is available, so his doctor relies on the patient to tell her what happened. Unfortunately the patient does not remember all the details. He does remember something about the problem being caused by an "infection in my stomach," and he also notes that he was taken off his warfarin. Worried that her patient might have a stroke if he remains off his anticoagulant and thinking her patient had a viral gastritis, the PCP restarts his warfarin. One week later, the patient develops melena and is readmitted to the hospital with a recurrent GI bleed.

1. What barriers might have prevented the patient from accurately remember-ing the details of his hospital stay?

2. What practices could prevent this type of medical error?

Answers

1. In the above scenario, there are several potential barriers. First and foremost, the patient was told vital information about his warfarin at the time of his discharge—a time during which his mind may have been on many other things: how he was going to arrange for transportation home, how he was going to pay for his new prescriptions, when the nurse would be along to take out his IV, etc. His advanced age and the fact that he was recovering from a significant acute illness also play a role in his ability to remember information—elderly patients can be significantly cognitively impaired when ill, and this impairment can be very hard to detect in the normal course of a conversation. Finally, this patient's educational status should alert us to the fact that he might have basic or below-basic health literacy status. Patients with low health literacy find it particularly difficult to understand and retain information given to them in a 1-time, verbal format.

2. One way doctors can be sure they have communicated effectively to patients is through the process of "teach-back." Teach-back involves discussing an issue with a patient, and then asking the patient to share with you what was understood about the concept being discussed. The process is then repeated until the patient demonstrates full understanding of the concept. Use of printed documents, drawings, and pictures can enhance the process. Engaging patients in this method of education over several days is often necessary when the issues are myriad or complex, so it is a part of the discharge process that cannot be done effectively at the last minute.

Aside from empowering patients through effective education, it is important that physicians working in the hospital master the skill of effective transfer-of-care communication. Prompt, accurate, and succinct communication with a patient's PCP is of paramount importance in preventing the type of miscommunication illustrated in the example above. Strong ties between the electronic health records used in hospitals and the systems used at outpatient referral sites can also help health care practitioners receive adequate and up-to-date information about their patients.

CASE REVIEW: TRANSITIONS OF CARE COMMON PITFALLS AT DISCHARGE

Physicians are often surprised at the paucity of information that patients retain, even after they "have been told" the details of their medical condition. It is important to remember that simply telling a patient something does not mean the patient will understand it or can remember it. As physicians, it is important to make sure we communicate effectively. Being aware of the barriers our patients have to retaining information can help doctors be more effective communicators.

Shift work, duty hour limitations, and the increasing disconnect between hospital-based and clinic-based physicians have conspired to make the time during and immediately after discharge from the hospital fraught with opportunities for medical error. Thus, the ability to discharge a patient according to the best practices outlined in the medical literature is a necessary skill for all medical residents.

Screening tools could be used to identify patients at risk of readmission. This would enable the discharging provider to focus on risk factors identified. One such tool proposed by the Society of Hospital Medicine is the 8Ps risk assessment tool. Resources are available for clinicians to improve safe transition of care. The Project BOOST website from the Society of Hospital Medicine has guidance to improve transitions of care. Another website is the Care Transitions Program. Certain features on this website are available in languages other than English as well.

In the next paragraphs, we discuss common areas for poor practice and propose a checklist at discharge to help avoid these pitfalls.

Availability of discharge documentation: Although it seems obvious that a patient discharge from the hospital would work best as a collaborative effort between the discharging hospitalist team and the receiving ambulist team, a true collaboration rarely happens. Only 3% of PCPs report that they are routinely involved in discussions about the discharge of one of their patients. Fewer than 20% feel that they are routinely informed in any way about one of their patients being admitted to or discharged from the hospital. Twenty-five percent of dictated discharge summaries never reach the intended PCP, and, not surprisingly, 66% of patients who arrive for a follow-up visit are seen without a discharge summary available to the PCP. A clear and ordered discharge process would improve these statistics.

First, discharging physicians must complete discharge documentation immediately upon a patient's discharge. Forward-looking hospital systems often require that a discharge summary be dictated, and status transcribed and signed, before a patient is allowed to leave the hospital. The second step is to make sure the PCP receives the information as soon as possible. Remember that although the patient may not see the PCP for 1 or 2 weeks, questions directed to the PCP may begin mere minutes after the patient leaves the hospital (ie, from a pharmacy questioning a drug dosage or interaction). PCPs find personal letters (as opposed to a copy of the discharge summary) and phone calls to be the most helpful way to communicate issues at discharge. While this may not be possible for all discharges, it is important to consider making personal contact with the PCP on complex or sensitive patient cases. Phone calls between providers at discharge can be immensely helpful, as it permits a two-way conversation about the patient. In our opening scenario, it is clear that the absence of a discharge summary when the patient presented for a follow-up began the chain of events that led to a poor patient outcome.

High-quality documentation: The data related to the quality of the discharge information that does reach the PCP suggest that there are many opportunities for better practice. Written paperwork is illegible at least 10% of the time, the main diagnosis is missing from the documentation 17.5% of the time, reasons for medication changes are clearly explained only 21% of the time, and the name of the main doctor caring for the patient during the hospitalization is missing in 25% of all discharge summaries. Recalling the opening scenario in this chapter, a legible discharge summary explaining why warfarin was being held would have eliminated the need for the PCP to make an educated guess about her patient's pathology (which, in this case, turned out to be wrong).

Pending laboratory tests: Tests that have been ordered and performed but not resulted by the time of discharge deserve special attention by the discharging physician. A full 75% of patients leaving the hospital have pending lab tests, 15% of which turn out to be abnormal. Most of these abnormal tests are seen by neither the hospitalist team after discharge nor the PCP's team, which is unaware that any testing has been done. The medical and legal liability of letting a patient "fall through the cracks" at discharge in this way is of significant concern. Few hospital systems have a foolproof way of making sure these results are seen by a physician who can take responsibility for acting on the results.

In order to avoid these common errors at discharge, it is important that physicians get into the habit of following a checklist of tasks when discharging a patient.

1. Make sure the patient and/or his or her caregivers understand the important diagnoses or issues that necessitated the admission to the hospital. Use the teach-back method to make sure the patient understands, and supply brochures, handouts, or illustrations to help reinforce the concepts. Make sure to dictate these diagnoses into the discharge document.

   It is important to involve family members in the discharge process of elderly patients, especially those with cognitive impairment. Education of family members also facilitates a safe transition.

2. Summarize the pertinent medical history and the key physical findings in discharge documentation. For instance, for a patient with CHF and pulmonary fibrosis, it would be important to note that even when the patient was clinically no longer in a CHF exacerbation, there were still crackles on the lung examination due to fibrosis.

3. Include the dates of hospital admission and discharge with a brief narrative of the hospitalization. Novice doctors often spend most of their time on this part of their discharge summary, when in reality it is the least read section. Be brief and problem oriented.

4. List the procedures done and key lab results in the discharge summary. Do not create an unreadable "data dump" by including all available information—make a decision about what to include based on the patient's active problems. For instance, that a patient's creatinine remained normal for 10 days only needs to be mentioned once, but the evolving INR and changing warfarin doses for new-onset atrial fibrillation should be mentioned in detail.

5. A proposed way of listing medications on the discharge medication list is new medications followed by continued medications and then discontinued medications. It is recommended to mention the indication for new medication, reason for any changes in dosing or frequency of the continued medications, and reason for discontinuation of a medication. Finally, make sure to "de-autosubstitute" medications. For instance, if your hospital automatically changes your patient's omeprazole to an equivalent dose of esomeprazole, make sure his or her medication list at discharge lists his or her home medication, omeprazole, as his or her PPI. Failure to do so can result in harmful (and expensive) medication class duplication.

6. If your patient was seen by specialists, include a list of them in the discharge summary. Make sure to list the names of the attending physicians and the

problem for which they saw the patient. "Patient was seen by Dr. Friend of GI for peptic ulcer disease" is much more informative than "Patient was seen by GI."

7. If you spent time educating a patient or family on a medical issue, indicate that in the discharge documentation. "Since patient was new to warfarin, we discussed eating a vitamin K–consistent diet and supplied a handout" can help the PCP know education needs remain for the patient.

8. Describe the patient's functional and mental status at discharge, so that the PCP knows if the patient's "baseline" has changed. If changes have been made in the DNR status or advance directives, make sure to describe them. If the patient is being sent to an extended care facility (ECF) or home with assistance, note that in the summary.

9. List all the follow-up appointments and recommendations in the discharge document so that both the PCP and the patient (who may receive this information by way of written prescription or a printed list at discharge) know future plans. By doing this, you make it easy for the PCP to be on the lookout for follow-up information, and you make it easier to help the patient comply with follow-up recommendations.

10. Call special attention to the patient's critical follow-up needs. The last section of the discharge document should be a bulleted list of important follow-up issues. Using the patient from our opening scenario as an example, it is clear that a summary statement in a discharge summary that said "Important Follow-up Issue: Per Dr. Friend of GI, this patient can re-start his warfarin therapy in 6 weeks barring further issues" would have prevented the medical error that was made.

11. Include the name of the attending physician in the hospital and contact information. Patients meet many new people during their hospital stays, and few can name their attending physicians. Providing this information is crucial to facilitating good communication between the hospital team and the patient's outpatient team.

12. Give or send the patient a copy of the discharge summary. This is vitally important for patients who have yet to establish with a PCP or who are from out of town. On a very literal level, the only way to ensure that a patient arrives at an outpatient appointment with all pertinent information is to place the information in the patient's hands.

TIPS TO REMEMBER

- Issues at discharge are myriad and complex. Work as a team to accomplish the tasks and remember that the patient's outpatient team (PCP, caregivers, family) should be included in the process.

- Prompt discharge documentation that lists pending labs and important follow-up issues is the most important piece of a successful transition from the hospital to home.
- Use a checklist approach to make sure your discharge work is complete and that your discharge summary gives important information to the patient's PCP.

COMPREHENSION QUESTIONS

1. Use the checklist of items to consider at discharge and turn them into workable "section headings" you can use in a discharge document.

2. List 5 problems that patients could have immediately following discharge that could result in a readmission to the hospital.

Answers

1. Although the hospital at which you work may suggest a template for discharge summaries, they can insufficiently address the complex discharges doctors in internal medicine must manage. In general, you can use a template of your own devising when dictating discharge summaries. Using the checklist discussed above, a template for discharge summaries could be:

> Primary and secondary diagnosis
> Pertinent history and physical findings
> Dates of hospitalization and hospital course
> Previous (home) medications
> Medication list at discharge
> Results of procedures and labs
> Subspecialists involved in care
> Educational issues addressed
> Patient's functional status/advanced directive at discharge
> Follow-up arrangements made
> Specific follow-up needs
> Name and contact information of discharging team

2. It is important to put yourself in the patient's shoes and think about the problems that might occur after discharge. These issues can be as likely as exacerbations of acute illness to result in a readmission. Common issues include:

- Medications:
  Inability to afford new prescription medication
  Interactions or severe side effects from new medications
  Mixing up old and new doses of medications
  Continuing to take medications that have been stopped

- Home environment:
Not having the keys to get back into the house
Being unable to climb the stairs to enter the house
Being alone with no access to food/telephone/toileting/heat/air conditioning
Family/caregivers who are unprepared for patient's needs
Needing equipment that has not been arranged/delivered (home oxygen, hospital bed)

- Follow-up:
Losing the papers listing follow-up appointments
Finding out about a scheduling conflict with 1 of the follow-up appointments
Not being able to arrange transport to a follow-up appointment

SUGGESTED READINGS

Halasyamani L, Kripalani S, Coleman EA, et al. Transition of care for hospitalized elderly patients—development of a discharge checklist for hospitalists. *J Hosp Med.* 2006;1:354–360.
Hesselink G, Schoonhoven L, Barach P, et al. Improving patient handovers from hospital to primary care: a systematic review. *Ann Intern Med.* 2012;157(6):417–428.
Kim CS, Flanders S. In the clinic. Transitions of care. *Ann Intern Med.* 2013;158(5 Pt 1):ITC3-1.
Kripalani S, Jackson A, Schnipper J, Coleman EA. Promoting effective transitions of care at hospital discharge: a review of key issues for hospitalists. *J Hosp Med.* 2007;2:314–323.
Kripalani S, LeFevre F, Phillips CO, et al. Deficits in communications and information transfer between hospital-based and primary care physicians: implications for patient safety and continuity of care. *JAMA.* 2007;297:831–841.
Moore C, Wisnivesky J, Williams S, McGinn T. Medical errors related to discontinuity of care from an inpatient to an outpatient setting. *J Gen Intern Med.* 2003;18:646–651.
van Walraven C, Dhalla IA, Bell C, et al. Derivation and validation of an index to predict early death or unplanned readmission after discharge from hospital to the community. *CMAJ.* 2010;182(6):551.

A Woman With Mild Dementia and a CHF Exacerbation

Christine Y. Todd, MD, FACP, FHM

You are an intern on the General Ward Service. Ms Brown, one of your patients, is a woman with mild baseline dementia who was admitted 2 days ago with a CHF exacerbation. For the last 2 nights in the hospital she has had agitation and confusion at night, which your team has attributed to "sundowning." She received quetiapine for these symptoms by the night resident, which worked well.

On hospital day 3, your team sees Ms Brown on rounds and decides, based on persistent crackles in her lung bases, elevated JVD, and continued shortness of breath, that continued diuresis is needed before discharge can be contemplated. Forty milligrams of IV furosemide is prescribed as a 1-time dose that morning, and when you check back on Ms Brown later in the day, she seems to feel better.

When handing your patients off to the night residents before your shift is over, you go over Ms Brown's case, explaining that her diagnoses are dementia and CHF and letting your teammates know that she is stable and hopefully will be discharged soon.

When you arrive to the hospital the next day, you see Ms Brown and find that she is not doing well. She complains of shortness of breath, has prominent JVD, and has bilateral lower lobe crackles. You see by her intake and output tally that she had quite a bit to drink the night before, and even though she had 1 L of urine after her morning dose of furosemide, she had 3 L of intake to only 2 L of output for the last 24-hour period. She is still in a CHF exacerbation and will not be able to be discharged today.

In addition, the night residents tell you that she was very agitated last night, and became even more agitated after they gave her a dose of benzodiazepines to calm her down. In fact, they had to restrain her arms in order to keep her from pulling out her IV line, which was very upsetting to her family, who had to be notified about the restraint order.

1. **What unintended consequences did Ms Brown suffer during her hospital course? What was the root cause of these errors?**

Answer

1. This case illustrates a few of the many mishaps that can occur when patients receive care from shifting teams of providers, as opposed to one provider who is responsible for them throughout a hospital stay. There are many good reasons why doctors and other health care providers must transfer the responsibility

for a patient's care among each other during a patient's hospital stay, but these transition points are also fraught with the opportunity for serious error. In this case, Ms Brown fell victim to 2 errors, both traceable to handoff issues.

Although Ms Brown was identified as a patient with CHF during the handoff, she was not classified as a patient in a CHF *exacerbation*. Thus, the night team did not know that the primary team intended for the patient to be in a negative fluid balance during their shift. Second, the information that Ms Brown's "sundowning" responded well to quetiapine was not relayed to the night team. Without this knowledge, they chose a medication to which the patient had unintended side effects when a superior medication for the patient was available. The combination of these 2 preventable unintended outcomes, or medical errors, will likely prolong Ms Brown's hospital stay.

CASE REVIEW: HAND-OFFS WITH ANTICIPATED COMMUNICATION

A high-functioning health care team puts best practices into effect in managing handoffs. The medical literature suggests a number of ways to ensure that handoffs happen seamlessly (discussed in detail below). In the scenario above, a handoff that made acute issues explicit by specifying that Ms Brown had a CHF *exacerbation and needed further diuresis* would have made it more clear to the night team that they needed to watch her Is and Os and possibly give her additional doses of furosemide.

Besides offering specific information about acute issues, good-quality handoffs also give recommendations about anticipated complications. In Ms Brown's case, her dementia makes her prone to nighttime delirium or "sundowning," and since it has happened on the first 2 nights of her hospitalization, it is very likely to happen again. Since there was a treatment that worked for her, a handoff to the night team should have included not only the warning that she might get delirious but also a specific recommendation for the medication that helped her.

Anticipated Problems

Poor-quality handoffs have been implicated in the medical literature as one of the most common sources of medical errors in the hospital. Even though everyone on a health care team feels responsible for the patients in the hospital, it remains difficult to "know" the patients you did not admit or for whom you do not have primary responsibility. Teams that aim to give excellent care to their patients work hard on avoiding the "voltage drop" of information at handoff by effecting succinct, accurate, and helpful communication at the point of transition. Chief among the skills it takes to do this is the ability to give specific tasks on active issues and specific recommendations about anticipated problems.

When asked to hand off a patient to a covering physician, many novice physicians will begin by relating the patient's narrative, starting with the events that led to the patient's illness and working in chronologic order through the events of the hospitalization. Although this type of handoff can impressively demonstrate how thoroughly you know your patient, it usually does not help the receiving doctor manage the patient's needs. More helpful is a non-narrative bulleted presentation of the patient's acute or active issues along with specific recommendations for anticipated problems. In this way, you can most efficiently pass your knowledge of the patient to your colleague. It is important to be as specific as possible—not just "give furosemide," but relay *how much* furosemide has worked in the past for the patient. Don't advise giving a patient blood "if he or she needs it." Rather, give specifics for the hemoglobin level at which you feel a transfusion is warranted, and why.

For novices, a good way to organize a bulleted list of acute issues is to work from the problem list you've generated as part of your SOAP note on the patient. You do not need to mention every issue on your problem list during your handoff, but you should mention the ones you feel are likely to need intervention. Your senior resident can help you develop your list of acute issues for handoff. The senior can also help you think of specific recommendations for actions on these acute issues until you are comfortable coming up with these on your own.

Table 45-1 lists common inpatient issues and suggests specific recommendations that may be needed to help covering residents take care of your patient when you are not on shift.

When handing off your patients to a colleague, be accurate, to the point, and specific about the issues facing your patient. It is equally important that you be engaged in the handoff process when you are the resident who will be covering a group of patients for a shift. Pay close attention to the information you are being given, and write notes to yourself so that you can remember the specific actions recommended to you by your peers. Be assertive in asking questions so that you get the type of information you need in order to take care of the patient. For instance, if you are told a patient may "need extra insulin," be sure to ask what kind of insulin is indicated and in what doses it is likely to work.

The course of a patient in the hospital is not always predictable, and surprises, emergencies, and generally unforeseen events occur frequently. It is impossible to account for every issue that may arise for your patient—covering residents will always have to keep an open mind, be flexible, and see the patient for themselves to decide on the best course of action for every situation. However, a succinct summary of active issues along with specific recommendations for action can help everyone on the health care team work together to create good outcomes for the patient.

Table 45-1. Common Inpatient Issues and Recommendations for Covering

Symptom or Diagnosis	Anticipated Issues
Chest pain	Do you suspect cardiac or noncardiac pain?
	What should be ordered if the pain recurs—ECG, chest x-ray, antacid, antianxiety medicine?
Dyspnea	What would be the most likely cause in this patient?
	What are the patient's baseline oxygen needs?
Oliguria	If this occurs, is it likely that the patient needs a diuretic or a fluid bolus?
GI bleed	Is the bleeding active, or has it clinically stopped?
	How likely is the patient to rebleed?
	When will the next hemoglobin be checked? What value is likely to represent further bleeding?
	What should be done if further bleeding is suspected—bleeding scan? Notify GI team?
CHF	What is your goal for diuresis in the next 24 h?
Infection	What should be done for a fever? Reculture or change in antibiotics?
Pain	What additional steps should be taken if the patient's pain is not controlled? Should the current analgesic be increased in dose or frequency? Should there be an additional workup as to the source of the pain?
IV access	How important are the IV medications the patient is on? If the patient loses IV access, can his or her medications be changed to oral equivalents, or should a central line be placed?
Advance directives	If this patient's status worsens, what steps should be taken? Should a transfer to ICU be contemplated, or does the patient wish to de-escalate care at that point?
	Who has the power of attorney, and what is the contact information?

TIPS TO REMEMBER

● The handoff is one of the few places in medicine in which a narrative approach to communication will not benefit the patient.

- Put work and thought into making a complete and prioritized problem list for your patient. This cannot be done "on the fly" and is the most important step toward a high-quality handoff.

- Think of patient care in terms of a 24-hours-a-day, 7-days-a-week cycle. What can you communicate at the point of handoff that will make sure that your patient's care will be advanced during the shifts in which you are absent?

- Incorporate unexpected events into updated action steps you include in the next handoff on the patient.

- If you are receiving a handoff that does not include specific tasks and delineates active issues, be assertive! Clarify vague recommendations, and make sure you clearly understand the active patient issues.

COMPREHENSION QUESTIONS

1. Your patient, Mr Brown, has end-stage COPD and is hospitalized with a COPD exacerbation. After a day of hospitalization, the IV steroids, antibiotics, and breathing treatments seem to be improving his symptoms. However, your senior warns you on rounds that he is "not out of the woods yet." You note that he is a full code, but wonder if resuscitation would be much of a benefit to him should his condition suddenly worsen. What is the best way to hand off this patient to your colleagues at the end of your shift?

2. Your co-intern is finished with her work and is ready to go home. During the handoff, she mentions that one of her patients has become more dyspneic this afternoon, and a CT angiogram of the chest to look for pulmonary embolism has been ordered but hasn't been done yet. She asks you to follow up on this test and start anticoagulation if it is positive. What kinds of questions would give you more specific information to help you take care of this patient?

Answers

1. It is important to discuss unresolved issues, such as goals of care in patients with serious illnesses, before handing off a patient's case to your colleagues. The time you have spent with your patient and his or her family establishes an important rapport and allows your patient the chance to have an informed conversation about the condition and make a clear-headed choice about care should the condition worsen. Without the benefit of this relationship, conversations between covering residents and patients done during a time of medical crisis can lead to decisions that all parties regret. By discussing end-of-life issues with your patient in preparation for handoff, you can offer your peers specific information and action steps in case your patient's condition deteriorates.

2. Although your co-intern has supplied you with a specific request—to follow up on her patient's CT scan—there are a few issues that bear further questioning so that the patient can get high-quality care. First, it would be a good idea to ask how strongly a PE is suspected—if the clinical suspicion is high, starting anticoagulation before getting the CT results back is warranted. Next, it would be helpful to know what other diagnoses the patient's primary team is contemplating for the patient's dyspnea. That way, you can continue a workup for the problem if the CT scan is negative for PE. Finally, asking if there are any relative contraindications or concerns for anticoagulation can help you be alert for concerning symptoms while you are caring for the patient.

SUGGESTED READINGS

Arora VM, Manjarrez E, Dressler DD, et al. Hospitalist handoffs: a systematic review and task force recommendations. *J Hosp Med.* 2009;4(7):433–440 [review].

Burton MC, Kashiwagi DT, Kirkland LL, et al. Gaining efficiency and satisfaction in the handoff process. *J Hosp Med.* 2010;5(9):547–552.

Riesenberg LA, Leitzsch J, Massucci JL, et al. Residents' and attending physicians' handoffs: a systematic review of the literature. *Acad Med.* 2009;84(12):1775–1787 [review].

A Patient in Respiratory Distress

Christine Y. Todd, MD, FACP, FHM

You are on call for the General Wards service, and it's late in the afternoon. One of your co-interns, Dr. George, went home a few hours ago. He sent you a text page telling you that a list of his patients is taped to the door of the resident's lounge and that "every one is stable." As you were busy admitting a sick patient when you got his text, you did not have time to call Dr. George back and ask for more detailed information.

Just as you are getting ready to eat supper, you get a page from a nurse. He tells you that one of Dr. George's patients is in respiratory distress and needs to be assessed. This patient is not on the list that Dr. George printed out for you, but when you check the patient's chart, you see that he has been seeing and writing notes on the patient daily. Unfortunately, his note in her chart from today is largely illegible. When you go to the patient's room to assess her and begin asking questions, the patient becomes irritated. "I already answered these questions a million times! Don't you people talk to each other?"

1. What are the communication challenges present in this scenario?

2. How can a handoff process be structured in order to mitigate the communication breakdowns present in the above case?

Answers

1. In the above scenario, there are many opportunities for improvement in communication of handoff information. First, and perhaps most importantly, the handoff does not occur in a face-to-face fashion. Since the giving and the receiving interns do not meet and discuss the patients, the only information shared is a list of names and the vague assurance that all patients are "stable." Because there is not an appointed time and place for the handoff to occur, the list ends up being posted in a potentially public area, and the receiving intern is too distracted by a new patient to be able to take the time to ask Dr. George important questions about the patients on his service. Lastly, the list of patients to cover is incorrect, leading to additional time spent by the covering intern gathering facts from the patient and chart, which is illegible. The patient's perception that this is a poor way to approach patient care is correct.

2. Although the focus on skills for successful transfers of care is relatively new, there are best practices advocated for and supported by a growing body of medical literature. It is important that your residency program provide a consistent structure for handoffs. A specific time and place for handoff, consistent written and verbal formats, content guidelines, and an insistence on legible, accurate charting should be strong elements of the resident culture around transfers of patient information and care. These items should be perceived as mandatory by

house staff and done as a matter of routine in order to create a safe environment for patients.

TRANSITIONS OF CARE—HANDOFFS

Handoffs, an ever more frequent occurrence in the course of hospitalized patient care, are a time when significant patient safety issues can occur. Residents working in today's compressed, shift-work-oriented environment must develop the ability to competently give and receive handoff information.

Novice house staff may think that poor-quality handoff communication occurs in a somewhat random fashion due to lack of experience. They may assume that as they gain confidence and general know-how, they will naturally produce high-quality transfers of care. In fact, errors in handoff communication are very predictable and can be largely avoided, even by novices, by adhering to a consistent structure for handoff. The Joint Commission, the national association that accredits health care organizations, lists a standardized approach to handoff communication as a mandatory National Patient Safety Goal.

There is no substitute for face-to-face handoffs. When you personally meet to transfer patient care, the quality of the information shared is higher. In addition, the person receiving the handoff has the opportunity to ask questions. For instance, in a patient with a complex illness and an involved family, a face-to-face handoff makes it more likely that ongoing treatment decisions and the vocabulary used to explain them will be consistent across caregivers. This leads to care that advances despite changes in staff and higher patient and family satisfaction.

There should be a consistent time and place for handoff communication. Handoffs that take place as each team finishes work and leaves for the day are inefficient, as they occur at random and unplanned times. Although the residents giving the handoff information may have tied up all loose ends and are ready to focus on the handoff, the receiving resident is frequently in the middle of a task. A distracted resident will not be able to listen and participate in the handoff process. A routine, specific time for handoff should be established so that both teams of caretakers can be ready to participate in the process. It's also important to choose a place for handoff that is quiet, private, and HIPAA compliant.

Participants should use a standard template for written and verbal handoffs. There are many popular templates to guide information transfer, such as SBAR and I PASS THE BATON. You should use the one endorsed by your institution, as it can be very helpful when both nurses and doctors use the same handoff template. Verbal handoffs that are accompanied by written prompts result in better-quality handoffs than verbal handoffs by themselves. Recent studies suggest that computer-generated printouts that autopopulate important fields can make handoffs more accurate. They also lead to fewer patients being forgotten and left off the list at handoff. These types of lists are increasingly available for use at hospitals that have instituted electronic health records with computerized physician order entry. In any case, when composing a written list or cards to pass along at handoff, remember the "garbage in, garbage out" rule. Written handoffs are only as good as the information they display, so it is important to update information such as code status, active problems, and medication lists.

It is important to create an environment during handoff that minimizes distractions. Participants should be seated so that they can take notes and focus on their task. The room should be quiet, with no side conversations taking place among house staff waiting their turn to sign out patients. Supervising residents should relieve the resident taking over patient care of the pager, so that the resident is not rushed and the handoff process is not fractured by frequent pauses while the on-call intern returns a page.

Lastly, remember that no matter how good a handoff is, it is impossible for all information to be transferred and all issues to be anticipated. In many cases, an issue evolving on a patient will require some time spent with the chart in order to make good clinical decisions. It is thus very important to maintain high standards of quality in written charting. Legible handwriting is mandatory. Legible signatures (or legible written names appended to signatures) are of utmost importance in terms of helping others know whom to contact for patient issues. For institutions that use a computerized record, remember that overuse of cut and paste in composing notes can lead to the perpetuation of outdated and incorrect information in a patient's chart. Original content, particularly in the assessment and plan area of your SOAP note, is a hallmark of quality care.

TIPS TO REMEMBER

- There is no substitute for a standardized approach to patient handoffs that includes a face-to-face conversation at a preestablished place and time and with a standardized informational template.
- Verbal handoffs that are accompanied by a written document lead to better outcomes.
- Prepopulated computer-generated sign-out documents can lead to more efficient handoffs and fewer missed patients.
- Handoffs are 2-way conversations. The resident handing off patients must be accurate and efficient, and the resident receiving the handoff should actively participate by asking questions clarifying complex issues.

COMPREHENSION QUESTIONS

1. Although handoffs are often discussed in the context of inpatient care, what are some scenarios where good handoff skills could be used to augment ambulatory care?

2. You are on call and realize that one of your co-interns has gone home without signing out her patients to you. You have handled a few straightforward calls on her patients but will be responsible for her patients until the end of your shift. What should you do?

Answers

1. The overall acuity of an outpatient panel is lower than that of a group of inpatients, but at any given point in time, there are patients in an outpatient practice who have important evolving issues. Outpatient practitioners should consider a formal handoff of this group of patients to one of their partners when they will be away from their practice for a substantial period of time—that is, vacation, educational leave, or medical leave. Residents might consider an inpatient handoff during training months during which their clinic time will be limited, as it may be during a month in the ICU or working night shifts. A short session where a verbal and written sign-out of patients with acute issues is discussed between colleagues (and potentially other staff, such as clinic nurses) would further patient continuity.

2. A handoff must occur so that patient care can be rendered safely, and it is your duty to purse the information you need to take care of patients for whom you are responsible. Unfortunately, due to work duty hour restrictions, you may not be able to page your co-intern to obtain handoff information. In this case, contacting either your co-intern's senior resident or attending for handoff information would be the advised course of action. Asking your program to establish a routine time and place where all teams gather for handoff (and the process does not start without all participants present) would alleviate this problem in the future.

SUGGESTED READINGS

Arora VM, Manjarrez E, Dressler DD, et al. Hospitalist handoffs: a systematic review and task force recommendations. *J Hosp Med*. 2009;4(7):433–440.

Joint Commission. *Critical Access Hospital: 2024 National Patient Safety Goals*. www.jointcommission.org/standards/national-patient-safety-goals/critical-access-hospital-national-patient-safety-goals. Accessed December 26, 2023.

Kripalani S, Jackson AT, Schnipper JL, Coleman EA. Promoting effective transitions of care at hospital discharge: a review of key issues for hospitalists. *J Hosp Med*. 2007;2(5):314–323.

Solet DJ, Norvell JM, Rutan GH, Frankel RM. Lost in translation: challenges and opportunities during physician-to-physician communication during patient handoffs. *Acad Med*. 2005;80:1094–1099.

Williams MV, Flanders SA, Whitcomb W, et al. *Comprehensive Hospital Medicine*. Philadelphia: Saunders; 2007.

A 78-year-old Woman Taking Multiple Medications

Beaux Cole, PharmD and Tiffany I. Leung, MD, MPH

A 78-year-old woman with hypertension, diabetes mellitus, and osteoporosis presents to the clinic for a hospital follow-up appointment. She had presented to the ED with unilateral weakness and garbled speech after being found on the floor at home after an unknown period of time. Her medicine list upon presentation to the ED was as follows: hydrochlorothiazide, candesartan, baby aspirin, metformin, and alendronate. At the ED, she presented with lethargy, slurred speech, and orientation to self only, but respirations were unlabored. Her blood pressure was 98/65 mm Hg with a heart rate of 128 bpm. Oxygen saturation was 97% on room air. Cardiac examination demonstrated an irregularly irregular rhythm. A thorough neurologic examination revealed a right-sided facial droop, and she was unable to lift her right arm or leg off the bed. A CT brain showed a left middle cerebral artery ischemic stroke. An ECG confirmed new atrial fibrillation. A pelvic x-ray showed a left pubic ramus fracture. Her laboratory data showed a blood glucose of 360 mg/dL and findings consistent with acute kidney injury and mild rhabdomyolysis. During hospitalization, she developed a right lower extremity deep-vein thrombus and was started on therapeutic anticoagulation.

She was discharged to her home less than a week ago, with assistance from her son and a hired caregiver. She now needs assistance with taking her medications. You review her medication list and find the following:

- Hydrochlorothiazide and metformin were discontinued.
- Alendronate was not given during hospitalization.
- Aspirin was continued during hospitalization.
- Candesartan was originally substituted with losartan but then changed to ramipril.
- New medications include insulin glargine, insulin lispro, metoprolol tartrate, diltiazem, warfarin, atorvastatin, pantoprazole, hydrocodone–acetaminophen, and calcium with vitamin D_3.

1. What are important next steps in managing this patient's medication list as you evaluate her during her first posthospitalization follow-up appointment?
2. What counseling should you provide to this patient and her caregivers?

Answers

1. A *comprehensive medication review* (CMR) (see definition in Table 47-1) must occur at every transition of care between health care settings. It is important to recognize that medication errors can compromise patient safety and contribute to increased rates of rehospitalization within 30 days after discharge. Medication reconciliation helps to reduce these errors. Medication changes must be clearly identified and appropriate counseling provided to the patient and caregiver in a patient-centered manner that is sensitive to both health literacy level and cultural background. Additionally, preparing for this transition of care should include direct communication of the recommended medication changes from the hospitalist to the patient's primary care physician.

2. Medication-specific counseling must be provided to ensure safe medication administration outside of the closely monitored setting of the hospital. For example, this patient began taking warfarin to reduce her risk of recurrent cardioembolic stroke and also to prevent additional deep-vein thrombosis. Warfarin administration requires appropriate counseling about diet because of the effects of variable vitamin K intake on INR, monitoring for symptoms and signs of potentially life-threatening bleeding, and the importance of regular INR follow-up to monitor and continue this medication safely. Similarly, skill-focused education is important to ensure that the patient and family understand how to safely administer the right insulin doses and types of insulin at the right times, check blood sugars with a glucometer, and monitor for signs of hypoglycemia. Additional counseling on possible adverse effects of all medications must be provided.

Table 47-1. Definitions

Medication reconciliation	The process of verifying that a patient's current list of medications (including dose, route, and frequency) is correct and that the medications are currently medically necessary and safe
Medical error	Failure of a planned action to be completed as intended. Errors during the transition from discharge to post-acute or outpatient care include medication errors and potential adverse drug events, test follow-up errors, and workup errors
Medication discrepancy	Lack of agreement (or incompatibility) between different medication regimens, which may be recorded (eg, in the medical record) or reported (eg, provided by the patient verbally or with medication bottles)

CASE REVIEW

Throughout this patient's hospital course, multiple medication changes were required to address her new and pre-existing medical problems. Additionally, she now has an increased need for assistance in performing activities of daily living, has impaired mobility, and is at risk for additional functional, cognitive, and communication impairments that would increase the complexity of her post-acute care and long-term recovery.

This patient's medication regimen has become increasingly complex but is clinically indicated given her multiple medical conditions. Safe prescribing practices involve accounting for the side-effect profile of each new medication and ensuring that the patient and caregivers are given appropriate medication education and counseling. Clearly and explicitly informing patients and caregivers of medications discontinued during the hospitalization also is important.

A comprehensive medication review can require a significant amount of time and effort, but there are clear care, quality, and patient safety benefits of a detailed medication review. An inaccurate or incomplete medication list obtained at admission will likely result in an inaccurate and incomplete list at discharge. Additionally, when the initial reconciliation is performed, medication adherence should be addressed. *Medication adherence*, rather than compliance, is preferred language regarding patients' medication usage because there can be external factors that may have led to a patient not taking medication as prescribed. Examples include access barriers such as cost or adequate insurance coverage for prescribed medications, or inadequate counseling about technique or other special instructions relating to self-administration of a prescribed medication. In some circumstances, discovery of barriers to medication adherence can reveal opportunities for treatment and continuing care management without having to add, discontinue, or change existing medication regimens.

Anticipating potential medication-related complications before discharge can help to prevent problems with medications after discharge from hospital to home. For example, when the patient returns home, medications reconciled on admission may still be available at home or to pick up from a pharmacy (from an old prescription), even if they may have been discontinued during a hospitalization with the intention to keep the medication discontinued after discharge. A patient who inadvertently continues taking home medications when they were to be discontinued may be at higher risk of experiencing an adverse event or a poorer health outcome. In the case presented, hydrochlorothiazide and metformin have been discontinued in the hospital, and, in the absence of sufficient counseling or systems of care that facilitate medication discontinuation, the patient may inappropriately continue to take these medications.

Another common source of errors and miscommunication about medications is the use of brand names and generic names. *Therapeutic substitution* of similar medications within a medication class is common during hospitalization—for example, candesartan and losartan are in the class of angiotensin II receptor blockers, and ramipril is an angiotensin-converting enzyme inhibitor—as was done in this case. Particularly in cases where substitution is done based on a hospital's pharmacy formulary, it is important to resume use of the admission medication on discharge to avoid *therapeutic duplication*, unless an alternative is indicated based on the clinical scenario.

The risks and benefits of each new or modified medication or dosing regimen must be considered at each transition of care. Warfarin in this patient provides an evidence-based benefit of secondary stroke prevention, given the presumed etiology was a cardioembolic thrombus related to undiagnosed atrial fibrillation, and also protection against a recurrent venous thromboembolic event. However, the patient is on both aspirin and warfarin, which increases the risk of significant bleeding complications. Such risk–benefit considerations must be carefully weighed before making the final decision to adjust the medication regimen on discharge from the hospital. The clinical scenario and diagnoses should always guide decision-making about appropriate use of medications.

GENERAL APPROACH

Epidemiology

Discharge from the inpatient hospital to a continuing care facility or to home is a time of increased patient vulnerability to medical errors and adverse clinical outcomes. Transitions of care become increasingly complex when additional factors are considered, including multiple chronic conditions, polypharmacy, vulnerable populations including geriatric patients, increased demands for patient self-management, complex follow-up care plans, and multiple medication and treatment changes. All transition of care processes also depends heavily on clear patient–clinician communication and communication between clinicians during handoffs, particularly between the discharging hospitalist and primary care physician.

As the number of persons over the age of 65 increase, so does the prevalence of *polypharmacy*. There are several interpretations of polypharmacy, but the traditional definition is the use of five or more chronic medications. Patients with multiple chronic conditions often are under care of multiple specialists prescribing multiple medications. There is a potential for a silo effect to occur, where communication between clinicians leads to unchecked polypharmacy and undesirable outcomes. Polypharmacy from multiple clinicians who are following single chronic disease clinical practice guidelines can result in unchecked medication combinations and lead to decreased functional status and negative outcomes. Consequences of polypharmacy include greater health care costs, increased risk of adverse drug events (ADEs), drug interactions, medication nonadherence, reduced functional capacity, and multiple geriatric syndromes. The 5 most commonly implicated drugs leading to rehospitalization, especially in the elderly, are digoxin, warfarin, insulin, oral antiplatelet agents, and oral hypoglycemic agents. Health care costs such as outpatient and hospital visits may increase nearly 30% when the patient is taking potentially inappropriate medications (PIMs).

In the outpatient setting, one study showed that 58.6% of older patients are taking 1 or more unnecessary medications. Older individuals are at a greater risk for ADEs due to metabolic changes, memory issues, frailty, coexisting medial problems, use of multiple prescribed and nonprescribed medications, and decreased drug clearance associated with aging. Outpatients taking 5 or more medications have an 88% increased risk of an ADE compared with those patients taking fewer. A contributing factor to ADEs is the prescribing cascade (Table 47-1), where the adverse effect of a medication is misdiagnosed for a new disease state that is then treated with a new medication. The adverse effects can easily be misinterpreted as an illness that is common in older adults. The common drug classes for ADEs include anticoagulants, NSAIDs, cardiovascular medications, diuretics, antibiotics, anticonvulsants, benzodiazepines, and hypoglycemic medications. One study showed that 80% of older adults with polypharmacy have a potential hepatic cytochrome enzyme–mediated, drug–drug interaction. These drug–drug interactions regularly cause preventable ADEs and hospital readmissions. Another study indicated that 7% of all deaths in a hospital setting are drug related, with drug interactions being a contributing factor. As the population ages and multiple chronic conditions become increasingly common, heightened awareness of drug–drug interaction risks is an essential competency for clinicians including pharmacists and physicians.

The use of multiple medications is associated with complicated medication regimens, leading to barriers to medication adherence. Medication nonadherence is associated with ADEs, potential disease progression, treatment failure, and hospitalization. Cognitive impairment has also been associated with polypharmacy as a contributing factor for medication nonadherence.

As the complexity of care increases and the number of older adults increase, the need for care management has also increased. In 2017, the Center for Medicare Services transitioned to a Quality Payment Program (QPP) as a way to change their fee schedule to one that rewards high-value, high-quality Medicare clinicians. One of the tracks of the QPP to choose is the Merit-based Incentive Payment System (MIPS), where clinicians report quality measures to CMS and are being scored on these quality measures; depending on the score a clinician will get either a positive or negative incentive. Many of the quality measures evaluate medication management as an integral part of outcomes. Polypharmacy negatively impacts patient outcomes through ADEs, drug–drug interactions, medication nonadherence, functional status, and cognitive impairment. Identifying strategies to manage polypharmacy in an effort to improve outcomes and leverage quality-based measures is crucial to receiving sustainable reimbursement.

Treatment

Comprehensive medication reconciliation (CMR) and *comprehensive medication management* (CMM) can increase patient safety and quality of care in each health care setting *and* across transitions of care between health care settings. When managing the care of an outpatient hospital follow-up patient, the CMR plays a vital role to identify how clinicians should effectively manage medication therapy. This includes assessment of each medication's dose, frequency, and route of administration. Medications should include prescriptions from different providers, non-oral medications, over-the-counter products, and supplements. CMR should be conducted at every hospital follow-up visit and at least annually to prevent unchecked polypharmacy and undesirable outcomes. Possible sources of medication information include the patient, the patient's caregiver or family members, nursing home personnel, a primary care physician or other clinicians, and pharmacies. Medical assistants, students and learners can assist with this process ahead of the visit. With a complete and accurate medication list for the patient, clinicians can focus on medication management and the strategies that help improve quality outcomes.

Medication management, while challenging to implement in a primary care setting with time constraints, can be more effective by focusing on monitoring medication use and pharmacovigilance (Table 47-1). Monitoring, prescribing, and adherence have been identified as major factors that contribute to adverse drug events in the outpatient setting. Monitoring medication therapy is not limited to laboratory monitoring drug levels, which is necessary for a medication like warfarin. Monitoring medication therapy is an effective way to identify ADEs and differentiate them from a potential new disease state, or adding a medication to treat the symptom. Verifying drug–drug interactions and drug–disease interactions, monitoring renal and hepatic clearance, ensuring the medication is effective, and being aware of cytochrome enzyme clearance interactions, in addition to laboratory monitoring, are important ways to identify and prevent problematic polypharmacy in patients.

Prescribing or deprescribing is an effective way to address and correct ADEs that diminish the functional status of a patient. With pharmacovigilance, we can minimize potentially inappropriate medications (PIMs) by utilizing resources such as the Beers criteria and the START and STOPP criteria. While the Beers criteria list PIMs in older adults, the majority of ADEs that cause hospitalization are not on this list. Patients on digoxin, warfarin, insulins, oral antiplatelet medications, and oral hypoglycemics were 35 times more likely to be hospitalized. The START and STOPP criteria were first developed in 2008 and revised in 2018. There are currently 114 criteria (80 STOPP and 34 START) that minimize

Table 47-2. Factors Contributing to Medication Discrepancies After Hospital Discharge

Patient-associated factors
Nonadherence (nonintentional or intentional)
Financial barriers
Did not fill prescription
Did not need prescription
Performance deficit
Adverse drug effect or intolerance
System-associated factors
Incomplete, inaccurate, or illegible discharge instructions
Conflicting information from different informational sources
Duplication
Prescribed with known allergies/intolerances
Confusion between brand and generic names
Incorrect label, quantity, or dosage
Cognitive impairment, sight/dexterity limitations, or need for assistance not recognized

inappropriate prescribing in older adults. STOPP refers to scenarios where a medication should be stopped or deprescribed, and START refers to scenarios where a medication should be added to a patient's treatment plan. Every criterion is evidence-based and literature-supported.

Another scenario where pharmacovigilance is necessary is when a new drug is brought to market. Most clinical trials list older adults in the exclusion criteria. Therefore, most ADEs from new drugs are reported in postmarket data. Clinicians must include heightened monitoring when a new drug to market is prescribed to an older adult.

Medication adherence is important to improve clinical outcomes and care quality measures, but it is challenging to address as a clinician. Some contributing factors to nonadherence include low health literacy, lack of patient involvement in decision-making, complex treatment plans, and socioeconomic barriers (discussed in another chapter of the book). While adherence to therapy is challenging, there are some strategies clinicians can use. Ensuring open communication with the patient at the outpatient visit can empower the patient to ask questions about the therapy to improve health literacy. Using the teach-back method, an iterative technique in which the clinician assesses patient comprehension, tailors important learning points in response to the patient's level of comprehension, and then reassesses patient comprehension until the patient has mastered the knowledge or skill taught. In essence, the clinician is "closing the loop" of communication to ensure that the intended message was received by the patient.

In the case of learning about appropriate medication administration, a clinician might assess patient comprehension in a nonjudgmental manner by stating, "I want to make sure I explained your medicines well. Please tell me how you plan to take each one." Other general rules to follow for clear patient communication include speaking slowly and in plain, nonmedical language, limiting the amount of information conveyed, and repeating or summarizing the information for clarity.

Closing the Loop of Communication

Step 1: Clinician explains new information or advice to patient.

Step 2: Clinician assesses patient recall and comprehension of new information shared.

Step 3: Clinician clarifies and tailors explanation, based on patient's response in step 2.

Step 4: Steps 2 and 3 are repeated iteratively until patient expresses comprehension of new information.

TIPS TO REMEMBER

- Comprehensive medication reconciliation must be performed carefully at every care transition, including hospital follow-up and at least annually, noting medication dosage, frequency, and route of administration.

- Discharge medication discrepancies include omissions, substitutions, commissions, incomplete prescriptions, and duplicate prescriptions.

- Clinical justification must be present to explain each medication change identified when performing the discharge medication reconciliation.

- Discharge medication changes must be communicated clearly to the patient, the patient's caregiver, and post–acute care provider, including the continuing care facility and the patient's primary care physician.

- Medication-specific counseling on hospital discharge can help to improve patient understanding, safety, and outcomes.

- Anticipate potential problems with medications and consider potential sources of error, including where and when errors might occur.

COMPREHENSION QUESTIONS

1. In addition to identifying the name of each medication, what are the 3 most important elements of each medication that must be collected in a detailed and accurate medication reconciliation?
    A. Dose, prescribing physician, and dispensing pharmacy
    B. Dose, route, and frequency
    C. Brand name, dose, and route
    D. Indication, dose, and frequency

2. On admission, a patient reports taking famotidine daily. When she is discharged from the hospital, she is given discharge instructions and a prescription for ranitidine. At her follow-up visit with her primary care physician, she is found to be taking both famotidine and ranitidine. What type of medication discrepancy best describes this scenario?
    A. Omission
    B. Commission
    C. Substitution
    D. Duplication

3. What communication techniques should be utilized in counseling patients about their discharge medications?
    A. Use nonmedical language.
    B. Speak slowly.
    C. Use teach-back.
    D. Summarize information.
    E. All of the above.

Answers

1. B. It is important to identify the dose, route, and frequency of administration of each medication when reconciling a patient's medications at each care transition. Care transitions include admission, interhospital or intrahospital transfers, and discharge.

2. D. This patient is taking two H2-receptor antagonists. Duplication, which is the administration of two medications of the same class, is the correct answer. If famotidine was omitted from the discharge medication list, and no anti-reflux medication was provided on the list when it was intended, then this would be an error of omission. If the intent was to discontinue antireflux medications, but famotidine was included on the discharge medication list, then this would be an error of commission. If the intent was to continue the patient's home antireflux medication but instead ranitidine was prescribed, then this would be an error of substitution.

3. E. All of the options are important communication techniques to use when counseling patients about new medications and potential adverse effects. Communication should also be nonjudgmental, culturally sensitive, and ideally performed in an environment where the patient and his or her caregivers can feel at ease asking questions and engaging in conversation with the physician about medical recommendations.

SUGGESTED READINGS

Bedell SE, Jabbour S, Goldberg R, et al. Discrepancies in the use of medications: their extent and predictors in an outpatient practice. *Arch Intern Med.* 2000;160:2129–2134.

Budnitz DS, Lovegrove MC, Shehab N, Richards CL. Emergency hospitalizations for adverse drug events in older Americans. *N Engl J Med.* 2011;365:2002–2012.

By the 2019 American Geriatrics Society Beers Criteria® Update Expert Panel. American Geriatrics Society 2019 Updated AGS Beers Criteria® for Potentially Inappropriate Medication Use in Older Adults. *J Am Geriatr Soc.* 2019;67(4):674–694.

Care Transitions Program. Health care services for improving quality and safety during care hand-offs. www.caretransitions.org. Accessed May 27, 2022.

Coleman EA, Smith JD, Raha D, Min SJ. Posthospital medication discrepancies: prevalence and contributing factors. *Arch Intern Med.* 2005;165:1842–1847.

Council NR. *Crossing the Quality Chasm: A New Health System for the 21st Century.* Washington, DC: The National Academies Press; 2001.

Council NR. *To Err Is Human: Building a Safer Health System.* Washington, DC: The National Academies Press; 2000.

Greenwald JL, Halasyamani L, Greene J, et al. Making inpatient medication reconciliation patient centered, clinically relevant and implementable: a consensus statement on key principles and necessary first steps. *J Hosp Med.* 2010;5:477–485.

Herrero-Herrero JI, García-Aparicio J. Medication discrepancies at discharge from an internal medicine service. *Eur J Intern Med.* 2011;22:43–48.

Kripalani S, Jackson AT, Schnipper JL, Coleman EA. Promoting effective transitions of care at hospital discharge: a review of key issues for hospitalists. *J Hosp Med.* 2007;2:314–323.

Maher RL, Hanlon J, Hajjar ER. Clinical consequences of polypharmacy in elderly. *Expert Opin Drug Saf.* 2014;13(1):57–65.

Moore C, Wisnivesky J, Williams S, McGinn T. Medical errors related to discontinuity of care from an inpatient to an outpatient setting. *J Gen Intern Med.* 2003;18:646–651.

O'Mahony D, O'Sullivan D, Byrne S, et al. STOPP/START criteria for potentially inappropriate prescribing in older people: version 2. *Age Ageing.* 2015;44(2):213–218. Erratum in: *Age Ageing.* 2018;47(3):489.

Paasche-Orlow M. Caring for patients with limited health literacy: a 76-year-old man with multiple medical problems. *JAMA.* 2011;306:1122–1129.

Persell SD, Brown T, Doctor JN, et al. Development of high-risk geriatric polypharmacy electronic clinical quality measures and a pilot test of HER nudges based on these measures. *J Gen Intern Med.* 2022;37(11):2777–2785.

Schillinger D, Piette J, Grumbach K, et al. Closing the loop: physician communication with diabetic patients who have low health literacy. *Arch Intern Med.* 2003;163:83–90.

Quality Payment Program. qpp.cms.gov. Accessed May 27, 2022.

A 63-year-old Man With an Inability to Urinate

Stephanie Bitner, PharmD, CACP and Tiffany I. Leung, MD, MPH

A 63-year-old man with benign prostatic hypertrophy and diabetes mellitus presents to the ED with gradual decrease in urine output for the past 1 week and inability to urinate today. Over this time, he has developed abdominal pain and fullness. His medical history is otherwise unremarkable. His only medications are finasteride, terazosin, metformin, and a baby aspirin daily. On examination, his temperature is 99.8°F, blood pressure is 138/86 mm Hg, heart rate is 97 bpm, respiratory rate is 14/min, and pulse oximetry is 99% on room air. He appears uncomfortable but in no acute distress. His cardiopulmonary examination is unremarkable. He has suprapubic pain to palpation and dullness to percussion in the same region. He does not have costovertebral angle tenderness. Laboratory evaluation demonstrates WBCs of 13,000 cells/mm^3. After repeated attempts to place a straight urinary catheter, a Coudé catheter is finally placed successfully with resultant 1 L of urine output. Urinalysis shows large hematuria, leukocyte esterase, and nitrites, with 10 to 50 WBCs/hpf. Serum chemistry is normal. Urine and blood cultures are drawn, and empiric ciprofloxacin is started intravenously.

He is admitted for observation and discharged in less than 24 hours with an indwelling urinary catheter, a prescription for oral ciprofloxacin, and instructions to follow up with his primary care provider (PCP) in 24 to 48 hours. He is lost to follow-up and presents to the ED 1 week later with fever, hypotension, and acute kidney injury. His urinary catheter is no longer draining, but he cannot recall when it stopped doing so. Review of his chart shows that the urine and blood cultures drawn 1 week ago grew *Escherichia coli* that was resistant to ciprofloxacin. He is admitted to the hospital and started on piperacillin–tazobactam intravenously for urosepsis.

1. **What type of medical error occurred?**

2. **How could this error have been prevented? What process changes could help to prevent rehospitalization?**

Answers

1. Test follow-up error occurred, in which a test result that was pending at the time of discharge was not followed up. Urine and blood cultures can take up to 5 days for a final result to be reported; preliminary results may be available in 24 to 48 hours. However, the best practice for ensuring a complete course of antibiotic treatment is to ensure that the treatment is aligned with the final culture and sensitivity results. This patient stayed in the hospital for observation only and

was discharged in less than 24 hours. The case does not provide enough information to determine if an adequate handoff regarding the pending test result occurred. There is also no information provided about the follow-up process and who would check the final culture and sensitivity results to tailor antibiotic treatment further if indicated. The culture results provided indicate that oral ciprofloxacin prescribed at discharge would not provide sufficient antimicrobial coverage to treat the patient's urosepsis. The result was potentially actionable, meaning that the result would have changed the plan of management or, more specifically, the antibiotic choice. Medical errors can be divided into two types: errors of omission and errors of commission. Errors of omission are caused by actions not being taken.

2. Many interventions are possible to prevent medical errors and promote patient safety during the transition from the inpatient setting to the outpatient setting. Identifying patients at high risk for error can help to reduce harm. For example, the greater the patient age the higher risk for error; increasing age correlates with more comorbidities and possible altered or impaired function of vital organs. Increased complexity of the patient's condition, multiple chronic conditions and the interactions between them, and/or their treatments can also lead to higher risk of error. With greater complexity comes potentially more interventions, which can include medication administration, diagnostic tests, procedures, or even surgery. Every intervention is a possible opportunity for error. Also, patients seen in the ED experience higher risk for medical error than patients already admitted to the hospital. Finally, low health literacy is associated with higher risk for error. Nearly 90% of adults have difficulty understanding medical information when it is not explained in nonmedical terms. Patients with low health literacy are more likely to have poor health outcomes, medication errors, and difficulty managing their chronic conditions, and they are less likely to seek preventative healthcare.

Patient engagement is positively associated with patient safety. Thorough, health literacy–sensitive patient education should be provided to the patient and their caregivers at every hospital discharge. Hospital discharge processes should include education that explains in simple language the reason for hospitalization, procedures performed, medication changes, pending appointments, and test results. Counseling patients using the teach-back or repeat-back method, using plain language, and utilizing translators are helpful tools to improve patient and caregiver understanding. Also, discussing social issues, including prescription cost, transportation, and access to home care prior to leaving the hospital can greatly reduce risk of harm to the patients.

The Joint Commission advises institutions to begin discharge planning and complete a discharge risk assessment within 24 to 48 hours of admission. The risk assessment highlights barriers to discharge and risk factors for readmission. When a patient is ready for discharge home or to another facility, the discharge summary should provide all relevant information needed for the next clinician. It is essential that the discharge plan be shared with not only the patient and the PCP, but also with all the patients' post-hospital healthcare team. This team can include rehabilitation facilities, home health agencies, and skilled nursing facilities. The transmission of the discharge summary to the PCP is an invaluable intervention in preventing medical error. The goal is to use the discharge summary to communicate pending tests, in addition to other key discharge information, to the PCP for postdischarge follow-up. The summary should also include other important information about the discharge care plan, such as diagnoses, medication changes, pending diagnostic tests or laboratory results needing follow-up, and recommended outpatient workup such as additional diagnostic or laboratory testing, or specialty referrals. This method provides, at a minimum, the passive transmission of information via a discharge summary to indicate issues that need to be addressed during the postdischarge follow-up period. A direct verbal handoff between clinicians and healthcare professionals is also highly recommended. Stakeholders in the transmission of patient discharge information include the inpatient or ED physician, both of whom are the providers of new information obtained during a hospitalization or emergency room visit, respectively, and the PCP, who is the receiver of this information. Pending issues must be adequately handed off at each transition of care from one provider to each subsequent care provider.

It is important to recognize that the patient is clearly the primary stakeholder, but the patient should not be solely relied on to be the courier or the retainer of important information regarding the care transition. A study showed that 40% to 80% of medical information given to patients is forgotten. Additionally, half of the information retained is incorrect. In an accountable care arrangement, it is not acceptable to rely on the patient as courier of such important information. The hospital, postdischarge care facility, and/or primary care physician may be accountable for the transmission of discharge information by establishing standards of service, developing a culture of patient safety, and providing supportive information technology systems. Effective methods of minimizing medical errors during this important transition should address the potential outcomes of poorly managed care transitions. Outcomes may include increased rehospitalization rates, adverse clinical outcomes, and patient and provider dissatisfaction with discharge care planning.

TRANSITIONS OF CARE: PENDING ISSUES AT DISCHARGE

After medication errors, the next most common errors in the postdischarge period include test follow-up errors and workup errors (Table 48-1). Adequate and timely communication between care providers during the transition from the inpatient setting to the outpatient setting is an important target in high-quality,

Table 48-1. Types of Errors Related to Discontinuity of Care From the Inpatient to Outpatient Setting

Medication continuity errors	Medication was documented in the hospital chart but not in the medication list of the first postdischarge PCP visit
Test follow-up errors	A test result was pending at discharge but was not acknowledged in the outpatient chart
Workup error	An outpatient test or procedure suggested or scheduled by the inpatient provider was not adequately followed up by the outpatient provider

safe patient care. In a health care system where PCPs are increasingly less likely to be a patient's hospital physician, the transition of care from the inpatient setting to the outpatient setting becomes a time of increased patient vulnerability to medical errors and adverse clinical outcomes. From a patient-centered perspective, the transition between care settings should occur as a smooth continuum of patient care, rather than discrete, punctuated care settings. Transition-of-care processes must be executed efficiently through clear communication between the inpatient providers and outpatient PCP during the patient handoff. Accurate, timely information exchange during this transition is recognized as the benchmark for a successful care transition.

The primary goal of all discharge planning processes is to ensure a patient-centered, well-coordinated care transition that minimizes readmission, medical errors, and adverse events, and promotes the timely execution of appropriate patient care (Figure 48-1). The Joint Commission's National Patient Safety Goals program recognizes the importance of care transitions in managing patient care and safety.

Epidemiology

Three main categories of medical errors exist that are unique to the inpatient-to-outpatient care transition (Table 48-1). Medication continuity errors are the most common of the three categories to occur during this care transition. Medication changes at discharge are a topic discussed in detail in another case and thus will not be addressed further here. In a study examining test follow-up errors, a retrospective review of charts of patients discharged over a 5-month period revealed that half of patients had pending tests at discharge. Of these test follow-up errors, 9% were considered potentially actionable, of which more than one-third would change the diagnostic or therapeutic plan, and 12.6% required urgent action.

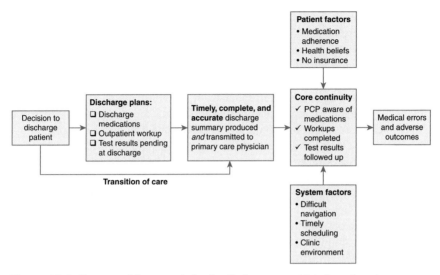

Figure 48-1. Conceptual framework for the discharge transition from inpatient to outpatient care.

Workup errors occur when an inpatient provider recommends outpatient tests or referrals but the recommended workup is inadvertently not completed (Figure 48-2). Approximately 27.6% of inpatients are recommended to have outpatient workups, of which only 35.9% are completed. In an observational study at an academic general internal medicine clinic, patients with at least 1 work-up

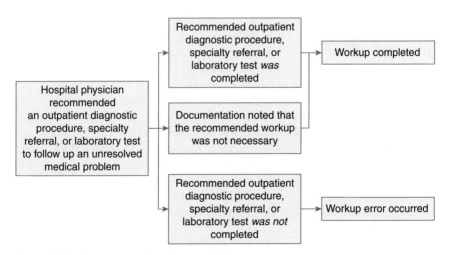

Figure 48-2. Assessment of workup completion.

error were more than 6 times as likely to be rehospitalized within 3 months after the first post-discharge PCP visit, compared with patients without workup errors. In the same study, medication continuity errors and test follow-up errors were less likely to lead to rehospitalization.

General practitioners surveyed about the care transition from the inpatient to outpatient setting described hospitalization of their patients as a "black box," in which inadequate communication led to lack of knowledge of the patient's clinical status and important continuity of care issues. The method of communication was far less important than the expectation that communication occurred at all. In an observational study, direct communication between hospital physicians and PCPs occurred only 3% to 20% of the time, and a discharge summary at the first postdischarge visit was available in only 12% to 34% of cases. Direct communication is arguably the most effective means to ensure adequate discharge communication between inpatient provider and primary care physician because it is more than simply a transfer of information—it provides an opportunity for 2-way dialogue.

Treatment

Various methods to achieve safe and efficient care transitions from the inpatient to outpatient setting have been studied. The foundation of the majority of proposed interventions depends on clear communication between providers in each of these settings. Clear communication skills about the care transition and appropriately detailed content of the transition should guide handoff etiquette (Table 48-2).

Another common method of ensuring appropriate content of a discharge summary is a checklist (Table 48-3). Implementation of a discharge checklist may be integrated into the hospital care process at various levels or may be the responsibility of different individuals. Multidisciplinary discharge teams are increasingly recognized as an important part of a well-coordinated discharge. Additionally, teams that continue care remotely in the postdischarge period prior to primary care follow-up are increasingly common. The impact of these and other interventions on medical errors and adverse outcomes is an active area of continuing research. Integration of health information technologies also can potentially enhance the discharge process, including production of an effective discharge summary that includes pending test results, recommended further workups, and medication changes. For example, many inpatient electronic health records (EHRs) have the capability to customize hospital discharge summary templates designed to ensure that all the discharge checklist items have been completed and effectively communicated to the patient, family, PCP, and other important postdischarge care providers, including home health care services and nursing homes.

However, health information systems (HISs) are not limited solely to EHR optimizations and new feature implementations. Pharmacy information systems

Table 48-2. Six Principles of the Inpatient-to-outpatient Handoff

Communicate, but do not irritate
The primary care physician should be sufficiently informed so that a question from a patient or family member can elicit an appropriate response. The hospitalist should select a communication method based on local primary care physician preference and patient population served, and can be by telephone, fax, or, increasingly, electronically.
Consult the primary care physician
The PCP can be an invaluable source of information about the patient, particularly when difficult circumstances arise—for example, discussions about code status. More importantly, the patient should not receive conflicting messages and the patient may be comforted to know that the primary care physician is in agreement with the plan of care.
Timeliness is next to godliness
Timeliness of primary care physician notification of patient admission to the hospital, involvement of the primary care physician at important decision points in care, and transmission of discharge summaries before the postdischarge follow-up visit are essential.
Partner with the patient
The patient should be empowered to be involved in his or her care, and the primary care physician can provide some insight into the patient's preferences regarding this process. The hospitalist's role is to develop rapport with the patient during a challenging time in the patient's continuum of care.
Make it clear that you are the patient's advocate
A hospitalist's institutional role in designing and implementing critical pathways, guidelines, and cost control measures cannot interfere with the hospitalist's role as a patient's doctor. The hospitalist should be the patient's advocate without conflicts of interest with his or her institutional roles.
Pass the baton as graciously as you received it (or even better, more graciously)
Ensure appropriate follow-up care is arranged and the patient is aware of whom to contact and how regarding problems in the postdischarge period.

dispense medications, manage inventory, and assist in clinical verification of orders. They flag patient allergies, drug utilization reviews, and high-risk medications. Electronic prescriptions (e-prescriptions, or eRx), electronic health records, prescription drug monitoring program databases, immunization registries, and telehealth patient interactions are some of the technologic innovations that reduce medical error and patient harm. HIS interoperability, or health information exchange (HIE), refers to the ability for different systems or databases to communicate with each other and exchange information. Improving HIE between pharmacy and prescribing information systems has long been a promising area of opportunity for improving patient safety and quality improvement, while also potentially reducing wasteful or duplicated care and medical errors.

While e-prescribing has become nearly universal in the United States, as well as non-US countries that have adopted EHR systems, unfortunately, electronic medication discontinuation (e-discontinuation) has lagged behind. A recent study showed that the rates at which discontinued medications continued to be dispensed to patients were as high as 4.94%. SureScripts, an e-prescribing system that facilitates HIE across different HISs that handle medication information, particularly many EHR systems, has a lesser-known functionality called CancelRx. This feature allows institutions to electronically cancel prescriptions in the same way electronic prescriptions are sent. However, this requires that both the sender and recipient of this information use this same platform for medication prescription information transmission and both have the CancelRx feature activated. As with any HIS, the additional feature comes with extra cost and has not yet been widely adopted. Furthermore, all HIS are subjected to appropriate usage by users in that system adoption should be seamless in everyday workflows for busy clinicians. For example, in addition to purchasing new HIS or new features of existing HIS, e-discontinuation workflows developed would need to consider who has access and permission to send eRx cancellations, when these cancellations should occur during routine processes of care, how transmission errors are handled, and more.

The adoption of HIS should not replace real-time medication reconciliation, which should always serve as the foundation for determining the actual medications a patient is using and how they are using them. Medication reconciliation involves the following:

(1) Encouraging patients and caregivers to bring all pill bottles to their doctor appointment, especially during a hospital follow-up visit

(2) Completing medication reconciliation by reviewing each pill and pill bottle

(3) Providing a current medication list to the patient and their caregiver at each visit, highlighting any changes that have occurred

(4) Providing the current medication list to the patient's pharmacy or sharing it with other physicians and clinicians also involved in the patient's care (or ensuring that the patient knows to keep the list with them at all times to be able to share with other clinicians they may see)

(5) Carefully monitoring and, if necessary, limiting drug quantity or refills on high-risk medications that may be time-limited from continuing to be dispensed

Table 48-3. Checklist for a Discharge Summary

Minimum Elements of a Transition Record	Ideal Additional Elements of a Transition Record
Main diagnosis or problem that led to hospitalization	Anticipated problems and suggested interventions, and contact number and person
Discharge medications, with reasons for any changes to the previous medication regimen	Proposed treatment and diagnostic plan
Name and contact information of transferring physician	Recommendations of subspecialty consultations
Discharge destination	Brief hospital course
Details of follow-up arrangements made	Pertinent physical findings and key findings, including results of procedures and laboratory tests
Pending laboratory work and tests	Information given to the patient and family, and documentation of patient education
Patient's cognitive status	Specific follow-up needs, including wound care, durable medical equipment, etc
	Advance directives, power of attorney, consent
	Assessment of caregiver status

TIPS TO REMEMBER

- Medication continuity errors, workup errors, and test follow-up errors are the three most common errors that occur during the discharge transition.
- Timely communication with the PCP, including transmission of a complete and accurate discharge summary, improves the coordination of care during a patient's discharge transition.

COMPREHENSION QUESTIONS

1. What is the most important foundational principle of an effective care transition?
A. Providing a detailed discharge summary to the patient and family
B. Communicating with the patient's PCP in a timely manner
C. Electronically transmitting a discharge summary to the patient's PCP
D. Calling the patient within 48 hours after discharge
E. Using teach-back to ensure patient understanding about the discharge

2. What information should be clearly communicated in a discharge summary or handoff to the patient's primary care physician to ensure pending issues are addressed after discharge?
>   A. Pending test results and procedure or radiology reports
>   B. Recommended outpatient workup, including tests and referrals
>   C. Medication reconciliation, changes, and timeline (eg, for antibiotics course)
>   D. All of the above

Answers

1. **B.** Communication with the PCP regarding pending issues is essential to a well-coordinated care transition from the inpatient to the outpatient setting. The discharge checklist helps to guide the discharge planner and/or hospitalist to ensure that all important clinical and follow-up information is provided in an efficient discharge summary.

2. **D.** Medication continuity errors, workup errors, and test follow-up errors are the three most common errors that occur during the discharge transition. Special attention to these components of the discharge summary will ensure that the handoff to the primary care physician is as well informed as possible. Scheduling and completing a follow-up appointment with the primary care physician for a postdischarge hospital follow-up visit within 30 days may reduce readmission for certain high-risk conditions, and it is one of the important drivers of the anticipated Medicare reimbursement penalty for hospitals that have higher-than-expected rates of readmissions.

SUGGESTED READINGS

Coleman EA, Williams MV. Executing high-quality care transitions: a call to do it right. *J Hosp Med.* 2007;2:287–290.

Goldman L, Pantilat SZ, Whitcomb WF. Passing the clinical baton: 6 principles to guide the hospitalist. *Am J Med.* 2001;111:S36–S39.

Hansen LO, Young RS, Hinami K, et al. Interventions to reduce 30-day rehospitalization: a systematic review. *Ann Intern Med.* 2011;155:520–528.

Joint Commission. *National Patient Safety Goals.* www.jointcommission.org/standards/national-patient-safety-goals. Accessed December 26, 2023.

Kessels RP. Patients' memory for medical information. *J R Soc Med.* 2003;96(5):219–222.

Kripalani S, Jackson AT, Schnipper JL, Coleman EA. Promoting effective transitions of care at hospital discharge: a review of key issues for hospitalists. *J Hosp Med.* 2007;2:314–323.

Kripalani S, LeFevre F, Phillips CO, et al. Deficits in communication and information transfer between hospital-based and primary care physicians: implications for patient safety and continuity of care. *JAMA.* 2007;297:831–841.

Moore C, McGinn T, Halm E. Tying up loose ends: discharging patients with unresolved medical issues. *Arch Intern Med.* 2007;167:1305–1311.

Moore C, Wisnivesky J, Williams S, McGinn T. Medical errors related to discontinuity of care from an inpatient to an outpatient setting. *J Gen Intern Med.* 2003;18:646–651.

Reason J. Human error: model and management *BMJ.* 2000;320:768–770

Roy CL, Poon EG, Karson AS, et al. Patient safety concerns arising from test results that return after hospital discharge. *Ann Intern Med.* 2005;143:121–128.

Snow V, Beck D, Budnitz T, et al. Transitions of Care Consensus policy statement: American College of Physicians, Society of General Internal Medicine, Society of Hospital Medicine, American Geriatrics Society, American College of Emergency Physicians, and Society for Academic Emergency Medicine. *J Hosp Med.* 2009;4:364–370.

Tandjung R, Rosemann T, Badertscher N. Gaps in continuity of care at the interface between primary care and specialized care: general practitioners' experiences and expectations. *Int J Gen Med.* 2011;4:773–778.

van Walraven C, Mamdani M, Fang J, Austin PC. Continuity of care and patient outcomes after hospital discharge. *J Gen Intern Med.* 2004;19:624–631.

White CL, Hohmeier KC. Pharmacy informatics: current and future roles for the pharmacy technician. *J Pharm Technol.* 2015;31(6):247–252.

WEBSITES

AHRQ Discharge Process Information for Clinicians and Consumers: www.ahrq.gov/patient-safety/resources.

Care Transitions Program: www.caretransitions.org.

Project RED (Re-engineered Discharge): www.bu.edu/fammed/projectred.

Society of Hospital Medicine's Project BOOST (Better Outcomes for Older adults through Safe Transitions): www.hospitalmedicine.org/globalassets/professional-development/professional-dev-pdf/boost-guide-second-edition.pdf.

Society of Hospital Medicine's Clinical Topics: Care Transitions: www.hospitalmedicine.org/clinical-topics/care-transitions.

A 27-year-old Woman With Fatigue and Unintentional Weight Loss

Mariam Murtaza Ali, MD and Michael Jakoby, MD, MA

A 27-year-old woman is referred for moderate fatigue, generalized body aches, and unintentional 7-kilogram weight gain over the past 6 months. She does not exercise or track her caloric intake. The patient reports loss of interest in activities she used to previously enjoy with her children and has had difficulty concentrating at her job. Her periods seem to last longer and are more painful than usual. She has no desire to be pregnant at this time. The patient takes no medications. Her mother had celiac disease, and a cousin was recently diagnosed with type 1 diabetes mellitus.

On examination, temperature is 98.6°F, blood pressure is 120/88 mm Hg, pulse is 60/min, and respiratory rate is 12/min. BMI is 33, and central adiposity is noted. Skin is dry and flaky but normally pigmented. Periorbital puffiness and mild lower extremity pitting edema are present. The thyroid gland is mildly enlarged and diffusely heterogeneous in texture. Biceps reflexes have 2+ upstrokes but delayed relaxation. She is able to squat and stand without difficulty. Thyroid-stimulating hormone (TSH) level checked prior to evaluation was 15.70 mIU/L (0.45–5.33). Subsequent measurements of TSH and free thyroxine (T4) were 14.24 mIU/L and 0.4 ng/dL (0.5–1.3), respectively.

1. What is the cause of the patient's symptoms?
2. How should the patient be treated, and what is the goal of management for this patient?

Answers

1. This is a young woman who presents with symptoms, examination findings, and a TSH level indicating primary hypothyroidism. Symptoms of hypothyroidism are usually nonspecific as in this patient's case. However, her strong family history of autoimmune endocrinopathies and examination findings including periorbital edema, dry skin, delayed deep tendon reflexes, and a small goiter are commonly found in cases of hypothyroidism, and unequivocally elevated TSH level confirms the diagnosis. Other etiologies to consider would be depression and Cushing syndrome.

2. The patient should be started on levothyroxine ("thyroxine"). There are other thyroid hormone preparations, including desiccated animal thyroid and liothyronine (triiodothyronine), but levothyroxine is adequate for the significant majority of patients with hypothyroidism and remains the standard of care. A full levothyroxine replacement dose for most adults is approximately 1.6 mcg/

kg/d, although dose requirements can range widely. In older patients (age >60 years) and patients with heart disease, a more conservative dose (eg, half of anticipated replacement dose) is started or patients are initially treated with 25 to 50 mcg daily. Thyroxine is adjusted to ameliorate symptoms of hypothyroidism and in most cases to achieve a TSH in the laboratory reference range (eg, 0.4–4.0 mIU/L or 0.5–5.0 mIU/L). However, in reproductive age women, the TSH target range is 0.5–2.5 mIU/L.

CASE REVIEW

Diagnosis

In areas of iodine sufficiency, such as the United States, the most common cause of primary hypothyroidism is chronic autoimmune thyroiditis (Hashimoto thyroiditis). Autoimmune thyroid disorders are estimated to be 5- to 10-fold more common in women than men. Globally, environmental iodine deficiency is the most common cause of hypothyroidism. Postablative hypothyroidism occurs after treatment of hyperthyroidism with radioiodine, and postsurgical hypothyroidism results after thyroidectomy to manage thyroid cancer, benign nodular thyroid disease, or thyroid enlargement causing symptoms of mass effect (eg, dyspnea or dysphagia). Hypothyroidism may complicate external beam radiation for nonthyroid head and neck malignancies, and several medications are known to cause hypothyroidism. The major etiologies of persistent primary hypothyroidism are presented in Table 49-1. Transient hypothyroidism may occur due to silent (painless) thyroiditis, postpartum thyroiditis, or subacute (painful) thyroiditis, or after thyroid lobectomy. Disorders that injure the pituitary or hypothalamus can result in secondary hypothyroidism due to a relative or absolute deficit of biologically active TSH.

Hypothyroidism may be overt (symptomatic) or subclinical (asymptomatic). Patients with subclinical hypothyroidism have an elevated TSH level, free (T4) level in the laboratory reference range, and no symptoms of hypothyroidism. In the third National Health and Nutrition Examination Survey (NHANES III), the overall prevalence of hypothyroidism was 4.6%, although only 0.3% of survey participants had overt hypothyroidism. There are no specific clinical manifestations of hypothyroidism, but common symptoms include fatigue, unintentional weight gain, dry skin, cold intolerance, myalgias, and menstrual abnormalities in women. Potential examination findings include goiter, delayed relaxation phase of deep tendon reflexes, dry skin, bradycardia, and diastolic hypertension.

Because there are no specific symptoms or signs of hypothyroidism, confirmation of the diagnosis requires laboratory evaluation of thyroid function. Since primary hypothyroidism accounts for the vast majority (>95%) of cases of hypothyroidism, TSH is the initial test of choice. If it is elevated, confirmatory testing with simultaneous measurements of TSH and free T4 is performed. Elevated TSH

Table 49-1. Etiologies of Primary Hypothyroidism

- Chronic autoimmune thyroiditis (Hashimoto thyroiditis)
- Thyroidectomy
- Radioiodine therapy
- External beam radiation
- Iodine deficiency
- Medications
  - Thioamides (methimazole, propylthiouracil, and carbimazole)
  - Lithium
  - Amiodarone
  - Tyrosine kinase inhibitors
  - Checkpoint inhibitors
  - Interferon a
  - Interleukin 2
- Infiltrative disorders
  - Sarcoidosis
  - Hemochromatosis
  - Fibrous thyroiditis
- Congenital thyroid disorders (agenesis and defects of hormone synthesis)

with low free T4 in the setting of provocative symptoms and examination findings confirms overt hypothyroidism. Subclinical hypothyroidism can be diagnosed if TSH is elevated but free T4 is in the laboratory reference range. Patients with concerning symptoms and signs of hypothyroidism but a TSH that is low or in the laboratory reference range should have free T4 checked; low free T4 indicates central hypothyroidism due to pituitary (secondary) or hypothalamic (tertiary) dysfunction.

Rare causes of elevated TSH include recovery from a serious nonthyroidal illness (NTI), resistance to TSH, resistance to thyroid hormone, and TSH-secreting adenomas. Elevations of TSH after NTI are transient, and patients usually recover normal thyroid function 4 to 6 weeks after documentation of an elevated TSH level. Most patients with TSH resistance have normal thyroid hormone levels and are euthyroid, although some may have reduced levels of thyroid hormone and hypothyroidism. Evaluation for TSH receptor mutations is required to confirm the diagnosis of TSH resistance. Patients with generalized thyroid hormone resistance are distinguished by elevated thyroid hormone levels but euthyroid status.

Patients with TSH-secreting pituitary adenomas have normal or elevated TSH levels, elevated thyroid hormone levels, and signs and symptoms of hyperthyroidism.

Antibodies to thyroid peroxidase (TPO) are elevated in more than 90% of patients with chronic lymphocytic thyroiditis, although TPO autoantibody titers are also elevated in approximately 10% of individuals with no functional or anatomical thyroid disorders. Due to the very high prevalence of chronic lymphocytic thyroiditis among patient with primary hypothyroidism and the somewhat low specificity of an elevated TPO autoantibody titer, checking anti-TPO antibody titer in most patients with newly diagnosed primary hypothyroidism is not indicated. Potential exceptions include patients with a goiter or to determine the likelihood of progression to permanent hypothyroidism in patients with postpartum or painless thyroiditis.

Hypothyroidism is characterized by a hypoechoic pattern on thyroid ultrasonography, but routine thyroid ultrasounds in the evaluation of patients with hypothyroidism are not recommended. Indications for thyroid ultrasound in patients with hypothyroidism include a palpable solitary nodule, multinodular goiter, difficult neck palpation, presence of cervical lymphadenopathy, history of head and neck radiation exposure, family history of thyroid carcinoma, and personal or family history of multiple endocrine neoplasia type 2 (MEN 2).

Immunoassays for TSH, free T4, and free triiodothyronine (T3) are vulnerable to factors that interfere with accurate measurements of these parameters and potentially confound clinical decision-making. The 6 most common types of interference are biotin, antistreptavidin antibodies, antiruthenium antibodies, thyroid hormone autoantibodies, heterophile antibodies, and macro-TSH. Both unfractionated and fractionated low-molecular-weight heparin may cause artifactual increases in free T4 levels, apparently by displacing T4 from binding sites on thyroxine-binding globulin (TBG) and albumin. Conditions that significantly affect TBG and albumin levels, such as pregnancy, severe acute illness, or chronic liver disease, also may impact the accuracy of free thyroid hormone measurements. Potential interference should be suspected if there is a significant discrepancy between clinical status and biochemical results. Investigation may require assistance from a laboratory medicine expert. Patients who take high-dose biotin should stop it for at least 48 hours before having blood drawn for thyroid function testing.

Screening asymptomatic individuals at risk of developing thyroid disease is controversial due to the lack of evidence that treating patients with subclinical hypothyroidism is beneficial. Routine screening of thyroid function is most cost effective in older women (age >65 years) in whom the prevalence of hypothyroidism has been reported at 5% to 15%. However, a study in the Netherlands of elderly women with both overt and subclinical hypothyroidism showed no impact of thyroid dysfunction on cognition, mental health, functional status, or mortality over 4 years of annual follow-up despite no treatment with supplemental thyroid hormone. Indications to check thyroid function in asymptomatic patients are presented in Table 49-2.

Treatment

Goals of treatment in hypothyroidism are to relieve or improve symptoms and achieve a TSH in a range appropriate for clinical status. For most nonpregnant adults, TSH in the range of 0.4 to 4.0 mIU/L or 0.5 to 5.0 mIU/L is acceptable. While most young, healthy, euthyroid adults have TSH levels in the range of 0.4 to 2.5 mIU/L, TSH increases with age and higher TSH targets are more appropriate for older patients, particularly over age 70 years. For reproductive-age women, a TSH goal of 0.5 to 2.5 mIU/L is considered most appropriate so that thyroxine is dosed adequately before early pregnancy is detected. Symptoms of hypothyroidism begin to resolve 2 to 3 weeks after starting treatment, although steady-state TSH levels take approximately 6 weeks to be achieved.

The treatment of choice for most patients with hypothyroidism is levothyroxine, or T4. It is a prohormone with little activity at the thyroid hormone receptor

Table 49-2. Indications to Check Thyroid Function in Asymptomatic Patients

- Laboratory abnormalities
  - o Hyperlipidemia
  - o Hyponatremia
  - o Increased creatinine kinase level
  - o Macrocytic anemia
  - o Hyperprolactinemia
- Clinical conditions
  - o Autoimmune disorders (especially endocrinopathies such as Addison disease)
  - o Pericardial or pleural effusions
  - o Bradycardia
  - o History of thyroid or head and neck surgery
  - o History of radioiodine treatment of external beam radiation to head and neck
  - o History of hypothalamic or pituitary disorders
- Medications
  - o Amiodarone
  - o Lithium
  - o Checkpoint inhibitors
  - o Tyrosine kinase inhibitors
  - o Interleukin 2

that is deiodinated in peripheral tissues to the biologically active form of thyroid hormone, T3. The plasma half-life of T4 is 5 to 7 days, and stable circulating levels of T4 and T3 can be achieved with daily dosing of levothyroxine. The majority of a thyroxine dose (70%–80%) is absorbed if the hormone is ingested with water and on an empty stomach, either 30 to 60 min before breakfast or at least 2 h after the last meal of the day. A recent meta-analysis found no difference in the effectiveness of T4 dosed in the morning or at bedtime. Factors that reduce absorption of thyroid hormone are presented in Table 49-3. Vitamin C (ascorbic acid) increases absorption of T4.

For most adults, the typical full replacement dose of T4 is approximately 1.6 mcg/kg/d. However, depending on the indication for treatment with T4 (eg, thyroidectomy vs chronic lymphocytic thyroiditis), degree of residual endogenous thyroid hormone production, patient age, and comorbid conditions (eg, ischemic heart disease), the range of ultimate T4 dose requirements is quite large. For patients under age 60 years without known cardiovascular disease (CVD), an initial full replacement dose of T4 can be started. If patients are older or have CVD, thyroxine is usually started at 25 to 50 mcg daily and then adjusted in 12.5- to 25-mcg increments every 4 to 6 weeks until TSH is at goal. In a small study comparing adults randomized to an initial full (1.6 mcg/kg/d) dose of T4 compared to

Table 49-3. Factors That Reduce Absorption of Thyroid Hormone

- Gastrointestinal disorders
  o Celiac disease
  o Lactose intolerance
  o Atrophic gastritis
  o *Helicobacter pylori* infection
- Dietary
  o Coffee
  o Soy products
  o Calcium supplements
  o Iron supplements
- Medications
  o Proton pump inhibitors
  o Bile acid sequestrants
  o Sevelamer
  o Lanthanum
  o Ciprofloxacin

25 mcg/d with dose adjustments every 4 weeks, target TSH was achieved faster in the full initial dose treatment arm but no differences in quality of life were measured between the groups.

Regardless of starting dose, TSH should be rechecked 4 to 6 weeks after initiating treatment for hypothyroidism. If TSH remains above goal, the dose of T4 should be increased and TSH rechecked in 4 to 6 weeks, with the process repeated until TSH is at target. Dose increases in older adults and patients with CVD or other significant comorbidities should be more conservative (eg, 12.5–25 mcg) than for younger, healthy patients. If a patient reaches a T4 dose greater than 2 mcg/kg/d without achieving clinical and biochemical euthyroidism, medication nonadherence or poor absorption should be considered. The patient's medication list should also be inspected for drugs that are known to increase microsomal clearance of T4 (eg, rifampin, carbamazepine, phenytoin, phenobarbital, imatinib). Exogenous estrogen may increase T4 dose requirement by increasing TBG level and reducing the fraction of unbound (free) T4. Progression of underlying autoimmune thyroid dysfunction, weight gain, pregnancy, and nephrotic syndrome also increase T4 dose requirements. The effects of bariatric surgery are variable, with reduced absorption potentially increasing T4 dose requirement but weight loss potentially reducing it.

Once a patient is on a stable maintenance dose of supplemental T4, TSH can be monitored yearly or as needed if changes to clinical status or medications occur that might affect T4 dose requirement. In patients with secondary hypothyroidism, TSH is an unreliable marker of the therapeutic response to T4 dose. The goal of treatment for most adults with secondary hypothyroidism is to maintain free T4 level in the upper half of the laboratory reference range. However, a free T4 level between the lower end and midpoint of the reference range may be more appropriate for older adults and patients with CVD or other significant comorbid conditions.

Although the significant majority of adults with hypothyroidism feel well on treatment with T4 alone, approximately 10% report a sense of impaired well-being despite achieving TSH levels at therapeutic goal. These patients may be candidates for combined therapy with T4 and T3 as liothyronine added to T4 or desiccated animal thyroid, particularly if they have a total T3 level below the reference range, have undergone thyroidectomy, or have a history of thyroid ablation with radioiodine. However, the combination of T4 and T3 should not be used routinely in management of hypothyroidism, and the latest American Thyroid Association (ATA) guidelines found insufficient evidence of benefit from combined T4 and T3 therapy in patients who perceive an inadequate therapeutic response to T4 monotherapy. For example, a meta-analysis of 11 randomized, controlled trials of T4/T3 combination therapy compared to T4 monotherapy found no measurable improvements in symptoms, body weight, or lipids for patients randomized to combined T4/T3 treatment. Clinicians should acknowledge a patient's symptoms but evaluate for alternative etiologies when patients are biochemically euthyroid on T4 monotherapy.

While there is a perception that changing thyroxine preparations—either from branded to generic or between generic manufacturers—complicates management of hypothyroidism, evidence indicates that most patients can switch between thyroxine preparations without adversely effecting control of hypothyroidism. A recent comparative effectiveness study of propensity-matched patients in the OptumLabs Data Warehouse demonstrated that switching among different generic T4 preparations was not associated with clinically significant changes in TSH level. In a study evaluating the impact of changing from branded to generic T4, TSH remained stable in comparable numbers of switchers and nonswitchers, although there was a difference when the thyroxine dose exceeded 100 mcg daily. Patients with dye sensitivities can be managed with multiples of dye-free 50-mcg T4 tablets, and patients with hypersensitivity to excipients (other than gelatin) can be managed with soft-gel T4 capsules.

A middle-aged woman with altered mental status and elevated TSH level
A 61-year-old woman is brought to the ED from a homeless shelter due to altered mental status. She is unable to provide a medical history. Examination is notable for BP 92/70 mm Hg, pulse 54/min, temperature 35°C, dry hair and skin, vitiligo, nonpitting edema of both lower extremities, and delayed deep tendon reflex relaxation. The patient's score on the Glasgow Coma Scale is 10 (moderate impairment). CT of the head shows no bleeding or masses. Initial laboratories are notable for mild hyponatremia and normochromic, normocytic anemia. TSH is 40.23 mIU/L (0.45–5.33), and simultaneously measured free T4 is 0.2 ng/dL (0.5–1.3). The patient is admitted to the intensive care unit for management.

1. What is the most appropriate next step in the patient's metabolic management?

2. How is hypothyroidism best managed?

Answers

1. Severe hypothyroidism leading to altered mental status and multiorgan system dysfunction is called myxedema coma. For patients with primary hypothyroidism, as in this patient's case, the possibility of coexisting primary adrenal insufficiency needs to be evaluated promptly. Vitiligo is a finding that indicates the patient has multiple autoimmune disorders. Starting the patient on thyroid hormone before treating adrenal insufficiency may accelerate cortisol clearance and lead to an adrenal crisis. A stress dose (4 mg) of parenteral dexamethasone should be administered and a cosyntropin stimulation test performed. If adrenal insufficiency is diagnosed, the patient can subsequently be treated with stress-dose hydrocortisone.

2. The optimal approach to providing thyroid hormone in myxedema coma is controversial because the condition is rare and there are no clinical trials comparing different regimens. Although there is debate on whether patients should receive

T4 alone or a combination of T4 and T3, thyroid hormone should be given parenterally until the patient is able to take medications by mouth safely. Thyroxine dose greater than 500 mcg daily and T3 dose greater than or equal to 75 mcg daily appear to increase risk of mortality.

CASE REVIEW

Diagnosis

Myxedema coma is severe hypothyroidism manifesting with altered mental status and dysfunction of multiple organ systems resulting in hypothermia, hypoventilation, bradycardia, hypotension, and hypoglycemia (often due to co-occurrence of adrenal insufficiency). Coarsened facial features, macroglossia, and nonpitting edema of the extremities are often present due to deposition of mucin in skin and other tissues. Myxedema coma may be the culmination of longstanding, poorly controlled or untreated hypothyroidism, or it may be precipitated by an acute event such as infection, myocardial infarction, trauma, or cold exposure in a patient with poorly controlled hypothyroidism. Cases of myxedema coma have been reported in the context of virtually all causes of hypothyroidism, including drug-induced hypothyroidism (eg, amiodarone and lithium). In a retrospective observational study of patients admitted to hospital in Japan from July 2010 through March 2013, myxedema coma was rare (149 cases out of approximately 19 million hospital admissions; estimated incidence 1.08 per million population) and affected primarily older (mean age 77 years) and female patients (two-thirds of cases). Mortality rate in this Japanese series was nearly 30% and unaffected by thyroid hormone regimen or dose. Older age and requirement for catecholamines were independent predictors of in-hospital mortality.

The diagnosis of myxedema coma should be considered in patients with altered mental status and concurrent hypothermia, hypercapnia, or hyponatremia. Manifestations of myxedema, a well-healed low-neck incision (indicating thyroidectomy), and delayed relaxation on evaluation of deep tendon reflexes are potential examination findings. TSH and free T4 should be checked promptly. The T4 level will be unequivocally low; TSH will be clearly elevated in cases of primary hypothyroidism, but it may be low, inappropriately in the laboratory reference range, or minimally elevated in cases of secondary hypothyroidism. Corticotroph axis function also should be evaluated quickly. A random cortisol level less than 3 mcg/dL is diagnostic of adrenal insufficiency, and a level greater than 15 mcg/dL indicates intact corticotroph axis function. However, an equivocal random cortisol result requires follow-up with a cosyntropin stimulation test.

Treatment

Key elements in management of myxedema coma are thyroid hormone replacement, glucocorticoid coverage until adrenal insufficiency has been excluded, and supportive measures for specific complications such as mechanical ventilation for respiratory failure, fluids and vasopressor agents to manage hypotension, passive rewarming for hypothermia, and IV dextrose to treat hypoglycemia. If T4 is used as monotherapy, it is administered as an initial IV loading dose of no more than 500 mcg (200–400 mcg typical) followed by daily IV boluses of ~1.6 mcg/kg/d until the patient is able to take T4 by mouth. In the event of no improvement in the first 24 hours after starting IV T4, parenteral T3 is added (10–25 mcg loading dose followed by 2.5–10 mcg every 8 h). If T3 is administered as part of the initial treatment regimen, the loading dose of T4 is reduced to 200 to 300 mcg. Treatment with T4 alone may be less effective than the combination of T4 and T3 due to impaired peripheral conversion of T4 to T3 in the setting of severe, acute illness, but treatment with T3 carries the risk of exposing organ systems to high levels of thyroid hormone that might lead to untoward effects such as tachyarrhythmias. One study found T3 levels to be twice as high in patients who died in hospital compared with patients who survived myxedema coma, and daily doses of T4 and T3 exceeding 500 mcg and 75 mcg, respectively, predispose to in-hospital mortality.

Dexamethasone, which does not interfere with assays for cortisol, can be dosed initially for empiric stress-dose (4 mg) glucocorticoid treatment while the test is performed. If adrenal insufficiency is diagnosed, stress-dose hydrocortisone (50–100 mg IV every 8 h) can then be started to provide both glucocorticoid and mineralocorticoid replacement. Mechanical ventilation may be required to support respiration, particularly when myxedema occurs with obesity. Patients should be rewarmed passively, as myxedema is characterized by peripheral vasoconstriction, and active rewarming may result in peripheral vasodilatation and hypotension due to volume depletion.

Volume expansion with isotonic fluids (eg, 0.9% saline) is often sufficient to treat hypotension, although patients may require pressor agents (eg, dopamine) if blood pressure fails to respond to volume expansion alone. Dextrose needs to be added to fluids when myxedema is complicated by hypoglycemia. In cases of severe hyponatremia and suspected hyponatremic encephalopathy, hypertonic (3%) saline should be administered and hyponatremia carefully corrected before an attempt at hydration with normal saline.

TIPS TO REMEMBER

● The overall prevalence of hypothyroidism is relatively high (4%–5%), but the significant majority of patients have subclinical hypothyroidism. Prevalence of hypothyroidism is highest in women over age 65 years. Chronic lymphocytic thyroiditis causes the significant majority of cases of hypothyroidism in the industrialized world.

- Levothyroxine is the preferred treatment for symptomatic hypothyroidism. A full replacement dose (1.6 mcg/kg/d) can be started in nonpregnant adults under age 60 years without CVD, but lower doses should be started in older patients and patients with CVD or other significant comorbidities. The goal for TSH in most adults is 0.5 to 5.0 mIU/L, but reproductive-age women are treated to a TSH goal of 0.5 to 2.5 mIU/L.

- Myxedema coma is severe hypothyroidism presenting with altered mental status and multiorgan system dysfunction manifesting as some combination of hypothermia, hyponatremia, hypercapnia, hypotension, and hypoglycemia. Coexisting adrenal insufficiency should be suspected and promptly evaluated, and empiric stress-dose glucocorticoids should be started while evaluation is in progress.

- Thyroid hormone must be dosed carefully in patients with myxedema coma. Daily thyroxine dose greater than 500 mcg and daily triiodothyronine dose greater than or equal to 75 mcg are associated with increased risk of in-hospital mortality.

SUGGESTED READINGS

Brito JP, Deng Y, Ross JS, et al. Association between generic-to-generic levothyroxine switching and thyrotropin levels among US adults. *JAMA Intern Med.* 2022;182(4):418–425.

Favresse J, Burlacu M-C, Maiter D, Gruson D. Interferences with thyroid function immunoassays: clinical implications and detection algorithm. *Endocr Rev.* 2018;39(5):830–850.

Flinterman LE, Kuiper JG, Korevaar JC, et al. Impact of forced dose-equivalent levothyroxine brand switch on plasma thyrotropin: a cohort study. *Thyroid.* 2020;30(6):821–828.

Grozinsky-Glasberg S, Fraser A, Nahshoni E, et al. Thyroxine-triiodothyronine combination therapy versus thyroxine monotherapy for clinical hypothyroidism: a meta-analysis of randomized controlled trials. *J Clin Endocrinol Metab.* 2006;91(7):2592–2599.

Gussekloo J, van Exel E, de Craen AJ, et al. Thyroid status, disability and cognitive function, and survival in old age. *JAMA.* 2004;29(21):2591–2599.

Hollowell JG, Staehling NW, Flanders WD, et al. Serum TSH, T(4), and thyroid antibodies in the United States population (1988 to 1994): National Health and Nutrition Examination Survey (NHANES III). *J Clin Endocrinol Metab.* 2002;87(2):489–499.

Hylander B, Rosenqvist U. Treatment of myxoedema coma – factors associated with fatal outcome. *Acta Endocrinol (Copenh).* 1985;108(1):65–71.

Jonklaas J, Bianco AC, Bauer AJ, et al. Guidelines for the treatment of hypothyroidism: prepared by the American Thyroid Association Task Force on Thyroid Hormone Replacement. *Thyroid.* 2014;24(12):1670–1751.

Laji K, Rhidha B, John R, et al. Abnormal free thyroid hormone levels due to heparin administration. *QJM.* 2001;94(9):471–473.

Mariotti S, Caturegli P, Piccolo P, et al. Antithyroid peroxidase autoantibodies in thyroid diseases. *J Clin Endocrinol Metab.* 1990;71(3):661–669.

Ono Y, Ono S, Yasunaga H, et al. Clinical characteristics and outcomes of myxedema coma: analysis of a national inpatient database in Japan. *J Epidemiol.* 2017;27(3):117–122.

Pang X, Pu T, Xu L, Sun R. Effect of L-thyroxine administration before breakfast vs at bedtime on hypothyroidism: a meta-analysis. *Clin Endocrinol (Oxf).* 2020;92(5):475–481.

Roos A, Linn-Rasker SP, van Domburg RT, et al. The starting dose of levothyroxine in primary hypothyroidism treatment: a prospective, randomized, double-blind trial. *Arch Intern Med.* 2005;165(15):1714–1720.

Saravanan P, Chau WF, Roberts N, et al. Psychological well-being in patients on 'adequate' doses of L-thyroxine: results of a large, controlled community-based questionnaire study. *Clin Endocrinol (Oxf).* 2002;57(5):577–585.

Vadiveloo T, Donnan P, Murphy MJ, Leese GP. Age- and gender-specific TSH reference intervals in people with no obvious thyroid disease in Tayside, Scotland: The Thyroid Epidemiology, Audit, and Research Study (TEARS). *J Clin Endocrinol Metab.* 2013;98(3):1147–1153.

Yamamoto T, Fukuyama J, Fujiyoshi A. Factors associated with mortality of myxedema coma: report of eight cases and literature survey. *Thyroid.* 1999;9(12):1167–1174.

A 72-year-old Man With Social Issues

Stacy Sattovia, MD, MBA and Harini Rathinamanickam, MD, FACP

The patient is a 72-year-old man with a past medical history significant for congestive heart failure with an ejection fraction of 25%. Your inpatient team is called by the ED to admit the patient, who has presented with decompensated congestive heart failure. Review of his records reveals 6 admissions in the past 4 months. Each time he is admitted he rapidly improves, and your team wonders why the patient requires so many hospitalizations.

1. **What social issues may be contributing to the patient's frequent hospitalizations?**

Answer

1. Readmissions often signal a failure to address aspects of a patient's social situation that might limit the patient's ability to comply with a complex medical regimen and thus hinder a successful recovery. Numerous social issues may exist for any patient.

CASE REVIEW

With this case, you further discover that while the patient's condition, medication regimen, and dietary restrictions seem standard to you, he doesn't understand it. His wife previously took care of him—she ensured that he took his medications correctly and prepared nutritious low-sodium meals for him; however, she passed away 8 months ago. In addition, the patient doesn't read very well and finds the small print on the bottles difficult to decipher. Even if he can read them, he doesn't always understand the directions. His meals consist mostly of frozen dinners and cans of soup, both of which tend to have a high sodium content. In general, the patient is very frustrated and beginning to feel hopeless about his medical condition, and he misses his wife terribly.

TRANSITIONS OF CARE: PATIENTS WITH SOCIAL ISSUES

Discharge is a complex transition of care that leaves a patient highly vulnerable to adverse events. The key to a successful transition from the inpatient to the outpatient setting begins at the time of admission. Numerous social issues might exist that can complicate patients' hospital stays and compromise their success during this critical transition of care.

The literature cites that up to 20% of US hospitalizations result in readmission within 30 days. The Medicare Payment Advisory Committee found that up to 76% of 30-day readmissions in Medicare beneficiaries are potentially avoidable. Similar literature states that unplanned rehospitalizations may signal a failure in hospital discharge processes, patients' ability to manage self-care, and/or the quality of care in the next community setting. Patients' ability to manage self-care is, in part, closely related to their social context.

Eliciting these social issues in the setting of medical illness requires the physician to think broadly—to move beyond symptoms, diagnosis, and treatment to inquire about aspects of the patient's life that may be quite personal. The physician may also need to obtain collateral information from family or other persons close to the patient.

Important factors to consider include:

1. Living situation:

    Where does the patient live?

    Does the patient live alone?

    Does the patient have family support?

    Is the support that exists healthy enough to care for the patient?

    Will the patient be able to return to independent living?

    Whom does the patient support? Will the patient still be able to do so?

    What are the physical attributes of the home, specifically related to the patient's functional status? For example, how many steps are required to move from the bedroom to bathroom?

    What durable medical equipment might help the patient remain as functional and independent as possible?

2. Finances:

    Does the patient have insurance coverage?

    Can the patient afford medications and follow-up care?

    Can the patient afford rent, bills, and food?

3. Transportation:

    How will the patient get home from the hospital?

    Can the patient get to follow-up appointments?

    If the patient used public transportation prior to hospitalization, is the patient still able to physically do this?

4. Health literacy:

    What is the patient's literacy level?

    Can the patient understand discharge instructions and medications?

5. Language barriers:

Are there any language barriers?

6. Other issues:

Does the patient have a primary care physician?

Does the patient know how to contact his or her primary care physician?

Are there substance abuse issues confounding the patient's health?

How to Assess

Eliciting this information needs to begin at admission. Begin with asking the patient about these issues—for example, "tell me about your life at home." Starting with an open-ended question can elicit factors that you may not consider asking about, particularly when you remember that everyone's social situation is unique. You may then move into specific questions to develop a more complete understanding of the patient's social context and the needs the patient might have.

There are typically resources that can be of tremendous benefit to the patient and the provider. Social workers possess the expertise to counsel patients and identify resources that might provide social and financial support. For example, there may be commercial or community programs that can help a patient afford medications. Some patients may qualify for help at home in the form of home health or senior support services, thereby allowing the patient to remain more independent. Social workers also may be helpful in the setting of homeless patients. Obtaining physical therapy and occupational therapy evaluations are particularly helpful in assessing a patient's functional status. These experts can then lend recommendations to provide a physically safe discharge plan for the patient. Using interpreters in the setting of patients who do not know English or are not fluent in English will help in safe transition of care.

The ultimate goal is to be able to formulate a plan at discharge that provides maximal support to the patient—this requires understanding not only the disease process and therapy but also the impact the social context has on each particular patient's overall health.

TIPS TO REMEMBER

- Patients' social situations are often quite complex. Asking about their lives at home can be very helpful to elicit barriers to adherence with the plan of care.
- Social service experts are typically available in the inpatient setting, and their expertise should be leveraged to help patients at the time of discharge.

COMPREHENSION QUESTIONS

1. The patient is an 89-year-old female who lives alone. She has had 6 admissions in the last 9 months, each for a different reason. At the time of the current discharge, she declines a short stay in a nursing home for continued rehabilitation, stating that her family will stay with her and provide 24-hour assistance. The family is in the room with her and they confirm this. However, the situation and solution do not seem that simple to you. What is a reasonable next step?

    A. Discharge the patient to the care of her family—you cannot force her to accept assistance.

    B. Ask social services to see the patient—perhaps she will qualify for some further assistance in her home.

    C. Ask the patient if you can speak with her alone to obtain further social history.

    D. Obtain a psychiatry consultation to assess decision-making capacity.

2. The patient is a 34-year-old male with a past medical history significant for schizophrenia that is well compensated. He has been admitted twice in the past 1 week for a lower extremity cellulitis. Each time he responded very well to IV antibiotics but worsened after discharge. You discover that he did not obtain his antibiotics at discharge and did not follow up with his primary care provider.

    He is again ready for discharge. How can you ensure his medical success?

    A. Consult psychiatry—they might be effective at helping him take his medications.

    B. Discharge him to an extended care facility to finish his IV antibiotics—this may represent oral antibiotic failure.

    C. Provide oral antibiotics at the time of discharge.

    D. Ask the patient what he needs to be able to comply with the recommended plan of care.

Answers

1. C. If something about the social situation seems unworkable to you, it is worth further exploration. On further discussion, alone with the patient, you discover that while she loves her family, she financially supports 2 of her adult children and there is concern that if she enters a nursing home, even for a short stay, she will not be able to provide this assistance to her children. Additionally, in the past, despite the recommendations of her providers, her children have not provided 24-hour care. She is scared she will not be able to meet her own medical needs.

This is a delicate, but not uncommon, social situation. At this point, enlisting the assistance of the social services experts will be helpful as you begin an important discussion with the family—the key is to place the patient's needs first.

2. **D**. Asking the patient what his needs are is an excellent way to help ensure his success. In this situation you would discover that he was unable to obtain his antibiotics because he was discharged over a holiday weekend and the pharmacy that he typically uses was closed and thus unable to deliver his medications. In addition, he did not attend his outpatient follow-up because the appointment was scheduled in the morning and the bus he takes to his appointments only runs in the afternoons. With attention to these 2 issues, you find that over the next few days, the patient did indeed obtain and take his medications appropriately and did attend his afternoon follow-up appointment with his primary care provider, with resolution of his cellulitis.

SUGGESTED READINGS

Berenson RA, Paulus RA, Kalman NS. Medicare's readmissions-reduction program—a positive alternative. *N Engl J Med*. 2012;366:1364–1366.

Cain CH, Neuwirth E, Bellows J, et al. Patient experiences of transitioning from hospital to home: an ethnographic quality improvement project. *J Hosp Med*. 2012;7:382–387.

Messerli AW, Deutsch C. Implementation of institutional discharge protocols and transition of care following acute coronary syndrome. *Cardiovasc Revasc Med*. 2020;21(9):1180–1188.

Mudge AM, Kasper K, Clair A, et al. Recurrent readmissions in medical patients: a prospective study. *J Hosp Med*. 2011;6(2):61–67.

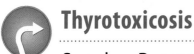

Thyrotoxicosis

Sanober Parveen, MD and Michael
Jakoby, MD, MA

A Young Woman With Fatigue, Weight Loss, and Palpitations

A 31-year-old female with no chronic health problems and taking no medications presents with 4 weeks of unusual fatigue, palpitations, unintentional weight loss, increased sweating, and poor sleep. The patient's mother and older sister take thyroid hormone for management of hypothyroidism. Examination is notable for a smooth, nontender, and modestly enlarged thyroid gland, resting heart rate 100 bpm, fine tremor with both arms extended, and brisk biceps tendon reflexes. Thyroid-stimulating hormone (TSH) level is less than 0.03 mIU/L (0.45–5.33), and simultaneously measured free thyroxine (T4) level is 5.0 ng/dL (0.5–1.3). Thyroid-stimulating immunoglobulin (TSI) level is 31.90 IU/L (<0.54). Subsequent thyroid scan and uptake study shows uniform uptake of radioiodine in the thyroid gland and a measured 6-h I-123 uptake of 33% (5–15).

1. What is the distinction between "thyrotoxicosis" and "hyperthyroidism?"

2. What are the potential etiologies of thyrotoxicosis?

3. What are clinical manifestations of thyrotoxicosis?

4. How should thyrotoxicosis be evaluated?

5. What are the management options for hyperthyroidism?

Answers

1. "Thyrotoxicosis" refers to the clinical state that results from increased thyroid hormone activity in peripheral organ systems due to high thyroid hormone levels. "Hyperthyroidism" is a form of thyrotoxicosis due to inappropriately high synthesis and secretion of T4 and triiodothyronine (T3) by the thyroid gland.

2. Thyrotoxicosis can be caused by endogenous overproduction of thyroid hormone, unregulated release of thyroid hormone (eg, from injury caused by

inflammation, "thyroiditis"), or consumption of excess thyroid, either prescription or surreptitiously obtained. A detailed list of etiologies is presented in Table 51-1. In this patient's case, the elevated TSI titer and findings on thyroid scintigraphy confirm Graves' disease as the cause of thyrotoxicosis. Female gender, young age, and family history of apparent autoimmune thyroid disease—chronic lymphocytic thyroiditis is the etiology of hypothyroidism in more than 95% of cases among iodine-replete individuals—are risk factors for Graves' hyperthyroidism in this case.

3. Thyroid hormone excess has effects on every organ system, resulting in multiple potential clinical manifestations. A list of symptoms is presented in Table 51-2. This patient's complaints of fatigue, unintentional weight loss, palpitations, excessive perspiration, and poor sleep are common in thyrotoxicosis.

4. TSH is the appropriate initial laboratory test for evaluation of potential thyrotoxicosis. Many thyroid experts also recommend obtaining a simultaneous measurement of thyroid hormone, typically free T4. A pattern of low TSH with

Table 51-1. Etiologies of Thyrotoxicosis

Increased thyroid radioiodine uptake

- Graves' disease
- Toxic multinodular goiter
- Toxic solitary adenoma
- Physiologic hyperthyroidism of pregnancy (due to β-hCG)
- Trophoblastic tumors (due to β-hCG)
- TSH-secreting pituitary adenomas
- Pituitary resistance to thyroid hormone
- Inherited nonimmune hyperthyroidism (TSH receptor and G protein mutations)

Low thyroid radioiodine uptake

- Thyroiditis
  Lymphocytic (eg, silent, postpartum)
  Viral or postviral (eg, subacute)
  Drug-induced (eg, amiodarone, lithium)
- Infectious
- Iodide-induced (Jod-Basedow syndrome)
- Iatrogenic
- Factitious
- Struma ovarii

hCG, human chorionic gonadotropin.

Table 51-2. Potential Symptoms of Thyrotoxicosis

Organ System	Symptoms
Eyes	Foreign body sensation, increased lacrimation, pain, photophobia, diplopia, blurry vision, loss color vision, decreased visual acuity
Skin and hair	Increased sweating, loose, soft nails, increased hair loss, thickened skin on shins (Graves' dermatopathy)
Cardiovascular	Palpitations, decreased exertional tolerance
Gastrointestinal	Hyperdefecation
Genitourinary	Increased urinary frequency, nocturia
Metabolic	Heat intolerance, hyperphagia, anorexia (older patients), weight loss
Musculoskeletal	Fatigue, muscle weakness
Neuropsychiatric	Tremulous, anxious, depression, psychosis
Reproductive	Irregular menses, decreased libido, erectile dysfunction
Respiratory	Shortness of breath, dyspnea on exertion

elevated T4 or T4 inappropriately in the laboratory reference range indicates thyrotoxicosis. An assay of TSH receptor antibodies such as TSI is obtained for serologic evidence of Graves' disease, although absence of an elevated TSI titer does not exclude the diagnosis. The pattern of radioiodine and pertechnetate uptake on thyroid scintigraphy is useful for distinguishing etiologies of endogenous thyroid hormone overproduction (eg, Graves' disease, toxic nodular goiter) from etiologies of unregulated thyroid hormone release (eg, a form of thyroiditis).

5. The 3 treatment options for hyperthyroidism are thioamides, radioiodine (I-131), and thyroidectomy. Most patients choose either long-term management with a thioamide (methimazole or propylthiouracil) or radioiodine ablation. A thioamide can be prescribed initially to treat symptomatic patients as in this case and then briefly held (5–7 d) to allow treatment with I-131 or surgery. Thyroidectomy is typically reserved for patients with very large goiters or those who are severely ill from hyperthyroidism.

CASE REVIEW

Diagnosis

Thyrotoxicosis has a strong female predominance, occurring in approximately 2% of women and 0.2% of men. Most cases of thyrotoxicosis are subclinical, with TSH less than 0.4 mIU/L but normal measures of thyroid hormone such as free

Table 51-3. Pathognomonic Signs of Graves' Disease

Manifestation	Prevalence (%)	Findings
Orbitopathy	25	Proptosis, periorbital edema
Dermatopathy*	1.5	Nonpitting, thickened, and well-defined nodules or papules, usually pretibial
Acropathy	0.5	Clubbing, swelling of hands and feet, periosteal reaction on plain films

*Almost all patients with dermatopathy have coexisting orbitopathy.

T4 level, no clinical manifestations of thyrotoxicosis, and absent or nonspecific symptoms. Symptoms of thyrotoxicosis are presented in Table 51-2. Potential findings on examination include goiter (smooth or nodular); stare; lid lag; tremor; hyperreflexia; tachycardia; irregularly irregular rhythm (atrial fibrillation); warm, moist, and smooth skin; and thinning hair. Signs specific for Graves' disease are presented in Table 51-3.

The diagnosis of thyrotoxicosis is confirmed by checking markers of thyroid function. All patients should have TSH checked, and measurements of T4 and T3 are obtained to assess the severity of thyrotoxicosis and facilitate determination of the cause of thyrotoxicosis. In almost all cases of overt thyrotoxicosis, TSH is low and thyroid hormone levels are elevated. T4 level may be in the laboratory reference range in cases of T3 toxicosis that present with elevations of only total or free T3 levels. Potential etiologies of T3 toxicosis include Graves' disease, toxic solitary adenoma, and ingestion of liothyronine (T3). Thyrotoxicosis due to amiodarone may present with a pattern of low TSH, elevated T4, and T3 level in the laboratory reference range due to anti-deiodinase activity of the drug. In rare cases of TSH-secreting pituitary adenomas, T4 and T3 are elevated but with TSH inappropriately in the laboratory reference range or increased.

High-dose consumption of biotin (5–30 mg daily) may interfere with thyroid function assays utilizing biotin-streptavidin affinity systems in their design. TSH measured by immunometric assays will be spuriously low, while measures of thyroid hormone (T4 and T3) using competitive binding assays can give falsely elevated results. The pattern of findings will appear to indicate thyrotoxicosis, although the patient will have no symptoms or findings to indicate the diagnosis. Spurious findings should resolve on repeat measurements of thyroid function after the patient has stopped supplemental biotin for at least 48 hours.

If patients have pathognomonic signs of Graves' disease (Table 51-3), no additional workup to determine the etiology of thyrotoxicosis is required. If the etiology of thyrotoxicosis is uncertain, next steps in evaluation are measurements of thyroid receptor antibodies (TRAb) or radioiodine uptake (RAIU). For patients with no evidence of nodular thyroid disease, measurement of TRAb (eg, TSI) is the appropriate initial step in evaluation; if TRAb is positive, the result indicates Graves' disease and measurement of RAIU is required only if treatment with radioiodine (I-131) is being considered. If TRAb is undetectable, RAIU is then measured. For patients with palpable or sonographically detected thyroid nodules, RAIU is measured to distinguish Graves' disease from toxic nodular goiter (multinodular or solitary adenoma) and determine the functionality of nodules Graves' disease patients. The finding of a nonfunctional ("cold") nodule in a patient with otherwise increased RAIU of Graves' disease requires fine-needle biopsy of the nodule to evaluate for thyroid carcinoma. Radioiodine is contraindicated in pregnancy, and pregnant women undergoing evaluation for thyrotoxicosis should have TRAb measured followed by thyroid ultrasound with measurement of thyroid blood flow if TRAb is undetectable.

Treatment

Priorities in management of thyrotoxicosis are prompt control of symptoms and manifestations of thyroid hormone excess and, in cases of hyperthyroidism, control of thyroid hormone over production. For all patients with thyrotoxicosis, beta blockers may be useful to mitigate adrenergic symptoms (eg, palpitations, tremor, anxiety) and control heart rate in patients with significant tachycardia or atrial fibrillation. Although propranolol has modest anti-deiodinase activity, the effect is only significant at high doses, is slow in onset, and does not significantly contribute to its therapeutic benefit, particularly when coprescribed with a thioamide. Medications with higher beta-1 selectivity, such as metoprolol or atenolol, also are effective in management of thyrotoxicosis. Selected beta blockers are presented in Table 51-4. Due to neonatal complications such as intrauterine growth restriction, hypoglycemia, bradycardia, and respiratory depression, beta blockers should be dosed conservatively and for the shortest possible duration if used to treat thyrotoxicosis in pregnancy.

For patients with hyperthyroidism, the 3 major treatment options are thioamides, radioiodine (I-131), and thyroidectomy. In the United States, methimazole (MMI) and propylthiouracil (PTU) are the available thioamides, and carbimazole, a prodrug of MMI, is available in many other countries. Although serious liver injury is rare, MMI is preferred to PTU for management of hyperthyroidism in nonpregnant adults due to a lower risk of drug-induced hepatic necrosis.. However, PTU is the drug of choice in the first trimester of pregnancy due to risk of fetal aplasia cutis from treatment with MMI. Thioamides are indicated for patients who require rapid clinical and biochemical control of hyperthyroidism, prefer antithyroid medications to surgery or radioiodine, have a high likelihood of remission of Graves' disease (eg, women, mild hyperthyroidism, small goiter, negative or low-titer TRAb), have moderate or severe Graves' orbitopathy, or have significant comorbidities or limited life expectancy, or during

Table 51-4. Beta Blockers for Management of Thyrotoxicosis

Drug	Treatment Considerations
Propranolol	Nonselective beta antagonist
	Most therapeutic experience
	Reduces T4-to-T3 conversion at high doses
	Preferred agent for nursing and pregnant mothers
Atenolol	Relative beta-1 selectivity
	Once-daily dosing improves medication compliance
	Avoid during pregnancy
Metoprolol	Relative beta-1 selectivity
	May be used in pregnancy
Nadolol	Nonselective beta antagonist dosed once daily
	Least experience with this agent
	May reduce T4-to-T3 conversion at high doses
Esmolol	Rapid-acting parenteral drug for treatment of severe hyperthyroidism in an intensive care unit

pregnancy. The starting dose of MMI is generally determined by the degree of thyroid hormone elevation (Table 51-5). Thyroid function should be monitored at 4- to 6-week intervals after starting MMI until biochemical euthyroidism is achieved. The dose of MMI may then be reduced by 25% to 50% and thyroid function monitored until a maintenance dose of medication has been confirmed. When patients have achieved euthyroidism on a stable dose of MMI, they can be monitored every 6 months.

The rate of prolonged remission of hyperthyroidism in patients with Graves' disease treated with a thioamide is approximately 40%. However, remission is unlikely to be an immunomodulating effect of thioamides but rather part of the natural history of Graves' disease as patients with mild hyperthyroidism treated

Table 51-5. Initial Dosing of Methimazole (MMI)

Free T4 Elevation (Above Upper Limit of Reference Range)	Starting MMI Dose (mg)
≥1.5-fold	5–10
1.5- to 2-fold	10–20
≥2-fold	20–40

with propranolol alone had a similar remission rate. After approximately 18 months of treatment, TRAb can be rechecked and cessation of thioamide treatment offered to patients with an undetectable titer. Patients with an elevated titer can continue thioamide treatment or proceed to management with radioiodine or thyroidectomy.

Rash, pruritis, urticaria, altered sense of taste, and nausea are minor side effects of thioamides that occur in approximately 10% of patients. Unfortunately, cross-reactivity between MMI and PTU is approximately 50%. In addition to hepatic injury, other rare but serious adverse events include agranulocytosis and antineutrophil cytoplasmic antibody (ANCA)-positive vasculitis. MMI-induced agranulocytosis appears to be dose dependent, with risk only at total daily doses exceeding 20 mg. Increased risk of ANCA-positive vasculitis has only been linked to PTU. Thioamide treatment should be stopped immediately if agranulocytosis or ANCA-positive vasculitis occurs.

Radioiodine (RAI) is safe and effective treatment for hyperthyroidism, although it is now chosen less often than antithyroid medications. A dose of I-131 determined by RAIU on a thyroid scan is administered as sodium iodide, and the I-131 is rapidly taken up and incorporated by thyroid tissue. Beta-emissions from the RAI cause ablation of thyroid tissue 6 to 18 weeks after treatment. Patients are candidates for RAI treatment if they prefer the option to thioamides or thyroidectomy, have experienced adverse effects during thioamide treatment or have contraindications to thioamides, failed to achieve euthyroidism during a trial of thioamide treatment, are poor surgical candidates, or lack access to an experienced thyroid surgeon. RAI is contraindicated in women who are pregnant or considering pregnancy within 6 months of treatment, are breastfeeding, or have moderate to severe Graves' orbitopathy.

RAI treatment, particularly for Graves' disease, may cause transient elevation of thyroid hormone levels and exacerbation of hyperthyroidism. Treatment with a beta blocker should be considered even for patients asymptomatic prior to dosing RAI, and pretreatment with a thioamide is indicated for patient's with significantly increased thyroid hormone levels and significant symptoms prior to RAI. The thioamide should be stopped no later than 2 to 3 days before RAI is administered. Thioamide treatment can also be resumed 3 to 7 days after RAI to limit the rise in thyroid hormone level that results from early thyroid ablation.

Thyroid hormone levels and TSH should be monitored at 4- to 6-week intervals after RAI is dosed until postablative hypothyroidism occurs and treatment with thyroxine is started. Most patients experience resolution of hyperthyroidism in 4 to 10 weeks. Free T4 is the best measure of the early response to RAI treatment because thyrotrophs may take several weeks or even months before becoming capable of a fully physiologic TSH response to changes in thyroid hormone levels. Factors that affect the success rate of RAI treatment in patients with Graves' disease include the absorbed dose of I-131, thyroid volume, and pretreatment with a thioamide. For patients with toxic nodular goiters, nodule volume and RAI dose, but not pretreatment with a thioamide, are the key factors that influence response to treatment.

Indications for surgical management of hyperthyroidism include very large goiter with or without substernal extension, goiter causing symptoms of mass effect (eg, dysphagia or dyspnea from upper airway obstruction), nonfunctional nodule with cytology indeterminate, suspicious, or positive for malignancy, moderate to severe Graves' orbitopathy, persistent hyperthyroidism despite treatment with a thioamide or RAI, coexisting primary hyperparathyroidism, pregnancy with intolerance to thioamides, and plans for pregnancy less than or equal to 6 months from treatment for hyperthyroidism. Patients choosing thyroidectomy should be treated with a thioamide to achieve normal thyroid hormone levels before surgery. Supersaturated potassium iodide (SSKI) is prescribed 7 to 10 days prior to surgery for patients with Graves' disease to reduce vascularity of the thyroid gland and reduce intraoperative bleeding. Treatment with the combination of glucocorticoids to reduce conversion of T4 to T3, iodide to reduce thyroid vascularity, and beta blockers to manage adrenergic manifestations of hyperthyroidism has been shown to safely prepare patients for urgent thyroidectomy.

A Middle-Aged Male With Severe Hyperthyroidism

A 47-year-old male with known Graves' disease is brought to the ED due to altered mental status and dyspnea. The patient is afebrile but tachycardic (HR 120) and hypotensive (BP 79/53 mm Hg). He requires mechanical ventilation and treatment with vasopressors shortly after arrival due to respiratory failure and hypotension. The person accompanying the patient suspects he has not been taking MMI as prescribed, and TSH less than 0.03 mIU/L (0.45–5.33) and free T4 4.3 ng/dL (0.5–1.3) are measured on admission laboratories. Proptosis and a goiter are apparent on limited examination.

1. What it the patient's diagnosis?
2. What are options for management?

Answers

1. This patient presents with a rare but life-threatening manifestation of severe hyperthyroidism called thyroid storm. The Burch-Wartofsky Point Scale (BWPS) provides a systematic approach to making the diagnosis of thyroid storm and is presented in Table 51-6. A total score of more than 45 is highly suggestive of thyroid storm, 25 to 44 supports the diagnosis, and less than 25 makes the diagnosis unlikely.

Table 51-6. Burch-Wartofsky Point Scale (BWPS) for Diagnosis of Thyroid Storm

Temperature: 5 points per 1° F above 99°F (maximum 30 points)
CNS dysfunction: 10 points for mild (agitation), 20 for moderate (delirium, psychosis or extreme lethargy), and 30 for severe (seizure or coma)
Tachycardia: 5 (99–109), 10 (110–119), 15 (120–129), 20 (130–139) and 25 (>140)
Presence of atrial fibrillation: 10
Heart failure: 5 for mild (pedal edema), 10 for moderate (bi-basilar rales), and 15 for severe (pulmonary edema)
GI dysfunction: 10 for moderate (diarrhea, nausea/vomiting or abdominal pain) and 20 for severe (unexplained jaundice)
Presence of Precipitating factor: 10 points
Diagnosis: A total score of >45 is highly suggestive of thyroid storm, 25–44 supports the diagnosis, and <25 makes the diagnosis unlikely

From Burch HB, Wartofsky L. Life-threatening thyrotoxicosis. Thyroid storm. *Endocrinol Metab Clin North Am.* 1993; 22:263–277.

2. Supportive care in an intensive care unit is required to manage life-threatening organ system dysfunction, and urgent and aggressive interventions are required to reduce thyroid hormone levels as quickly as possible. A combination of thioamides, beta blockers, glucocorticoids, iodide, and the bile acid sequestrant cholestyramine may be required to reduce thyroid hormone production and release from the gland, peripheral conversion of T4 to T3, and enterohepatic recycling of T4. Details for management are presented in the case review.

CASE REVIEW

Diagnosis

The incidence of thyroid storm is quite low at approximately 5 cases per 100,000 hospitalized patients annually, although the mortality rate is 10%–25%. Thyroid storm is almost always a complication of Graves' hyperthyroidism, but it may also occur in patients with toxic nodular goiters and has been reported in patients with checkpoint inhibitor induced thyroiditis. It is often triggered by events such as trauma, thyroid or nonthyroidal surgery, infection, parturition, or an acute iodide load. Cardiovascular comorbidities—extreme tachycardia, atrial fibrillation, and heart failure—are most common in thyroid storm, although patients also frequently have hyperpyrexia (≥104°F) and altered mental status ranging from agitation to coma. All patients have a pattern of low TSH and elevated levels of T4 and

T3, although the magnitude of thyroid function abnormalities in thyroid storm is not more severe than patients with uncomplicated hyperthyroidism.

Treatment

Management of thyroid storm consists of supportive measures ranging from supplemental oxygen, acetaminophen, IV fluids, and cooling blankets to mechanical ventilation and vasopressors. Potential precipitating factors, such as infection, should be treated if possible. Interventions to address hyperthyroidism in thyroid storm are presented in Table 51-7. The same medications (ie, thioamides, beta blockers, and SSKI) used to manage uncomplicated hyperthyroidism are used to treat patients with thyroid storm but at higher and more frequent doses. Treatment with beta blockers may need to be initially deferred or invasive cardiovascular monitoring with a pulmonary artery catheter may be required if patients are hypotensive or have severe heart failure. High-dose glucocorticoids are used to reduce peripheral T4 to T3 conversion, and cholestyramine may be used as an adjunctive treatment to reduce enteric reabsorption of thyroid hormone.

Thyroidectomy is required for thyroid storm patients who cannot be treated with thioamides. Beta blockers, glucocorticoids, potassium iodide, and cholestyramine are used for 5 to 7 days to reduce thyroid hormone levels and vascularity of the thyroid gland prior to surgery. Surgery should not be delayed more

Table 51-7. Interventions for Hyperthyroidism in Thyroid Storm

Category	Medications	Mechanism
Thioamides*	PTU 200 mg q4h MMI 20 mg q4–6h	Reduce production of new thyroid hormone
Potassium iodide†	SSKI 5 drops q6h Lugol solution 10 drops q8h	Reduce production and release of thyroid hormone (Wolff-Chaikoff effect)
Beta blockers	Propranolol 60–80 mg q6h Esmolol 0.25–0.5 mg/kg bolus, then 0.05–0.1 mg/kg/min infusion	Control manifestations of increased adrenergic tone
Glucocorticoids	Hydrocortisone 100 mg IV q 8 h	Inhibit peripheral T4 to T3 conversion
Bile acid sequestrants	Cholestyramine 4 g q6h	Reduce enterohepatic recycling of T4

*May be specially prepared for administration IV or by rectal enema.

†Administer no sooner than 1 h after the first dose of thioamide.

than 7 days due to concern that patients may escape the Wolff-Chaikoff effect and resume organification of iodide. Plasmapheresis removes thyroid hormone from plasma, and there are case reports of plasmapheresis significantly reducing thyroid hormone levels and preparing patients for emergent thyroidectomy when traditional treatment options have been unsuccessful.

When there is clear evidence of clinical improvement such as resolution of fever, control of cardiovascular complications, and improvement in mental status, potassium iodide can be stopped and glucocorticoids tapered off. A beta blocker should be continued until thyroid hormone levels are in their laboratory reference ranges. If PTU was chosen for initial treatment, it should be changed to MMI. Treatment with RAI or thyroidectomy is recommended for long-term management of hyperthyroidism to eliminate the potential for recurrence of thyroid storm.

TIPS TO REMEMBER

- Thyrotoxicosis may be caused by endogenous overproduction of thyroid hormone (eg, Graves' disease and toxic nodular goiter), unregulated release of thyroid hormone (thyroiditis), or consumption of excess thyroid hormone.

- TSH is the best single test of thyroid function. Free T4 and total T3 measurements help to determine severity and etiology of thyrotoxicosis. Clinical features such as exophthalmos, periorbital and conjunctival edema, and infiltrative dermopathy (pretibial myxedema) occur only in patients with Graves' disease.

- An elevated TSI titer indicates Graves' disease, but the absence of a high titer does not exclude the diagnosis.

- The pattern of radioiodine and pertechnetate uptake on thyroid scintigraphy is useful for distinguishing etiologies of endogenous thyroid hormone overproduction. Diffusely increased uptake is observed in Graves' disease, localized increased uptake with suppression of surrounding tissue is characteristic of toxic nodular goiters, and generalized decreased uptake is indicative of thyroiditis.

- The finding of a nonfunctional ("cold") nodule in a patient with otherwise increased radioiodine uptake of Graves' disease requires fine-needle biopsy of the nodule to evaluate for possible thyroid carcinoma.

- Treatment of hyperthyroidism includes control of adrenergic symptoms (eg, palpitations, tremor) with beta blockers for patients with moderate to severe symptoms until euthyroidism is achieved with thioamides (methimazole or propylthiouracil [PTU]), radioiodine (RAI, I-131), or thyroidectomy.

- Methimazole is preferred over PTU due to lower risk of drug-induced hepatic injury. PTU is preferred during first trimester of pregnancy and during treatment of severe hyperthyroidism ("thyroid storm").

- RAI is contraindicated in women who are pregnant or considering pregnancy within 6 months of treatment, who are breastfeeding, or who have moderate to severe Graves' orbitopathy.

- Thyroid storm is a rare life-threatening manifestation of severe hyperthyroidism. The Burch-Wartofsky Point Scale (BWPS) provides a systematic approach to making the diagnosis of thyroid storm. Management requires admission to an ICU for appropriate supportive care in addition to thioamides, high-dose glucocorticoids, SSKI, and beta blockers. Bile acid sequestrants (eg, cholestyramine) may be required to reduce enterohepatic recycling of thyroxine.

SUGGESTED READINGS

Akamizu T, Satoh T, Isozaki O, et al. Diagnostic criteria, clinical features, and incidence of thyroid storm based on nationwide surveys. *Thyroid.* 2012;22(7):661–679.

Baeza A, Aguayo J, Barria M, Pineda G. Rapid preoperative preparation in hyperthyroidism. *Clin Endocrinol (Oxf).* 1991;35(5):439–442.

Bahn RS, Burch HS, Cooper DS, et al. The role of propylthiouracil in the management of Graves' disease in adults: report of a meeting jointly sponsored by the American Thyroid Association and the Food and Drug Administration. *Thyroid.* 2009;19(7):673–674.

Balavoine AS, Glinoer D, Dubucquoi S, Wémeau JL. Antineutrophil cytoplasmic antibody–positive small-vessel vasculitis associated with antithyroid drug therapy: how significant is the clinical problem? *Thyroid.* 2015;25(12):1273–1281.

Brito JP, Payne S, Singh Ospina N, et al. Patterns of use, efficacy, and safety of treatment options for patients with Graves' disease: a nationwide population-based study. *Thyroid.* 2020;30(3):357–364.

Burch HB, Wartofsky L. Life-threatening thyrotoxicosis. Thyroid storm. *Endocrinol Metab Clin North Am.* 1993;22:263–277.

Codaccioni JL, Orgiazzi J, Blanc P, et al. Lasting remissions in patients treated for Graves' hyperthyroidism with propranolol alone: a pattern of spontaneous evolution of the disease. *J Clin Endocrinol Metab.* 1988;67(4):656–662.

Hollowell JG, Staehling NW, Flanders WD, et al. Serum TSH, T(4), and thyroid antibodies in the United States population (1988 to 1994): National Health and Nutrition Examination Survey (NHANES III) *J Clin Endocrinol Metab.* 2002;87:489–499.

Kahaly GJ, Bartalena L, Hegedüs L, et al. 2018 European Thyroid Association Guideline for the management of Graves' hyperthyroidism. *Eur Thyroid J.* 2018;7(4):167–186.

Li D, Radulescu A, Shrestha RT, et al. Association of biotin ingestion with performance of hormone and nonhormone assays in healthy adults. *JAMA.* 2017;318(12):1150–1160.

Peters H, Fischer C, Bogner U, et al. 1997 Treatment of Graves' hyperthyroidism with radioiodine: results of a prospective randomized study. *Thyroid.* 1997;7(2):247–251.

Ross DS, Burch HB, Cooper DS, et al. 2016 American Thyroid Association Guidelines for diagnosis and management of hyperthyroidism and other causes of thyrotoxicosis. *Thyroid.* 2016;26(10):1343–1421.

Sabri O, Zimny M, Schulz G, et al. Success rate of radioidine therapy in Graves' disease: the influence of thyrostatic medication. *J Clin Endocrinol Metab.* 1999;84(4):1229–1233.

Saki H, Cengiz, A, Yürekli Y. Effectiveness of radioiodine treatment in toxic nodular goiter. *Mol Imaging Radionucl Ther.* 2015;24(3):100–104.

Sherif IH, Oyan WT, Bosairi S, Carrascal SM. Treatment of hyperthyroidism in pregnancy. *Acta Obstet Gynecol Scand.* 1991;70(6):461–463.

Stan MN, Durski JM, Brito JP, et al. Cohort study on radioactive iodine-induced hypothyroidism: implications for Graves' ophthalmopathy and optimal timing for thyroid hormone assessment. *Thyroid.* 2013;23(5):620–625.

Swee du S, Chng CL, Lim A. Clinical characteristics and outcome of thyroid storm: a case series and review of neuropsychiatric derangements in thyrotoxicosis. *Endocr Pract.* 2015;21(2):182–189.

Törring O, Tallstedt L, Wallin G, et al. Graves' hyperthyroidism: treatment with antithyroid drugs, surgery, or radioiodine—a prospective, randomized study. Thyroid Study Group. *J Clin Endocrinol Metab.* 1996;81(8):2986–2993.

Van Dijke CP, Heydendael RJ, De Kleine MJ. Methimazole, carbimazole, and congenital skin defects. *Ann Intern Med.* 1987;106(1):60–61.

van Staa TP, Boulton F, Cooper C, et al. Neutropenia and agranulocytosis in England and Wales: incidence and risk factors. *Am J Hematol.* 2003;72(4):248–254.

Vyas AA, Vyas P, Fillipon NL, et al. Successful treatment of thyroid storm with plasmapheresis in a patient with methimazole-induced agranulocytosis. *Endocr Pract.* 2010;16(4):673–676.

Wiersinga WM, Touber JL. The influence of beta-adrenoceptor blocking agents on plasma thyroxine and triiodothyronine. *J Clin Endocrinol Metab.* 1977;45(2):293–298.

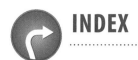

INDEX

Page numbers followed by *f* or *t* indicate figures or tables, respectively.